PHARMACY

Career Planning and Professi

PHARMACY

Career Planning and Professional Opportunity

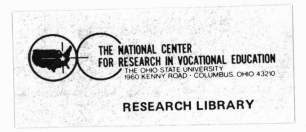

T. Donald Rucker, Editor

AUPHA PRESS
Washington, D.C.—Ann Arbor, Michigan

Library of Congress Cataloging in Publication Data
Main entry under title:

Pharmacy: career planning and professional
    opportunities.

    Bibliography: p.
    Includes index.
    1.   Pharmacy—Vocational guidance—United States.
I.   Rucker, T. Donald.
RS122.5.P476   615'.1'02373   80-21716
ISBN 0-914904-52-3

AUPHA Press is an imprint of Health Administration Press

Health Administration Press   Association of University
School of Public Health   Programs in Health Administration
The University of Michigan   One DuPont Circle
Ann Arbor, Michigan 48109   Washington, D.C. 20036
313-764-1380   212-659-4354

To the authors of your readings, who sustained personal sacrifices in order to record their experiences in pharmacy, and to those publishers whose cooperation made it possible to share these insights with young persons interested in this profession.

Contents

Preface

This guide has been designed to serve as a self-study reference for students who wish to consider pharmacy as a college major and as a professional career. Nearly 150,000 men and women with pharmacy training are employed in our society, while over 23,000 students are enrolled in American colleges of pharmacy. These data imply that pharmacists represent an important group among the professionals who serve patients in our health care delivery system.

Pharmacists are specialists who possess particular knowledge about the chemical composition and appropriate use of pharmaceutical products—their names, active ingredients, actions in the body, possible side-effects, and roles in the treatment of medical problems. In addition, society has granted pharmacists legal authority to dispense drugs according to formal instructions issued by prescribers. Given these qualifications and responsibilities, pharmacists act as a resource for many physicians and patients who require technical information concerning how drug therapy can help to control the health problems of individuals.

Contrary to popular opinion, pharmacy is not a simple area in which professional contributions are limited to the filling of prescription orders. Rather, it is a complex field and one with many different opportunities for dedicated graduates. This book will help you to explore these possibilities.

Chapter One introduces the world of pharmacy and the role of the professionals who function in this environment. Chapter Two outlines the methods used to compile the readings, and suggests various steps that you can follow to improve the reliability of your investigation of pharmacy as a potential career choice. The heart of this volume, though, is found in Chapters Three through Five. They provide detailed examples of what pharmacists do both as practitioners and as non-practitioners. In order that you may better understand the framework within which pharmacy is practiced, additional references describe current problems and future directions which the profession seems to be taking.

The next two chapters review educational routes and the licensure requirements that are necessary to achieve professional status. The concluding chapter discusses techniques to facilitate your successful entry into the job market. For most readers, this decision is at least four years away. Nevertheless, an appraisal of pharmacy as a career option would be incomplete without some guidance concerning how professional training can be translated into employment opportunities.

This survey should be of particular value to both high school seniors and college freshmen who are in the process of examining career alternatives and setting personal goals. In addition, counselors may wish to retain or recommend this compilation when advising students about a possible career in pharmacy, including the selection of an appropriate institution for study.

If you are enrolled in a college of pharmacy already, this guide can serve as a basis for (a) selecting a track within the pharmacy curriculum, (b) determining which elective courses should be taken, (c) deciding on the kind of job you will seek upon graduation, and/or (d) establishing whether additional training may be essential in order to meet your career objectives. Some readers may shudder, and a few may panic, at the thought of advanced study, when their undergraduate program has only just begun. However, in our age of specialization, job opportunities seem especially favorable for many of those who are willing to make such an investment. Pharmacy represents a very good example of this principle. If you decide to continue your studies, this guide can minimize the time you will need to achieve additional qualifications as well as suggest areas with the greatest potential for professional service.

Finally, instructors with responsibility for a course covering an introduction or an orientation to pharmacy may wish to consider this reference as a supplement to, or in lieu of, an assigned text.

In preparing this manuscript, I have made a special effort to reflect the actual and potential contributions of pharmacy graduates, without neglecting the limitations that are to be found in current methods of practice. Since a sound career decision should be based on the whole picture, this aim of "telling it like it is" seems essential.

Pharmacy is an integral part of a $230 billion health care system that is subject to change through the influence of various economic and political forces. In addition to these external factors, many leaders and practitioners within the field of pharmacy are striving to develop better ways to improve the beneficial results of drug therapy while minimizing the expense of achieving this goal. Students desiring to escape problems of this nature should consider positions outside the health care delivery system. However, those with a combined interest in basic science areas such as chemistry and mathematics, patients and their medical problems, the role of drug therapy in treating illness conditions, and the efficient use of scarce resources, may find a challenge in pharmacy that could consume their energies for a lifetime. In attempting to establish your best career opportunity, it should be noted that this field has one characteristic in common with many occupational outlets—pharmacy can be as dull or as exciting as you make it.

Your perspective on careers in pharmacy has been enriched by the contributions of W. Ray Burns, Virginia B. Hall, and Frank Kunkel, who prepared especially commissioned papers, as will be noted below. Further, the research assistance of Richard A. Grover, M.S., R.Ph., a doctoral candidate in pharmacy administration, set a high standard of scholarship in helping to ensure that this guide would meet the needs of thoughtful readers.

Any errors of fact and judgment that remain must be ascribed to the undersigned.

T. Donald Rucker
Columbus, Ohio

Chapter One

An Introduction to Pharmacy

The term pharmacy has several meanings that are important for the purposes of career planning. This brief overview, therefore, will provide a foundation for your readings by describing pharmacy both as a place of employment and as an integrated system for producing and distributing pharmaceutical products. Because these chemical agents are a key responsibility of pharmacists as practitioners, the types of drug products that are legally available in our society also will be reviewed.

Most students are interested in pharmacy as a profession—how these experts serve the therapeutic needs of patients. Consequently, the next section treats this general subject. Finally, we will conclude with an outline of how prescribed medications fit into the health care delivery system as a whole. With this background in mind, you will be ready to embark on your exploration of pharmacy as a possible career.

Pharmacy as a Location

One way of considering pharmacy is to view it as a physical facility where prescription drugs are stored, prepared, and released for patient use. The two major types are (a) institutional pharmacies, which serve bed patients, and (b) outlets that serve ambulatory patients, individuals whose medical problems enable them to maintain functional activity outside institutional settings. In terms of numbers, community pharmacies are most common; there are some 50,000 units. Moreover, they are distributed so widely that only 48 counties in the United States (of 3,044) do not have a pharmacy.

Within the community pharmacy category, independent (self-owned) stores are the most prominent, but recently chains (four or more units under a common ownership) have been experiencing the greatest growth. Although most of these firms sell non-drug merchandise, over 1,000 prescription centers are operative where nearly all the revenue is generated by the sale of pharmaceutical products. While the sole proprietorship and partnership have traditionally dominated the community scene, the recent success of chain operations has raised the number of stores controlled by private and public corporations to more than 10,000. One consequence of this development is that over 65 percent of all active practitioners hold status in the work force as employees.

Ambulatory patients also may obtain prescribed medications from the approximately 1,200 hospitals that operate outpatient pharmacy departments. These units, along with the more numerous community pharmacies, account for nearly 90 percent of the prescriptions received by such patients. The remainder are provided by dispensing physicians, mail-order firms, military installations, clinics (both public and private), health maintenance organizations, prisons, and ships.

Pharmacies are also found in many facilities that provide acute or long-term care for bed patients. This category includes more than 6,500 general hospitals, about 2,000 specialized hospitals, and over 16,500 nursing homes. In the largest hospitals, the pharmacy may have an annual budget for drug products alone that reaches five million dollars; thus, the director of such a pharmacy department assumes a financial responsibility that exceeds the sales volume of most retail establishments. In the smallest facilities, however, the size of the organization often makes it uneconomical to maintain a pharmacy on the premises. As a consequence, the medication requirements of patients confined to several thousand hospitals and over 15,400 nursing homes are furnished by community pharmacies. This function involves over one quarter of the community pharmacists. Indeed, some even restrict their practice to the service of individuals receiving care in such institutions.

Pharmacy as an Integrated System

The distribution of prescription products at the retail level does not take place without the contribution of other productive and supportive organizations. Thus, it is necessary to expand our perspective and consider pharmacy as a vertical structure involving the roles of these related firms. Let us start at the beginning of the industrial process by identifying over 350 manufacturing firms responsible for the discovery, production, and distribution of pharmaceutical preparations. In addition, it is necessary to include certain subcontractors* and 1,500 repackagers who facilitate this activity. The structural approach also embraces 750 drug wholesalers who are the primary suppliers of the inventory carried in the prescription department of the typical pharmacy (about 33 percent of the stock is obtained directly from the manufacturer). Of course, all retailers, including even non-pharmacist owners, form the basis for a view of pharmacy as an integrated system. Indeed, the ties between drug production and distribution are so great that it is difficult to discuss any single component of pharmacy without appreciating the interdependence that exists among these suppliers.

Within the past decade, this broader view of pharmacy has become even more complicated, due to the growth of drug insurance coverage in both public and private plans. The proportion of all prescriptions protected by these third-party programs nationwide currently hovers between 15 and 20 percent. In one chain with 159 units, however, over 50 percent of the prescription sales are subject to contractual agreements with various insurance organizations. These specifications are noteworthy because they determine the method of compensation for both product cost and professional services. Consequently, certain prescription prices and a portion of pharmacy income may be influenced by external forces in the form of third-party programs. Moreover, it seems likely that the percentage of prescriptions covered by private and public drug insurance plans will increase significantly in the future.

Our description of pharmacy as a system, however, is still incomplete. There are many supporting organizations and agencies that ultimately influence the scope of practitioner activities and the quality of the care that is rendered by pharmacists. First, each state has established a Board of Pharmacy which examines applicants seeking a license to practice pharmacy. The Board also licenses pharmacies and periodically inspects them, as well as their professional dispensing procedures, to ensure that patient health and safety are not jeopardized. Moreover, at least 21 states now require that pharmacists keep up to date on new drug products and drug uses in order to maintain their licenses. The task of determining the type and amount of continuing education programs that are essential for this purpose currently represents another important responsibility exercised by the State Board.

Second, the United States Drug Enforcement Administration (DEA) classifies especially dangerous drugs according to their

---

*Manufacturers and subcontractors produce pharmaceuticals in 3,600 "establishments." The industry concept also includes 200 quality control testing laboratories which are operated as distinct units, separated from the establishment.

potential for abuse. Thus, pharmacists must be alert to special conditions such as maximum quantity and number of refills for prescriptions falling in one of the five categories of drugs that have been established by the DEA.

Third, all drug products dispensed by the pharmacist are subject to the general control that is exercised by the United States Food and Drug Administration (FDA). This agency enforces laws which require that manufacturers, as a condition for marketing a new pharmaceutical preparation, demonstrate that the drug is (1) safe and (2) effective for the medical problem(s) for which it is intended. Once the new product goes into production, FDA regulations also require that the supplier follow procedures to ensure the purity, potency, and correct labeling of these medications.

Other organizations also affect the structure of pharmacy as a broad system. These are manifest in the 71 colleges of pharmacy

in the United States, at least 18 professional organizations and 10 trade associations, and over 100 scientific, professional, and trade publications. Contributions by these sources often represent a vital underpinning in support of the role of the modern pharmacist.

This brief review of pharmacy as a system may seem to have little relevance to the question of whether pharmacy may be a good choice for a professional career. However, we will pause to summarize our findings: (1) Pharmacy may be practiced in a number of different delivery settings. (2) The pharmacist's discretion in both professional and business matters may often be influenced by factors external to the direct relationship that exists between practitioner, patient, and prescriber. (3) Pharmacy training provides an ideal foundation for seeking employment outside the practice setting—for example, in many of the structural and supporting areas noted above. This principle is illustrated by the data in Table I-1, which indicate that

Table I-1

**Active Pharmacists by Place
of Employment, U.S.A., 1973**

Place of Employment	Number	Percent
Independent community pharmacy	54,884	47.0%
Large chain	17,929	15.4
Small chain	13,144	11.3
Private hospital	10,798	9.3
†Pharmaceutical manufacturer	5,119	4.4
Clinic or medical building pharmacy	4,438	3.8
Government: Non-federal hospital	3,622	3.1
Government: Federal and military hospital	2,100	1.8
†College of pharmacy	1,418	1.2
†Other state and local government	1,300	1.1
Nursing home	498	0.4
†Pharmaceutical wholesaler	443	0.4
†Other federal government	340	0.3
†Other	533	0.5
	116,566	100.0

Source: "A Report to the President and Congress on the Status of Health Professions Personnel in the United States." DHEW Pub. No. (HRA) 78-93. August, 1978. p.VII-15.

†The vast majority of these positions involve the pharmacist in non-practitioner responsibilities.

over 9,000 pharmacists held positions in non-practice environments in 1973. Since national manpower studies cannot readily follow a pharmacy graduate who does not hold a license to practice, this figure may be understated by as much as 20 percent.

Classification of Drug Products

A major responsibility of the pharmacist as a practitioner usually involves control over pharmaceutical preparations. In order to facilitate your understanding of such duties, these chemical agents will be examined briefly in terms of their legal status, restrictions on availability, and source of supply.

With respect to legal status, all drug products can be classified as either licit or illicit substances. Chemical agents are legally certified for medical use when it is established that they can mitigate disease conditions or otherwise help individuals maintain functional activity. Illicit agents, on the other hand, lack medical properties sufficient to warrant their use in patient treatment programs. Pharmacists, of course, are specialists in the handling and use of licit substances. Because their academic training covers chemical actions within the human body, pharmacists may provide both patients and community organizations with information on the use and abuse of illicit preparations as well.

Licit drugs are divided further according to a two-part classification covering general availability. Since 1952, all such products have been designated by the United States Food and Drug Administration as either legend or over-the-counter (OTC) items. Legend pharmaceuticals, due to their relative potency and potential danger, cannot be given to a patient legally unless they have been formally authorized by a doctor. Moreover, society restricts their ultimate distribu-

tion to specific channels, that is, those supervised by pharmacists or physicians.

On the other hand, OTC products—chemical agents judged to be less dangerous than legend items—do not require the order of a doctor, nor is their sale restricted to a pharmacy. As a result, about one half of the OTC purchases are made outside a pharmacy.* From the point of view of both the typical independent pharmacy and the small chain pharmacy, legend products are more significant because they account for nearly 75 percent of the dollar value of all pharmaceuticals sold. For the large chain, however, this ratio falls to under 40 percent.

Our third basis for classifying drug products involves the source of supply. Since patents protect newly developed pharmaceuticals from competitive forces for up to 17 years, most of these agents are sold exclusively by the originating firm during this period. The pharmacist's ability to purchase such products economically, therefore, is limited because of this market situation. Sole-source items account for about 70 percent of the drugs on the market and approximately 60 percent of all prescription orders dispensed.

The balance are multiple-source products. If agents of this type have been ordered by their established (generic) names, the pharmacist may select the supplier. Moreover, 46 states now give the pharmacist expanded authority even when the prescriber has designated such products by their brand (trademark) name. Consequently, the task of selecting suppliers of high-quality products, while giving due attention to relative product cost, represents an increasing responsibility of the pharmacist in his role as a practitioner.

The Pharmacist: Practitioner and Professional

Several steps must be followed by a person

*The discerning reader will quickly perceive that a comprehensive study of drug distribution could be expanded to embrace these non-pharmacy outlets as well.

who intends to become a pharmacist. The first requirement is graduation from an accredited college of pharmacy. (The minimum duration of training is five years.) Approximately 90 percent of individuals who hold degrees in pharmacy subsequently enter the practice environment, where they provide pharmaceutical products and related services to patients—hence the term "practitioner." The rest follow a variety of careers, as will be described in Chapter Five.

In order to become practitioners, graduates must satisfy a practical experience requirement and then pass a licensure examination. Both provisions are controlled by the Board of Pharmacy established in each state. To continue in that status, the individual must renew the license annually and fulfill other requirements, such as continuing education, that have been established by the Board. Many non-practitioners also maintain their licenses, but they are excluded from our definition of active members of the profession.

Once employed, pharmacists in their role as practitioners serve patients in a manner somewhat similar to that of physicians who diagnose their complaints, and, when appropriate, order medications. The primary basis for pharmacist participation in the medical care process is the prescription order generated by a prescriber. (Figure I-1 illustrates its components.) According to law, such orders can be authorized only by a physician, surgeon, dentist, or podiatrist. In some states, though, others such as physician's assistants have recently acquired limited responsibility to carry out this function. Written prescription orders are seldom typed, while many original and refill orders are placed by telephone. (Regulations issued by the State Boards, however, require that verbal instructions be transcribed to written form within a short period of time.) Thus, considerable technical knowledge and skill is required on the part of the pharmacist to ensure that the patient receives the proper drug, dosage form, and strength.

The formal prescription order is a legal document which serves as the official communication between doctor and pharmacist. Despite this close relationship between these practitioners, and the physician's authority to order drugs, these medical experts are not regarded as part of pharmacy when viewed as either a profession or an integrated system.

Over the next several decades, however, this distinction may be weakened. Two pilot projects were started recently in California to permit pharmacists to prescribe drugs for patients previously diagnosed by physicians. Further, clinical pharmacists in some teaching hospitals serve as therapeutic advisors to the doctors before they write the prescription orders. If these trends become important, perhaps by the end of this century the current division between medicine and pharmacy as discrete disciplines in patient care may be more difficult to substantiate.

Although most retail pharmacies are owned and managed by pharmacists, a few are controlled by persons who have other qualifications. These individuals also fall outside our definition of pharmacy as a profession. Nevertheless, they influence the conditions under which some staff pharmacists perform their duties.

The pharmacist is faced with several basic choices in applying his professional training. One involves the emphasis placed on the traditional control function over drug products. This approach is illustrated in the definition of pharmacy practice that appeared as recently as 1964:

> Pharmacy is a profession that deals with the preparation and distribution of medicinals and their identification, storage, preservation, standardization, intended use, and administration, and requires an understanding of economics, law, and public and interprofessional relations.*

*Gable, F. B. *Opportunities in Pharmacy Careers.* New York: Vocational Guidance Materials, 1964. p. 13.

Figure I-1

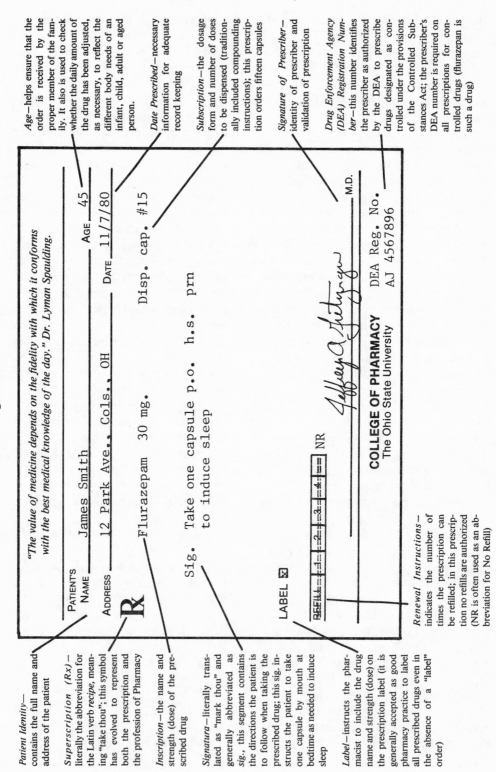

Patient Identity— contains the full name and address of the patient

Superscription (Rx)— literally the abbreviation for the Latin verb *recipe*, meaning "take thou"; this symbol has evolved to represent both the prescription and the profession of Pharmacy

Inscription— the name and strength (dose) of the prescribed drug

Signatura— literally translated as "mark thou" and generally abbreviated as *sig.*, this segment contains the directions the patient is to follow when taking the prescribed drug; this sig. instructs the patient to take one capsule by mouth at bedtime as needed to induce sleep

Label— instructs the pharmacist to include the drug name and strength (dose) on the prescription label (it is generally accepted as good pharmacy practice to label all prescribed drugs even in the absence of a "label" order)

Renewal Instructions— indicates the number of times the prescription can be refilled; in this prescription no refills are authorized (NR is often used as an abbreviation for No Refill)

"The value of medicine depends on the fidelity with which it conforms with the best medical knowledge of the day." Dr. Lyman Spaulding.

PATIENT'S
NAME ___James Smith___ AGE __45__
ADDRESS __12 Park Ave., Cols., OH__ DATE __11/7/80__

℞ Flurazepam 30 mg. Disp. cap. #15

Sig. Take one capsule p.o. h.s. prn
      to induce sleep

LABEL ☒

REFILL ☐1☐2☐3☐4☐ NR

COLLEGE OF PHARMACY   DEA Reg. No.
The Ohio State University   AJ 4567896

M.D.

Age— helps ensure that the order is received by the proper member of the family. It also is used to check whether the daily amount of the drug has been adjusted, as necessary, to reflect the different body needs of an infant, child, adult or aged person.

Date Prescribed— necessary information for adequate record keeping

Subscription— the dosage form and number of doses to be dispensed (traditionally included compounding instructions); this prescription orders fifteen capsules

Signature of Prescriber— identity of prescriber and validation of prescription

Drug Enforcement Agency (DEA) Registration Number— this number identifies the prescriber as authorized by the DEA to prescribe drugs designated as controlled under the provisions of the Controlled Substances Act; the prescriber's DEA number is required on all prescriptions for controlled drugs (flurazepam is such a drug)

These functions reflect a valid historical summary of the role of the typical pharmacist. Within the last several decades, though, the nature of professional services has been altered by a major change in the kind of pharmaceutical products supplied by the industry. Prior to the 1940s, most prescriptions were prepared by extemporaneous compounding carried out in the pharmacy. In this task, the pharmacist takes basic chemicals from containers on the shelf and combines them in a unique formula as specified on the doctor's prescription order. Under these conditions, the preparation of each patient's medication requires a great deal of manipulative skill, time, and technical knowledge. Prescriptions of this type have become so infrequent that they now account for less than 1 percent of the total number of prescriptions filled nationally. Compounding is not obsolete, though, since some physicians, dermatologists, for example, may order such preparations for 5 to 10 percent of their patients. If a pharmacy happens to be located in close proximity to one or more of these specialists, the dispensing duties of the pharmacist will reflect this situation.

For the nation as a whole, though, 99 percent of the prescriptions sold require only the provision of finished dosage forms (tablets, capsules, creams, etc.) as processed by the pharmaceutical manufacturer. With this shift in function from retail pharmacy to remote producer, some observers contend that the pharmacist's time is consumed largely by what I have heard called "counting and pouring, licking and sticking."

Consequently, the last decade has been characterized by a growing emphasis on clinical pharmacy—the provision of unique drug-related information and services that help patients maximize their health status. Among others, the factors accelerating the movement toward clinical pharmacy include the following:

1. The potency of drugs marketed in the past 20 to 30 years. If these chemical agents are prescribed outside the boundaries established for their safety and effectiveness, intervention by the pharmacist often becomes essential and even life-saving, for patients who are at risk.

2. The proliferation of therapeutic choices in the form of unique drug products, names, dosage forms and strengths. Although relatively few of the some 54,000 market alternatives will be applicable in treating a single patient afflicted with a particular medical problem, both the prescriber and the dispenser are often confronted with a task of unusual complexity.

The difficulty of selecting a "best" prescription is illustrated by the number of choices found in Table I-2, which depicts options for one drug category, antihistamines. These chemical preparations are used to control patient response to allergic reactions. Since our data cover only single-entity agents, expansion of the model to include preparations with multiple ingredients would raise the number of alternatives from 18 to more than several hundred.

Once the prescriber has identified the drug to be ordered, it is then necessary for him to consider the most appropriate dosage form, product strength, and duration of therapy. Guidelines for making many of these judgments are found in the "package insert," an official descriptive document which must, according to law, accompany every container marketed by the distributing firm. (After completing your readings in Chapters Three through Five, you may wish to visit your local pharmacy and request a copy of such a package insert. While any insert will illustrate the technical complexity of pharmaceutical products, I suggest that you ask for the one pertaining to ampicillin, the most frequently prescribed multiple-source product.) Ironically, the law requires that the dispenser, usually the pharmacist, receive the package insert. However, this information is appropriate for the prescriber, since he decides which drug will be used by the patient. The United States Food and Drug Adminis-

Table I–2

**Major Single-Entity Antihistamine
Products Sold, U.S.A., 1978**

Generic Name of Product	Number of			
	Suppliers	Dosage Forms*	Strengths for Tablet or Capsule Only	Package Sizes
Methapyrilene	9	6	3	7
Chlorpheniramine Maleate	57	5	3	5
Brompheniramine Maleate	22	4	3	7
Promethazine	43	5	3	10
Diphenhydramine HCl	69	5	2	7
Carbinoxamine Maleate	1	3	3	7
Bromodiphenhydramine HCl	1	2	1	2
Doxylamine Succinate	1	2	2	3
Tripelennamine HCl	26	5	2	6
Pyrilamine Maleate	10	3	2	5
Diphenylpyraline HCl	2	2	2	2
Dexchlorpheniramine Maleate	1	3	3	4
Dexbrompheniramine Maleate	1	1	1	1
Dimethindene	2	2	2	1
Triprolidine HCl	1	2	1	2
Cyproheptadine HCl	1	2	1	2
Trimeprazine	1	3	2	5
Methdilazine	1	3	2	3

Source: 1978 Red Book, Litton Industries.

*This category includes 16 different forms: ampule, capsule, chewable tablet, cream, dosette, elixir, expectorant, injectable-intramuscular, injectable-intravenous, injectable-subcutaneous, opthalmic, powder, suppository, syrup, tablet, and unit dose.

tration is now considering regulations to require that suppliers prepare an additional insert for distribution to patients, to aid them in taking their medications properly. The duties and professional responsibilities of the pharmacist will be influenced by the ultimate resolution of this proposal.

3. The problem of polypharmacy, that is, the use of more than one chemical agent (legend and/or OTC) concurrently. Because certain drugs interact with each other in undesired ways, patients may sustain harmful side effects or even find that the intended actions cancel each other. A major portion of the pharmacist's training involves the recognition of these problems, including, of course, the scientific knowledge necessary to recommend alternative preparations.

4. Numerous studies documenting irrational prescribing and dispensing, as well as instances where patients disregard the instructions for consuming their medications.

5. Decreased time needed to prepare compounded prescriptions, coupled with the possibility that pharmacists can allocate more time to consultation with the patient and the physician.

6. The availability of drugs for multiple purposes—diagnostic, preventive, acute, and chronic care.

7. Awareness of the above on the part of many educators, practitioners, and leaders in pharmacy.

In order to recognize the convergence of such forces, and the role of pharmacists in

Table I-3

Average Data for Selected Characteristics of Community Pharmacies, Based on a Voluntary Sample of Establishments Reporting to the Lilly Digest, 1977

Pharmacy Characteristic	Type of Pharmacy	
	Independent† (N=1,712)	Chain* (N=1,472)
Total Sales	$322,755	$1,295,213
Prescription Sales	$162,631	$ 244,558
Number of Prescriptions Dispensed: Total	26,649	43,742
New	12,931	22,882
Renewed	13,718	20,860
Average Prescription Charge	$ 6.10	$ 5.59
Inventory Value: Total	$ 53,382	$ 195,234
Prescription	$ 19,471	$ 24,133
Non-Prescription	$ 33,911	$ 171,101
Proprietor's or Manager's Salary	$ 22,622	$ 22,789
Size of Area (Square Feet)		
Prescription	371	385
Other	2,131	8,286
Number of Hours Open per Week	65	83

†Lilly Digest 1978.

*NACDS-Lilly Digest 1978.

confronting them, the American Pharmaceutical Association has defined pharmacy practice as

a patient-oriented health service that applies a scientific body of knowledge to improve and promote health through assurances of safety and efficacy in drug use and drug-related therapy.*

The first major choice for the pharmacist, therefore, involves a decision either to limit professional duties to the conventional tasks of product handling and prescription preparation, or to broaden this role by including the interpretative services that lead to the more beneficial results in the application of drug therapy.

The second basic question for the practitioner concerns the prominence that will be given to non-pharmaceutical merchandise. A slowly expanding minority of the profession feel that clinical (patient-oriented) services are best provided through prescription (pharmaceutical) centers which carry a limited amount of non-drug items. A strong majority, on the other hand, continue to operate more traditional pharmacies where front-end merchandise (photographic equipment, beauty aids, etc.) is sold in addition to drug items. These pharmacists hold that this secondary activity does not impair the delivery of professional services when prescriptions are filled. Indeed, they contend that front-end business helps to keep prescription prices down, because the overhead cost of operating the pharmacy will be spread over a larger sales volume. Interpretation of the data in Table I-3 shows that prescription

*apharmacy weekly 17 (March 18, 1978):3.

department sales account for only 50 percent of the total business in the typical independent community pharmacy and less than 20 percent in the typical chain store.

While the critical choices for pharmacists that I have discussed here provide a useful point of reference, readers contemplating pharmacy as a career may feel they need more details. Fortunately, a scientifically designed national survey was conducted recently in which 1,402 practitioners responded to a questionnaire covering 71 of their most important activities. A summary of these findings has been compiled and is furnished in Table I-4. Although the report does not account for pharmacist time allocated to such categories as "travel" or "idle,"

it does reflect the multiplicity of duties and their relative importance, as they are experienced by community practitioners. What is of equal significance, the study reveals a remarkable consistency in the way pharmacists spend their time. Minor differences, however, appear with respect to practice setting and number of years an individual has been in pharmacy. You may wish to refer to Table I-4 from time to time in order to keep these functions and their related percentages in perspective.

Another view of professional activities is provided in a statement on competency, which is reproduced below, that was prepared by the California State Board of Pharmacy. You will note that this descrip-

Table I–4

Functions of Pharmacists as Practitioners, by Type and Percent of Time Required, U.S.A., 1977–1978

Percent of Practitioner Time Currently Spent	Practitioner Duties	
	Functional Category	Illustrative Responsibilities
48%	I. Processing the Prescription Order	Receives prescription, verifies authenticity, prepares the order, labels the container, certifies that the contents and instructions are correct, and issues the prescription (see Figure 1-1).
33%	II. Management and Administration of the Pharmacy	Selects and supervises professional and non-professional staff, determines pricing structure, prepares budget and reviews financial statements, negotiates with vendors, controls inventory, receives merchandise.
12%	III. Patient Care Responsibilities	Clarifies patient understanding of how to use the medication, checks for allergic reactions to the prescription and for potential drug interactions, refers patients to other health centers for treatment, monitors patient response to the prescription, maintains competency in disease knowledge and appropriate drug use.
7%	IV. General Health Education of the Public	Supplies general information and literature about medical problems, drug use, and drug abuse to other pharmacists, health care practitioners, and the public.
100%		

Source: Rosenfeld, M., Thorton, R. F., and Glazer, R. *A National Study of the Practice of Pharmacy*. (A study sponsored jointly by the American Pharmaceutical Association and the American Association of Colleges of Pharmacy.) Princeton, N.J.: Educational Testing Service, 1978.

tion focuses on clinical skills and overlooks one third of the typical pharmacist's time, which is devoted to the management of the physical, financial, and human resources that are employed in the pharmacy. Nevertheless, it captures the spirit of patient orientation by identifying key services furnished by pharmacists.

Professional Competency in Pharmacy*

A competent pharmacist is capable of conferring with a physician concerning the care and treatment of his patient. He should appreciate the essentials of the clinical diagnosis and comprehend the medical management of the patient. He should have a knowledge of the drugs that may be used in the treatment of the patient's disease state, their mechanism of action, their commercial drug combinations and dosage forms, the fate and disposition of the drugs (if known), the factors which may influence the physiological availability and biological activity of the drugs from their dosage forms; how the age, sex, or secondary disease states might influence the course of treatment, and how other administered drugs, foods, and diagnostic procedures may interact to modify the activity of the drug.

A competent pharmacist is one whose overall functions result in optimum drug therapy. He should know the appropriate use and dosage regimen for the drug therapy being undertaken, the contraindications and potential untoward reactions which may result during therapy. He should be informed as to what proprietary products might interact adversely with such therapy or may be useful adjuncts to improve the convenience of administration or the overall patient care.

A competent pharmacist must know the proposed therapeutic actions of proprietary medication, their composition, and any uniqueness or potential limitations of their dosage forms. He should be capable of an objective appraisal of the advertising claims for the product. When requested by the patient, he should be capable of ascertaining the probable therapeutic usefulness of available proprietary medication in relation to the patient's complaints.

A competent pharmacist should be able to review a scientific publication and be able to summarize the practical implications of the findings as they may relate to the clinical use of drugs. He should be able to analyze a literature report of a clinical trial as to the appropriateness of the design of the study and of the statistical analysis made of the data. He should be able to prepare an objective summary of the significance of the data and the author's conclusions.

A competent pharmacist is a specialist on the stability of characteristics and storage requirements of drugs and drug products, on the factors that influence the release of drugs from dosage forms, how the site of administration or environment within its location in the body may influence the absorption of a specific drug from the administered dosage form, and most importantly, how these may interact to influence the onset, intensity, or duration of therapeutic action.

A competent pharmacist should be precisely informed of the legal limitations on procurement, storage, distribution, and sale of drugs. He should be informed of the approved use of a drug as specified by federal authorities and acceptable medical practice and his legal responsibilities to the patient in the use of drugs in experimental therapeutic procedures.

A competent pharmacist should be capable, with the availability of appropriate source material, of recommending which drug product and/or dosage form may be potentially most useful for a particular therapeutic need, and he should be able to support objectively his choice. He should also be capable, within a reasonable time, of identifying a drug product on the basis of its described color and shape, and possibly its proposed use, using appropriate source material.

A competent pharmacist, on the basis of the symptoms described in an interview with the patient, should be aware of what additional information he should attempt to gain from the patient concerning his condition. Based on this information he should be able to refer the patient to the

California Pharmacist 25 (April 1978):46–47.

proper medical practitioner, specialist, or agency which may be of most help to him in his case.

A competent pharmacist should have a knowledge of the toxic manifestations of drugs and the necessary measures which are best available means of treatment of these toxic symptoms.

A competent pharmacist should be able to communicate effectively with a patient on the instructions for proper administration of prescription and proprietary drugs. He should know the limitations which should be placed on food intake, other medication, and physical activity.

A competent pharmacist should be able to communicate with other health professionals or to laymen on appropriate drug subjects. He should be able to make the recipient understand the contents of the message being communicated.

A competent pharmacist should be capable of compounding appropriate drugs or combinations in acceptable dosage forms.

Finally, a competent pharmacist is a person who undertakes appropriate measures to maintain his level of competency in each of the above areas.

Prescription Drugs in Medical Care

How important are prescription drugs in patient care? While there are several ways to approach the question, your understanding of pharmacy will be facilitated by a consideration of a short statistical profile that covers drug use in our society.

According to a 1976 survey taken by the National Center for Health Statistics, prescription drug orders were most often initiated by doctors of medicine and osteopathy who were engaged in office-based practice, in comparison to those engaged in any other type of service. Consequently, the frequency of prescribing was nearly equal to the use of all other therapies (counseling, office surgery, etc.) combined. Because of the major role that pharmaceutical products play in the treatment of ambulatory patients, about 60 percent of all office visits result in

the individual's receiving an order for one or more prescriptions. Nearly 10 percent of this population, however, neglect to have these drug order(s) filled. Nevertheless, community pharmacists serve some 130,000,000 patients each year.

As noted above, polypharmacy is a common occurrence. A survey sponsored by the Upjohn Company found that 23 percent of the households with drug users include three or more prescribed medications that are currently being consumed. In fact, some surveys have discovered single individuals taking as many as 15 to 18 drugs at one time. The typical hospitalized patient, according to one study, receives 9 different prescriptions during confinement. Another investigation, carried out in Houston, Texas, found that the average mother consumes 19 different medications during the nine months of pregnancy and delivery. As you will learn in your readings, the professional training of the pharmacist can be employed to help minimize the drug interactions that are likely to occur when multiple medications are consumed.

These illustrative data depicting the frequency of prescribing, when added together on a national basis, reveal that an estimated 2.8 billion orders are dispensed each year to patients in the United States. The total economic value of all prescriptions, including product cost and the expense for professional services in various treatment settings, is estimated to have reached nearly 20 billion dollars in 1979.

Sometime during the early part of the 1980s, the number of prescriptions ordered in all health care environments—inpatient and outpatient, private and government—will probably exceed an annual rate of three billion. This total is likely to be composed of more than two billion orders for ambulatory patients and nearly one billion for institutionalized bed patients. The role of government relative to the private sector in paying for these medications, however, cannot be predicted at this time. If a National Health

Insurance program with drug benefits is enacted, there is no question that the proportion of prescriptions subject to third-party regulations will rise.

In order to accommodate a demand of this magnitude, one Department of Health, Education, and Welfare report predicts that the number of active pharmacists will grow from 117,000 in 1973 to 185,000 by 1990—an increase of almost 60 percent in less than twenty years. Another manpower study has placed pharmacy among the top ten professions for growth in terms of employment potential. A more detailed assessment of the supply and demand factors affecting job opportunities for pharmacists is provided in Chapter Eight.

This overview indicates that prescription drugs represent one of the cornerstones of the health care delivery system. Since pharmacists play a major part in effecting both their distribution and their rational use, many readers may wish to consider the information furnished below.

Chapter Two

Using This Guide Efficiently

This chapter explains the methods that were used to select your readings. It also includes tips on how to improve the accuracy of your perceptions about pharmacy as a possible career. Since the implications of your choice are likely to extend for more than 40 years after graduation from college, these procedures and recommendations merit careful consideration.

How Your Readings Were Selected

The 77 readings in this compilation were drawn from a survey of 13 major pharmacy periodicals that cover the period 1975–1978.* We have supplemented this foundation with a review of other sources in order to ensure that a representative picture of pharmacy developed. Despite the short time frame of four years, the search process generated more than 4,000 potential entries. From this base, over 385 selections were marked initially as worthy of your attention. After an intensive review of these items, nearly 100 were discarded. The balance, which form the basis for this book, were classified in terms of their relative value as either Readings or Bibliography.

The final determination governing which entries would be reproduced was based on a number of criteria. First, because this volume is designed to help students appraise pharmacy as a career option, it seemed important that most articles describe the actual or proposed duties of pharmacy graduates. These descriptions of what pharmacists do have been augmented by studies or essays pertaining to problems of general concern to professionals. This strategy reflects the fact that practitioners do not operate exclusively within a treatment setting, but are influenced often by a host of such external forces as government regulations pertaining to drug distribution, third-party reimbursement, licensure, and continuing education.

Preference has also been given to shorter rather than longer articles and to elementary rather than complicated analyses. As a result, each reading should be especially useful for beginning students who are appraising various opportunities that exist for personnel who are trained in pharmacy.

Moreover, emphasis has been placed on current trends and future possibilities for professional contribution. Thus, your readings stress where pharmacy seems to be headed and the issues that may be encountered as new role models evolve. Since it is ordained that you will spend the rest of your life living in the future, this orientation seems sound. You should recognize, though, that various institutions (academia and government, for example) and commercial activities (such as the sale of non-drug items) may act as a brake on new developments. It is essential, therefore, to obtain some understanding of the contemporary forces that could facilitate or impede the more effective delivery of prescription products and professional services.

Some students may develop an interest in newly emerging specialty areas such as medical oncology or pediatric pharmacy. How-

---

*This general cut-off may result in some useful references being overlooked. For most decisions related to career planning, however, such a limitation is not thought to be critical.

ever, the actual relationship between job openings and applicants a decade or two from now is not easy to predict. Readers are cautioned, therefore, that employment opportunities will not necessarily be proportional to the number of articles used to describe a given function or problem area. Thus we must distinguish clearly between the romance and social utility of new frontiers and the willingness of our nation to support the pharmacist's discretion in undertaking innovative methods related to the medication needs of patients.

This guide has also endeavored to reflect a wide range of communication formats— among others, it includes research reports, testimonials, interviews, job descriptions and essays. In addition, depth of understanding has been sacrificed in favor of a broad overview and you should be alert to this limitation. Further, several readings outline pharmacist activities in general as illustrated in numbers 1, 20, 25, 39, 40, 43, 44, 45, 46, and 50. Many, though, focus on functions that involve only a portion of the typical pharmacist's responsibilities. Numbers 2, 7, 8, 9, 10, 11, 13, 14, 17, 21, 26, 27, 28, 29, 32, 33, 34, 35, 37, 38, 42, 48, 49, 51, 60, and 62 represent the latter type. While several of these selections may depict the duties of a full-time specialist, most portray only a small portion of the functions assumed by a staff (general) pharmacist. When you have completed this volume, check to make sure that your interest pattern has not been built exclusively on such part-time activities.

The nature of the author's background is another factor that was employed in the selection process. Pharmacists employed as practitioners were afforded priority over experts found in academia. Because of the paucity of studies conducted by the former, a large proportion of the readings still emanate from college faculty. In addition, since hospital based pharmacists are represented in the literature more frequently than community practitioners, the readings mirror this bias.

The professional literature also includes important statements by physicians who discuss the role of pharmacists in the treatment of a particular medical condition such as hypertension or diabetes. With one exception, a priority was established to let the pharmacist describe his own contribution in such programs. If you wish to examine the views of persons outside pharmacy, the bibliography at the conclusion of each reading unit will direct you to these sources.

In general, no effort has been made to update statistical data, excise repetitious material, or reconcile conflicting points of view. Indeed, several articles and references have been selected because they reflect disagreement among the experts. Further, over 40 percent of the readings appeared originally in a journal that relied upon peer review before the editor accepted the manuscript for publication. This process of anonymous evaluation by professional specialists does not guarantee the scientific validity of the data or the objectivity of the author's interpretation. It does tend to raise the probability that the findings warrant your attention.

Finally, this overview does not purport to suggest the multiple facets of pharmacy training or all opportunities for a professional career. The former requires that a student spend four or more years in pharmacy school, while the latter may consume much of a lifetime during which a practitioner explores alternative employment options. Nevertheless, this volume should provide you with a strong foundation for making a wise selection.

Testing Your Impressions

Let us assume that your initial interest in pharmacy as a means of professional expression is favorable, but some doubts remain. Uneasiness of this type is not uncommon, regardless of which career you pursue, whether medicine, law, prize fighting, or politics. Indeed, for a few individuals, confirmation of a vocational preference may not appear until after between 10 and 20 years of actual experience. There are, however, seven basic steps that you can follow over the next several months to help maximize the probability of your making a good choice. If a few hours each weekend, or the major part of a week's vacation, can be salvaged from your schedule, I urge that you investigate several of the following possibilities.

First, identify those readings that have generated the greatest initial appeal. (You can use the Pharmacy Scorecard at the back of the book.) Now supplement your first impressions by exploring these topics more deeply. The college of pharmacy library or community library should be able to help you locate the following:

1. one or two of the most important references from among those that often appear at the conclusion of each reading.
2. several selections from the specially compiled bibliography that follows each section. Should you desire more information on a given subject, don't hesitate to consult a book or monograph when one is listed at the conclusion of the bibliography. Keep in mind that you are not examining these works for a grade but simply to establish whether your career objectives might be reflected in the professional activities that are described.

By reading more intensively, you should be able to improve the accuracy of your interpretation and confirm the level of interest in a particular aspect of pharmacy.

Second, read more extensively. One way of applying this guideline is to read several pharmacy periodicals for at least four months. The special, abbreviated list below has been compiled to help you pursue this goal. Selection of a journal from one or preferably both categories should help to expand your understanding about the many dimensions of pharmacy practice. If the desired periodicals are not available in your public or college library, ask your closest pharmacist to borrow his old copies for several weeks. Indeed, an expenditure of $20 or $30 for a personal subscription to two of the most interesting journals might represent the soundest investment that a freshman could make during his or her entire year in college.

Reviewed Journals
American Journal of Hospital Pharmacy
The Apothecary
Contemporary Pharmacy Practice
Drug Intelligence & Clinical Pharmacy
Hospital Pharmacy

Other Journals
American Druggist
American Pharmacy
Drug Topics
NARD Journal
Pharmacy Times
U.S. Pharmacist

Third, review some of the selections that did not rate highly at the time of your initial reading. This extra effort may help to clarify your assessment of certain aspects of pharmacy practice.

Fourth, visit several community or hospital pharmacies and request permission to observe the pharmacist carry out a variety of professional responsibilities. If your arrival coincides with a period of low prescription demand, the practitioner should be able to answer your questions about his or her duties and to help you evaluate the choice of a career in pharmacy.

Fifth, write or visit faculty members at one or preferably two colleges of pharmacy. Since the faculties are composed of both basic scientists and experts in the applied aspects of professional practice, you should try to contact representatives from both areas. Most instructors will be flattered to recommend one or two important readings, especially if he or she is the author.

In addition, a number of colleges hold an annual Pharmacy Day Open House to acquaint interested students (and parents) with their educational requirements and program. Plan to attend one or more of these sessions. If scientific exhibits dominate the activities, however, you will want to keep in mind that many of these demonstrations may be more representative of the educational curriculum than of duties performed by practicing pharmacists.

Sixth, consider pharmacy training as a stepping stone for an advanced degree in one of the health, biological, physical, administrative, or social sciences. For example, it can be held that pharmacy is an excellent foundation for subsequent practice as a physician, dentist, or podiatrist. Moreover, with the probable growth of drug insurance programs, a pharmacist with a Ph.D. in pharmacy administration or preventive medicine would seem to have a very bright future, especially if specialization in evaluating the quality of prescribing, dispensing, and drug compliance is pursued.

Seventh, consider pharmacy training as a second degree. In certain western institutions, nearly 50 percent of the students admitted to their six-year programs have already received a bachelor's degree in another field. While dual degrees at this level are not needed by all pharmacy graduates, unique opportunities for professional contribution could arise for those who possess the "right" combination of academic backgrounds. For example, computer science, economics, or business administration could serve as a useful foundation for handling problems that often are slighted in the pharmacy curriculum. If your interest lies in the clinical area (patient care) a prior degree in biology or communications might be preferred.

The graduate degree route will probably require a total educational investment of 7 to 12 years, while the dual degree route may take from 7 to 10 years. The former could be preferable, however, because employment opportunities are likely to be greater, while lifetime earning power may be enhanced as well. Although manpower studies do not indicate precisely how many pharmacy graduates might be absorbed through the sixth and seventh options, it seems probable that attractive employment opportunities will still be present even if the current proportion of such graduates (perhaps 5 to 6 percent) were doubled or even tripled. Regardless of which of these alternatives is preferred, consultation with appropriate faculty and specialists should be undertaken prior to and during the formulation of a student's academic program.

In addition to the seven steps outlined above, you may elect to devise an eighth or ninth of your own. One of these approaches might include weekend or summer employment in a local pharmacy. Alternatively, you may wish to consider first whether working in the field of health care, with the challenges of improving patient health status and containing costs, seems important. Society thinks so because health care as an industry is currently one of the nation's largest.

Regardless of the path you choose for your investigation, be systematic and diligent in your pursuit of pharmacy as a career option. It seems far better to allocate some 50 hours to this task during the next few months than to discover three or ten years later that another profession should have been selected. The tradeoff from undertaking this homework assignment now will be at least 156:1 in your favor, just considering the time, to say nothing of the dollar amount, if it can be established that pharmacy seems to be the preferred educational route for your talents and interests.

In summary, this section has stressed that learning about pharmacy is not a passive process. While your guide has been constructed to serve as an efficient means of probing the multiple aspects of pharmacy, you can get a more accurate impression primarily by putting more personal time into the discovery process. The summer before you enter college could represent an ideal period for exercising this responsibility.

Finding Your Area(s) of Interest

There is no best (that is to say, not misleading) way of classifying the material that will provide your introduction to pharmacy. At least eight methods of organizing the readings might have been employed.* Exclusive reliance on one or two systems, however, would tend to present a distorted view of how pharmacists function in our society. A multiple classification scheme, therefore, has been used, as is indicated by the detailed index presented at the beginning of Chapter Three (see Table III-1).

The application of this or other classification systems will enable an individual to become acquainted with the opportunities for graduates in pharmacy. Since many students may require additional aid in choosing a career, a unique Pharmacy Scorecard has been prepared (see inside back cover) which should be marked after each reading. In addition, the text includes three decision-making tables where your Scorecard can be applied to help pinpoint those professional responsibilities and educational choices that seem to be consistent with your interests (see Tables II-1, VI-4, and VI-5).

In order to illustrate how your Pharmacy Scorecard should be compiled, a hypothetical example of a completed form is reproduced below. The results for each reader will, of course, be unique.

When you finish reading each article in this volume, record your rating on the Scorecard, as shown above. In some instances, you will wish to check the bibliographical references before making a final entry. If a majority of the selections appear in the final column, pharmacy may be a poor

choice as an area for your college education and professional expression.

Classification of Numbered Readings

Interesting or Very Interesting	Moderately Interesting	Little or No Interest
1, 2, 3, 7, 8, 9	4	5, 6
10, 11, 14, 16, 17, 18, 19	12, 15	13
20, 22, 28, 29	21, 23, 24, 27	25, 26
33, 34, 35, 36, 37, 38	30, 31, 39	32
40, 45, 46, 47, 49	41, 42, 43, 44, 48	
52, 53, 54	50, 55, 59	51, 56, 57, 58
61, 64, 65, 66, 68, 69	60, 62	63
71, 72, 76, 77	70, 73	74, 75

On the other hand, if most numbers appear in the first two columns, then you will want to proceed to Table II-1. Using a pencil, transfer the ratings on the Scorecard to the Table as indicated below:

Rating You Assigned Reading	Code for Numbered Selection
Very interesting/interesting =	0
Moderately interesting =	(No mark)
Little or no interest =	X

Once Table II-1 has been marked with your summary impressions, the concentration of circles and unmarked readings will provide a working hypothesis to indicate the type of activity that seems most important as you begin your educational program. Repeat this transcribing process for Tables VI-4 and VI-5. Visual inspection of each modified table will furnish an accurate picture of the educational and career objectives that are most likely to reflect your interests at this time.

Since a year or two of study, coupled with some work experience, could lead to a change in your professional goals, it may be useful to reread the entire guide sometime

*This general issue is discussed by Bruce R. Siecker in "Pharmacy Specialties: The Unresolved Dilemma," *California Pharmacist* 23 (October 1976):36–40.

during the second or third year of enrollment in pharmacy school. Moreover, it will be necessary to create a new Pharmacy Scorecard. If this additional review yields a profile similar to the first, it would appear that you are on the right track and going in the right direction. If a sharp disparity arises, however, discussion with your academic adviser and parents is probably desirable.

Table II-1

Paired Alternatives to Help Establish Your Place in Pharmacy

In order to test your interest in a given area below, investigate the readings in the opposite column.	If a majority of the readings in a particular block have been circled, your area of primary interest is indicated in the column on the left. If a heavy concentration of X's appears, however, you should proceed with caution.
Community Practice	1, 2, 4, 5, 6, 7, 10, 12, 13, 14, 15, 16, 20, 23, 24, 35, 39, 40, 41, 42, 44, 49, 50, 51, 54, 60, 62
Institutional Practice	6, 8, 9, 10, 11, 13, 17, 20, 21, 25, 26, 27, 28, 29, 31, 32, 33, 34, 35, 36, 37, 38, 43, 45, 46, 47, 48, 51
Private Sector of the Delivery System	1, 2, 4, 5, 6, 7, 9, 10, 11, 12, 13, 14, 15, 16, 17, 21, 23, 24, 25, 27, 28, 29, 31, 32, 33, 35, 37, 39, 40, 41, 42, 44, 45, 46, 47, 48, 49, 50, 51
Government Sector of the Delivery System	1, 6, 7, 8, 9, 10, 11, 12, 13, 14, 17, 21, 23, 24, 25, 26, 27, 28, 29, 31, 32, 33, 34, 35, 37, 38, 43, 45, 46, 47, 51
Practitioner Serving Patients	1, 2, 4, 5, 6, 7, 8, 9, 10, 11, 12, 13, 14, 15, 16, 17, 20, 21, 23, 24, 25, 26, 27, 28, 29, 31, 32, 33, 34, 35, 37, 38, 39, 40, 41, 42, 43, 44, 45, 46, 47, 48, 49, 50, 51
Non-Practitioner	5, 27, 29, 42, 51, 57, 69, 70, 71, 72, 73, 74, 75, 76, 77,

Note: (1) A few readings have been excluded from certain paired combinations because they do not enhance your power of discrimination. (2) If a code appears simultaneously in the upper and lower cell of a paired alternative, this situation simply illustrates that the professional function usually is common to both. (3) With respect to the non-practitioner cell, numbers 5, 27, 29, 42, 51, and 57 indicate that these practitioner roles, for some, could lead to full-time specialization without direct responsibility for patient care.

Chapter Three

Pharmacists as Practitioners

The 63 readings that follow this introduction depict the wide variety of professional responsibilities exercised by pharmacists in their role as practitioners. Despite the length of this compilation, it still is somewhat incomplete due to either gaps in the literature or the inability of published works to satisfy the selection criteria specified above. (This problem, though, is a minor one, as is indicated by the material in Appendix A.) Nevertheless, the insights gained from your readings as a whole, coupled with the enhanced perspective obtained by pursuing several of the additional steps recommended in Chapter Two, will provide you with an informed basis for appraising pharmacy as a career option.

In order to facilitate your understanding of what pharmacists do when they serve patients, you should take a few moments to review the adjacent table. This outline defines the organizational framework that has been used to classify your readings. The primary levels of classification represent three ways of describing different aspects of pharmacy practice. Within each category, functional responsibilities have been presented in alphabetical order. As you move from the first, "Type of Professional Service," to the second, "Place of Treatment," you will perceive some duplication. This material has been included because certain practitioners

develop a strong preference for working in one location in contrast to another. Moreover, differences in personal satisfaction have even been reported within a given setting. The third heading, "Other Perspectives," furnishes readings on broad issues that apply to pharmacy practice regardless of function or place.

Since a majority of active pharmacists are engaged as generalists, the readings begin by describing major components of general practice.* The next subsection, "Specialized Services/Medical Problems," lists functions where more than 50 pharmacists, in the opinion of the author, are likely to be engaged in full-time practice by 1990. This employment threshold has already been crossed in Clinical Pharmacy, Drug Information, and perhaps other areas as well. While some of the possible occupational specialities noted here may not have achieved formal certification by that date (only Nuclear Pharmacy is recognized currently), this subsection† is recommended as a starting point for students seeking a practice environment and/or responsibilities different from those of the general practitioner. The last subsection, "Primary Care," describes a role in which pharmacists act mainly as physicians' assistants, where they also diagnose and treat certain acute illnesses and manage patients with specific chronic conditions. Most employ-

---

*In reviewing selections numbered 6 through 17, you should note that the number of pages represented by each reading unit is not proportional to the actual duties of the average pharmacist. (See Table I–4.)

†Formal speciality status usually is determined by a unique professional contribution, not merely by place of employment. Students should anticipate, therefore, that some of the positions cited here may fail to gain speciality certification. However, they do represent differentiated job opportunities, and this is the major focus of your guide.

Table III-1

Pharmacists as Practitioners: Classification System and Reading Units

	Reading Number
Type of Professional Service	
1. General Practice	
a. An Overview	1–5
b. Adverse Reactions and Interactions	6
c. Contraception	7
d. Diabetes	8
e. Drug Abuse	9–10
f. Drug Utilization Review	11
g. General Health Education/Preventive Services	12–13
h. Hypertension	14
i. Over-the-Counter Preparations	15–16
j. Terminal Illness	17
2. Specialized Services/Medical Problems	
a. Clinical: Overview	18–20
• Drug History Taking	21
• Drug Therapy Adviser	22
• Patient Counseling	23–24
• Therapeutic Monitoring	25
• Therapeutic Management	26
b. Clinical Pharmacokinetics	27
c. Critical Care	28
d. Drug Information	29
e. Geriatrics	30
f. Intravenous Drug Therapy	31–32
g. Medical Oncology	33
h. Mental Illness	34
i. Nuclear Pharmacy	35
j. Pediatrics	36
k. Poisoning	37
3. Primary Care	38
Place of Treatment	
1. Community Pharmacy	39–42
2. Federal Facility	43
3. Group Medical Clinic	44
4. Hospital	45–47
5. Long-Term Care Institution	48–49
6. Rural Area	50
Other Perspectives	
1. Computers in Pharmacy	51
2. Minorities in Pharmacy	52
3. Problems and Issues	53–62
4. Women in Pharmacy	63

ment opportunities of this nature are likely to be found in government-operated clinics and hospitals.

In order to derive maximum benefit from the articles below, you should keep the following three points in mind:

1. At the conclusion of each reading unit, supplemental aids, when appropriate, have been supplied in the following sequence:

  a. a code number indicating related readings that appear in this volume. Since the material in a given unit may focus on only a portion of the practitioner's total responsibilities, these cross-references can be used to expand your comprehension of the duties associated with a particular activity. In some instances you may wish to check these supporting selections before making a final entry on your Pharmacy Scorecard.

  b. a bibliography identifying important articles that appear elsewhere. Moreover, items have been ranked to reflect their potential utility for your purpose—thus the first and/or second citation should be of greater incremental value that those that follow.

  c. monographs, books, or, in a few instances, specialized journals.

While each type of aid will not appear at the end of every reading unit, students interested in such sources should be alert to their availability.

2. The classification scheme adopted for your readings has been designed to highlight the unique services that may be provided by pharmacists. As noted above, this format, from time to time, results in some functional overlap within and between sections. For example, the role of the clinical pharmacist is outlined in sections 18 through 26. However, competency in this area also serves as the basis for rendering professional service in even more specialized areas such as geriatric (30) or medical oncology pharmacy (33). Further, pharmacists trained in clinical programs are likely to be proficient in performing most of the professional tasks carried out

by generalists. On the other hand, general practitioners may offer certain clinical services (for example, patient counseling) interspersed with traditional dispensing duties and managerial activities.

This flexibility in responsibilities arises, in part, because regulations issued by state licensure boards specify minimum rather than maximum standards of performance. Consequently, the ultimate contribution of the pharmacist is seldom set exclusively by his work place, but it may depend more on individual initiative in determining the scope of services furnished to patients. Your readings should be regarded, therefore, as examples of pharmacy practice rather than as efforts to produce a precise definition of any single role model.

3. Several articles contain scientific terminology that probably will require external help from a dictionary, a pharmacist, or an instructor. If you are simply considering pharmacy as a career, many of these technical terms can be skipped as you focus on the general content of the article. On the other hand, if you are already enrolled in a college of pharmacy, it seems essential that resources be consulted to build up your vocabulary and your understanding of the topic. Since this book has been prepared for persons without a background in pharmacy, communication barriers of this type should be at a minimum.

If your level of comprehension still seems inadequate, selections 1, 2, 15, 24, 41, 42, 43, and 49 may be read first. Alternatively, bypass the more difficult numbers for the time being—27, 29, 31, and 46—and return to them after you have completed all other material. For most students, an examination of the readings in their normal sequence should prove to be the most efficient way of exploring their interest in pharmacy.

Finally, in approaching the information below, you may wish to develop a personal plan to ensure that your appraisal of pharmacy as a career option is as accurate as pos-

sible. First, prepare a schedule that will facilitate your keeping the various roles of pharmacists clearly in mind. The following example should be modified to reflect your own preferences and discretionary time.

Approximate Allocation of Time by Week	Recommended Study Schedule
1	Chapters One and Two; Chapter Three, at this point
2	Readings 1–17
3	18–38
4	39–63
5	64–68
6	Chapter Five
7	Chapters Six and Seven
8	Chapter Eight and Appendixes

When picking up this volume, set aside enough time to review each reading unit as a whole. In certain instances (such as with Readings 37 and 69), only four or five minutes will be required. In other cases (such as with Readings 18–20 and 53–62), an hour may be needed. Whatever plan is adopted, it should exclude an attempt to digest the entire volume in a single week.

Second, note the heading and, as appropriate, the subheading where each selection appears. Since new territory is being examined, it is important to recall whether your point of reference is that of a generalist, a specialist, or problem in pharmacy that may apply to most practitioners.

Third, use the Pharmacy Scorecard to record your summary impression as soon as you have completed each reading. If it seems desirable to return to a particular reference a second time, or to obtain more data from one of the special bibliographical citations, your original rating can be changed, when necessary, to reflect this broader perspective.

The Pharmacy Scorecard concept has been derived from research studies which indicate that the primary basis for choosing a career is the anticipated enjoyment of one's work. This device should not be regarded as infallible. Nevertheless, when the Scorecard is used in conjunction with the three decision-making tables that are found in Chapters Two and Six, it can serve as an interim guide until additional and possibly contrary evidence about pharmacy has been accumulated.

GENERAL PRACTICE

An Overview

1—What Are Comprehensive Pharmacy Services?

Peter P. Lamy and Donald O. Fedder

It is truly fortunate that in this age of management-engineering studies, economic restrictions, and demands for cost-cutting, Pharmacy has embarked on a program of restating its role in health care. No longer are Pharmacy services focused only on the product. No longer is the pharmacist solely the counting-and-pouring "dispenser of drugs." Pharmacists and the patients they serve are learning that pharmacy can effectively cut the cost of health care and, at the same time, contribute greatly to its quality.

Furthermore, the patient's well-being is no longer the single responsibility of the physician. Efforts in preventive, acute, and chronic care of the patient are now a joint responsibility of many health professionals, including the pharmacist.

It is important, therefore, that we define pharmacy practice in terms of services provided to the patient. The authors have drawn on the experience of practitioners in all areas of Pharmacy in preparing these practice parameters, and commend these parameters to those groups studying standards of practice as well as to the schools of pharmacy, the boards, and the profession itself.

Comprehensive Pharmacy Services

Our definition would encompass, in outline form, those tasks that are vital in providing Comprehensive Pharmacy Services (CPS). This definition is based on the concept that Pharmacy has changed and continues to change. "Dispensing" of the prescription (i.e., the receipt of a prescription, the unquestioned response to the physician's directions, the packaging of the drug, the writing of the label, and the handling of the finished product) was at one time the basis of pharmacy practice.

This "dispensing" process has now become a part, and *only one part*, of the overall CPS. This service continues to begin with the selection of quality drugs to be dispensed. This requires, on the pharmacist's part, a thorough knowledge of the pharmaceutical literature (including drug recalls) and manufacturer's information available. (See outline, Table 1.1.)

Better Understanding of Pharmacy

In this CPS effort, we are attempting to focus on the need for a better understanding of the practice of Pharmacy. This understanding requires acceptance in some form of these concepts by the profession, by the public, as well as by government and also by 3rd party payors.

In defining this aspect of pharmacy service, no effort was made by the authors to limit practitioners in other levels of service. Therefore, such functions as drug information to physicians, patient counseling where no dispensing is involved, home health care services, and others are not included in this particular report.

We do not delineate which of the tasks in the dispensing process are to be performed by a pharmacist and which could be performed by a technician.

The tasks that are outlined in this article are those that, in the authors' opinion, are essential in providing CPS—Comprehensive Pharmacy Services—to the patient.

Table 1.1

These 16 Separate Steps Outline Comprehensive Pharmacy Services

1 **Receive prescription**
   a. written
   b. oral

2 **Check prescription for**
   a. authenticity
   b. legality

3 **Identify patient clearly and update patient medication profile**
   a. review patient's disease state
   b. review current therapy
   c. review age, sex, weight, allergies, idiosyncracies, dietary restrictions

4 **Decide on therapeutic appropriateness of prescription**
   a. drug
   b. dosage regimen
   c. administration regimen
   d. route of administration

5 **Decide on economic appropriateness of prescription**
   a. quantity
   b. drug product selection

6 **Make appropriate recommendations to physician, patient, and/or patient's family**

7 **Assemble correct drug and select appropriate container**
   a. decide on patient's ability to handle child-proof container
   b. decide on patient's ability to store drug correctly at home

8 **Measure, weigh, count, compound, and package medication**

9 **Prepare label instructions and attach**
   a. specific administration directions

   b. appropriate auxiliary labels
      1) storage   2) refill authorization
      3) cautionary   4) therapeutic warnings

10 **Determine cost and appropriate fee**

11 **Patient consultation and dispensing**
   a. reinforce all label instructions
      1) special consideration of patient's ability to comprehend written and oral instructions
   b. add more instructions as necessary
      1) special consideration of a patient with impaired sight or hearing
      2) special consideration of patient's physical impairment
      3) special consideration of patient's age (pediatric, geriatric)
   c. consider the need for special instructions to the patient's family
   d. point out need for compliance with all instructions
   e. dispense the prescription

12 **If patient is not present**
   a. follow procedure 11
   b. select additional method (telephone, written instructions) to address patient personally

13 **Complete patient record**

14 **Return product to storage area; reorder, if necessary**

15 **If patient fails to pick up prescription**
   a. contact patient
   b. if patient does not respond
      1) adjust the patient record
      2) notify the prescriber

16 **Notify patient of impending refill (where appropriate, as in chronic care medications)**
   a. if no response, follow procedure 15b

2—Serving the Woodstock Nation

Joseph J. Forno

Woodstock, New York, population 7,000, is nestled in the Catskill Mountains, 100 miles north of New York City. The town might be termed a "case history" of the American art colony, having hosted successive waves of avant-garde artists since the days of the Bohemian movement early in this century.

In recent years, Woodstock has become famous as a musicians' retreat. Bob Dylan, The Band, the Rolling Stones, and other players have found something in Woodstock to inspire an entire generation that bears the town's name.

Woodstock offers a rich mixture of rural community spirit, scenic beauty and sophisticated culture. Two statistics make today's Woodstock unique among the rural communities of upstate New York:

• 32 percent of the population earns more than $15,000 per year;

• 50 percent of the working population consists of management and professional people.

This unusual setting has provided me with an opportunity to practice community pharmacy in a uniquely receptive environment.

I practice in Woodstock Colonial Pharmacy, a modern, yet physically traditional, family-owned corporation founded by my father in 1947 that is far from being the typical rural pharmacy. Our patients represent a cascade of personalities and life experiences, which have stimulated me to offer much more than traditional pharmacy services. Through working in such a creative community I have found that the boundaries of community pharmacy are broad but well within the reach of today's younger pharmacists.

My gradual involvement in "extracurricular" pharmacy began in 1974, when I served on the Woodstock Narcotics Guidance Council. That year I produced a video film entitled "What Do You Do for Pain?" which included on-the-street interviews as well as discussions by physicians and dentists. The former revealed many alternative approaches to emotional and physical pain, while the latter concentrated on more traditional drug therapy for pain and anxiety. For many Woodstock residents, acupuncture, biofeedback, and massage, as well as herbal, chiropractic, and homeopathic medicine, are a part of the healing process.

Through this experience, as well as in the pharmacy, I learned that my patients are of above-average intelligence. They also have a keen sense of body awareness, often asking probing drug information questions such as "Can I breast-feed while taking Flagyl (metronidazole)?" A patient being treated for a convulsive disorder with phenobarbital asked whether the skin rash she had developed could be iatrogenic. "Is Gyne-Lotrimin (clotrimazole) more effective for monilia than Mycostatin (nystatin)?" was another question.

'Fact Sheets'

In response to these and other queries I developed my first "fact sheets" in 1974.

These handouts describe drug effects, side effects and precautions and offer instructions for instilling eye and ear medicaments. Patients receive these sheets with prescriptions for such drugs as phenylbutazone, metronidazole, and antibiotics. Other handouts explain conditions such as hypertension, genital herpes, scabies, and urinary tract infections.

Our pharmacy staff, which also includes Frank Damis and Paul Rode, uses patient profiles and auxiliary labeling to increase the efficiency of our drug delivery.

Clearly, the best way to encourage patient compliance is to combine written and verbal instructions. I have attempted to "spread the word" around the community in the local newspapers, offering my opinions on such topics as Medicaid, generic drugs, flu vaccines, and drug abuse. In addition to articles and editorial comments, I have placed professionally oriented advertisements describing the fact sheet program, hypertension, poison prevention, and drug product selection laws.

Pharmacy Bulletin

Patients are not the only people asking questions. The four local physicians and six dentists often come up with challenging inquiries of their own. Among them: recent research on genital herpes, new uses for *l*-tryptophan, the controversial use of N2 root canal paste in dentistry, and the use of mebendazole in whipworm infections.

In responding to questions on these topics, I found myself augmenting the pharmacy library to include several medical and drug journals, as well as the latest editions of many popular textbooks. I began to publish the results of my research in a bimonthly pharmacy bulletin, which is now distributed countywide to 100 physicians, dentists and pharmaceutical salespeople. The bulletin also covers recently available or soon-to-be marketed drugs and discusses laws affecting both pharmacist and physician.

The bulletin has received an excellent response. Many readers have expressed disbelief that they were receiving such a publication, at no charge, from a local pharmacist. Since I do most of the layout for the fact sheets and bulletin myself, my only costs are photocopying and postage, a minimal investment for such worthwhile projects.

Going from print to public speaking has been a natural progression for me. Five years ago I was invited to speak to the health class at Onteora High School, whose district boasts a 62 percent college placement. Working with health educator Robin Sears, I helped develop a progressive drug awareness unit taught each semester. Topics range from recent marijuana research to OTC drugs.

In 1975 I began conducting training workshops for area drug abuse agencies, which started my association with Family of Woodstock, a well-known state-funded crisis intervention center, which operates a 24-hour telephone hotline for Ulster County. Currently, I am working with second-level drug training and have just received funding for a comprehensive 12-week alcohol and drug abuse course to be taught with other Family staff in spring 1979.

I also serve on the board of advisors for Family House, a home for runaway children operated by the same organization. As unofficial drug consultant for Family, I was recently overwhelmed with calls about paraquat contamination of Mexican marijuana and began selling testing kits shortly after the spraying program became front-page news.

Elsewhere in the community, I have organized workshops for the Ulster County Drug Task Force and for a subsequently videotaped crisis intervention course at State University of New York (New Paltz). I have lectured on various drug-related topics before community forums at local churches, the Ulster County Police Chiefs Association and the Senior Citizen Action Council.

Pharmacology Course

Last spring, pharmacist-colleague Ed Ullmann and I taught a credit-free continuing education course in pharmacology for area nurses. The six-week course, given at Ulster County Community College, was filled within a week to our maximum of 45 registrants. Our lectures dealt with introductory pharmacology, antidepressants, antipsychotics, antibiotics, cardiovascular, and over-the-counter drugs and hypertension. The course will be repeated during UCCC's spring 1979 session. Because of other commitments, Ed and I had to turn down a request that we teach an undergraduate pharmacology course for the college nursing program, but we are excited at the possibility of such an opportunity in the future.

Most recently, I was appointed to the medical advisory board of the local Planned Parenthood chapter. This group of physicians and staff personnel meets several times a year to discuss protocol changes in birth control and related drug therapies.

Although a great deal of work is required, I have found it easy to become more involved in "extracurricular" pharmacy. I have found this work to be not only personally exciting and rewarding, but also beneficial to the community in which I live and work.

In my opinion, too many of my fellow pharmacists have lost touch with their ability to be something more than good businessmen. Contemporary practitioners must realize that they can profit by being more patient oriented.

3—Code of Ethics

American Pharmaceutical Association

Preamble

These principles of professional conduct for pharmacists are established to guide the pharmacist in his relationship with patients, fellow practitioners, other health professionals and the public.

A Pharmacist *should hold the health and safety of patients to be of first consideration; he should render to each patient the full measure of his ability as an essential health practitioner.*

A Pharmacist *should never knowingly con-* *done the dispensing, promoting or distributing of drugs or medical devices, or assist therein, which are not of good quality, which do not meet standards required by law or which lack therapeutic value for the patient.*

A Pharmacist *should always strive to perfect and enlarge his professional knowledge. He should utilize and make available this knowledge as may be required in accordance with his best professional judgment.*

A Pharmacist *has the duty to observe the*

law, to uphold the dignity and honor of the profession, and to accept its ethical principles. He should not engage in any activity that will bring discredit to the profession and should expose, without fear or favor, illegal or unethical conduct in the profession.

A Pharmacist *should seek at all times only fair and reasonable remuneration for his services. He should never agree to, or participate in, transactions with practitioners of other health professions or any other person under which fees are divided or which may cause financial or other exploitation in connection with the rendering of his professional services.*

A Pharmacist *should respect the confidential and personal nature of his professional records; except where the best interest of the patient requires or the law demands, he should not disclose such information to anyone without proper patient authorization.*

A Pharmacist *should not agree to practice*

under terms or conditions which tend to interfere with or impair the proper exercise of his professional judgment and skill, which tend to cause a deterioration of the quality of his service or which require him to consent to unethical conduct.

A Pharmacist *should strive to provide information to patients regarding professional services truthfully, accurately, and fully and should avoid misleading patients regarding the nature, cost, or value of the pharmacist's professional services.*

A Pharmacist *should associate with organizations having for their objective the betterment of the profession of pharmacy; he should contribute of his time and funds to carry on the work of these organizations.*

*Approved by APhA
Active and Life members
August 1969
Amended December 1975*

4—An Analysis of The Office Practice of Pharmacy

Eugene V. White

Although I had very little encouragement (and many skeptics openly predicted an early demise when I removed all vestiges of commercialism from my practice), the experience of the past 18 years has clearly demonstrated that society *will* support the pharmacist as a practitioner in a professional office setting.

Public Acceptance of the Concept

In the overall plan, it was essential that the public accept and support the *concept* of the office-based family pharmacist—because it was the only avenue in *community* practice that would enable the pharmacist to step up eventually into a new and major role on the

Included in this article are excerpts from publications entitled *The Office-Based Family Pharmacist* (copyrighted 1977) and *The Office Practice of Pharmacy* (copyrighted 1978), both written by the author.

health care team. The pharmacist could never accomplish this goal—nor ever expect to be on a par with the physician on the health team—without first *restoring* his professional and patient-oriented image.

The plunge of the pharmacist, from one skilled in the "art of the apothecary" to a retail merchant or "operator of a store," evoked a grave professional identity crisis. The development of the office setting was the first step on the long journey to restore his (or her) professional image.

And, at the same time it also prepared a proper setting in the *community* for Doctors of Pharmacy to practice and function in their new role as the community experts in pharmacotherapeutics.

Professional Environment

The concept of the private family practice of Pharmacy demands a professional environment where the pharmacist can create an office setting that conveys to his patients an "I care" approach—an attitude of warmth, empathy, and welcome. It implies a sense of personal concern. It provides an atmosphere that is serene, dignified, and professional. It creates a setting that is unencumbered with activities unrelated to professional services. It emphasizes the dedication of the pharmacist to his profession and to the best interests of his patients. It projects a patient-oriented image of a reliable source of professional advice and counsel. It engenders an aura of professionalism in which the expertise of the pharmacist is enhanced so that patient confidence and trust in him can grow.

Patient Profile Paved the Way

However, it was my introduction of the patient medication profile record that provided the *core* of this concept which has

helped to change Pharmacy's direction. Development of the profile opened new vistas for Pharmacy as it enabled the pharmacist to perform a new function—that of ensuring the safe and appropriate use of drugs by patients. It helped to transform the pharmacist into a vital and responsive member of the health care team, and it provided him with added opportunities to exercise his *professional judgment*. The medication profile record also revealed to the pharmacist significant instances of irrational or inappropriate prescribing that he could ill-afford to ignore, and projected him into new involvement in pharmacotherapy, as well as new involvement in pharmacist-patient and pharmacist-physician relationships.

During the 18-year-interval since the implementation of the first patient pharmacotherapy monitoring system in a pharmacy practice, I suppose nothing has been more rewarding to me than to witness its acceptance by the patient, the pharmacist, and the allied health professions—as well as by legislative and judicial bodies. Its value has been cited in judicial opinions as supportive evidence that pharmacists render a professional service.[1] Proposed Congressional legislation (i.e., the Veterans Health Care Amendments of 1977) recognizes its value in certain federally-funded, health-related programs, and it is a required subject in pharmacy school curricula.

Inappropriate Prescribing

The patient pharmacotherapy monitoring system revealed to the Task Force on Prescription Drugs the *extent* of irrational and inappropriate prescribing by the medical profession, very little of which could have been proved prior to pharmacists' use of this monitoring system. There is no question that it has been of immense value to the patient, physician, and pharmacist during the past 18

[1] A.Ph.A. Legal Division, "Washington Spotlight," *The Virginia Pharmacist*, 58 (January 1974):4.

years. Today, take away the patient medication profile record as a working tool of the pharmacist and only a shell remains, because the practitioner would lose the basis for his monitoring, counseling, and consulting roles.

I also think that once pharmacists discover that they can create their own office practice setting, we will witness an exodus from the "commercial" environments. Those seers who predict that commercial conglomerates will eventually engulf the private practitioners are simply not observing the profound changes in pharmacy school curricula toward patient orientation (so-called "clinical pharmacy"). These changes are bound to have a pronounced effect on the future *direction* and *practice setting* of community pharmacy.

In a pharmacy publication[2] in 1962, I predicted that the office-type practice would dominate the American pharmacy scene by 1975. It is obvious that it did not proliferate to the degree that I had hoped for—and many of my predictions of the early 1960s were also wide of the mark. Though the timing was off, I feel the office practice concept will one day be as widely accepted by the community pharmacist practitioner as the patient medication profile record is today. My 22-year-old typist, who was reared in Berryville [Va.], has no recollection of the old "drug store." She disclosed to me that it was years before she realized that the office practice of pharmacy was *not* commonplace in the American scene.

Reasons for Slow Growth

One reason for the slow growth of the office practice may be due to the unrelenting brainwashing and haranguing of pharmacy students and pharmacists by commercial propagandists over the past few decades.

I think the people of Clark County, Virginia, have proved over the past 18 years that the pharmacist can separate himself from commercialism. The abrupt cessation in my practice (in November 1960) of *all* commercial activities—including those related to marketing and merchandising—did not provoke my clientele to flee the premises or to avoid my practice.

In hundreds of pharmacy office practices across the nation, society has clearly demonstrated that it will support the pharmacist who wishes to concentrate on his own field, without "sidelines" of any kind. The successful pharmacy office practitioner needs no greater degree of *business* acumen than any other office practitioner in the health care field. The same "outsiders" who are attempting to control the destiny of Pharmacy today were also declaring, as late as the 1950s, that no pharmacy could succeed without a soda fountain!

Similar to the family physician and to the family dentist, the family pharmacist can freely choose one of 3 modes of office practice: solo, group, or joint practice. I am firmly convinced that once pharmacists begin thinking for themselves, society will witness major and profound advances in the profession—all to the benefit of the patient.

The community pharmacist in the primary care role is destined to become a major point of entry into the health care system. Ultimately, in his role as consultant and educator, he will be responsible for the drug treatment of his patients. Involvement to this extent in pharmacotherapy will require a private consultation room environment.

Transition Requires Education

In the evolution of the pharmacist's practice setting in the community, it is highly doubtful that society would have accepted, in 1960, the giant, one-step transition directly from commercial emporium to the

[2] Eugene V. White, "An Interesting Pharmacy," *The Virginia Pharmacist*, 46 (March 1962):24.

consultation room/office practice environment—with its abrupt abandonment of the historic pharmacist-patient relationship at the front counter. As it was, our sudden transition from a traditional "corner drug store" to an office without a cash register and one that was devoid of shelves, islands, or displays of merchandise *in view*, was an enigma to many people—even though the front counter arrangement was retained. That transition required some educating—as to *why*. Although retaining the front counter was a definite barrier to *complete* professionalization, it enabled the public to adjust to something radically new by keeping something they felt comfortable with—something to which they were accustomed. It was simply a matter of conditioning the public.

Convincing a Minority of Pharmacists

Although it appears that the strictly-professional pharmacy office setting has not been as readily adopted by the profession as has the patient medication profile record, I believe it will eventually evolve from a "radical innovation" to an accepted standard of pharmacy practice—similar to the patient profile record. It is only necessary to convince a *minority* of the profession about the merits of the office-based family pharmacist concept; once convinced, they will change the profession.

Dissatisfaction, disillusionment, and frustration with what they see in contemporary community pharmacy practice will instill in pharmacists the enthusiasm, motivation, and challenge to aspire to a better way. Those who thirst for an office practice must first have the desire, will, courage, determination, and stamina to fight hard to attain their goal. Once that goal is achieved, the future of community pharmacy will take on a new perspective. One cannot realize the exhilaration, contentment, and happiness in achieving an office practice until he has experienced it. The key to a rewarding life's work is to focus on the patient and his total health.

5—The Implementation of a Uniform Cost Accounting System

Janet MacMurphey

A uniform cost accounting system (UCAS) has become a reality in one pharmacy in California. Bell Pharmacy of Sacramento has fully implemented UCAS, possibly the first pharmacy in the nation to do so. The implementation of this system was brought to fruition after an interesting phase of research for documenting pharmacy's economic dimensions.

This research project and field study took place in California and Ohio during 1976. The study, under the auspices of the California Pharmaceutical Association and American Pharmaceutical Association, involved a field evaluation of a proposed uniform pharmacy accounting scheme. Sixteen stores were examined for their recordkeeping, accounting, and business operation procedures. A cost accounting system was adapted from the UCAS model for each store, with accompanying procedural changes required for implementation. Actual implementation was not a part of this phase of the study.

Upon completion of the fieldwork at the 16 sites, the results, evaluations, and recommendations were submitted to the project director, Dr. Bruce R. Siecker at the Ohio State University College of Pharmacy in Columbus. A two-part report evaluating the use of the proposed system in the 16 stores, including results and recommendations, was written by Siecker and published by the American Pharmaceutical Association.

The management of Bell Pharmacy decided to implement this cost system as soon as possible. The system offers numerous sources of information useful to pharmacy management in the short run. Management can use the accumulated cost data for operational planning and control purposes, special management decisions, and product costing. In the case of a community pharmacy, product costing refers to the cost of filling a prescription, which in turn assists in determining prescription charges. The system also has some very important consequences for the economics of pharmacy in the long run.

UCAS is a double-entry accounting system which records all transactions of a business with two or more self-balancing entries. The built-in controls automatically call attention to errors and facilitate the recording and accumulation of accurate data.

Accrual method of accounting is used as distinguished from the cash basis of accounting. Revenue is recognized when it is realized and expenses are recognized when incurred, whether or not such transactions have been finally settled by the receipt or payment of cash or its equivalent. This enables a better matching for each reporting period of revenue and the necessary costs or expenses incurred to generate that revenue.[1]

The prescription department of each pharmacy is a separate operating department from the rest of the store. By segmenting the prescription department economically from the remainder of the pharmacy, the cost of providing prescription department goods and services can be measured. This is the main emphasis of the uniform cost accounting system for pharmacy. The old question that has plagued the pharmacy profession— "How much does it cost to dispense a prescription?"—can finally be answered.

UCAS offers guidelines so that the accumulation of accounting data takes place in a comprehensive and uniform manner. Procedures have been developed to determine how expenses are charged to each operating department. For example, delivery expenses are accumulated in a delivery cost center and then allocated to the prescription department (and to other departments if they also provide delivery service). UCAS deals with all expenses, including rent and other occupancy costs, manager and owner's salaries, employees' salaries, and general overhead. With widespread adoption, efforts to accumulate data of numerous pharmacies will produce comparable results, since the recording of this data would be handled in a uniform and consistent manner.

The UCAS potential and the genuine interest in this whole project were the two decisive factors that led to this pharmacy's management decision for early implementation. In late spring of 1976, the necessary steps for the conversion to UCAS were initiated and full-scale adoption was undertaken at the beginning of the fiscal year, Nov. 1, 1976.

Before the uniform cost accounting system could be implemented, several procedural changes were required. Medicaid and other third-party billings had been accounted for on a cash basis and had to be converted to an accrual basis to conform to UCAS procedure. A new set of books was established at the beginning of the fiscal year using the new chart of accounts with the uniform numbering system of UCAS (*see Table 5.1*).

Table 5.1

Chart of Accounts

Classifications	Numbering Sequence
ASSETS	(1000–1999)
Current assets	(1000–1499)
Fixed assets	(1600–1699)
Intangible assets	(1700–1799)
Deferred assets	(1800–1899)
Other assets	(1900–1999)
LIABILITIES	(2000–2999)
Current	(2000–2399)
Long-term debt	(2500–2699)
EQUITY	(3000–3999)
REVENUE	(4000–4999)
EXPENSES	(5000–7999)
Cost of sales	(5000–5999)
Operating expenses	(6000–7999)
OTHER INCOME AND DEDUCTIONS	(8000–9999)

The area of major change and the one that required the most work centered around the departmentalization of the store. UCAS requires that the pharmacy be divided into a minimum of two departments—the prescription department and the nonprescription or general department. Management wanted better information and control over the front end of the store, which accounted for approximately 40% of the total sales volume. The front end was divided into three departments: cards and stationery, cosmetics, and general. The general department was further divided into three subcenters: tobacco-candy, photo, and other front-end merchandise (*see Table 5.2*).

After the departments were categorized, the procedures to record sales, cost of goods and direct expenses by these departments were organized. Four steps were taken:

1. A cash register was purchased with the capacity for recording the six sales classifications.
2. Employees were trained to identify purchases of merchandise by departments and subcenters.
3. A physical inventory by department was taken at the beginning of the fiscal year.
4. A daily cash reporting form was designed to record sales by departments.

Through experimentation, management found that a color-coding system helps facilitate the departmentalization of sales and purchases. The keys on the cash register are color-coded by department. This same color is used to price-tag merchandise. Purchases are identified by department and circled on invoices with the same color coding. For example, the general department key on the cash register is blue. Merchandise for the general department is price-tagged in blue and purchases of front-end merchandise are identified on invoices by circling the extended amounts in blue. This is easy with the use of colored felt-tip pens.

A crossover log had been established to record the sale of merchandise purchased in one department but sold in another. An example of this type of transaction is an over-the-counter vitamin. This item would customarily be purchased and sold through the nonprescription department. If, however, the vitamins are dispensed on a physician's order as a prescription, the merchandise is then sold through the prescription department. The cost of this item needs to be recorded in a crossover log so that the cost of sales can be charged to the appropriate department. This adjustment is necessary to accomplish an accurate and precise measurement of the prescription department's gross margin.

A time survey was conducted to determine where employees spend time according to

Table 5.2

Bell Pharmacy's Six Sales Departments

	General Department				
Prescription Department	Tobacco, Candy Subcenter	Photo Subcenter	Other General Subcenter	Cosmetic Department	Cards, Stationery Department
Prescriptions	Cigarettes Cigars Pipe Tobacco Candy Gum	Finishing Film Flashbulbs Batteries	Vitamins Dental needs Foot products Hair care products Deodorants Skin care products Feminine hygiene First-aid supplies Men's grooming aids Baby needs Hosiery Jewelry Clocks, watches Giftware	Treatment lines Make-up Perfumes Colognes Dusting powders Gift sets	Greeting cards Gift wrap Boxed stationery School supplies Pens

the various departments, delivery duties, and general and administrative duties. The results of this study were used to determine the percentage of each employee's wages to be charged directly to each of the four departments and the delivery and general and administrative cost centers.

These procedural changes took place over a three-to-four month period. Some areas required only a minimum of time and effort to complete while other areas were more involved. Taking the physical inventory by department was completed in one day. The employee time survey took place over a one-week period. Training employees to ring sales and mark purchases by departments required the most effort. This was to be expected, however, since the new system with six sales classifications is considerably more sophisticated than the one-department approach.

Until the next physical inventory, quarterly financial statements necessitate a determination of a gross profit percentage for each department. This was not difficult for departments with a fairly standard markup. For the prescription department, a monthly record was kept of the actual cost of goods sold and selling price of all prescriptions. The percentages established are used in preparing financial statements until the next physical inventory.

The only unexpected situation that arose as the final plans for implementation were completed was a lack of cooperation by the pharmacy's accountant.[2] It appeared that the accountant was more interested in generation of tax reports than in developing an accounting system which would provide meaningful management information. Therefore, management hired a new accountant who showed more interest in UCAS and understanding of its benefits. Hopefully, this was an isolated instance.

The new accounting system is functioning well. It is producing accounting information which was previously unavailable to management. The most important benefit of this system is the departmentalized, comprehensive income statement (*see Table 5.3*).

Table 5.3

Bell Pharmacy's Statement of Departmental Income

(For the 12 Months Ended October 31, 1977)

General Department = Tobacco and Candy, Photo, Other

	Prescription Department	Tobacco and Candy	Photo	Other	Total General	Cosmetics Dept.	Card Dept.	Occupancy Cost Center	Delivery Cost Center	Genl. & Adm. Cost Center	Total Store
Sales, Net	$ X	$ X	$ X	$ X	$ X	$ X	$ X				$ X
Cost of Sales:											
Beginning Inventory	X	X	X.	X	X	X	X				X
Purchases	X	X	X	X	X	X	X				X
Less ending inventory	(X)	(X)	(X)	(X)	(X)	(X)	(X)				(X)
Cost of goods sold:	X	X	X	X	X	X	X				X
Gross Profit:	X	X	X	X	X	X	X				X
Direct Operating Expenses:											
Salary, pharmacist manager	X										X
Other salaries	X				X	X	X		X	X	X
Payroll taxes	X				X	X	X		X	X	X
Employee benefits	X				X	X	X		X	X	X
Operating supplies	X				X	X	X			X	X
Communication	X					X	X			X	X
Travel & prof. development											
Advertising										X	X
Bad debts & collection										X	X
Professional attire, laundry	X										X
Professional & outside services									X	X	X
Equipment rental & repair	X								X	X	X
Licenses, dues & donations	X									X	X
General insurance										X	X
Taxes										X	X
Depreciation	X				X	X	X	X		X	X
Other occupancy expense								X			X
Miscellaneous operating					X			X		X	X
Purchase discounts	(X)				(X)	(X)	(X)			(X)	(X)
Total direct expense	X				X	X	X	X	X	X	X
Direct Profit Contribution	X				X	X	X				X
Indirect Operating Expense (allocated):											
Occupancy cost center	X				X	X	X	(X)		X	
Delivery cost center	X					X			(X)		
General & administrative cost center	X				X	X	X			(X)	
Total indirect expense	X				X	X	X	—	—	—	X
Income (Loss) from Operations	X				X	X	X				X
Other Non-Operating Income											X
Other Deductions: Interest expense											(X)
Life insurance premiums											(X)
Federal income taxes											(X)
CA franchise taxes											(X)
Net Income (Loss) for the Period											X

This income statement provides management with valuable economic information for each department in sales performance, inventory turnover and control, direct and indirect expenses, and net profit. In addition, further interpretation and analysis are possible. In the prescription department, the cost of dispensing can be determined. Pricing structures can be evaluated after periodic prescription costs are determined. The prescription department's profitability can be compared with that of the rest of the store. In the nonprescription section, profitability can be identified for the various departments. Problems in the front end can be determined with more accuracy. This information has been found to be invaluable for effective and efficient store management.

UCAS is a powerful managerial tool for the individual pharmacy. Its usefulness, however, is not confined to the individual pharmacy. The pharmacy profession is facing major problems. Economic survival in the marketplace is becoming more difficult, consumer criticism of drug pricing is becoming louder, and external pressures from third-party drug programs are becoming greater. It is not likely these trends will decrease or reverse themselves in the future, so the profession faces the problem of responding.

Adequate economic documentation and cost-finding data need to be produced on a profession-wide level in a comprehensive, uniform, and comparable manner in order to assure economic survival. The uniform cost accounting system for pharmacy is the method which can accomplish this.

The management of Bell Pharmacy decided it was time to act, and the results are becoming apparent in this operation. However, the ability of the profession to respond to the economic challenges confronting it is dependent upon wide acceptance and implementation of UCAS.

References

1. Siecker, Bruce R.: "The Uniform Cost Accounting Approach for Pharmacy Pricing Decisions," *JAPhA*, NS 17:208–212; April 1977.
2. Siecker, Bruce R.: "A Multi-Site Implementation and Evaluation of the Uniform Cost Accounting System for Pharmacy," American Pharmaceutical Association Foundation, Washington, DC; 1976, p. 43.

Related Readings in This Volume

Readings for a Broader Perspective

1. Dolan, M. "Pharmacy By the Bay," *American Pharmacy* NS 18 (November 1978):28–30.
2. Valentino, J. G. "How Pharmacists Report to the USP Drug Product Problems," *Pharmacy Times* 44 (March 1978):39–43.
3. Kalman, S. H., and Schlegel, J. F. "Standards of Practice for the Profession of Pharmacy," *American Pharmacy* NS 19 (March 1979): 21–35.
4. Hussar, D. A. "Pharmacy Practice—The Importance of Effective Communications," *American Journal of Pharmacy* 148 (September/October 1976):136–47.
5. "For the First Time, R_x Account for Over Half of All Sales Dollars," *Pharmacy Times* 44 (November 1978):63.
6. Smith, M. C. "The Prescription: Everything You Wanted to Know But Didn't Think to Ask," *American Pharmacy* NS 18 (June 1978): 31–33.
7. Smith, M. C., and Knapp, D. A. *Pharmacy, Drugs and Medical Care* (3rd ed.). Baltimore: The Williams & Wilkins Co., 1981. 322 pages.

Adverse Reactions & Interactions

6—Drug-Induced Disease

William A. Parker

Almost any manifestation of illness may be mimicked by an adverse drug reaction (ADR). For every pharmacist this should suggest awareness of a patient's present and past history of drug use. Familiarity with the adverse pharmacologic effects of therapeutic agents and the manifestations of illness associated with different agents should facilitate recognition of their potential etiological role in causing or aggravating disease.

Seventy-five percent of all patients leave the physician's office with a prescription.[1] As the last link in the health care chain, the pharmacist must be aware of the possible patient responses to these agents. Patient complaints of illness should always raise the question, "Could this be drug-related?"

A widely accepted definition of an adverse drug reaction is "any undesired or unintended response to medication that requires treatment or alteration of therapy." Such responses constitute a significant health care problem that has been estimated to account for about five percent of patient admissions to hospital general medical services.

In addition, 10 to 30 percent of all patients admitted to medical wards will acquire an adverse drug reaction during their stay.[2] Fatality rates of these reactions generally ranged from three to 13 percent, averaging about five percent. The accurate identification of adverse drug reactions is difficult because they usually present no unique clinical or laboratory findings demarcating them from manifestations of concurrent illnesses. The uncertainty is often compounded by variable patient compliance with medication orders and self-medication habits.

20 Percent Unavoidable

Approximately 20 to 30 percent of adverse drug reactions are believed to be unpredictable and unavoidable—such as idiosyncratic and hypersensitivity reactions.[1] The remaining 70 to 80 percent of drug reactions are predictable and preventable. They consist of overdosage and underdosage, drug interactions, and secondary drug effects. It seems clear that pharmacists should offer physicians and patients direct and ready access to their drug expertise.

The concern is not how many reactions occur, but how we may implement systems to detect and *prevent* them, while *educating* the public and health professionals to decrease drug therapy risks.

Most Common ADRs

Certain drug groups are more likely to cause adverse drug reactions than other drug groups. These drug groups and their primary reactions include:

1. cardiac drugs, particularly digitalis—cardiac arrhythmias;
2. anticoagulants—bleeding;
3. antihypertensive drugs—hypotension;
4. antibiotics—allergies;
5. immunosuppressive and chemotherapeutic drugs—bone marrow suppression;
6. diuretics—fluid and electrolyte imbalance; and
7. psychotropic drugs, including sedatives and tranquilizers—confusion and disorientation.

Besides reactions *per se*, drug therapy of symptoms may delay disease diagnosis and possibly prevent appropriate therapy for a potentially curable disorder. The inappropriate drug also may cause a disorder to which the patient would otherwise not be exposed.

Causes of ADRs

A number of causes of adverse drug reactions have been identified:

1. *Multiple prescribers*—The number of physicians a patient sees correlates directly with the adverse drug reaction rate. Almost 50 percent of patients receive medication from more than one physician at a time.[3] About 35 percent of patients seen by one physician have a potential drug interaction from their medication while nearly 70 percent of patients seen by more than two physicians are at risk.[3] A major contributing factor is poor communication between patient and physician.

2. *Multiple prescriptions*—The number of prescriptions received by a patient correlates directly with the adverse drug reaction rate, and the benefit-to-risk ratio for each drug decreases as additional drugs are taken. The average hospitalized patient receives between six and 10 drugs simultaneously, with

an adverse reaction rate of seven to 10 percent. Patients receiving 20 or more drugs, seen in the geriatric population, have at least a 40 percent risk of having an adverse reaction.[1] Use of fixed-dosage combinations of drugs similarly increases the reaction rate. Only when specific objectives have been established should drugs be added to an existing regimen.

3. *Lack of monitoring parameters*—Another cause of adverse drug reactions is the failure to establish therapeutic endpoints for drug therapy. When therapeutic objectives are not defined, one encounters a significant increase in unrecognized toxic and subtherapeutic effects. Two additional problems related to the lack of therapeutic endpoints include unreasonable expectations of drug therapy, often causing the therapy to be "pushed" beyond rational limits, and failure to modify drug therapy as the condition being treated changes.

4. *Physiologic variables*—Among the important determinants of the effects of a drug, both desired and undesired, are the physiologic state of the patient and the pathophysiology of his or her disease. Adverse drug reactions are nearly twice as common in the pediatric and geriatric populations as in the adult age group.[1] Pathologic states also modify drug response, contributing to adverse drug reactions. There are several diseases, such as psychiatric disorders and disorders of the cardiovascular system, in which multiple drug therapy is often unavoidable. There are also a number of diseases that primarily affect the organs of absorption, metabolism and/or excretion which must be anticipated and adjusted for.

5. *Lack of drug education*—The public appears unsophisticated, at the very least, concerning the proper use of prescription and nonprescription drugs. In general, nonprescription drugs are considered totally safe "or they wouldn't be on the market." Prescription drugs are considered safe because "a physician would give nothing that

would harm a patient." Many patients also "swap" or "borrow" prescription drugs, or compromise their therapy and health by not adhering to their dosage regimens. Physicians are frequently confronted by a wide variety of new drugs on which they need responsible drug information. Lack of understanding of pharmacology, pharmacokinetics and chemistry of these drugs may contribute to poor prescription practices and drug-induced disease. Down-playing of side effects and adverse reactions in promotional literature can give clinicians a low index of suspicion toward drug toxicity and iatrogenic disease.

Pharmacist's Role

What role should the pharmacist take in the detection, prevention and management of drug-induced disease?

First, an active drug-use control and drug-use surveillance program should be conducted. The routine monitoring of drug orders for discontinuation or reduction of drug dosage or antidotes for treating adverse drug reactions may offer early detection. Definitive action thus occurs before the condition progresses.

Second, the pharmacist may make a major contribution through the acquisition of drug histories and the maintenance of patient medication profiles. The determination of which prescription and nonprescription drugs the patient has taken recently is critical in identifying the agents which may be incriminated as a cause of an adverse drug reaction. The information will also prove invaluable in determining past drug intolerances, medication habits and compliance patterns, predisposing factors and drugs to avoid in the future.

Here the pharmacist's knowledge of drug chemistry and structure-activity relationships may prove beneficial in minimizing cross-reactivities between drug groups. The

maintenance of patient medication profiles gives the pharmacist an unequalled vantage point in monitoring the patient's *total* drug therapy, irrespective of the number of physicians treating the patient. Such profiles may be the most complete means for detecting drug interactions, past drug intolerances and compliance problems.

Third, pharmacists should contribute to the education of their patients and other health professionals. Patients must be adequately counseled concerning their proper use of both prescription and nonprescription drugs. They must be made aware of the precautions to exercise while using specific drugs, proper storage and early warning signs for common adverse reactions.

Reporting and Identifying

Patients experiencing these reactions should be counseled to report to their physician and to avoid certain drugs in the future. They should also be helped to obtain proper Medic-Alert identification to minimize future rechallenge risks and counseled to inform any physician treating them of the medication they are taking. The advantages of obtaining all of an individual patient's medication (prescription and nonprescription) from the same pharmacy should be explained.

Last, pharmacists should actively assist in the validation and reporting of adverse drug reactions. Through regular reading of the pharmaceutical and medical literature, pharmacists can gather information concerning the clinical incidence, manifestations, significance and management of adverse drug reactions, making such information readily available to their medical colleagues.

Additionally, an understanding of the mechanism involved is essential for providing alternative treatments. Validated adverse drug reactions should be reported to the physicians concerned, the pharmaceutical manufacturers involved and the Food and Drug Administration. By so doing, more reliable statistics and information will be available for future evaluations.

The greatest asset to detection and prevention of drug toxicity is a high index of suspicion. Virtually every drug has a potential to induce a reaction, even in "normal" doses. It has been said that "the pharmacist is at the strategic interface between a patient and his drug; an interface which may lie between a patient and his disease."[4]

References

1. Melmon, K. L.: "Preventable Drug Reactions—Causes and Cures," *N Engl J Med*, 284: 1361–1368, June 17, 1971.
2. Stewart, R. B.: "Fatal Drug Reaction Debate," *Drug Intell Clin Pharm*, 9:382–383, July 1975.
3. Cluff, L. E.; Caranasos, G. J.; and Stewart, R. B.: *Clinical Problems With Drugs*, W. B. Saunders, Philadelphia, 1975.

4. Maudlin, R. K.: "Drug-Induced Diseases," *J Am Pharm Assoc*, NS.13:316–322, June 1973.

Related Readings in This Volume

12. Pharmacist and Preventive Medicine
16. Over-the-Counter Medications
59. Drug Therapy in the Elderly

Readings for a Broader Perspective

1. Bergman, H. David. "Drug-Induced Diseases and Disorders," *The Apothecary* 89 (July/August 1977):16–18, 56.
2. Bennett, J. A. "Drug-Food Interactions: A Guide for the Community Pharmacist," *The Apothecary* 89 (May/June 1977):8.
3. Lamy, P. P. "The Food/Drug Connection in Elderly Patients," *American Pharmacy* NS 18 (July 1978):30–31.
4. Cacace, L. G., Schweigert, B. F., and Gildon, A. M. "Erythromycin Estolate Induced Hepatotoxicity," *Drug Intelligence & Clinical Pharmacy* 11 (January 1977):22–25.
5. Shue, M. E., and Parker, H. E. "If You're Pregnant, Tell Your Pharmacist," *American Pharmacy* NS 19 (October 1979):25–27.

Contraception

7—The Pharmacist and Family Planning: Review and Report of a Study

Mickey C. Smith, Helen Wetherbee and Thomas R. Sharpe

Pharmacists located near doctors' offices do have rush periods during the office hours of the doctors, but these are usually limited to two or three hours during the normal working day, which lasts eight to ten hours. Thus, during most of the day, pharmacies are relatively empty and their proprietors are more than willing to spend time conversing with customers or other visitors at great length. Many pharmacies have actually become informal social centers. Almost every pharmacy in the country is furnished with benches or chairs providing a seating capacity for several visitors or customers at one time. Such a setting is ideal for the dissemination of family planning information. The surrounding is one of health-related activity. Business is carried on in an unhurried manner, and open conversations frequently take place anyway. The pharmacist, or another family planning worker, could easily turn these discussions in the direction of birth control. Also, information sessions could be deliberately organized to take place in the pharmacy during those hours when the pharmacist is not normally busy. Thus, the pharmacies definitely are able to provide suitable facilities for family planning activities. Their willingness to cooperate in such activities depends upon their present knowledge and attitudes about contraception and birth control, plus the ability of family planning innovators to convince them to cooperate in these matters.[1]

Although these views refer to pharmacy in Afghanistan, we feel they are equally applicable in the United States.

Proposals to involve pharmacists in family planning are consistent with data cited in an editorial in the *American Journal of Public Health* indicating that one-third or more of American couples obtain birth control supplies through "non-medical" sources.[2] This editorial pointed out that "research is urgently needed on ways to expand the present non-medical delivery of contraceptives."

Review

Dr. Audrey Bingel, associate professor at the University of Illinois College of Pharmacy, told an annual meeting of the Student American Pharmaceutical Association that there are an estimated one to one and one-half million teenage girls who risk unwanted pregnancies and who do not have the opportunity to learn about available contracep-

tives.[3] Moreover, about half the women of all age groups in the United States are not practicing any form of family planning to limit pregnancies. The reason is not a failure of technology, but rather embarrassment, lack of education, and inaccessibility of contraceptives. Although sex education is being taught in the schools today, it was not offered when the child-bearing population was in school. For women between the ages of 18 and 40, the physician traditionally has been the source of family planning information; however, those who most need family planning information are often those who can least afford it.

Evidence that many young women are unlikely to consult a physician was presented in a report of the Joint Working Group on Oral Contraceptives, a British governmental committee.[4] Whether this was due to fear, ignorance, or financial limitations, the committee reported that many women were prevented from receiving effective contraception because oral contraceptives were available only on a physician's prescription. Single women reportedly were reluctant to seek services because they feared being asked about their sexual behavior, or having moral judgments made. Many women expressed a fear of a pelvic examination as well. Family involvement, lack of transportation and problems of child care posed additional problems.

The committee's recommendation was to allow nurses, midwives, health visitors and pharmacists to assume a greater role in the delivery of family planning services. It was recommended that they function as non-physician prescribers following specific training in taking medical histories, monitoring patients' blood pressure and recognition of adverse reactions associated with oral contraceptives. Direct consultation with physicians and a government registry of authorized prescribers also were included in the recommendations. By using non-physician prescribers, it was felt that women would have greater accessibility to these services, thus fulfilling their need for family planning.

A Canadian government committee of physicians and lay persons also determined that certain non-physicians trained in family planning counseling should be allowed to prescribe oral contraceptives.[5] Pharmacists were included in a recommendation for the following reasons: (1) the pharmacist is a "drug expert" and would know the possible drug interactions and any adverse reactions; (2) the pharmacist is presently active in counseling patients about medication which has been prescribed; and (3) the pharmacy is easily accessible to those who need family planning services.

Both in the United States and Canada, pharmacists who previously did little more than display some over-the-counter contraceptive products are beginning to become more active in patient counseling and in advising local agencies about family planning. Sales of vaginal spermicides—foams, creams, jellies, gels—account for about $70 million in annual sales volume.[6] The majority of these sales take place in community pharmacies and account for 75% of the non-prescription birth control devices sold. Condoms make up the other 25% of this market. Until recently, most states had laws against the open display of condoms in the pharmacy. Presently, 44 states allow such open display. In these states, approximately 60% of the pharmacies, or about 26,000, have open displays.[7] Eighty percent of these pharmacies with open displays are the self-service variety. Since utilizing these open displays, sales of condoms have increased about 37%. The proportion of women purchasing condoms is about 12% nationally. However, in pharmacies with open displays, purchases by women have increased to about 15%.

Reflecting an apparent change in attitude, pharmacists in New York are now openly displaying these devices. The New York State Pharmaceutical Association would prefer to restrict sales to pharmacies, citing the pharmacist's role as advisor and counselor as the reason. The courts, however, have not supported this sales restriction.[8]

Shewfelt of the California Pharmaceutical Association reported that pharmacists in his state have been actively promoting condom use for some time.[9] As early as 1969, educational efforts were being organized to inform the public about the use of the condom in prevention of venereal diseases. The California prophylactic law had to be changed, however, as it was interpreted to mean that no one could purchase condoms without a physician's prescription. Through efforts of community-minded pharmacists, the law was changed in 1970. Also, public display of condoms was allowed. In 1972, a law was passed to permit non-public school faculty to give instruction in venereal disease treatment and prevention in schools, thus opening the door for qualified pharmacists to participate in such programs. Although pharmacists had accomplished much in California, the state Public Health Department called on them to find ways of promoting condoms for birth control as well as for venereal disease prevention. Current efforts to accomplish this include continuing education on family planning counseling, education of the public on the value of the pharmacist as a family planning counselor, and the use of advertising and marketing techniques to promote sales and information about condoms and other birth control devices.

The pharmacist's role in family planning need not be limited to non-prescription methods of contraception. Under FDA regulations, pharmacists disseminate patient package inserts when they dispense oral contraceptives. Furthermore, if patients' questions remain unsatisfied, they are required to provide the more technical package labeling itself. While the literature is prepared by the pharmaceutical manufacturers, it is the pharmacist who delivers it and who is in a position to explain the information and counsel the patient.[10]

For both prescription and non-prescription contraceptives, the pharmacist is in the unique position of being able to educate the public while he is dispensing his products. Furthermore, the pharmacist traditionally has been regarded as a respected source of pharmaceutical and medical knowledge who is both visible and accessible to the community. Finally, the pharmacist is the major source of contraceptive products.

A few studies have investigated the feelings of pharmacists toward family planning counseling and toward the adequacy of their education and training for such a task.

In 1970, a survey of the entire membership of the Washington State Pharmaceutical Association was conducted.[11] The survey instrument included demographic questions, followed by items about selling, displaying, counseling and controlling contraceptives in the pharmacy. Ninety-eight percent of the respondents sold contraceptives in the pharmacy. The most significant difference between those who did and those who did not sell contraceptives related to religion. Fewer Roman Catholic pharmacists sold contraceptives. An interesting reverse double standard was noted in the fact that *all* the respondents stated they displayed either foams, creams or jellies, but only 5% displayed condoms or diaphragms, and only 2% displayed oral contraceptives. (The reason for displaying the prescription products was not given.)

The Washington pharmacists were asked several questions about who should be allowed to purchase birth control products. About two-thirds favored sales to unmarried minors; one-third opposed such sales. Age and religion were the most significant factors in these differences. More Catholic pharmacists (57%) opposed sales to minors, and younger pharmacists were more in favor of these sales than was the older group. Phar-

macists reported that 21% of the male clients and 19% of the female clients asked for information on contraception. Female pharmacists were asked less frequently than male pharmacists about contraception; however, female patients did ask female pharmacists slightly more frequently.

In their conclusion, the researchers in Washington pointed out an interesting paradox in the results of this study. Pharmacists display many products utilizing sex appeal as the advertising agent. Yet, they allow personal factors such as religion, age and sex to affect their behavior with regard to the sale and display of contraceptives. This is unfortunate, since the pharmacist could be leading the way in informing and educating the public about family planning.

Rumel *et al.* conducted a similar study of pharmacists in the entire state of Hawaii.[12] The majority of the respondents were Japanese-American males. Ninety-seven percent said they had had no formal training in family planning or counseling in pharmacy school, but most (94%) agreed that families should be planned. Ninety-four percent approved of contraceptive use by unmarried persons. Most of the pharmacists were concerned with the problem of overpopulation. However, only about 1% of the pharmacists displayed condoms in the pharmacy, and 85% said they dispensed condoms only upon request. On the other hand, female non-prescription contraceptives were displayed in 58% of the pharmacies. In Hawaii, twice as many female as male patients asked pharmacists for contraceptive information. When these results are compared to those of the Washington survey, it is apparent that Hawaiian men were less likely to ask the pharmacist about this information than were men in Washington. From these two surveys, it seems the pharmacist could be, but is not, engaged in the role of family planner.

Later, in 1973, an "action study" was started in Hawaii by Solomon and Pion because many pharmacists started openly displaying nonprescription contraceptives.[13] Preliminary findings show that condom sales have increased considerably. The study hopes to provide pharmacists, manufacturers and family planning organizations with information on marketing techniques which will greatly increase the use of contraceptives.

In October 1970, a Pennsylvania survey similar to the Washington State study was conducted.[14] Most pharmacists (97%) sold contraceptives, but 41% did not display them for sale. One-fourth of the pharmacists felt that unmarried minors should not be allowed to purchase contraceptives and 10% of the respondents believed married minors should not be allowed to make such purchases. Eight times as many pharmacists displayed jellies, foams and creams as displayed condoms in their pharmacies. Very few pharmacists had been asked questions about family planning. Sixty-six percent of the pharmacists responding felt there should be some control over the sales of birth control devices. The authors observed a lack of cooperation between pharmaceutical manufacturers and the pharmacists in providing family planning information.

Another study focused on the attitudes and the practices of pharmacists with regard to distribution of contraceptives and birth control information in Utah.[15] The majority of respondents were members of the Church of Jesus Christ of Latter-Day Saints.

Most pharmacists felt that both married and unmarried adults should be allowed to purchase contraceptives. The attitudes of the pharmacist toward the sale of contraceptives to unmarried minors were somewhat equally divided. Older pharmacists felt that such sales lead to an increase in promiscuity and venereal disease. Many felt that sales were against the church's position on premarital sexual relationships. Younger pharmacists or those who had recently graduated from pharmacy school approved such sales to minors as a means of decreasing the number of

illegitimate births. The question of sales of condoms to minors brought a variety of responses from the pharmacists, probably because condom sales are prohibited by Utah law to unmarried persons under the age of 21. Some pharmacists told minors they were out of stock, while others required proof of age. However, if the minor looked mature and asked to purchase condoms, he usually received them. The survey showed that the pharmacists had an inconsistent viewpoint on birth control. All the Utah pharmacists who replied indicated they had advised patients on family planning at one time or another, but only infrequently. The factors influencing the pharmacist's practice were religion, background, and experience as a pharmacy intern. The authors suggested several steps to guide pharmacists into the role of patient counselor in family planning:

1. Pharmacy schools should offer courses emphasizing family planning and contraceptive devices.
2. Guidelines should be formulated to effectively market contraceptive products to the patient.
3. All governmental agencies—local, state, and federal—should be actively involved in counseling the public on family planning.
4. The pharmacist should be involved in family planning as a part of his professional practice.
5. The medical community should be educated about the needs of the public in family planning.
6. Programs should be developed for the pharmacist to motivate the public toward greater utilization of family planning.[15]

Roffman *et al.* conducted a survey of Maryland pharmacists in 1973.[16] The general findings of this study, in comparison to those of earlier studies in Hawaii, Pennsylvania, Washington and Utah, were that Maryland pharmacists were more liberal in their attitudes regarding sale of contraceptives to minors. The researchers felt this finding reflected a "liberalizing trend" toward family planning for minors and premarital sexual activities in general. Evidence of these liberal attitudes was found in the higher percentage of respondents willing to display contraceptives.

However, Maryland pharmacists reported they were infrequently used as a source of birth control information. One explanation suggested for the discrepancy between display practices and counseling was insecurity resulting from lack of knowledge about contraceptive methods. Nevertheless, more than 80% of the respondents did feel that the pharmacist should become active as a family planning counselor in order to meet the needs of society by helping to combat unwanted pregnancies and overpopulation. Only a small percentage felt that pharmacists should not be involved in family planning or that they should be limited to selling contraceptive products. Seventy-six percent of the pharmacists said they could provide educational material to their patrons. Also, most (65%) felt the pharmacist should supply information about cost and effectiveness; however, only half considered giving instructions about the use of contraceptives, or dispersing information about the physical and psychological advantages and disadvantages of the different contraceptives, to be the duty of the pharmacist. On the other hand, half the pharmacists requested information about family planning and agreed that there should be a list available in the pharmacy of referral agencies which deal with family planning. The researchers believed that Maryland pharmacists were similar to other pharmacists nationally in their involvement with family planning.

Grindstaff surveyed about 24,000 Canadian pharmacists in 1975 and reported several significant findings about the pharmacist and family planning.[5] Fifty percent of those surveyed were in favor of advertising contraceptive products through mass media. However, only 8% actually advertised the products in this manner.

The survey also posed questions regarding information provided to the patient by the pharmacist. Ninety-six percent of the pharmacists stated they would like to provide this type of information, while 54% of the pharmacists actually did provide such information. Very few pharmacists (8%) displayed informational material in the pharmacy. Rather than counsel their patients, twothirds of those surveyed referred their patients to physicians for family planning information. Ten percent of the pharmacists referred their patients to birth control clinics or public health agencies. Only 10% of the respondents made two or more referrals in a year's period. Those pharmacists who displayed birth control devices received an increased number of inquiries. There also was evidence that male patients preferred to ask male pharmacists, and females preferred female pharmacists. In addition, neither males nor females considered pharmacists a primary source of birth control information; and patrons did not ask questions about birth control on a regular basis. Ninety percent of the pharmacists felt that family planning counseling is a part of their professional practice.

From the studies reviewed, a few general conclusions may be reached. Pharmacists appear to feel that family planning is an appropriate part of their practice, although some feel religious, moral or legal constraints. At the same time, the studies suggest that pharmacists are not frequently sought as providers of family planning services and do not necessarily feel adequately educated for this role. A trend toward recognition of the necessity of family planning has led to reduction of legal barriers to the sale of birth control products, and reduced reluctance to sell such products to unmarried people or minors. The studies suggested the need to assess the pharmacist's level of knowledge in Mississippi and to identify any moral or religious barriers to the pharmacist's function as a family planning counselor. Such research can provide the necessary basis for development of programs to train pharmacists for an expanded role in this area.

Mississippi Study

The sample used in our study in Mississippi consisted of all pharmacists in community practice in an eight-county study area. A list of these pharmacists was obtained from the mailing list of the Bureau of Pharmaceutical Services at the University of Mississippi School of Pharmacy. This mailing list describes all practicing pharmacists in the state and is regularly updated. Pharmacists were contacted by a letter informing them of our interest in their involvement in family planning activities and advising that they would be contacted at a later date to arrange an interview. After pharmacists had received the letter, research assistants contacted them by phone and arranged for a convenient interview time.

Interviewers received two full days of training. The first day was devoted primarily to the purpose of the study and the survey instrument involved. The second day was concentrated on practice interviewing both with the investigators and between interviewers. Questions concerning the instrument were discussed and every effort was made to anticipate possible problems in the administration of the instrument. The instrument had been pretested previously in a county outside the study area.

The interview instrument was developed by the investigators based upon information requested in previous work performed by other investigators. The interview was intended to determine the degree of involvement of the pharmacist in family planning counseling, his attitudes toward possible expansion of this involvement, and his willingness to participate in special training and publicity programs aimed at expanding his role in family planning counseling.

Results

One hundred and eleven pharmacists were identified as active community practitioners in the study area. Of these, 108 agreed to participate in the study. The other three declined on the basis of health or inconvenience. The characteristics of the participating pharmacists are described in Table 7.1.

Table 7.1

Pharmacist Characteristics

Age	
0–29	34%
30–39	31%
40–49	17%
50–59	13%
60+	5%
Total Years in Practice	
0–10	56%
11–20	21%
21–30	20%
31+	3%
Sex	
Male	98%
Female	2%

Only 8% of the respondents felt it was not appropriate for a pharmacist to function as a birth control counselor, and most said they at least responded to questions from clients. The type of questions asked by clients varied. Seventy-two percent indicated they received questions about specific products. Sixty-four percent said clients asked questions concerning safety and efficacy. Only 36%, however, were asked questions concerning desirability, e.g., esthetic problems.

More than 95% of the respondents felt comfortable when discussing birth control information with clients of both sexes and of any race, including clients known personally by the pharmacist. Exceptions were clients known to be unmarried (85% were comfortable) and minors (72% comfortable with males, 68% comfortable with females).

Eighty-one percent of the pharmacists believed there was a need in their community for more family planning services, but one-third felt they were not adequately prepared to counsel clients on this subject. Nevertheless, nearly all (97%) felt confident about the accuracy of the information that they did provide.

There were variations in the opinions of pharmacists concerning the appropriateness of counseling clients on specific family planning methods. As Table 7.2 shows, pharmacists indicated their counsel was much more appropriate with regard to products they normally distribute.

Table 7.2

Appropriateness of Pharmacist Counseling on Specific Methods

Methods	Percentage of Pharmacists Believing it Appropriate
Vaginal cream	95
Vaginal foam	95
Condom	93
Vaginal jelly	91
Oral contraceptive	91
Diaphragm	70
Douche	65
Basal thermometer	61
Suppository	56
Abstinence	46
IUD	43
Withdrawal	42
Vasectomy	41
Rhythm	41
Tubal ligation	32

When pharmacists were asked about a future role, a clear interest in expanded activities emerged. Eighty-four percent indicated a willingness to expand their family planning role, and 90% indicated they would partici-

pate in pertinent continuing education efforts, if available.

Less than 20% felt that local physicians might oppose an expanded family planning role for pharmacists; about 85% believed that local physicians would support such a role. Eighty-six percent felt *their* clients would be receptive, but slightly less (77%) felt their clients would *seek* such counseling from them.

If pharmacists in general were to provide family planning counseling, 84% of the pharmacies felt it should be publicized. Similarly, three-fourths felt that participation in continuing education programs should be publicized. Only 35% indicated they would advertise such services. Only 22% felt pharmacists should be paid a separate fee for family planning counseling, and even fewer (14%) would charge such a fee.

Conclusion

It is clear from this review, and the Mississippi study further confirms, that pharmacists presently are involved to some degree in providing birth control products and information. Expansion of this role to full-scale family planning counseling would seem to require more formal efforts. These efforts could be incorporated into expanded continuing education as well as better training in the pharmacy curriculum.

There is a clear and documented need for accessible, inexpensive family planning counseling in this country, particularly in rural areas. By every criterion, with the possible exception of formal training, the community pharmacist is a logical choice to help meet this need. We hope that professional pharmacy organizations, manufacturers, and social and government agencies will recognize these facts and take the steps necessary to bring pharmacists into this area of health service.

References

1. Stone, R. A., Graham S., Kerr, G. B.: Commercial distribution of contraceptives in Afghanistan: actual and potential use of the pharmaceutical marketing system. *Studies in Family Planning 3:* 477 (Nov.), 1972.
2. Anon: Non-medical birth control—a neglected and promising field. *Am J Public Health 63:* 473 (June), 1973.
3. Anon: Rx for pharmacists: a call for greater involvement. *Family Planner 6:* 1 (Nov./Dec.), 1974.
4. Anon: Permit nurses, midwives, health visitors, and pharmacists to prescribe the pill, official British committee recommends. *Family Planning Perspectives 9:* 30–31 (Jan./Feb.), 1977.
5. Grindstaff, C. F.: The Canadian pharmacist and family planning. *Family Planning Perspectives 9:* 81–84 (Mar./Apr.), 1977.
6. Family planning and the pharmacist. *Chain Store Age* (Supplement by Ortho Pharmaceutical Corporation) *51:* 52 (Apr.), 1975.
7. The condom comes out of hiding. *Am Drug 173:* 26–38 (Jan.), 1976.
8. Carey v. population services, 45 LW 4601, 1977.
9. Shewfelt, E. R.: The pharmacist as the primary distribution agent for condoms. In Redford, M.vH., Duncan, G. W., Prager, D. J., Eds.: *The Condom: Increasing Utilization in the United States*, San Francisco Press, San Francisco, 1974, pp. 71–82.
10. Women will be given full details on pill side effects, contraindications in leaflet accompanying each packet. *Family Planning Perspectives 9:* 34–35, (Jan./Feb.), 1977.
11. Wagner, N. N., Millard, P. R., Pion, R. J.: The role of the pharmacist in family planning. *J Am Pharm Assoc NS10:* 258–260 (May), 1970.
12. Rumel, M. J., Reich, L., Stringfellow, L. C., Pion, R. J.: The pharmacists' neglected role. *Family Planning Perspectives 3:* 80–82 (Oct.), 1971.
13. Solomon, D. S., Pion, R. J.: Pharmacist and condoms: a preliminary view from Hawaii. In Redford, M.H., Duncan, G.W., Prager, D.J., Eds.: *The Condom: Increasing Utilization in the United States*, San Francisco Press, San Francisco, 1974, pp. 194–198.
14. Chez, R. A.: The role of the pharmacist in family planning: a Pennsylvania survey. *J Am Pharm Assoc NS12:* 464–466 (Sept.), 1972.
15. Hastings, D. W., Provol, G.E.: Pharmacists' attitudes and practices toward contraceptives. *J Am Pharm Assoc NS12:* 74–81 (Feb.), 1972.
16. Roffman, D. M., Speckman, C. E., Gruz, N. L.; Maryland pharmacists ready for family planning initiative. *Family Planning Perspectives 5:* 243–247 (Fall), 1973.

Related Reading in This Volume

Readings for a Broader Perspective

1. Marshall, C., and Schulze, A.L. "The Male Pharmacist as a Contraceptive Counselor: The Woman's View," *The Apothecary* 90 (March/April 1978) 10–11, 14, 57.
2. D'Angelo, A.C. "Psychological Effects of Pregnancy and Contraception," *J. Am. Pharm. Assoc.* NS 14 (December 1974): 667–70.
3. Huff, J.E., and Hernandez, L. "Contraceptives Available by Prescription," *J. Am. Pharm. Assoc.* NS 14 (May 1974): 244–51.
4. Smith, M.C., and McDaniel, P.A. "The Contraception Consultant," *American Pharmacy* NS 19 (July 1979): 23–24.

Diabetes

8—Pharmacy Program for Monitoring Diabetic Patients

Karl W. Schilling

Pharmacists within the Indian Health Service (IHS) are involved in the provision of primary care to patients with chronic diseases and minor acute diseases. Since the pioneering work reported by the Cass Lake Indian Hospital,[1] other IHS stations have developed similar programs.[2] Most stations now have some type of chronic care program and the means for monitoring the usage of nonprescription medicines, although the clinical functions performed by the pharmacist at each of these facilities vary greatly.

Most of the stations have established guidelines, such as those used at Cass Lake or the Shiprock Indian Hospital,[3] to aid them in following patients being treated for chronic illnesses. These guidelines were established jointly by the pharmacy and physician staffs at each station and allowed the pharmacist to provide primary care for up to 50% of the patients seen at these facilities. (Usually, less than 20% received care from the pharmacy; higher figures often reflected the absence of a full-time physician and very active nonprescription programs.)

However, most of the chronic care guidelines stipulated that only the stabilized patient be followed by the pharmacy. Patients experiencing symptoms or adverse effects, no matter how minor, were referred to a physician. Often the pharmacist would know the proper therapy to remedy the problem, but a physician consultation was required. This could be inconvenient for all involved—the physician was interrupted during busy clinic days, the patients had to wait for the consultation or even to be seen by the physician, and the pharmacist was being underused. This restriction was probably imposed because of the newness of the situation when these programs were started. Both pharmacists and physicians were uncertain of just what abilities the pharmacist did have in providing primary care.

However, as these programs spread throughout the IHS, more pharmacists gained experience and demonstrated their competence in providing this care.[2-4] It soon became apparent that in certain situations or disease states, the pharmacist could make independent therapeutic decisions within expanded guidelines. The logical expansion of the pharmacist's responsibilities within these programs was to allow him to monitor and treat the unstabilized patient who had certain chronic diseases. This was the step taken by the pharmacy service at the Pine Ridge Indian Hospital in establishing its program for monitoring diabetic patients.

The hospital is a 58-bed, acute-care facility located in southwestern South Dakota and serves approximately 12,000 Indian patients, mostly Oglalla Sioux. When fully staffed, there are nine physicians, three pharmacists and one pharmacy technician, plus nursing, mental health, social services, laboratory, x-ray, and other services. In addition to the busy clinic duties and field clinics, pharmaceutical services include unit dose drug distribution, preparation of i.v. admixtures, prefilling syringes, reviewing charts, attending weekly physician rounds, participating on the cardiac arrest team and providing drug information.

During fiscal year 1975, there were 42,727 outpatient visits to the hospital and 16,171 visits in the field. Pharmacists provided primary care (refills of chronic medication and treatment of minor acute problems) in 12.2% of these visits. All prescriptions were dispensed from the patient's chart and all nonprescription drugs dispensed by the pharmacy were recorded in the chart. The problem-oriented method of record keeping was used. Of the total visits to pharmacists, both in the field and at the hospital, 946 (17.3%) were for diabetes.

Procedure

Most of the diagnosed diabetic patients are monitored in the diabetic clinic, which is held every Tuesday morning from 8:00 a.m. until noon. Patients with problems not related to diabetes are usually not seen during this time. Establishment of this clinic has allowed a concentrated effort by all of the involved staff with a resulting increase in the efficiency of care delivered to the patient. Staff involvement includes the services of one physician, a registered nurse, a licensed practical nurse, a clinic aide, laboratory technicians, a dietician and two pharmacists. The regularity of the clinic makes it easier for patients to attend.

Patients are requested to arrive as early as possible for their clinic visits. Appointments are not used because past experience showed

that patient response to this system was very poor. After signing in at the medical records department, the patient goes to the clinic area where vital signs (blood pressure, pulse, weight) and a urine sample are taken. The nurses or clinic aide do dipstick tests for urine glucose, ketones and protein. A fasting blood sugar may be ordered if the patient is in a fasting state. Results are usually available within 30 to 60 minutes.

During this time the patient will usually indicate to the nurse if he wishes to see a physician. All patients are seen at least once yearly by a physician and always have the option of being seen by him. When the program was started, pharmacists would screen all patients, but as they began spending more time in direct patient care, this became impractical. Now, the clinic nurse does a general screening and directs obviously ill patients or those with grossly elevated blood sugars to the physician. Newly diagnosed diabetics are usually seen by a physician.

Many patients seen by the pharmacist are well controlled and are complying with their treatment regimens (diet, medication). Using established guidelines (see Appendix), the pharmacist interviews the patient to check for any problems; if there are none, he refills the medications. However, the pharmacist also sees a number of patients who are not adequately controlled, even using a liberal definition of control (asymptomatic and having a fasting blood sugar of about 200 mg/100 ml or below). Few Indian patients would be classified as "ketosis-prone" diabetics. Most tolerate wide variations in blood sugar and it is not uncommon for patients with a fasting blood sugar above 300 mg/100 ml to be asymptomatic.

A room adjacent to the pharmacy is used for the patient interview. If a problem is found that requires further data collection or physical examination, or both, the pharmacist orders the appropriate lab tests or refers the patient to a physician. The pharmacists at Pine Ridge have not received training in physical examination, so this function must be performed by physicians or physician extenders. If the problem appears to be a result of inadequate control of the disease, the pharmacist will initiate corrective action. This will usually be done independently, although a physician is readily available for consultation and referral.

Often the lack of control is because of noncompliance with prescribed treatment. Lack of compliance is one of the main problems in treating diabetes faced by the practitioners at Pine Ridge.

If compliance does not seem to be the reason for a lack of control, the reason must be determined. Acute illnesses, changes in dietary habits, emotional stress or a number of other factors may be responsible. If it appears that the problem is not just an acute episode that can be treated or corrected, then alteration of the patient's treatment regimen is indicated.

Once this assessment is completed, the plan of therapy is determined and fully explained to the patient. Medication and supplies are dispensed to the patient along with proper instructions. An entry is made in the chart using the problem-oriented record format. If no changes in therapy are made, the chart is returned to medical records. If a change is made, the chart is set aside for physician review and countersignature.

Controlled patients are usually asked to return at two- or three-month intervals. Uncontrolled patients are requested to return at one- or two-week intervals, although this may vary with the patient's ability or willingness to return this often. When the patient returns, the procedure is repeated. Therapy is continued or alterations made as is appropriate under the guidelines. In a few cases it has become obvious, after repeated attempts, that control cannot be obtained on an outpatient basis. Referral has then been made to the physician for evaluation and admission.

Program Experience

During the period from November 1973 until May 1975, 230 diabetic patients were identified. One hundred and ninety-three charts were reviewed to determine which providers were primarily treating these patients and what the status of their disease was during the 18 months since the beginning of the program. (The remaining charts involved patients who were also being treated elsewhere.) Ninety-six (50%) of these patients were monitored a majority of the time by a pharmacist, 85 (44%) by a physician and the remainder equally by each.

One hundred and nineteen (62%) of these patients were considered controlled at the time of the review, that is, no complaints at the last visit, a fasting blood sugar of less than 200 mg/100 ml, and urine glucose negative or one plus. However, 39 of these 119 patients (33%) were over two weeks late for scheduled prescription refills. Of the 77 patients considered uncontrolled, 57 (77%) were over two weeks overdue for prescription refills. Fifty percent of all the diabetic patients were over two weeks late for their scheduled refills.

Discussion

Treatment compliance continues to be a major problem. Many patients do not attend clinic unless they are symptomatic. The expanded responsibilities of the pharmacist result in care for a much larger group of patients than would be possible if all symptomatic patients had to be seen by a physician. By relieving the physician of having to see all noncompliant patients, he has much more time to deal with patients who have acute problems or more serious complications of their disease. The pharmacist can also spend more time with the remaining patients in an attempt to improve their understanding of the disease and their compliance with prescribed therapy.

The pharmacist is in an excellent position to serve as an educator to the patient. It is the pharmacist who gives the patient his medication and can explain its purpose while the patient can actually see what "pill" is being talked about. The pharmacist also dispenses the urine testing strips to be used at home and can ensure that the patient understands their use. Additionally, many patients need continuing education on their disease state, assuming they have ever received this education in the past.

The establishment of a regular diabetic clinic has appeared to improve compliance and also the continuity of care. Previously, patients were seen in general clinic, usually by a different physician at each visit. Because of the large number of people seen during clinic hours, care was often superficial and fragmented. For many patients it was difficult to even find chart entries concerning their diabetes, other than an occasional refill of medication. Patients were often reluctant to come to the clinic because of the superficial attention they received.

The establishment of the diabetic clinic and its active promotion by the pharmacy staff showed patients that they could expect more interest in their problems. A better patient-provider rapport was achieved since the same pharmacists could be seen at each visit.

An additional advantage of the regular clinic has been an improvement in routine health maintenance. Several patients have been discovered with elevated blood pressure, and two patients with severe renal disease, who had been lost to follow-up, were detected by pharmacists.

One of the major differences between the Pine Ridge program and that of other facilities is that changes in therapy are initiated independently by the pharmacist with retrospective physician review. This concept is not new. Streit[1] predicted progression to this type of program in his paper. The Report of Task Force on the Pharmacist's Clinical Role[5] details how pharmacists have been performing a prescribing function.

Patient and physician acceptance of the program has been excellent. Although a small number of patients do request to see a physician at each visit, most are satisfied with a pharmacy visit and some even prefer seeing a pharmacist. Physicians have been pleased with the efforts of the pharmacist and this has aided in developing closer working relationships between these professionals.

Perhaps one of the greatest drawbacks to the program has been the pharmacists' reluctance to become directly involved with patients. The lack of formal training in patient interviewing and how to respond to various patient problems has caused the pharmacists a certain amount of insecurity. There was also some uncertainty by the pharmacists concerning the adequacy of their understanding of the disease and its therapy. These problems have decreased as the pharmacists became more familiar with their new role.

Conclusion

The pharmacists have demonstrated their ability to monitor and treat patients with chronic diseases, including those not stabilized. They have demonstrated that they have the knowledge and responsibility to carry out the prescribing function while working closely with other members of the health care team. They have also proved to be a good resource for patient education.

The success of this program has opened the way for continued expansion of pharmacy involvement in the care of other chronic diseases at Pine Ridge. Guidelines for the care of hypertensive patients have been established and pharmacists are following an increasing number of patients with this disease. Further expansion will depend on adequate staffing and facilities. Additionally, continued education and training of the pharmacist in disease states, therapy, diagnostic techniques and even physical examination will be of great benefit in expanding the pharmacist's responsibilities.

References

1. Streit, R. J.: A program expanding the pharmacist's role, *J Am Pharm Assoc NS13:* 434–436, 443 (Aug) 1973.
2. Anon: Annual report—pharmacy branch, FY 1974, Department of HEW, Public Health Service, Indian Health Service, unpublished.
3. Ellinoy, B. J., Mays, J. F., McSherry, P. V., Solomon, A. C., Hoag, S. G., and Kloesel, W. A.: A pharmacy outpatient monitoring program providing primary medical care to selected patients, *Am J Hosp Pharm 30:* 593–598 (Jul) 1973.
4. Johnson, R. E., and Tuchler, R. J.: Role of the pharmacist in primary health care, *Am J Hosp Pharm 32:* 162–164 (Feb) 1975.
5. Anon: Report of task force on the pharmacist's clinical role, *J Am Pharm Assoc NS11:* 482–485 (Sep) 1971.

Appendix

Guidelines for Pharmacy Diabetic Program

Goals of Therapy
—Lack of symptoms or complications, or both.
—Urine negative for glucose and ketones.
—Fasting blood sugar (FBS) in "normal" range.
Treatment and Follow-up
Subjective
—Blurred vision.
—Cardiovascular—shortness of breath, chest pains, edema, headaches.
—Genitourinary—nocturia, frequency, dysuria, thirst, vaginitis.
—Extremities—sores, numbness or tingling.

Objective
—Urine (Clinistix), blood pressure, weight and pulse on each visit.
—FBS, blood urea nitrogen or other lab values deemed necessary.
Assessment
—Controlled or not controlled.
Plan
—Patient education on disease, diet, self care and medications.
—Continue current regimen or change.

Changes made by the pharmacist should be countersigned by the physician assigned to the clinic. A physician will be available to see patients who request to see him, whom the pharmacist refers or on whom a pharmacist requests consultation.

If objective information other than the above is needed, the patient may be referred to the clinic nurse or laboratory for certain procedures, or to the medex or physician for specific physical findings that cannot be obtained through consultation with the patient.

The goal of this program is to improve patient care, follow-up and education. It will also allow more time for the physician to devote to more seriously ill patients, while others are followed by the pharmacy.

Readings for a Broader Perspective

1. Phelps, M. R., and White, S. J. "The Pharmacist's Role in a Team Approach for Diabetic Education," *Hospital Pharmacy* 12 (February 1977): 78–80.
2. Gans, J. "What the Patient Needs to Know About Drugs in the Management of Diabetes Mellitus," *American Journal of Pharmacy* 149 (July/August 1977): 97–105.
3. Solomon, A. C., Hoag, S. G. and Kloesel, W. A. "A Community Pharmacist-Sponsored Diabetes Detection Program," *J. Am. Pharm. Assoc.* NS 17 (March 1977): 161–63.
4. Sesin, G. P. "Understanding Diabetes," *The Apothecary* 89 (September/October 1977): 22–23, 26, 50.
5. Campbell, R. K. "The Pharmacist's Role in the Treatment of Diabetes," *American Pharmacy* NS 19 (July 1979): 36–43.

Drug Abuse

9—The Pharmacist's Role in a Community Drug Addiction Treatment Program

Ken Burleson

The need for a treatment program to deal with drug addiction exists in many communities today, even in small cities and towns. Establishing a drug addiction treatment program involves the skills of many health professionals to coordinate the therapy. For this professional staff considerable financial outlay is required for salaries. In metropolitan areas, funds usually are available to establish a treatment program. However, in smaller communities the necessary funding may not be available. Yet an effective program can be established through community cooperation and support. I will explain the approach taken by one such community, High Point, North Carolina, where a largely volunteer staff is used to coordinate an effective program.

Types of Treatment Programs

There are numerous approaches to treatment of drug addiction. In some of these only psychotherapy is used, while in others a combination of psychotherapy and drug substitution therapy is used. In the latter approach methadone usually is used as part of the drug therapy.

There are two types of methadone treatment programs, detoxification and maintenance. Detoxification is designed to return an addict (also referred to as a client) to a drug-free state within a short period of time. Presently, methadone is the drug of choice for detoxifying a client, since it can substitute for the client's addictive drug, and the dose of methadone can be reduced daily without the client experiencing physical withdrawal symptoms. The client is started on a daily dose of methadone sufficient to prevent withdrawal symptoms. Usually, 40 mg or less per day is enough. The dosage is reduced over a 21-day period until no drug is being taken. At this point, the addict has been withdrawn from his physical addiction without having suffered severe withdrawal symptoms. To qualify for admission to a detoxification program, the addict need only to prove true physical addiction to a narcotic drug.

In maintenance programs the client receives a daily dose of methadone which is high enough to prevent withdrawal symptoms, as well as to block the euphoric effects of any other drugs which he might ingest. This effect is referred to as "blockading," and discourages the client from further drug use. A client may remain in a maintenance program for years, although the aim of the program is to eventually return him to a drug-free state. The usual dose of methadone in such treatment is 40 to 100 mg/day or more. To gain admittance to a maintenance program, the addict must have at least a two-year documented history of addiction, and repeated attempts at detoxification must have failed. Documentation is usually done through medical and/or legal records.

Both forms of treatment programs are regulated by the Food and Drug Administration. In these guidelines, established in December of 1972, methadone is listed as a drug approved for use in treatment. Inclusive regulations for the operation of such programs are provided. These are necessary to insure that all programs in the U.S. meet minimum standards of care and that they function in the best interest for both the client and the general public. The regulations also prevent indiscriminate prescribing of methadone, because the prescribing of the drug on a long-term basis is primarily limited to physicians involved with treatment programs.

The programs must provide the client with supportive therapy and rehabilitation, both of which are essential to the successful treatment of the addict. The physical need for narcotics can easily be cured with detoxification, but the psychological need must be compensated through supportive therapy if the addict is to overcome the physical addiction.

A Community-Coordinated Approach to a Treatment Program

In the spring of 1971, it became apparent to a number of concerned citizens in High Point, N.C., that drug abuse and narcotic addiction existed on such a scale that a treatment program was necessary. In a city of 60,000 persons with a surrounding rural population of 30,000, there was an estimated 300–350 narcotic addicts, most of whom were addicted to heroin. However, it was realized that the funds for hiring a full-time professional staff for the program were not available. It was decided that trained professionals from various existing agencies in the town could be coordinated to provide an effective treatment program.

A volunteer board of directors, consisting of health professionals, legal and law enforcement professionals, businessmen, housewives and others, was set up to coordinate the organization and operation of the program. With this coordinated approach the program was set up, with a psychiatrist from the local mental health agency as medical director. Psychological counseling for selected clients is provided by a local mental health agency and a psychologist on a part-time basis. A program director and a project director together operate the program's office on a day-to-day basis, providing most of the counseling and rehabilitative treatment. The local vocational rehabilitation office provides job training and placement. The hospital pharmacist administers medication, provides a drug abuse information service, and functions as a liaison between the medical director and the client on a daily basis.

The only salaried staff members are the program and the project directors. The psychiatrist and the psychologist receive small fees for service. All others on the staff donate their time and efforts.

Funding comes from various sources. Much money comes from community action agencies, local civic groups and churches. The clients are expected to pay for much of their treatment.

Initially, the program was set up for detoxification only, and continued as such until 1974, when maintenance was offered to selected clients.

Treatment of a Typical Client, with Emphasis on the Pharmacist's Role

Clients come to the program from various sources, including word-of-mouth through former clients, judicial and social agencies referrals, medical referrals, and contact with former addicts who are case workers.

Each potential client is screened before admission for treatment to determine if he is truly addicted to narcotics. His motivation for treatment is also evaluated, so as to exclude those addicts who are interested only in obtaining medication to sustain their habits.

If he is admitted to the program, he is seen by the medical director, who interviews and counsels the client. The medical director also examines the client for physical evidence of long-term drug use to substantiate addiction. Based on the information gathered, the medical director sets up a methadone dosage schedule for the client. Each client's dosage schedule is individualized to his need.

Following this, a staff member of the treatment center accompanies the client to the hospital pharmacy, where positive identification is established for pharmacy personnel.

The client reports to the pharmacy daily for medication, twice a day if he is on detoxification, and once a day if he is on maintenance. The methadone, available as soluble tablets, is suspended in water or juice and taken by mouth.

The liquid formulation has two advantages over oral tablets. First, the client cannot conceal the liquid in his mouth, thus we are sure that all of the drug has been taken. Second, we have found that if a client knows the amount of methadone he receives, as he does when taking oral tablets, he psychologically feels that it is not enough to prevent withdrawal symptoms. When he takes the drug in liquid form, he does not know the dose; we have found that he will respond better to treatment if we use this bit of psychology.

All methadone is taken at the hospital pharmacy under the scrutiny of the pharmacist. No methadone is taken home by the client. The pharmacist refers to the dosage schedule prepared by the medical director to determine the amount of drug to be given at each dose. As he receives the dose, the client signs a log, verifying that he received the dose. He may miss one dose, but if two consecutive doses are missed, treatment is terminated.

Because the medical director is unable to see each client on a daily basis, the pharmacist is the only health professional who sees the clients daily. Thus, he functions as a liaison between the medical director and the client. Each day, the pharmacist talks to the client, questioning him about his progress and problems, if any. If in the pharmacist's professional judgement the client needs medical or psychiatric attention, the pharmacist contacts the medical director and tells him of the situation. Back-up medical care is also available through the hospital emergency room physicians, if necessary.

The pharmacist routinely treats many of the complaints of the clients himself. We have found that clients, especially those undergoing detoxification, suffer more than usual from common complaints such as constipation, nausea, vomiting and insomnia. The pharmacist may administer nonprescription drugs for these complaints. For nervousness and insomnia, he may also administer prescription tranquilizers to selected clients, with the prior knowledge of the medical director.

All clients must submit to random urinalyses while in the program. The urinalysis, done by thin-layer chromatography, can test for all drugs of abuse. This insures that the client is not abusing drugs while in treatment. Urine samples, which are taken at least twice weekly, may be collected by the treatment center or the pharmacist.

We can also test for heroin abuse with a heroin detection kit. This kit gives a positive color reaction in the presence of morphine, which is the urinary metabolite of heroin. If evidence of drug abuse is found, treatment is terminated immediately.

At one time, the hospital pharmacist performed the urinalyses, using a Chromat/O/ Screen Kit by Eastman Kodak. However, the time required for this service became burdensome, and the results from the tests were not always accurate. Now a commercial laboratory performs the tests.

Other Roles for the Pharmacist

Although the primary daily activities of the pharmacist in a treatment program usually involve medication administration and counseling of clients, his unique knowledge of pharmacology and drug therapy allow him to expand his role into other areas as well.

In our program, the pharmacists serve as drug information consultants, providing information to the medical director and the treatment center staff. We have also expanded our information center to other members of the medical community, who use our service when dealing with drug-abusing patients. The emergency room staff relies on the pharmacist to keep them abreast of the latest drug abuse problems in the area, so that they are aware of this in dealing with overdose cases. The pharmacist many times is relied upon for information in treatment of various drug overdoses.

The pharmacists are also important in dissemination of drug abuse information to the public. We have presented many programs on the topic to community groups, in conjunction with other members of the treatment team.

Conclusions

In our program, we have detoxified over 200 drug-dependent persons, many of whom had received treatment more than one time. A select few have been admitted to the maintenance program after repeated failures in detoxification. Our overall cure rate has been low, as it is in many other programs. However, approximately 10% of our clients have maintained a drug-free state for more than one year. Even with the low overall cure rate, we believe that the program has been beneficial to both the community and the client, and justifies its continued operation.

Methadone programs are not the total answer to drug addiction, but they are a step in the right direction. As more and more communities are faced with the problem of treatment, the hospital pharmacist should step in and take his proper place on the treatment team. His unique knowledge in the areas of pharmacology, drug use and abuse and pharmacy laws makes him an ideal person to contribute significantly to the treatment program.

References

1. Bensel, J. J.: Methadone maintenance of narcotic addicts. *J. Am. Pharm. Assn.* NS11:372, 1971.
2. Canada, A. A., and Flinkow, S. P.: Narcotic addiction: A methadone program. *J. Am. Pharm. Assn.* NS11:368, 1971.
3. Chappell, J. N.: Attitudinal barriers to physician involvement with drug abusers. *JAMA* 224:1011, 1973.
4. Cuskey, W. R.: Methadone use in the outpatient treatment of narcotic addicts. *Bull. Narcotics* 23:23, 1971.
5. Gearing, F. R.: Methadone maintenance: Six years later. *Contemp. Drug Prob.* 1:191, 1972.
6. Jackson, R. A., et al: The potential of the pharmacist to serve as a drug abuse consultant. *J. School Health* 42:536, 1972.
7. Lennard, H. L., et al: Methadone: The cure becomes a new problem. *Smithsonian* 4:51, April 1973.

8. Ruiz, P.: Community approach to addiction problem. *NY State J. Med.* 970, 1972.
9. Wieland, W. F.: Narcotic substitution therapy. *Int. J. Clin. Pharmacol.* 4:462, 1971.

10. U.S. Department of Health, Education and Welfare: Methadone, listing as a new drug. *Federal Register* 37:26790, Dec. 1972.

10—Drug Abuse Education: The Pharmacist's Role

Michael Dolan

"A significant number of pharmacists don't know diddly about street drugs," says Thomas Milne, RPh. "And I think that's a shame."

Tom Milne feels that drug abuse is drug abuse, whether you're talking about an addict firing up impure heroin, a truck driver eating handfuls of amphetamines, or a housewife gulping too many Valiums. Pharmacists have always informed patients about the potential for abuse of certain prescription and over-the-counter products. Milne would like to see more of his peers take the next logical step of learning about illicit drugs of abuse, as well.

Milne, 37, manages the support/special services division of the Multnomah County (Oregon) Department of Human Services. He recently spent a year developing and directing a demonstration street drug analysis program in Portland, and for the past seven years has worked with Freedom House, a therapeutic community for heroin addicts.

Milne's involvement in community health work began when he signed on as an "outreach pharmacist" with the now-defunct federal Office of Economic Opportunity neighborhood program, run by the Kaiser Foundation. Milne found his community work a valuable, sometimes shocking experience.

"I didn't know what 'community health' meant until I started visiting people's homes, talking with them, and getting laughed at for my naive ideas.

"So I started hanging out, meeting addicts, spending time in court. I learned from these experiences; they have been my textbook."

Milne feels that for many pharmacists drug use and/or abuse is strictly a chemical, clinical affair. He tries to bring an element of socioeconomic understanding to his work as well.

"Too many pharmacists turn people off by giving non-useful information," said Milne, who has attempted to correct that imbalance by running an "experiential seminar" for health science professional students in the Portland area.

"It was a 10-week course, during which we visited the courts, seeing how they're administered, how the legal system works, and how a person is influenced by that experience," added Milne. "If pharmacists are going to open their mouths about drug abuse, they should be sure of themselves."

Tony Tommasello is sure of himself. The 27-year-old pharmacist and faculty advisor of the University of Maryland Student Committee for Drug Abuse Education spends between three and five hours a week giving presentations on drug abuse all over his home state. In addition to his work on a master's degree in pharmacology, Tommasello is helping to develop a series of drug abuse education lectures aimed specifically at health and legal professionals who will graduate from the University's nursing, law, medical, dental and pharmacy schools.

"I think that the pharmacist's unique education enables him or her to peruse and interpret scientific information on drugs, then disseminate that material in lay language to the people," said Tommasello, who does not feel that such community awareness work should stop at drug abuse.

"I'd like to think that my fellow pharmacists would make time, if necessary, to do the reading, digest the material, and go out and talk to people, to specific community groups like diabetics and the aged, about the drugs they take. Older people, for example, use a lot of drugs, and some of them need to understand better about interactions and compliance."

Tommasello, a native of Baltimore, did his undergraduate work at the College Park campus of the University of Maryland, went to the pharmacy school in Baltimore, and began his professional life as an assistant to the medical director of the state Drug Abuse Administration. He then worked as a resident assistant in Baltimore City Hospital, and upon returning to his pharmacy studies was offered the opportunity to develop an education program for health professionals. Tommasello also directs the efforts of the 11-year-old student committee, which works to spread the word on drug abuse throughout Maryland.

"Every pharmacist should be involved," says Tommasello.

Salvatore Di Masi's community involvement has been more as a concerned human being than as an expert on drug interactions, but he feels that he has made a valuable contribution nonetheless.

Di Masi, 30, owns two pharmacies in the Chicago area, and since 1971 has worked with Metro Help, a 24-hour crisis intervention/reference telephone service. "Hot lines" such as Metro Help offer troubled people an opportunity to talk about themselves and their problems; upon request the services often provide information on drug abuse, birth control, and psychotherapy.

"The main thing is to be a resource for the person calling in," said Di Masi. "We try not to deal with someone judgmentally; we offer information, not advice. You have to let them decide for themselves."

Di Masi estimates that 25 or 30 percent of his work with Metro Help is directly dependent on his pharmacy background, and the rest "has come experientially." A 1970 graduate of the school of pharmacy at St. Louis University, Di Masi joined Metro Help as a volunteer in November 1971. He underwent a special training program, and spent eight hours a week "on the phones" until April 1976. Selected to serve on the board of directors of the organization in 1972, he still holds that position.

While he feels that his managerial experience and his education have been of immeasurable help in his work with Metro Help, Di Masi feels that his deepest satisfaction comes from "the personal relationships I've gotten going with people, the philosophy of caring for my fellow human being. I'm also glad to be able to use that wonderful knowledge I've had stuffed in my head for something other than making a good living.

"I'm nobody special . . . any pharmacist could do it."

H. R., and Schooff, K. G. "Pharmacy Involvement-Polydrug Detoxification Unit," *Drug Intelligence & Clinical Pharmacy* 9 (December 1975):638–47.

2. Jackson, R. A., Elkins, J. C., and Smith, M. C. "The Potential of the Pharmacist to Serve as a Drug Abuse Consultant," *The Journal of School Health*, 42 (November 1972):536–39.

Drug Utilization Review

11—Drug Usage Review in a Community Hospital

William N. Kelly, Jaxon A. White and *Douglas E. Miller*

The primary goals of drug usage review should be to increase the quality of drug therapy and to assure the safety of prescribing and administering medication to patients. Any reductions in the cost of prescribed drugs should be considered an additional benefit to these two primary goals.

It has been stated that drug usage review has become necessary because first, there is increasing evidence that the current level of physician understanding of clinical pharmacology falls short of optimal standards; second, the current level of prescribing is very costly; and third, there is a clear mandate from the public to establish and continually monitor quality health care performance.[1] Recently passed legislation concerning Professional Standards Review Organizations (PSROs) and the development of national health insurance proposals support the fact that the public is demanding better, safer and less expensive medical care than what is currently provided.

Background of Program

Hamot Medical Center is a 550-bed voluntary, nonprofit, general, community teaching hospital located in Erie, Pennsylvania. In the fall of 1972, the medical staff, having identified a need for quality assurance review processes, incorporated into the medical staff bylaws, rules and regulations, a charge to the pharmacy and therapeutics committee to establish and maintain an ongoing drug usage review program.

During the process of developing this program, the literature was surveyed to identify what types of procedures were being used in other institutions. It was soon discovered that there were only a few other hospitals involved in the drug usage review process and that there were many shortcomings in the present "state of the art." Most reports were of one-time drug usage studies which only identified some of the problems (i.e., cumulative data on which drugs and routes were being used the most and for what purposes).[2-5] Many of these studies offered no solutions to problems associated with drug prescribing.

Comprehensive drug usage reviews were being accomplished with the aid of sophisticated data processing equipment with the obvious advantages of securing complete objective data and being able to maintain an ongoing program with relative ease.[6] However, many shortcomings were also evident. Gathered data only reflected the basic facts concerning the circumstances under which the drugs were prescribed. For example, the acuteness of the disease, the patient's past medical history, and associated laboratory tests were never taken into consideration. No protocols were established to make sound decisions concerning the appropriateness of therapy. Evidence of influencing prescribing patterns because of the review processes was not reported. In addition, no one accepted responsibility for reporting to the prescriber the potential legal liabilities of the questioned practices discovered by the review process. One thing was evident: The use of data processing equipment for drug usage review was expensive.

With the aforementioned disadvantages and shortcomings in mind, a drug usage review process, which we consider simple yet effective, was developed and implemented in May 1973.

Procedure

Each month 10–15 patient charts are randomly selected by the medical records department for drug usage review. The only criterion for selection is that discharge has occurred within the past 60 days. The quantity of 10 charts was selected because it was a reasonable number for one person to review

in one afternoon. The quantity was increased to 15 charts per month in order to shorten the time it would take to review at least one chart of every physician at Hamot; this also makes the review more complete. Fifteen charts represents approximately 1% of the total number of new charts generated each month.

There are three parts to the review process: (1) an initial screen; (2) a secondary screen; and (3) a committee review (Figure 11–1).

Figure 11–1

Flow chart of the procedure for drug usage review

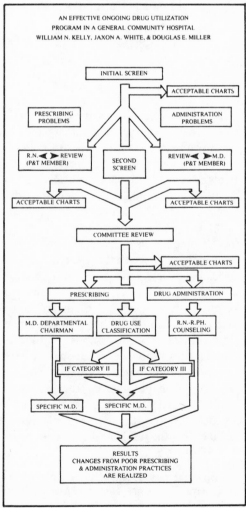

Table 11.1

Criteria Used for Screening Charts During Drug Usage Review

Drug Prescribing	Drug Administration
Was drug therapy indicated?	Was drug ordered/not given?
Optimal drug for situation?	Was drug given/not ordered?
Optimal route for situation?	Was drug administered by proper schedule?
Optimal dosage for situation?	Was the correct dose administered?
Proper course of therapy?	Was the correct route used?
Was therapy properly monitored?	Was drug given on schedule?
Was order properly written?	Was drug properly charted?
Approved indication?	
Therapeutic incompatibilities?	
Overlapping therapy?	
Efficacious use?	
Culture and sensitivities taken?	

Initial Screening. A drug information pharmacist who is a member of the pharmacy and therapeutics committee screens each chart for a variety of potential problems using the criteria listed in Table 11.1. Charts posing no questions are placed back into the medical records library. Questionable charts are held and reported in writing to a physician member of the pharmacy and therapeutics committee as shown in Figure 11.2. Charts questioned for possible problems relating to the administration of drugs are referred to the nursing member of the committee.

Secondary Screening. Both physician and nurse committee members are responsible for further screening of the questionable charts. Following this screening, and any investigation necessary, the physician and nurse present such cases as they feel deserve further review to the entire committee.

Committee Review. Review by the committee consists of a discussion of the circum-

stances under which the prescribing or drug administration problem or question occurred. As needed, material abstracted from the literature by the drug information service is brought into the discussion. In addition, drug use is classified into one of three categories:

Category I —Drug is being used as approved by the Food and Drug Administration (FDA).

Category II —Drug is being used in a manner not approved by the FDA; however there is substantial documentation in the literature (including the *American Hospital Formulary Service*) to justify such use.

Category III—Drug is being used in a manner not approved by the FDA and no documented evidence in the literature exists to support such an "unapproved use."

All factors associated with the problem in question are considered before a decision is made by the committee to either approve or disapprove the drug usage in question.

Action. A record of all charts reviewed is maintained by the drug information pharmacist member of the committee. A record of the second screener's action and committee action is maintained in the committee minutes.

When the committee determines that improper drug administration has taken place, nursing or the pharmacy and drug information service, or both, are obligated to follow-up the circumstances under which the improper event took place. The head nurse is informed and the specific nurse involved is counseled by the associate director of nursing, either with or without the director of the pharmacy and drug information service, depending upon the situation.

In those cases in which basic principles of drug therapy (taking cultures and sensitivities when indicated, proper monitoring of therapy, etc.) are violated, letters are sent to

Figure 11–2

Sample report generated by initial screening of drug usage.

Hamot Medical Center

PHARMACY & DRUG INFORMATION SERVICE

DATE: March 13, 1974

MEMORANDUM

TO: R. E. Miller, M.D., Chairman
                             Pharmacy and Therapeutics Committee

FROM: William N. Kelly, Pharm. D., Assistant Director
                             Pharmacy & Drug Information Service

SUBJECT: Drug Utilization Review for March, 1974.

On March 10, 1974 fifteen randomly selected charts were reviewed with regard to drug utilization. The following charts were found to be in order:

Surgery	Pediatrics	Urology	Family Practice	Medicine
1-628717	1-629237	1-628249	1-628815	1-627697
1-627300	1-629247	1-626516		
1-628701				

Orthopedic Surgery	Cardiovascular Surgery
1-628204	1-627618

The following charts are being held for your review in the Medical Records Library as they may have potential for review by the Pharmacy and Therapeutics Committee.

Chart Number	Service	Patient	Admitting Dx.	Item in Question
1-626506	Orthopedic Surgery	46 y.o.w.m.	back pain	Patient given (IV) 0.1% procaine in 1000cc of D5W; efficacy?
1-624976*	Medicine	16 y.o.w.f.	hypothyroidism	No medication ordered; Valium (po) charted 2 times on 2/5/74 and 2/6/74.
1-628204	General Surgery	28 y.o.b.m.	Valium overdose	Admitted 2/9/74/ (7A.M.). Progress note states: "patient in semi-stuperdous state". Patient rec'd Valium, Dalmane, and Tofranil.
1-627622	Urology	31 y.o.w.f.	severe abdominal pain	Temperature (2/7/74-2/11/74) ranged from 100.0-101.8; WBC (2/7/74) 16,500. No C & S or antimicrobial therapy ordered.

* cc: N. McCreary, R.N.

the physician's departmental chairman stating the problem identified by the committee.

When instances of Category II drug use are identified by the committee, letters are sent directly to the attending physician informing him that he is working in a "gray area," and indicating the amount of support he would have from the literature should liability be incurred.

In cases of Category III drug use, letters

are sent by the chairman of the pharmacy and therapeutics committee, to the attending physician and appropriate department chairman, stating the facts and requesting that the physician either work with the pharmacy and drug information service to submit an application for investigational use to the FDA or discontinue the "unapproved" practice.

In the two latter cases, follow-up with the appropriate department chairman is pursued as necessary.

Results

During the first two years of the program (July 1973–July 1975), 341 charts were screened for drug usage. . . . Of these 341 charts initially screened, 80 (23.5%) required further examination. From these 80 charts, 62 were further referred to the pharmacy and therapeutics committee for review. The committee review process resulted in four letters being sent to attending physicians. All four instances involved Category II drug use. In 16 cases, letters were sent to the physician's department chairman. In 16 separate instances (4.7%), the committee found questionable drug administration practices which were referred to nursing administration for investigation and appropriate counseling.

Discussion

The major advantages of this type of drug usage review process are that it is ongoing, simple and effective.

An ongoing program provides a continuing opportunity for physicians to learn about the implications of their prescribed therapy. At the rate of reviewing 15 charts each month, virtually all physicians will shortly be affected by the review process. During the first two years of the program, the charts of 128 different physicians were reviewed.

The procedure involved in this type of review process is simple since it takes only three to four hours per month of one pharmacist's time. An additional benefit of the program is that there is team involvement and commitment, involving nurses, physicians, pharmacists, the drug information service and the medical records librarian.

The third, and by far the most important aspect of any drug usage review program, is that there is an action phase. The program is effective because people are counseled for unsatisfactory drug usage. It is useless to spend time collecting data to define problems concerning misuse of drugs without proper procedures to take care of those problems. In questionable cases to date, physicians, as indicated, have either discontinued the practices in question or have filed appropriate papers with the FDA. In most cases, the chairmen of the various medical specialties have followed through with their counseling of the physicians using questionable prescribing identified by the review process. We have found that this part of the review process is more effective if each department chairman also is informed of the number of charts from their department that passed the review process.

Where questionable prescribing practices are common, an awareness of the problem is created among the physicians by writing well-documented articles in the pharmacy newsletter for physicians, a publication which has been found to be actively read by a majority of our physicians.

One valid criticism of this type of drug usage review process may be that a limited number of charts are reviewed when compared to the total number of charts generated each month. However, it must be remembered that the same type of therapy is normally prescribed by the same physician for all patients who have the same diagnosis, and implications of the random review can be quite significant.

Legal Considerations. It has been our experience that, in general, physicians like to know whether their prescribing practices are in accord with FDA approved labeling. Although we have had limited experience in advising physicians by letter concerning Category II drug use, the response has been favorable. A typical letter notes that a particular drug use is not currently listed in the labeling approved by the FDA. Furthermore, the letter also informs the prescriber about the role of the drug manufacturer in a civil suit for damages based upon an unfavorable experience with the drug in question. Thus, it is unlikely that a pharmaceutical company could lend evidentiary support for a drug use that is not listed in the approved labeling. However, it is also stated (in the case of Category II drug use) that the literature may provide a basis upon which the prescriber can defend a medical decision to employ the drug for a use unapproved by the FDA. A drug use not listed in approved labeling but presented in recent monographs of the *American Hospital Formulary Service* and other current literature is acceptable for such use at Hamot Medical Center. Accordingly, the physician is advised that professional liability for an unapproved drug use is minimized by careful monitoring of drug therapy consistent with the findings and controls reported by other practitioners.

The *American Hospital Formulary Service (AHFS)* is used as part of the evaluation process because it has high recognition in the health care field as a drug information service. Should it be necessary to defend a prescribing practice in litigation, the *AHFS* could be introduced as evidence to support a therapeutic decision. Although not conclusive, a current *AHFS* monograph (within five years) setting forth therapeutic information outside the approved labeling would demonstrate professional acceptance of certain drug therapy not, as yet, incorporated into FDA approved labeling.

The value to the institution of notifying physicians concerning Category III drug use cannot be underestimated. Physicians are asked in writing either to discontinue the questioned prescribing practice or to undertake an FDA approved clinical investigation. In this manner, the institution establishes a record that it will not be a party to unproven or unsanctioned use of certain drugs in patient care. In addition to the letter, the pharmacy and drug information service is directed not to honor any subsequent Category III drug orders for the prescribing practice attributed to the physician. The committee believes that these professional and administrative procedures establish a policy which eliminates the possibility of joint responsibility with the physician for inappropriate drug therapy.

Conclusion

We have presented what we feel is a simple, yet effective ongoing drug usage review program. It can be particularly useful in hospitals that do not have data processing equipment available, yet have the desire to increase the quality, safety and efficacy of drug prescribing and administration in their institution. The system not only defines problems in the misuse of drugs, but also incorporates a three-step approach to solving these problems. The program is effective because it gets desired results; changes from questionable or poor prescribing habits are realized.

As with this program, however, most drug usage review processes scrutinize the medication practices of only physicians and nurses. It will not be long before quality assurance will be an expected part of the practice of pharmacy. Two possible areas that we are considering in this regard are retrospective reviews of answers given to drug information questions and drug therapy decisions made by our pharmacists.

References

1. Pierpaoli, P. G. and Bowman, G. K.: Drug utilization review/implementation, *Hospitals* 46:95–104 (Jun 16) 1972.

2. Muller, C., Herbst, M. and Westheimer, R.: Use and cost of drugs for inpatients at four New York City hospitals, *Med. Care 5*:294–312 (Sep–Oct) 1967.
3. Lamy, P. P. and Kitler, M.E.: Drug use in hospitals, *Drug Intell 2*:302–304 (Nov) 1968.
4. Alexander, W. E., Humenchuk, R. J. and Keeping, D.: A drug usage study, *Drug Intell 3*:6–13 (Jan) 1969.
5. Kistler, S. B. and Kough, R. H.: Antibiotic acquisitions, *Am J Hosp Pharm 26*:680–685 (Dec) 1969.
6. Maronde, R. F., Burks, D. II, Lee, P. V. et al: Physician prescribing practices—a computer based study, *Am J Hosp Pharm 26*:566–573 (Oct) 1969.

Related Readings in This Volume

Readings for a Broader Perspective

1. Kabat, H. F., Marttila, J., and Stewart, J. "Drug Utilization Review in Skilled Nursing Facilities," *J. Am. Pharm. Assoc.* NS 15 (January 1975): 34–37.
2. Keys, P. W., Lech, J. G., and Gonzales Duffy, M. "Drug Audits and In-Service Education as Functions of a Drug Information Center," *American Journal of Pharmacy* 150 (May/June 1978):89–93.
3. Bergman, H. D. "Prescribing of Drugs in a Nursing Home," *Drug Intelligence & Clinical Pharmacy* 9 (July 1975):365–68.
4. Greenlaw, C. W. "Antimicrobial Use Monitoring by a Hospital Pharmacy," *American Journal of Hospital Pharmacy* 34 (August 1977):835–38.
5. Gregory, J. M., and Knapp, D. E. "State-of-the-Art of Drug Usage Review," *American Journal of Hospital Pharmacy* 33 (September 1976):925–28.

Health Education/Preventive Services

12—The Pharmacist and Preventive Medicine

Mickey C. Smith and J. Tyrone Gibson

It seems hardly necessary to attempt to demonstrate again here the need for and value of good preventive medicine practices. Evidence of growing national concern has appeared in efforts (admittedly unsuccessful) to establish a government-financed "Preventicare" program.[1] Preventive services have been identified as an essential element of "comprehensive health care."[2] A number of studies has been conducted which indicate the favorable cost-benefit ratio for preventive practices.[3] It has even been suggested that special "preventia" be established, not only to provide needed preventive services, but also to give preventive medicine a separate identity.[4]

It is the intent of this paper to examine the proposition that the nation's community pharmacists might be enlisted into a program of preventive medicine. The positive possibilities as well as acknowledged barriers will be explored.

Rationale

What are the reasons that preventive medicine has, so far, not been as effective as it promises to be? One of these must be found in the widely publicized shortage of health manpower, particularly physicians. Given the choice in choosing how to spend professional time which is already inadequate, the physician can be expected to spend it in obviously needed treatment, rather than the not-so-obvious prevention. Given also the already cluttered waiting rooms, and less than optimal awareness of its value, the consumer can hardly be expected to *initiate* a visit for preventive purposes. (What sort of crisis would result if everyone did get a "checkup" twice or even once a year?). At that a substantial proportion (20 percent) of patient visits to physicians in a recent study of general practitioners was for checkups.[5] In that same study nearly one out of four patients saw the physician for "nonsickness" reasons. An earlier study of rural Missouri general practitioners found them spending 28 percent of their professional time in "preventive medicine" (10.9 percent) and "health information and counseling" (17.2 percent).[6]

Some possibility to "stretch" the physician by use of nonphysician personnel does, of course, exist. A demonstration of this technique in Pittsburgh found such personnel performing 41 percent of total health services in a general medical practice.[7] Such a technique has its limitations, however, particularly in the rural setting where the nonphysician personnel may, themselves, be in short supply.

Added to the time problem is one of attitudes. It has been pointed out that preventive medicine has had a lack-lustre history as a medical specialty, and that this history still, apparently, impedes its progress in the medical schools.[8] Such an atmosphere cannot but hamper efforts to "sell" preventive medicine to the medical student. James has pointed to the failure to supply departments "sufficient quality and numbers of personnel and facilities to permit them to compete for the students' interest against the glamor of cardiac surgery, organ transplant and microneurosurgery".[9] It would be understandable if these attitudes were ultimately translated into practice.

What possibilities does the pharmacist offer? One is his availability/accessibility. A study in Colorado is probably fairly typical of the U.S. generally. It found "drug stores" in 76 percent of incorporated places in Colorado (compared with 63 percent for physicians, 45 percent for dentists and 32 percent for hospitals).[10] In Mississippi 81 percent of the towns greater than 500 in population have a pharmacy.[11] Ironically, at a time when the "store front" has become the fashion for health and legal facilities, pharmacy's traditional store front (and, of course, the frequent jumble of merchandise within) has become a barrier to a professional image. Many pharmacists, in addition to being on the scene, apparently have available idle time. Data on this subject are sparse, but Smith, in a limited rural study, found one-third of the professional time available for reallocation.[12] Rodowskas and Gagnon, in a more comprehensive study, identified approximately 15 percent of pharmacists' time as "idle."[13] Without addressing the problems of scheduling, there does seem to be the possibility of finding time for the pharmacist to participate in preventive medicine activities.

Is the pharmacist willing to participate? The answer to this question would seem to be "yes." At any rate, the pages of pharmacy journals and the halls of pharmacy meetings have recently been filled with discussions of pharmacy's "new roles." Silverman recently anticipated some of these, commenting that " . . . (the pharmacist) can make a truly heroic contribution to the improvement of health care, to the prevention of needless drug expenditures, to the prevention and control of needless, destructive, costly illnesses."[14] It should be noted that this last comment is one of only a few which deals specifically with a role for the pharmacist in preventive medicine. New roles proposed have not treated this role extensively except indirectly, e.g., health advisor, health educator.

What are the pharmacist's capabilities? Among health care professionals the pharmacist graduate of today receives training more extensive than any other except the physician. Nearly all schools have incorporated some clinical training in their programs, although these vary markedly in length and content. Among pharmacists, approximately 70 percent received four or more years of pharmacy training, with only 30 percent being graduates of training programs of three years or less. [15] The specific applicability of this training to preventive medicine remains in question and is discussed further.

Drug Abuse

The pharmacist can contribute to limiting drug abuse in essentially two environments. The first is the environment within the pharmacy in which the pharmacist has a good probability of face-to-face and consequently personal contact. The second is in an impersonal environment away from the pharmacy.

Within the pharmacy, activities can be divided into those directed towards curbing abuse of drugs obtained legally and those obtained illegally. The method of dealing with the former may considerably affect the response to the latter.

The pharmacist will be most effective in minimizing drug abuse of prescription and non-prescription drugs by maintaining an efficient and yet comprehensive family and patient record system. This can be further enhanced through pooling of patient drug consumption information by local pharmacists. An increasing number of pharmacists is maintaining such records for prescription drugs but rarely are o-t-c drugs included. Through such a record a pharmacist can monitor consumption and detect abuse or the first signs of possible abuse. For example, if, from review of the patient record, the pharmacist notes that a patient is repeatedly receiving a sedative medication, he would review the case and possibly call attention to the patient of the hazards of potentially securing a sedative habit. By counseling the patient (in an appropriate environment), the pharmacist can explain to the patient the particular hazards of the drug. If the message is provided in a clear and understandable manner, a rational person would likely accept the pharmacist's advice and counsel. The pharmacist could refuse to dispense medication to any person refusing to supply enough information to allow him to make a rational decision regarding a given drug (the family record would usually suffice for this purpose).

To curb abuse of drugs obtained illegally, the pharmacist should be sensitive to those drugs most likely to be sought by potential abusers. He should verify the authenticity of both written and oral prescriptions. He should maintain his "most attractive" drugs in suitably protected areas such as double-locked, heavy, metal, storage cabinets.

Many of the problems associated with the obtaining of drugs illegally would be resolved through the use of the record described above. The sale of over-the-counter drugs would have to be restricted to pharmacists in order for the system described to function.

In the environment external to the pharmacy the pharmacist can offer his services to the public as a drug expert. He can publicize his readiness and willingness to dispense his knowledge to listeners. Through the local pharmaceutical association, a speakers and information bureau can be maintained. Pharmacists should inform schools, colleges, churches and other local organizations of their efforts and availability. A challenging and worthwhile contribution to drug abuse education can be made in orphan homes, reformatories, prisons and similar institutions. In all but the first, high concentrations of drug abusers are likely to be found. If a sane, rational, truthful approach is taken regarding drug abuse, these inmates should respond in much the fashion as have health professionals through their own education. The latter statement also would apply to the vast number of youth who are potential abusers of drugs. The pharmacist must first accept drug abuse as a sociologically defined problem. He must be willing to cope with the paradox of the legal availability of a proven potent drug—e.g., ethanol—and the unavailability of legal marijuana.

Drug Misuse

The area between drug abuse and drug misuse is gray and uncertain. Perhaps they can best be viewed as points along a continuum. It is far from clear which represents the "worst end" of the continuum. Drug abuse clearly gets the most publicity, while at the same time drug misuse tends to be insidious and pervasive in nature due in part to being cloaked in the garb of legitimacy.

The pharmacist can reduce drug misuse by both health professional (those directing the consumption of drugs by others) and layman alike by encouraging rationality in drug use. He can encourage adhering to the uses listed for a drug in its "package insert" (full disclosure information) and make departing from the tenets of the package insert the exception rather than the rule.

Pharmacists in Houston, Texas, in cooperation with physicians, have demonstrated an apparently effective means of restricting consumption of legal amphetamines. They have accomplished this by agreeing through the local pharmaceutical association to dispense medications for this class of drugs only in rare and life-threatening cases. (This is consistent with the out-right banning of amphetamine sales in some countries.) For

example, pharmacists should emphasize that amphetamines are accepted as valuable drugs only in the treatment of narcolepsy and that their anorectic effect lasts only for a few weeks.[16] The foregoing is really a call for pharmacists to be the leaders in instilling a greater element of rationality in drug consumption patterns.

Perhaps the single greatest area in which pharmacists can contribute to reducing drug misuse is the o-t-c area. Pharmacists should strive individually and collectively to ban advertising (in its *present* form) of all o-t-c drugs. (Other countries already have taken steps in this direction.) Advertising, especially as seen on television, tends to encourage maximization of drug consumption. It does this by encouraging a "drug culture" where the consumer is led to believe that what is wrong with him can be corrected through consumption of *some* drug. Moreover, it appears that many of these advertisements tend to encourage the belief that a consumer is afflicted with a given condition. The best example of this is probably the laxative ads. In this case using the "cure" may give the consumer the disease, whether he had it originally or not, a truly wonder drug (in sales terms) for almost everyone but the patient.

The family and patient record system already discussed would function just as effectively, if not more so, in limiting drug misuse. If, for example, a patient has not returned to secure scheduled medication, the pharmacist should take appropriate action to resolve the apparent problem. This would frequently involve contacting the patient, ascertaining the facts of the situation, and providing remedial instructions to the patient or his representatives. To function as he should to curtail drug misuse, the pharmacist must advise patients against taking drugs as well as for taking drugs. He must be prepared to convince the patient that no drug at all is needed in many cases. The hazards encountered by those consuming drugs is made clear by enumeration of many drug-induced conditions in a number of reference works devoted to iatrogenic diseases of drugs. The pharmacist must strive towards encouraging optimization of drug use; he must at the same time discourage maximization of drug use.

Drug Reactions and Interactions

Extensive documentation of the literature supporting the high incidence of drug reactions and interactions will not be presented. The pervasiveness of drug reactions can be most readily appreciated by reviewing almost any package insert. Therein one finds a usually impressive array of adverse drug reactions one may encounter from consumption of a drug. Visconti,[17] Brodie,[18] and Lasagna,[19] among others, have documented the drug reaction problem. Although considerable variation is reported pertaining to the incidence of drug reactions, it appears to be the consensus of informed sources that drug reactions represent a serious health problem. Indeed, in an older study, adverse drug reactions ranked eighth (out of 17) in reasons for which patients are hospitalized.[20]

Drug interactions (mainly drug-drug) have recently received wide attention. Although still a problem, their clinical importance may have been overstated.[21] The pharmacist is the drug expert and should do all he can to prevent adverse drug reactions and interactions. He can probably best do this through an educational program aimed at optimization of drug consumption. At the same time, he should stress and encourage the desirability of simply reading the label (for non-prescription drugs in particular) and following the directions given thereon. The simplicity involved in reading a label may obscure the results. For example, an automobile accident due to falling asleep at the wheel may be avoided by heeding the warning on antihistamine labels pointing out that drowsiness may occur when the drug is taken.

Venereal Diseases

Provision of venereal disease services by the pharmacist can best be achieved through two routes. The first of these would be a program directed towards supplying information that prevents venereal diseases by assisting people in avoiding exposure to these diseases. The second route would involve supplying appropriate prophylactic materials to reduce the possibility of acquiring a disease through personal contact.

The pharmacist's educational role could best be achieved through a cooperative effort with the state department of health and the local department of health. For example, in Texas the department of health will provide free of charge large quantities of venereal disease prevention pamphlets and brochures. In addition, it will provide free printing services to print copies of a pharmacist's own venereal disease prevention materials. A pharmacist can disseminate this information through the pharmacy itself. Also, he can display this information on a public health information rack. This information should be located in such a fashion that the person acquiring the information (pamphlets, brochures, leaflets) would not feel that his purpose was suspect. Moreover, it is quite likely that merely communicating an obvious fact regarding the etiological origin of the disease to the person would be adequate in many cases to prevent the disease. Likewise, syphilis and other venereal diseases might best be prevented by merely explaining to the public how the disease is transmitted. The details can be presented in such a fashion that the person gets the message clearly and unambiguously without offending his sense of morality and dignity.

The program outlined above could probably best be achieved through a cooperative effort of the local pharmaceutical association; this applies to local hospital pharmacy societies as well as community pharmacy associations.

Venereal disease could be combated in the

environment outside the pharmacy by supplying public health information to local schools, colleges, prisons, orphan homes and other institutions having concentrated numbers of people. The pharmacist in each case would not necessarily have to present the program himself. He might provide the information to school teachers, for example, thus allowing them to present the information to their own students. Indeed, a public health venereal disease prevention program might best be achieved through a program aimed at educating the local school teachers. The pharmacist might arrange to present a weekly or other periodic training session to the local junior high and high school teachers. He must keep in mind that frequently and especially in rural areas the pharmacist is the most (formally) educated health care provider (and in many communities the most educated person).

Family Planning

Family planning is an area in which the pharmacist can make a major contribution. Since pharmacies are widely distributed and usually evenly distributed, one usually finds at least one pharmacy in each county. Therefore, the pharmacist is well located for the distribution of family planning information and family planning products (for example, condoms, foams, diaphragms). Likewise, he could offer a pregnancy testing service. Those pharmacies located in low income areas having a government agency providing health services have unusually attractive opportunities for service. Frequently, these agencies already are involved in family planning programs of one kind or another. In the income areas just described or in higher income areas, a pharmacist can set aside a portion of his pharmacy for family planning services. This portion of his pharmacy should be located in an area that is suitable for private consultation.

As far as distributing products is concerned the pharmacist appears to be opti-

mally located. He has high exposure to the public and is easily accessible via automobile. He could provide condoms on a demand basis and could inform the potential user of the proper use of these devices (at the user's option, of course). In the case of oral contraceptives, it appears that the pharmacist must provide this type of medication on a prescription basis. The very least he should do is provide the user information suggested by FDA at the time of dispensing.

The possibilities for provision of family planning information by the pharmacist would appear to be enormous. A tremendous asset for the pharmacist is his frequent contact with a cross-section of the population; this is especially important regarding family planning. By providing birth control information that has been written so that persons of all social classes can understand it, he has the possibility of achieving a great impact on patient family planning practices. By letting patients know that he is available for supplying birth control and family planning information, patients can be encouraged to seek out the pharmacist when special or specific advice is needed or sought. Again, the pharmacist has an obligation as well as opportunity to provide family planning information for the schools if this becomes necessary (and it appears necessary). The oft-cited figure that one out of every four pregnancies occurs in an unwedded female matched with the estimate of unwanted children running as high as 50 percent of those born, would suggest that much needs to be done in the family planning area.

Screening and Diagnostic Testing

The pharmacist can and should provide services in this area. It would appear that marginal pharmacies may be particularly well-suited for providing this type of information (by marginal pharmacies we mean those pharmacies having to include products other than health care products in order to achieve enough volume to support the pharmacy economically). This is true because in these areas there is frequently a great need but little availability of screening and diagnostic testing services. With funding through the local health department or state health department a portion of the pharmacy could be set aside for providing screening and diagnostic testing for the population at large.

One might logically speculate that the pharmacist could maximize his contribution by working towards stimulation of demand for screening and diagnostic testing. Demand could be stimulated through the distribution of public health information materials and public health audio-visual materials such as live lectures, TV lectures or audio-lectures via appropriate telephone hook-ups. For example, the pharmacist might author a periodic newsletter and as a part of this newsletter include information relevant to screening and diagnostic testing of the population. The pharmacist could easily within his existing pharmacy conduct large scale screening tests for diabetes mellitus detection. Likewise, perhaps in conjunction with the local optometrist, he might conduct a glaucoma screening test for the most susceptible age groups. Somewhat related, the pharmacist might direct his patrons to the local health department informing them that a particular screening program is being conducted by the local health department. Clearly, since the pharmacist is exposed to a cross-section of the public including low income as well as middle and upper income persons, he conceivably could make a significant contribution by merely making people aware of an on-going screening and diagnostic program of the local health department or other organization.

Immunizations

The pharmacist could be the local health practitioner who provides large-scale immunization programs to various population groups. For example, the pharmacist could arrange to have an injection provided for a preschooler upon presentation of the child in the pharmacy. Again, the pharmacy area reserved for various public health activities could be used for this immunization program. Indeed, if Rh-disease is used as an example, then the making known of the availability of a preventive drug can be a worthwhile and humanitarian achievement.

Animal Feed Manufacturing

The problem of contamination of animal products consumed by people has in the past been given less attention by the Food and Drug Administration and others than is desired. Dairy cattle consuming penicillin-contaminated feed will provide penicillin-contaminated milk. This could lead to penicillin sensitization and possibly even anaphylactic shock. Other examples can be cited. These instances of contamination of animal products by the presence of drug residues frequently arise from a gross misunderstanding of how well manufacturing is done by a local feed manufacturing firm with a low level of drug and manufacturing knowledge. The pharmacist, by volunteering his services and knowledge of drugs to the local feed manufacturer, could instruct the manufacturer in procedures to be followed which are likely to avoid contamination of feeds with drugs. That is, he should strive towards helping the local feed manufacturer to produce feeds containing only those drugs indicated on the labeling, and feeds containing no drugs in the case of nonmedicated feeds. Almost every county in predominantly agricultural areas has such a feed manufacturing establishment which could utilize the services of a pharmacist in the manner described.

Nutrition

Many counties and a large fraction of those counties with a high percentage of indigent population have the services of a home economist available. As part of her training and education she is prepared to offer nutritional services to the public. As a minimum, the pharmacist could advertise the availability of this person's services to his patrons and potential patrons.

The pharmacist could suggest diets that insure adequate vitamin intake in lieu of the usual practice of dispensing vitamins. All too frequently money spent on vitamins deprives lower income families of money to pay for an adequate diet.

Hazardous Substances Handling

Each time a purchase of a hazardous substance is made in a pharmacy, the pharmacist could personally, or through his employees, caution the purchaser of the importance of reading the label on the container. He also could attach a piece of paper to the container encouraging adherence to the information listed on the label. As part of his general role as health educator, the pharmacist should encourage the public to use hazardous substances cautiously.

For substances not meeting the legal definition of hazardous substances, the pharmacist should provide a "flyer" to be placed in the bag with the substance, encouraging care in usage, handling, and especially storage.

Automobile Accident Prevention

The pharmacist should personally dispense all drugs that have the potential of reducing the ability of a person to drive. He should caution the purchaser of the hazards of driving while consuming these drugs; this especially applies to antihistamines. Incidentally, in Texas it is a crime for driving under the influence of *any* drug.

Barriers and Proposed Solutions

If the foregoing discussion has been presented successfully, the obvious question

must be, "Why are these things not already being done?" The answer, as seems to be the case with so many questions involving health care delivery, is a complex one with behavioral, economic, attitudinal, educational and legal components.

Before the patient can be expected to seek preventive services from the pharmacist, he must first be moved just to seek such services. Years ago it was pointed out that it was useless to distribute answers to people who were not asking questions.[22] Weisbrod, among others, has pointed out that preventive services have traditionally been underutilized.[23] Today's better educated consumer activist seems certain, however, to begin to demand such services, particularly as financial barriers are removed. Indeed, education toward such demands is an integral part of the practice of preventive medicine.

At least two kinds of economic barriers exist. The first, just mentioned above, has "prevented prevention" by the consumer. Adoption of the "health care as a right" concept, and implementation of the concept through current and proposed health programs may be expected to effectively remove this barrier. (Most current proposals for national health insurance recognize formally the importance of preventive medicine.) The second economic barrier involves the pharmacist. Is he to be compensated for these activities, and, if so, how? Pharmacists have, as noted previously, participated to some extent without compensation. They cannot and should not be expected to perform the comprehensive range of services described without pay. The public is accustomed to paying only for merchandise in the pharmacy. The only preventive medicine for which the public is accustomed to paying in the pharmacy also involves products—the various types of condoms and other contraceptives. (Pharmacy's contention, while valid, that the public pays a fee for professional services in connection with the prescription is not widely known or recognized by the public.) The only alternative to fee-for-service would, it seems, have to flow from official recognition by Medicaid, national health insurance or other financial schemes.

The next barrier is found in the pharmacist's training. Although, as previously pointed out, the education of the pharmacist is extensive, it has, almost by definition, been treatment-oriented. A national seminar on Public Health in the Curricula of Colleges of Pharmacy, held in 1965, resulted in agreement that schools and colleges of pharmacy should "upgrade the public health component(s) of their curricula."[24] Mention of the importance of preventive medicine in public health was made by some, "implying that pharmacists, as well as physicians, might contribute to the prevention of disease and to the promotion of health instead of dealing only with those who were seeking the relief of symptoms and a cure for their illness."

In spite of the emphasis in this meeting, it should be noted that a syllabus for a course in public health had appeared in the report, *The Pharmaceutical Curriculum*,[25] in the 1940's. Implementation was slow, but Froh reported in 1970 that 73 percent of the colleges of pharmacy offered courses in public health.[26]

It is expected, but by no means assured, that the developing clinical orientation in pharmacy education will include at least an exposure to preventive medicine concepts.

Legal barriers exist, varying from state to state, which could also hinder the development of the pharmacy as a center for preventive medicine. Obviously, many of the activities called for in the pursuit of true preventive health care could be construed to involve "practicing medicine without a license." Any major efforts would require substantial modification of practice laws and regulations. Similar modifications are already underway in many areas to accommodate some newly developing health practitioners, however, and it is believed that this barrier is not immovable.

Backing up the legal barriers is the barrier which involves physician attitudes, particularly when one considers the informal power which physicians have in many areas over all types of health-related legislation and regulation. It is not presently known how physicians would react to a greater role for pharmacists in preventive medicine. Freidson provided a clue: " . . . the solution of the physician's problem (competition from other professions) was . . . by gaining from the state control over those occupations' activities so as to limit what they could do and to supervise or direct their activities."[27]

Physicians have, on the one hand, accepted, indeed *promoted*, a more responsible role for other nonphysician personnel, while on the other opposing repeal of anti-substitution laws, which would have the effect of expanding the pharmacist's responsibility in drug selection. It is not known whether this latter reaction represents a reaction specific to pharmacy or if the former reflects a willingness to share responsibilities so long as authority is not similarly shared.

For this discussion the final barrier, and, of course, ultimately the most important one, involves the attitude and behavior of the public. If the people can be moved to seek preventive care, if a payment mechanism can be worked out, would the public be willing to trust their preventive health care (or parts of it) to a pharmacist? Knapp and associates in two studies found, respectively, that the lower limit on pharmacist advice acceptable to the public still ranks rather low and that efforts to educate the public concerning his capabilities met with only limited success.[28,29] Nevertheless, these studies did not deal with preventive medicine practices specifically. While other studies have demonstrated that the public does come to the pharmacist for advice, the desire for non-traditional services has been shown to lag behind acceptability,[30] and it remains to be seen how acceptable he would be in a preventive medicine role.

Conclusion

Preventive medicine is a major, unmet need in this country, particularly among the poor. The likelihood of meeting this need is dimmed by manpower shortages and lack of emphasis among the traditional providers. The demand for such services may be expected to increase.

The potential for pharmacy to assist in meeting this need is enhanced by pharmacy's accessibility, search for new roles, and the level, if not the emphasis, of pharmacy education. There is some evidence that many pharmacists have the time to become involved in preventive medicine, and evidence of ability in some applications has been seen.

It remains to be seen whether the potential, which seems to exist here, can be exploited or whether the attitudinal, legal and economic barriers will deny it and new, separate programs be developed.

References

Note: *It would have been possible to cite numerous references in many of the instances below (e.g., the value of preventive medicine, new roles for pharmacists). Therefore, these should be viewed as representative rather than exhaustive.*

1. Congressional Record, 114, S10340 (Sept. 5, 1968)
2. Somers, Anne R., *Health Care in Transition*, Am. Hospital Assoc., Chicago (1971)
3. cf. Hanlon, John J., *Principles of Public Health Administration*, C. V. Mosby Company, St. Louis, Mo., 123 (1969)
4. Chapman, A. L., "Concept of Preventia," *Public Health Reports*, 82, 115 (1967)
5. Brown, J. W., *et al.*, "A Study of General Practice in Massachusetts," *JAMA*, 216 (2) (April 12, 1971)
6. Baker, A. S., Parrish, H. M., and Bishop, F. M., "What Do Rural General Practitioners in Missouri Really Do in Their Offices?," *Missouri Medicine* (March 1967)
7. Rogers, Kenneth D., Mally, Mary, and Mar

cus, Florence L., "A General Medical Practice Using Nonphysician Personnel," *JAMA*, 205 (8) (Nov. 18, 1968)
8. Ellingson, Harold V., "The Specialty of Preventive Medicine," *JAMA*, 207, 1899 (March 10, 1969)
9. James, George, "The Teaching of Prevention in Medical and Paramedical Education," *Inquiry*, VII (1) 37 (March 1971)
10. Wanderer, Jules J., and Smart, George R., "The Structure of Service Institutions in Rural and Urban Communities of Colorado and Sweden," *Rural Soc.*, 34 (3) 368 (Sept. 1969)
11. Smith, Mickey C., "Rural Pharmacy Practice in Mississippi," *Bulletin of the Bureau of Pharmaceutical Services*, 8 (Sept. 1968)
12. Smith, Mickey C., "Independent Pharmacy Practice in Rural Communities," *JAPhA*, NS10 (4), 200 (April 1970)
13. Rodowskas, C. A., and Gagnon, Jean P., "Personnel Activities in Prescription Departments of Community Pharmacies," *JAPhA*, NS12 (8) (Aug. 1972)
14. Silverman, Milton, "Now It's Their Turn," *JAPhA*, NS11 (7), 374 (July 1971)
15. *Proceedings*, National Association of Boards of Pharmacy, Chicago (1970)
16. "Amphetamine Abuse" *Medical Letter*, 16, 63 (Aug. 9, 1968)
17. Visconti, J. A., "An Epidemiologic and Economic Study of Adverse Drug Reactions in Patients on the Medical Service of a University Teaching Hospital," Unpublished PhD Thesis, University of Mississippi (1969)
18. Brodie, D. C., "Drug Utilization and Drug Utilization Review and Control," National Center for Health Services Research and Development, Rockville, Md. (1971)
19. Lasagna, L., "The Diseases Drugs Cause," *Perspectives in Biology and Medicine*, Summer, 458 (1964)
20. Cluff, L. E., "Problems With Drugs," *Proceedings, Conference on Continuing Education for Physicians in the Use of Drugs*, Sponsors: Committee on Continuing Education, Drug Research Board, National Academy of Sciences–National Research Council, Food and Drug Administration, Department of HEW, Regional Medical Programs, Health Services and Mental Health Administration, Washington, D.C. (Feb. 5, 1969)
21. Visconti, J. A., "An Epidemiological Study of the Clinical Significance of Drug-Drug Interactions in a Private Community Hospital," *Am. J. Hosp. Pharm.*, 28 (4) 247 (April 1971)
22. Percy, D. M., "Taking Up the Slack," *Canad. J. of Publ. Health*, 51, 400 (Oct. 1960)

23. Weisbrod, Burton A., *Economics of Public Health*, University of Pennsylvania Press, Philadelphia, (1961)

24. *Public Health in the Curricula of Colleges of Pharmacy*, Washington, American Association of Colleges of Pharmacy, 172 (1965)

25. Blauch, L. E., and Webster, G. L., *The Pharmaceutical Curriculum*, American Council on Education, Washington, D. C. (1952)

26. Froh, Richard, "The Teaching of Health Services Organization in Colleges of Pharmacy," *Am. J. Pharm. Educ.*, 35 (1) (Feb. 1971)

27. Freidson, Eliot, *Profession of Medicine*, Dodd, Mead and Company, New York, 47 (1970)

28. Knapp, D. E., Knapp, D. A., and Edwards, J. D., "The Pharmacist as Perceived by Physicians, Patrons, and Other Pharmacists," *JAPhA*, NS9 (2) 80 (Feb. 1969)

29. Jang, Raymond, Knapp, D. E., and Knapp, D. A., "Reactions of the Public to the Pharmacist as a Drug Advisor," Paper presented to the Academy of the General Practice of Pharmacy, Washington (1970)

30. Galloway, Sydney P., "Poverty Area Residents Look at Pharmacy Services," *Am. J. Public Health* 61 (11) 2211 (Nov. 1971)

13—Pharmacists Can Serve as Educators of These 8 Audiences

Byron R. Strickland

Interaction with the community can be most productive when pharmacists use their expertise to address various consumer audiences on topics related to health, disease, and drugs. Within every community, there are several groups with unique interests related to these topics. (See Table 13.1 . . . which also includes medical associations.) The pharmacist's interest plus a desire to find, and help, these community groups is required for this service. In such a program of community education, the pharmacist can fulfill his (or her) capabilities as a true professional.

Not each and every pharmacist is capable of providing these community educational services. The pharmacist must not only be competent and interested, but he must also maintain a professional level of discipline in order to perform properly in this challenging area.

The efficacy of the pharmacist's role in community education is, therefore, biphasic:

- One phase meets the needs of the people in the community;
- The second phase simultaneously creates community awareness and trust in the pharmacist's role in health care delivery.

Tragic Flaw

The real tragic flaw of modern pharmacy, and of pharmacists themselves, is the prevailing "inert" attitude towards total commitment for improving health care in the community. The role of the pharmacist as a community educator will certainly eradicate the notion of those who assess him as "overtrained and underutilized." Moreover, such

Table 13.1

**Topics for Pharmacists Based on the
Type of Audience**

Type of Audience	Topics for Discussion
Parent Organizations	Drug use during pregnancy Drug abuse and misuse Contraception Poison prevention Nutrition Hypertension
Youth Groups Church Groups	Drug abuse Venereal disease Pharmacy as a career Drugs in the Scriptures
Environmental Interest Groups	Environmental pharmacology and toxicology Industrial pollution Effects on human and animal life
Medical Associations	Bioavailability Generic and therapeutic equivalency & economic factors
Television, Radio, and Newspapers	Public service announcements Newspaper "by-line" on drugs
Community Colleges and Adult Education Classes	Self-medication Drug abuse Venereal disease Nutrition Hypertension
Free Clinics	Venereal disease Drug abuse
Geriatrics Handicapped	Self-medication safety Nutrition

educational activities could stimulate a positive community reassessment of the efficacy and potential role of the pharmacist—as a health information resource.

In connection with this, Albert Einstein once said: "It is high time that the ideal of success should be replaced by the ideal of service." *How true for Pharmacy!*

Related Readings in This Volume

7. Pharmacist and Family Planning
9. Pharmacist and Treatment of Drug Addiction
10. Drug Abuse Education
14. Hypertension Patients in Community Pharmacy
50. Pharmacies in Rural Areas

Readings for a Broader Perspective

1. Remes, N. "How Our Chain's Employees Back up the 'We C.A.R.E.' Program," *Pharmacy Times* 44 (September 1978):88–90.
2. Silver, E. N. "How Community Pharmacists Can Provide Dental Health Information," *Pharmacy Times* 43 (July 1977):36–39.
3. McKenney, J. M., Jenning, W. B., and White, E. V. "Blood Pressure Screening in a Community Pharmacy," *J. Am. Pharm. Assoc.* NS 16 (April 1976):187–93.

Hypertension

14—How We Screen & Monitor Hypertension Patients in Our Community Pharmacy

Emil W. Baker

In August of 1972, we opened Kentucky's first pharmaceutical office practice in Mt. Sterling (population 5,000). This was accomplished by converting a 20' ×40' traditional corner drugstore into a beautiful professional pharmacy which featured the following:

- Attractive patient waiting area
- Receptionist unit
- Patient medication profile system
- Professional library
- Professional fee system
- Private consultation room
- No merchandise on display
- Family health information literature
- Direct patient-pharmacist relationship.

Our attractive facility was mistaken for a physician's, dentist's, or a lawyer's office—or even a bank branch; and we soon found that practicing Pharmacy in this environment gave us a much more clinical and patient-oriented approach, because we were not spending valuable time putting up displays, buying non-health related items, and performing other non-professional duties. We had more time to devote to patient consultation, drug interactions, study of drug literature, etc.—and we still had ample time to serve our patients' prescription needs.

Almost two years after we remodeled our pharmacy, Mt. Sterling's local service clubs sponsored a community effort to screen for hypertension in supermarkets, banks, and department stores. The public responded very favorably to this program, and many of our patients expressed their appreciation and their hope that it would be repeated annually. Their enthusiastic response caused us to evaluate the community's need for an ongoing hypertension screening program—and we made the decision to provide that service from our pharmaceutical office.

Screening Equipment and Training

We purchased a sphygmomanometer, a blood pressure cuff, and a physician's stethoscope, choosing the best equipment we could find from a surgical supply house. We allowed ourselves an ample training period to study the available literature, to learn the technique of measuring blood pressure (from local nurses and physicians), and to practice on one another until we were entirely competent. We began our program in May, 1974—choosing that month because it had been designated as National High Blood Pressure month.

In order to promote our screening program, we ran newspaper and radio announcements in May, educating the public to the facts about high blood pressure, and stressing the importance of early detection in order to avoid possible cardiovascular damage, strokes, or kidney disease. We concluded our announcement by urging people to have their blood pressure checked by their own physicians—or to come to us for a screening at no charge. We also placed a sign about the program on one of our front desks, making it clear that it was open to the entire community, including residents of our county (Montgomery) which has a population of approximately 16,000, and to people in surrounding counties.

Screening Procedure

For our screening program, we used a small office at the rear of our pharmacy which was completely private when the door was shut. To facilitate accurate readings, we kept background noise as low as possible. Staff members spoke quietly, and radios were turned down or shut off.

We weighed our patients on a medical scale, asked what medications they were taking, and questioned them about their family blood pressure history. In speaking to the public, we deliberately avoided using the word "hypertension," because many people mistakenly believe that term refers only to "nervousness."

Our experience has shown that the left arm usually records the highest blood pressure reading—perhaps because of its proximity to the heart. In any event, the patron's blood pressure was taken at least twice in each screening, and we recorded the last reading. Both systolic and diastolic measurements were recorded and given to the patient, reflecting our belief that he should be knowledgeable about his own blood pressure.

Monitoring Hypertensive Patients

We soon realized that many persons who came through our screening program were already diagnosed as hypertensives—people who simply wanted to have their condition monitored between visits to their physician. Although we had not intended to sponsor more than a simple screening program, we sensed a public need for monitoring hypertensive patients, and we altered our plans to provide both screening *and* monitoring to people in our area.

Our extended service became a valuable aid both to patient and physician, because we could help determine patient response to drug therapy in between regularly-scheduled visits to the physician. We emphasized to patients the importance of continuing to see their physician regularly and regarding our pressure readings only as a helpful interim service.

Before we began our initial screening program, we designed a simple "Blood Pressure Screening Report" . . . to record individual readings—one copy to be given to the patient and another to be retained in our files.

The Hour of Blood Pressure Reading

Beyond the routine identifying information, this form provides space to record the *hour* of the blood pressure reading, because a patient's pressure may vary during the day commensurate with his periods of rest, work, and/or mental stress. Our form also provides space to indicate which arm was tested. (If we take readings from both arms, both results are recorded.)

Because the *position* of the patient may also cause blood pressure variance, there is a space on the form to insert the words "sitting," "standing," or "supine"—although most of our readings are taken with the patient in a sitting position.

Our screening report provides a space to record all prescription and non-prescription medications which the patient may be currently taking—an important consideration because some drugs will affect the blood pressure reading. We have learned that many patients are taking such non-prescription drugs, and without their physician's knowledge. This situation gives the pharmacist an opportunity to counsel the patient about the effects of non-prescription drugs containing sympathomimetics and about sodium-containing drugs.

The space reserved for "Recommendations" is important, because it allows us to record valuable reminders for the patient. If a blood pressure is normal, we simply recommend a periodic, or yearly, recheck of blood pressure. If a reading is "borderline hypertension," we recommend at least two more follow-up readings, 3 to 7 days apart. If a patient's blood pressure is hypertensive—whether it be mild, moderate, or severe—we advise an immediate visit to a physician. If we discover really severe high blood pressure, we telephone the physician immediately for advice—and we have actually sent such patients directly from our office to the hospital, on the physician's orders.

The signature space on the screening report is necessary to authenticate it, and to indicate that the reading has been made by qualified, trained personnel. If it is necessary for us to refer a patient to a physician, we always request that our "Blood Pressure Screening Report" be shown to the doctor.

Permanent Hypertension Record

After our program evolved to include both screening and monitoring, we decided we needed another, more permanent record of the patients we served. To meet this need, we designed the "Hypertension Record". . . . In addition to the information shown on the screening report, this form also records the patient's age, date of birth, and phone number, as well as the name and address of his physician. There is space to record the patient's weight, his medication and dosage regimen (if any), a limited personal and family medical history, and associated medical problems such as asthma and diabetes.

Perhaps the most helpful feature of this permanent record is the blood pressure scale (from 60 to 240 mm Hg) which permits cumulative blood pressure readings to be charted graphically, reflecting the results of diet, weight loss, and drug therapy. We retain these forms—and file them alphabetically—to give us a permanent record of patients' visits.

Occasionally, a patient will come in for a reading, complaining of headache, dizziness, flushing, or other symptoms often associated with high blood pressure. However, after taking the pressure, we find it to be normal. In such cases, we still refer the patient to his physician, even though the symptoms are apparently unrelated to hypertension.

To protect our patients and ourselves, we have established the following criteria to guide us in referring patients to physicians:

- Patients under 40 years of age with a blood pressure reading (either systolic or diastolic) of 140/90 or more are referred to the physician.

- Patients over 40 years of age with a blood pressure reading (either systolic or diastolic) of 160/95 or more are referred to the physician.
- For patients over 40, with a blood pressure ranging between 140/90 and 160/95, we recommend at least two more readings (at 3- to 7-day intervals)—either from the physician or at our screening office. If all of these readings—or 2 out of 3—fall within the same range, the patient is referred to his doctor for advice. If only one reading is in that range, we recommend a recheck in 3 months.
- Patients 12 years or over, with a pressure below 90/50, are referred to the physician as being possibly *hypo*tensive.

Current Patient Load

The number of patients we see for blood pressure screening and monitoring averages out to 10 per week. Some weeks, we may see only 4 or 5, but other weeks the patient load may run as high as 15 or 16. The most readings we have had in one day is 10—and there have been days when we had none.

In our experience, patients always come at varying times of the day, and we have never had more than one patient waiting at a time. We average approximately 20 minutes with each patient, from the time he enters the office until he is ready to leave. We are sometimes interrupted by phone calls or prescription work while we are taking a patient's blood pressure, and this may result in a short delay. But we have found most patients to be very understanding and aware that our blood pressure readings are an extra service, whereas prescription service is our primary pharmaceutical responsibility.

Patient Education

An essential part of our screening program is *patient education about high blood pressure*. Making no distinction between hypertensive and non-hypertensive patients, we educate them in the following areas:

- Systolic blood pressure—what it is,
- Diastolic blood pressure—what it is,
- Value of weight reduction in relation to hypertension & cardiovascular disease,
- Why moderate exercise, such as walking briskly, is beneficial in hypertension,
- Why hypertensive patients should ingest less salt and less saturated fats,
- Why antihypertensive medicine must be taken *daily* as prescribed,
- Why hypertension—a chronic disease in most cases—can't be cured like a cold.

When we are monitoring a patient who is being treated by a physician we ask that patient what his physician advised him to do. Once we learn the therapy pattern, we explain the reasons for it—a step at a time. We have discovered many people do not follow drug therapy, because they just *don't understand* its importance.

Some patients knowingly fail to follow their physician's orders—and then come to us to see how their pressure is doing. If we find a high reading in these uncooperative patients, we explain the dangers of ignoring proper therapy, and urge their compliance with drug therapy. Other patients complain that they feel worse when taking pills than they did with high blood pressure—thus excusing themselves from continuing to take their medicine. To them, we explain that if the side effects of their medication are too uncomfortable, they should tell their physician who can possibly recommend different drug therapy for them.

We also provide excellent high blood

pressure literature to assist us in our task of educating the patient. The major manufacturers of antihypertensive medications—and the American Pharmaceutical Association—have put out some very fine booklets on the subject. We offer these to patients coming in for screening or monitoring, and also place them in strategic locations where they can be readily picked up by any patient.

Patients' Acceptance of Program

From its inception, our hypertension screening program has been successful. With very little newspaper and radio promotion, we performed approximately 60 blood pressure measurements in our first month of operation. Our publicity emphasized the importance of blood pressure readings—either at the physician's office or at our screening office—so we have no way of knowing how many may have had their blood pressure checked at facilities other than ours. We also stressed the fact that our screening program was year-round, and not just for the month of May.

Our program has now been operating for over 3 years, and it continues with only month-of-May promotion—sustained mainly by word-of-mouth referrals. We are often the first to discover a hypertensive patient, because many people prefer to come to us, rather than pay for an office call and wait in a physician's waiting room. Of course, once we discover a patient *is* hypertensive, we immediately refer him to his physician for evaluation, diagnosis, and therapy.

Physicians' Acceptance of Program

As pharmacists, we were understandably concerned about the reaction of physicians to our screening program—although we had cleared it with two local physicians who (1) agreed it was an excellent community service, (2) advised us on testing techniques, and (3) helped us establish the proper criteria for referral of patients to physicians.

But there were 9 other physicians in our community, and we felt some anxiety about their reaction. However, now that the medical community has seen the results of our program, we believe that most of them approve what we are doing. Some, in fact, have accepted our program to such an extent that they send their patients to us for preliminary (3 in a week) screenings, asking that our reports be returned to them. Still other physicians have directed their patients to us for blood pressure monitoring while they are away on vacation or when they have to be absent from their offices for any length of time. And we, of course, are continuing to refer to local physicians those patients whose disease might not have been detected until a serious problem developed.

Sometimes our patrons visit doctors located in Lexington, or Louisville, or some other city—and they often tell us of their physician's appreciation of our between-visits monitoring service and our reports which give physicians authentic data on which to evaluate the results of their prescribed therapy.

Not only do we feel that we have very good acceptance of our program by physicians, but we have progressed to the point where we are working closely with them toward a better control of high blood pressure. Most physicians are very busy, and they really appreciate our phone calls when we uncover an exceptionally high blood pressure. Depending on the reading, the physician will either change the medication and/or dosage, or order the patient to go directly to his office or to the hospital. Some of these high-risk patients have come to us at times when their physicians' offices are closed—and our service and referral have resulted in immediate treatment which may have precluded serious complications had there been further delay.

Professional Fee for our Services

From the beginning of our screening program, many patients offered to pay us for our services, some even leaving $1 to $5—against our wishes. These people said that our time was worth something and that they wanted to pay us.

Although pharmacists have traditionally been paid for prescriptions rather than for services, per se, we decided in January, 1976, to experiment with a service fee of $1 for each patient visit. Somewhat to our surprise, no one complained. Many said that our service was worth much more than that sum, and they were glad we were making a nominal charge. If a patient does not have cash or a check with him, we will "charge" the fee; of course, we have never refused to take a blood pressure reading because someone could not afford the dollar service fee.

Actually, we have come to believe that charging a nominal fee for such a service may be a very small milestone for Pharmacy as it exists today. It indicates that the public _is willing to pay a pharmacist for clinical professional services_, and not just for medication. Perhaps future pharmacists will earn an increasing share of income from such clinical services, thus eliminating their traditional dependence on selling a variety of non-health-related merchandise.

Because of the legal liability involved, many pharmacists might not consider a program of this type. It is true that if a pharmacist is proved negligent in taking a patient's blood pressure—and if the patient is injured in some manner—he can be sued. Or, if a pharmacist gives a patient erroneous advice or information that results in patient injury, he can be sued.

These possibilities make it imperative that pharmacists who are considering a hypertension screening-monitoring program should thoroughly study the testing techniques, the criteria to be used for physician referral, the disease itself, and the pharmacology of the drugs used in treating hypertension. The effects of stress, diet, and weight reduction should also be studied by the pharmacist. Many publications, educational tapes, and continuing education programs are available to the pharmacist to help prepare him for this service.

We think a pharmacist should provide all the professional service within his capability —based on his education, training, and experience. If legal liability were the only consideration, pharmacists would never have instituted patient medication profile systems, drug consultation service, drug information counseling, poison control advice, and other professional services. Of course, each of these efforts increases a pharmacist's legal liability. Yet, if we are to be considered health-care _professionals_, we must assume a certain amount of liability.

Physicians, nurses, and dentists make mistakes and are sued, but that does not keep them from performing professional services. Pharmacists will make mistakes, also, and some will be sued. But, just as do our colleagues in the health care field, we must continue to provide as much service as we can perform _competently_.

Program is Worthwhile

We recommend that pharmacists—before starting a hypertension screening-monitoring program—consult with their professional liability insurance agent to make sure that such services are covered by their policy.

After over 3 years of screening and monitoring patients for hypertension, we have concluded that the program is very worthwhile—for our patients, the physicians, and the community.

Based on figures available from the first 33 months of our screening program, we recorded a total of 1,320 blood pressure readings on 637 patients. Within that group, we detected approximately 120 patients with hypertension, and referred them to physicians for evaluation, diagnosis, and therapy.

In our monitoring program, we have helped the patient and physician control hypertension by providing blood pressure measurements between regular medical office visits.

Through our hypertension program, we believe physicians have come to accept the pharmacist as a partner in helping to detect and control high blood pressure—thus strengthening the professional team concept and providing better health care for the community. Likewise, the patient and the community have accepted the pharmacist in the new role of detecting and monitoring hypertension—a role that makes him more involved in the health care of his patients.

The pharmacist has long been called overtrained for what he does. The highest court in the land places the pharmacist in the same category as a seller of law books. If the pharmacist is ever to be thought of as a true *health care professional*, he must accept new professional responsibilities. We believe that a program such as hypertension screening and monitoring can help the pharmacist solve one of his major problems—the building of a more professional image.

Readings for a Broader Perspective

1. McKenney, J. M. "Pharmacy Management of Hypertensive Patients," *J. Am. Pharm. Assoc.* NS 14 (April 1974):190–95.
2. Mattei, T. J., Balmer, J. A., and Gonzales Duffy, M. "A Hypertensive Patient Needs?" *J. Am. Pharm. Assoc.* NS 14 (April 1974):186–89.
3. Williams, R. L. "Needed: Pharmacists in High Blood Pressure Control," *American Pharmacy* NS 18 (May 1978):32.
4. Levy, R. I. "What You Should Know About Treating Hypertension," *Pharmacy Times* 44 (May 1978):39–44.
5. Kayne, R. "Perspectives on Essential Hypertension," *California Pharmacist* 24 (May 1977):6–10.

Over-The-Counter Medications

15—Self-Medication: Whose Responsibility?

Jacob W. Miller

The responsibilities of pharmacists in self-medication are among the most important duties of the practitioner. Among others, these involve stocking those over-the-counter (OTC) preparations that are both safe and effective and supported by reasonable claims concerning their therapeutic effects. They also include an obligation to provide accurate advice to patients regarding the selection and use of the most appropriate OTC product.

Many pharmacists have the notion that

Excerpted from a presentation before the Ohio Pharmaceutical Seminar, sponsored by the Pharmacy Extension Service, College of Pharmacy, The Ohio State University, Columbus, Ohio. April 24, 1978. Printed with permission of the author.

they should carry every OTC drug that a patient might demand or that they feel will "sell" as a result of national advertising or in-pharmacy promotion. APhA has challenged that point of view for many years, feeling that a pharmacist should carry only those OTC drugs that the pharmacist feels, based on his *own* professional evaluation, merit his implicit approval. I believe the public expects no less of pharmacists. I have heard this sentiment expressed by consumers on numerous occasions so I know it's valid. It is also implicit in the findings of the Dichter Report which APhA commissioned in 1973.

The pharmacist communicates something about himself through the type of products he makes available in his pharmacy. As a result, I feel that if pharmacists have any sense of self-worth about themselves and their professional image, they should pay special attention to the types of nonprescription medication which are offered to the public in their pharmacies. To do so requires an evaluation based on the claims which are made on the product labels as well as the advertising and promotion that go along with those claims. The evaluation should be simple and straightforward: does the pharmacist believe that the claims contained in the labeling of the product are justified based on his knowledge of the ingredients and the conditions the product is claimed to treat? Is the advertising for the product truthful and fair in that it does not overstate claims and expected benefits of use?

The evaluation of an individual patient's request for a nonprescription medication is far more complex. It involves first the establishment of a patient/pharmacist relationship; secondly, the application of the principles involved in achieving rational drug therapy; and thirdly, the performance of clinical pharmacy functions. All of these activities must usually take place within the space of just a few minutes and yet it is vitally important to the success of the professional service which is rendered and the health of the patient who is seeking advice that these steps occur.

Achieving rational drug therapy is another way of saying that the pharmacist has the responsibility to the patient for assuring that the right drug is given to the right patient, at the right time, in the right dose, for the right diagnosis, and with due consideration for cost.

The functions involved in the clinical pharmacy approach include: 1) data gathering, 2) patient assessment, 3) establishing therapeutic goals, 4) designing therapeutic regimen, 5) implementing therapy, 6) monitoring patient progress.

While the functions and terms described under rational drug therapy and clinical pharmacy functions may seem esoteric, they all apply in one way or another as the pharmacist provides professional service to a self-diagnosing and self-medicating patient.

The self-medicating patient is a day-to-day reality for most pharmacists. In certain respects, the self-medicating patient can represent the most challenging and demanding portion of the pharmacist's professional responsibilities. The self-medicating patient is most frequently a self-diagnosing patient. Such patients enter the pharmacy having already determined (a) the nature of their problem, (b) its probable resolution with nonprescription drugs, and (c) perhaps the product or product type they intend to use. The pharmacist then must not only answer specific patient questions but must also help the patient retrace the steps taken to arrive at the "self-diagnosis," and, if appropriate, recommend a product and provide adequate instructions and warnings.

The first responsibility of the pharmacist in counseling the self-medicating patient is to help the patient determine if the problem requires other professional medical attention. The pharmacist's general knowledge of disease and specific knowledge of the patient are important factors in fulfilling this responsibility.

The second responsibility of the pharmacist is assisting the self-medicating patient who does not require professional medical attention in choosing the most suitable alternate course of action, e.g., let the condition run its course, recommend an OTC product, or suggest methods to reduce or eliminate the problem. Third, if the pharmacist decides that an OTC product is indicated, the best available product must be recommended from among the many that may be claimed to be effective.

Such recommendations necessarily must consider other drugs (both prescription and OTC) that the person is concurrently taking, and the general condition of the patient, i.e., age, weight, activity, concurrent medical conditions, and so on.

The fourth and final area of responsibility involves being sure that the patient has all of the essential information that is needed for the safe and effective utilization of the product chosen, e.g., instructions for use, possible side effects, when to discontinue, how long to wait before seeking other professional medical attention, or when to check back with the pharmacist.

The elaboration of these clinical pharmacy concepts over the last decade has emphasized the clinical functions of pharmaceutical service, particularly regarding the pharmacist's understanding of minor illnesses, the OTC drugs available to treat them, and the reactions of patients to these drugs.

As the public becomes more aware of its own responsibilities in self-care, it will look more frequently to the pharmacist for advice in this area. Hence, the clinical aspects of self-care will grow as a challenge to pharmacy practice. The exercise by the pharmacist of professional judgment is the key factor in the patient/pharmacist interaction relating to advice for self-medication.

The entire range of functions relating to the pharmacist's clinical role in serving the self-medicating patient revolves around the recommendations that pharmacists make to the patient. Our continuing education, experience, knowledge of specific products and of individual patients all affect our final decision regarding the course of action recommended to patients in pursuing their self-care programs.

The responsibilities inherent in self-medication apply to everyone, the user, the physician, the manufacturer, government and the pharmacist. As I see things developing, self-care, along with self-medication, will increase substantially through the next generation. Provider-oriented health care is simply becoming too expensive. This trend indicates that the responsibilities we have discussed will become far more meaningful, far more ponderous.

Pharmacists, as the primary custodian of drugs in the community, and as the professional most knowledgeable about drugs, will continue to exercise a major role in maintaining responsibility for the nonprescription medications utilized by self-medicating patients. The opportunities are good for pharmacists to exercise clinical judgments for the benefit of patients they serve and those opportunities will be even better tomorrow. The challenge for pharmacy is to accept this responsibility and to turn that challenge into opportunities for professional service. It is not an easy challenge today and it will not be an easy challenge tomorrow. But it is a challenge which must be accepted. After all, while self-medication is everyone's responsibility, primarily it is our duty as responsible professional pharmacists.

16—Bigger Role for Pharmacist Advocated in Use of OTC's

Solomon Huriash

Much has appeared in the literature regarding the use of patient profile records and systems to detect interactions. Proper use of such records is a professional service that reflects on the expertise of the pharmacist in protecting the patient's health.

Much has also been written about the use of over-the-counter medications by the public. Radio, newspapers, and television are used by proprietary manufacturers to promote their use.

A Hollywood star, whose credibility is unquestioned because of his masterful portrayal of a hero or lover, reaches millions of people at a sitting to advise of the perfect headache remedy, cold tablet, laxative or whatever.

Assumptions

Safety is assumed because the federal government does not require a prescription for the items in question. Safety is assumed because such items are readily available in the supermarket. Safety is assumed for the user who will show enough interest to read the instructions and warnings on the label.

It is the purpose of this article to make a case that OTC's are not safe for many consumers to use on their own; also, that self-medication, without checking it out against the conditions and prescription items on a patient's profile, makes the use of that profile nearly ineffective.

OTC's are not to be considered an innocuous class of drugs. They are a vital and respected part of the physician's armamentarium, as are his prescription drugs.

Study

In the winter of 1977, I did a study of medications at a private hospital in Broward County, Florida, to compare the use of OTC items in relation to prescription items. For the 22 patients in the intensive-care-unit, of the 133 medications prescribed for that day, 93 were prescription items and 40 were OTC. Thus, OTC constituted 30 per cent of the patients' medications.

For 16 patients in the surgical area, of 66 drugs used for the day, 40 were prescriptions and 26 were OTC—for an OTC percentage of 39.

For 20 patients in the pediatric and general section, of 98 medications used for that day, 70 were prescription and 28 were OTC—for an OTC average of 29 per cent.

For 21 patients in the orthopedics and dialysis sections, for the 72 medications used that day, 46 were prescription and 26 were OTC—for an OTC average of 36 per cent.

For 28 patients in a general wing there were 151 medications dispensed for that day; 117 were prescription and 34 were OTC—for an OTC average of 22 per cent.

For 21 patients in the cancer and another surgery section, of 102 medications dispensed for that day, 68 were prescription and 34 were OTC—for an OTC average of 33 per cent.

In the coronary care section, for seven patients and a total of 36 medications issued for the day, 29 were prescription and 7 were OTC. Thus, OTC's accounted for 19 per cent of the medications.

In the urology section, for the 23 patients present, a total of 88 medications were dispensed for the day. Of those, 58 were prescription items and 30 were OTC—for an OTC share of 34 per cent.

The position of OTC's in the total prescribing picture thus becomes apparent.

Detection

It is the basic purpose of a patient profile to detect potential interactions. These interactions include prescription drugs *vis à vis* each other, any prescribed drug—even vitamins—*vis à vis* a medical condition, and, of course, OTC drugs. The chemicals in OTC drugs can react with the same degree of potency with a prescription chemical as the latter with another Rx drug. Example: aspirin and coumadin.

The pharmacist cannot detect a possible interaction if the patient is getting a salicylate chemical via some OTC product that was not cleared with him. In itself that OTC could be considered safe; but if it constitutes an improper combination as described above, it could prove quite harmful to that patient.

For instance, a patient being treated for parkinsonism with levodopa buys a B complex vitamin on sale at the supermarket. If there is 5 mg. or more of pyridoxine taken daily, the beneficial effects of the levodopa are either reduced or abolished completely.

Tetracycline absorption is decreased if the patient takes aluminum, calcium, or magne-

sium ions. A mineral combination containing ferrous sulfate may interfere with the absorption of tetracycline from the gastrointestinal tract.

A cancer patient taking methotrexate treats himself with a salicylate product. This creates a potential for methotrexate toxicity.

Avoidance

These and other problems could have been avoided if the pharmacist had been consulted for all OTC products given to patients on whom he maintains profiles.

The proper maintenance of a patient-profile requires mechanical aids to help the pharmacist detect potential interactions. This is no reflection on the pharmacist. The myriad of potential interactions make spot detecting almost impossible. Permit me to quote some statistics from a paper I am working on that shows numbers of potential interactions:

If a patient has one medical condition and is taking four different drugs, there is a possibility of 10 potential interactions. If an extra chemical entity is added, 15 potential interactions exist. If yet another drug is added, 21 potential interactions face the patient.

If a patient has two medical conditions and is taking a total of four drugs, 14 potential interactions exist. If one more drug is added, potential interactions rise to 20. Addition of yet another drug raises the number of potential interactions to 27.

If a patient has three conditions and is taking three drugs, there are 12 interaction potentials. Addition of another drug raises the interaction potential to 18.

Only with proper use of a patient profile can medications be properly and safely taken. This must include all OTC preparations. Ideally, they should be taken only after consultation with the pharmacist.

Related Readings in This Volume

Readings for a Broader Perspective

1. Knapp, D. A., and Beardsley, R. S. "Put Yourself into the OTC Picture—Profession-ally," *American Pharmacy* NS 19 (September 1979):37–39.
2. Lee, V. H., and Rowles, B. "O-T-C Diuretics," *J. Am. Pharm. Assoc.* NS 16 (July 1976): 417–19.
3. *The Medicine Show*. Mount Vernon, N.Y.: Consumers Union of the United States, 1976. 432 pp.
4. American Pharmaceutical Association. *Handbook of Nonprescription Drugs*. Washington, D.C., APhA, 1979. 488 pp.

Terminal Illness

17—Patient Needs Come First at Hillhaven Hospice

Pharmacy Services Essential for Pain Control

Maxine I., Hammel and Carl E. Trinca

Traditionally, a hospice was known as a way station for travelers. During the Middle Ages, many hospices existed throughout Europe, places where food and refuge were provided for travelers. The term "hospice" has since been adapted to describe a way station for the dying, an organized program that provides palliative and supportive care to terminally ill patients and their families. The entire family is considered the unit of care, and the care provided extends through the mourning process.

The hospice also can be thought of as a concept for all to identify with in considering care for the dying patient. Hospices with this definition originated in England in the 1950s. Perhaps best known is St. Christopher's Hospice, where Dr. Cicely Saunders, the author of numerous articles on the hospice concept, is the medical director. It was not until the early 1970s that hospices were first tried in the United States. More recently, however, there appears to be an accelerated interest in hospice care in this country.

It has been speculated that the reasons for the gain in favor of hospices include:

" . . . a curious amalgam of reactions and responses—a reaction against isolation or the 'cure at any cost' syndrome that hospice advocates see as the terminally ill patient's only options in an acute care hospital; a reaction against hospital regulations that often keep patients and families apart in times of crisis; a reaction, perhaps, against certain of society's attitudes about death that may be standing in the way of providing the best care, both medically and humanely, to the dying and a response to the slowly emerging wish for death with dignity and the search for alternatives to institutionalization."[1]

For these reasons, as well as others, hospice programs are rapidly appearing throughout the United States.

The hospice movement provides a call to pharmacists to be active participants in the care of the dying patient. Many aspects of hospice care, for example, pain control and the alleviation of other distressful symptoms incurred by the dying patient, are relevant to the practice of pharmacy. This paper will share one pharmacist's involvement in a hospice program at Hillhaven Hospice in Tucson, Arizona, which is jointly funded by Hillhaven Foundation in Tacoma, Washington, and the National Cancer Institute.

As many levels of pharmacist involvement with hospice programs and patients may exist as do variations in the hospice programs. Pharmacists should not allow the level of formal affiliation between themselves and a hospice to affect the provision of services to the dying patient and family members. Pharmacists can take the hospice concept and apply it in all pharmacy settings.

The Hillhaven Program

Hillhaven Hospice offers a complete program of care to terminal cancer patients. Currently, it is the nation's only freestanding hospice. Its range of services includes care in the home, day care in the facility, inpatient care and a bereavement service for the family following the death of a patient.[2] The staff of Hillhaven Hospice works as an interdisciplinary team reviewing applications, developing care plans and providing care. The pharmacist is an integral part of this team, which also includes a medical director, the nursing staff, a facilitator, a social worker, a physical therapist, an occupational therapist, a chaplain, a volunteer coordinator, the patient's attending physician and consultants.

The applications reviewed by members of the interdisciplinary team for admission to the program are from dying patients with cancer for whom active therapeutic treatment is no longer being aggressively pursued or deemed appropriate.[3] If the patient is admitted, a care plan is developed with the goal of making the patient's remaining life as comfortable and meaningful as possible.

On admission to Hillhaven Hospice a patient ideally would enter the home care program. Members of the hospice team visit the patient/family unit at home, providing direct care as well as teaching the family to care for the patient. The family may be taught, for example, to change dressings and administer medications, so that the patient can remain at home as long as possible.

An option for the patient at home is the day care program, where the patient may spend some hours every day or every few days in the facility. A patient could enter the facility, for example, for eight hours per day while the family member caring for the patient is at work.

If the patient cannot remain at home, admission is made to the inpatient program. Sometimes a patient admitted as an inpatient will be discharged later to the home after the pain has been controlled. The pharmacist participates in all phases of care, in the home and in the facility.

The pharmacist is responsible for developing, coordinating and supervising all pharmaceutical services for the hospice program. Duties include the development of policies and procedures, monitoring medication administration and record keeping and assuring the control and accountability of all medications. In addition, the pharmacist becomes involved with the primary care of the patient. The control of pain, nausea, vomiting, constipation and other distressful symptoms is of specific interest to the pharmacist.

Pharmacist's Role in Pain Control

The hospice pain control program has been quite successful, and its method of operation needs to be shared so that pharmacists working with dying patients in pain can be part of an organized program aimed at controlling pain. Many cancer patients have an overwhelming concern that their cancer will cause pain and that it will be uncontrollable at the end. The hospice staff, including the pharmacist, discuss this fear with the patient and family members, pointing out that pain does not always occur with cancer and that if it does occur it can be controlled. Statistics show that approximately 50 percent of patients with cancer have little or no physical pain, 10 percent have only mild pain and the remaining 40 percent need help with severe pain.[4]

To date, the hospice inpatient program has been represented disproportionately by cancer patients with pain; some pain is mild, but the majority experience severe pain. This slanted representation of cancer patients with pain is due in part to the success the hospice has had in controlling pain. Word of this success has spread, and physicians, patients and families who have experienced pain treatment failures call on the hospice for its expertise.

When a patient is admitted to the hospice, the interdisciplinary team evaluates the pain. No change in a patient's regimen is recommended if there is no pain or if the pain is controlled with an oral analgesic. However, if the pain is being treated with an injectable analgesic and the patient can take oral medications, a recommendation is made to the patient's private physician to change to the hospice analgesic protocol. Other patients placed on the hospice analgesic protocol

include those with uncontrolled pain or patients who develop pain after being in the hospice program.

Use of Modified Brompton's Mixture

Why is pain control successful in the hospice but not in the previously and still available avenues of medical care? The hospice pain control program uses basic pharmacological and pharmacokinetic principles for available analgesics as well as the availability of a concerned staff.

Following a research of the literature and personal communication with physicians in hospices in England, a modified version of Brompton's Mixture became the basis for the treatment of pain in Hillhaven Hospice. The modified Brompton's Mixture consists of morphine sulfate, 2 mg/ml, in water with a flavoring agent.

This formula was based specifically on recent findings by Dr. Robert Twycross. Twycross found that morphine is as effective as diamorphine, diamorphine being about twice as potent; cocaine does not increase alertness significantly, and the patients find the traditional "cocktail" too strong or complain of its alcoholic "bite."[5,6] For these reasons the hospice does not include cocaine or alcohol in the mixture, nor are there currently any regrets that diamorphine for oral administration is unavailable for use in the United States.

The advantages of using the mixture are that it is an oral dosage form, it is liquid and easily swallowed, it allows for easy increase or decrease in the amount of analgesic without the patient being unduly concerned about the change in number, color or shape of tablets and it can be mixed with other liquids, either medicated or nonmedicated.[7]

The hospice efforts to control pain would be to no avail if they did not take into consideration the many aspects of its administration. In treating chronic pain, a preventive schedule is used: the duration of action of the morphine sulfate is allowed for, and the medication is given at intervals that prevent the pain from occurring. The use of a PRN schedule is avoided.

The chronic administration of the modified Brompton's Mixture is not without undesirable effects. Constipation may occur, made worse by poor dietary intake, dehydration and decreased exercise. Daily use of stool softeners plus the intermittent administration of a laxative or enema to prevent impactions is incorporated into the regimen of those receiving the modified Brompton's Mixture. If constipation is allowed to develop, it not only causes discomfort, but may in turn lead to nausea and loss of appetite.

The nausea and vomiting due to the use of the morphine sulfate usually are associated with the initiation of the therapy and often subside spontaneously. In patients where these effects do not subside the prophylactic use of prochlorperazine syrup or another antiemetic is often successful. The antiemetic is administered either at the same time as the morphine mixture or before meals.

In addition to controlling pain, constipation, nausea and vomiting, the pharmacist also helps evaluate, monitor and provide information on the treatment of pressure sores, mouth care and infections in the mouth and the use of steroids and other medications prescribed for concomitant chronic diseases. Again, the goal of the program is to keep the patient comfortable.

There is actually a double goal: the patient should be not only comfortable, but also mentally alert. The hospice has found that only a transient sedation may occur in the first 48–72 hours following initiation of the modified Brompton's Mixture. Following this period, most patients are quite alert, even with very high doses of morphine. Problems of mental clouding do occur, however, with the misuse or overuse of sedatives or tranquilizers. The cases of oversedation that have occurred are due in part to the disease process itself adversely affecting the degree and duration of drug activity.

Conclusion

In summary, the pharmacist at Hillhaven Hospice has an ideal setting for direct involvement in care of the cancer patient, and parts of this involvement can be extrapolated to other pharmacy settings. In the home the pharmacist is available to either the home care or the day care patient and family to monitor treatment protocols and educate family members on the medications used by the patient. A thorough discussion of the medication treatment plan is made, including personal reinforcement and instructions on how to obtain, store and administer the medications.

The education and discussion of drug treatment plans are also available to patients and family members while in the facility. During these discussions the pharmacist can evaluate subjectively and objectively both favorable and adverse effects of medications being used and can coordinate this information with other members of the staff, either directly or in the weekly patient care conferences. Interwoven with all of these activities is the opportunity for pharmacy students to learn about the hospice concept, dying patients and the process of dying and, of great importance, how to communicate with the terminally ill patient.

The pharmacist at Hillhaven Hospice is one of the few pharmacists in the country actually working within the hospice concept. As the concept of the hospice and the care of terminally ill patients who are no longer pursuing active therapeutic treatment emerges, the pharmacy profession must be prepared to participate in similar programs and work with dying patients, their families and friends.

References

1. Plant, J.: Finding a Home for Hospice Care in the United States, *Hospitals 51*:53 (July 1) 1977.
2. Hackley, J. A.: Full-Service Hospice Offers Home, Day and Inpatient Care, *Hospitals 51*:84 (Nov. 1) 1977.
3. Hillhaven Hospice Brochure, 1978.
4. Saunders, C.: Control of Pain in Terminal Cancer, *Nursing Times* 1133 (July 22) 1976.
5. Twycross, R. G.: Choice of Strong Analgesic in Terminal Cancer: Diamorphine or Morphine? *Pain 3*:93, 1977.
6. Twycross, R. G.: Personal correspondence (Nov. 2) 1977.
7. Farr, W.: Oral Morphine for Control of Pain in Terminal Cancer, *Ariz. Med.* 167 (March) 1978.

Readings for a Broader Perspective

1. Lipman, A. G. "Drug Therapy in Terminally Ill Patients," *American Journal of Hospital Pharmacy* 32 (March 1975):270–76.
2. Wagner, J., and Goldstein, E. "Pharmacist's Role in Loss and Grief," *American Journal of Hospital Pharmacy* 34 (May 1977):490–92.

SPECIALIZED PHARMACY SERVICES/ MEDICAL PROBLEMS

Clinical: Overview

18—Evolution of the Clinical Pharmacy Concept

Donald C. Brodie and Roger A. Benson

Social change takes place in a variety of ways. It may come about as a result of long-identified needs which require a mandated social action at the highest level of authority. This type of change came about in the United States with the passage of the Social Security Act in 1933 and such amendments that have taken place subsequently, such as Titles 18 and 19 (Medicare and Medicaid, respectively). Another example of change of this type is the Hill-Burton legislation of 1946 (The Hospital Survey and Construction Act), which initiated an organized program of increasing the hospital bed capacity in the United States.

Change at the state and municipal levels in the health field also may come about because of enacted statutory and regulatory requirements. The latter may deal with licensure, certification and registration requirements of institutions and personnel designed to benefit the public welfare through some form of consumer protection.

Another type of change is seen in the voluntary system, a prime example of which was the report of Abraham Flexner in 1910, which caused a turn-around in the medical education in the U. S. during the early part of the twentieth century. In the area of health care standards, the American College of Surgeons, acting voluntarily, initiated its program of Hospital Standardization in 1917–18, a program that evolved into the Joint Commission on Accreditation of Hospitals in 1952. The introduction of an organized program for establishing and maintaining standards in pharmaceutical education came about voluntarily with the incorporation of the American Council on Pharmaceutical Education in 1939, which climaxed the efforts of the National Association of Boards of Pharmacy to evaluate colleges of pharmacy throughout the United States.

Emergence of Clinical Pharmacy

Whatever the nature of a social change, its origin may be traced to an idea or a concept.

The idea or concept becomes a forerunner or precursor to change. An idea in itself does not generate change, but it may initiate a series of events leading to organized planning that will envelop and embrace the concept. Planning, in turn, may lead to implementation of experimental programs designed to demonstrate and test hypotheses that evolve as the original idea or concept is translated into "action." This series of events has been unfolding in the field of pharmacy as the clinical pharmacy concept emerged, and has been carried forward through planning in both practice and educational settings, and has now developed into what are identified in the profession as operational clinical pharmacy programs. For purposes of this discussion, Parker's definition of clinical pharmacy is appropriate: "Clinical pharmacy is a concept or a philosophy emphasizing the safe and appropriate use of drugs in patients. . . ."[1]

Usually it is not possible to pinpoint a precise time when a concept first becomes visible. Gloria Francke, in her review of the literature, pointed to the University of Washington experiment of 1944 as the probable origin of the clinical pharmacy concept, although one would be hard pressed to associate Professor Wait Rising's experimental program with implementation of the clinical pharmacy concept as it stands today.[2,3,4] More than likely it was an attempt to meet the criticisms by practicing pharmacists that graduating pharmacists were lacking in practical pharmacy training, with the emphasis on "practical." Parenthetically, no one seemed to be able to explain precisely what the deficiencies were.

In the mid-60's, individual researchers in pharmacy education were far from inactive in producing conceptual thought about the future of pharmacy, and in defining its role in society. Writing in the Report of the Commission on Pharmaceutical Services to Ambulant Patients by Hospitals and Related Facilities, 1965, Brodie stated: "The ultimate goal of the services of pharmacy must be the safe use of drugs by the public. In this context, the mainstream function of pharmacy is clinical in nature, one that may be identified accurately as *drug-use control*,"[5] where drug-use control is defined as " . . . the sum total of knowledge, understanding, judgments, procedures, skills, controls, and ethics that assures optimal safety in the distribution and use of medication." In these remarks, Brodie has crystallized the concept of clinical pharmacy by giving the concept the essential form in which it could be further developed. By way of predicting the future of clinical pharmacy, he stated: "In the future, pharmacists will have increasing opportunities to participate in the distribution of drugs in a clinical situation. Emerging patterns of drug distribution in hospitals place the pharmacist on the floor, interpreting chart orders for medication, preparing the medication for the nursing staff, and providing consultative drug information when required."[6] And the concept was not restricted to only the hospital environment: "If drug-use control is the mainstream component of pharmacy service, it should apply to community pharmacy practice as well as to institutional practice."[5]

Soon after these concepts were stated, a pilot program was instituted at the University of California, San Francisco Medical Center, in September 1966, which placed the pharmacist in the clinical setting of a teaching hospital. The program, the "Ninth Floor Project," described by Smith[7] in 1967, was staffed on the surgical service on a 24-hour basis, and employed many advanced concepts of clinical pharmacy, including the decentralized pharmacy, the unit dose concept, the use of pharmacy technicians, a drug information center, and the use of patient drug profiles. Impetus for the program was a nursing activities study, performed in 1961, which indicated that 20 percent of nurses' time was devoted to the procurement, preparation, administration and charting of medications. "The broad purpose of the pharmacy pilot project was to characterize and study the pharmacist's clinical role on the hospital-based patient care team and to determine the spectrum of his contribution in a team approach to patient care."[8] This early experience in clinical pharmacy showed that the pharmacist, when properly trained and motivated " . . . can function as a contributing member of the health care team. Furthermore, his contributions can lead to improvement in the quality of patient care."

When the Pharmacy-Medicine-Nursing Conference on Health Education was held in connection with the 75th anniversary of the founding of the College of Pharmacy at the University of Michigan in 1967, there was ample evidence that a change in thinking was taking place in pharmacy education.[9] In reflecting upon the previous Planning Conference held in 1966, Pelligrino stated that the education of the pharmacist was a major concern at this time. Major directions included: " . . . patient orientation instead of drug orientation, better general education, closer functioning in the clinical setting, greater contiguity with the bedside, and assuming a more meaningful place on the health team."[10] The need for a clinical component in the curriculum emerged in these discussions. "Pharmacy practice and pharmaceutical education must be related to comprehensive medical care. In order to do this, pharmacists must be educated and trained to serve both in illness and wellness. To accomplish this goal, pharmacy service must become patient-oriented, thereby requiring the development of a clinical component in pharmaceutical education."[11] It is now eight years since that conference was held, and an opportunity is at hand to view retrospectively how the "clinical pharmacy concept" has been interpreted. It is too early to evaluate the "new" educational and practice programs that are intended to embody the clinical pharmacy concept. One can conclude with reasonable assurance, however,

that "clinical pharmacy" emerged in mid-20th century American pharmacy, and by the mid-1960's the concept has developed to the point where it could be seen but not necessarily understood.

Is Clinical Pharmacy Really New?

The time has come when an attempt should be made to understand what the clinical pharmacy concept, as implemented, actually is. Is pharmacy practice being transformed? Does pharmacy education have a new character? What is the impact of clinical pharmacy on health care? Have pharmacists' contributions in a new role met an unfulfilled social need? Is clinical pharmacy *really* new?

Normally, reading the history of a profession will reveal the relationships of past to present, showing how new expansions are extensions of traditional practices. Only rarely does a branch of knowledge exhibit the quantum jump phenomenon which has been experienced in some areas of the sciences, particularly in physics. A greater part of the literature generated by pharmacy educators during the past 10 years would seem to indicate that clinical pharmacy is such a phenomenon, and not a normal expansion of that which has constituted a major effort in pharmacy since its inception.

The fact that changes take place within a profession may be indicative of growth within that profession. If this were not true, a profession would soon lose its vitality and its value to society. Major changes in a profession, however, sometimes involve territorial expansion or retreat, and when these occur, the effects on the profession, and to be sure on society itself, are often dramatic. Pharmacy has undergone such changes, and is undergoing them now, and the effects are becoming visible. For example, the development of the pharmaceutical industry and the mass production of drugs caused a major change in pharmacy practice, resulting in a concomitant reduction in compounding activities, as well as in activities relating to supplying physicians with drug information. The industry's detail men have assumed the latter role. To ensure financial survival, the pharmacist has increased his merchandising efforts in areas of non-drug items, and in so doing has, in the opinion of some observers, reduced his professional image in the eyes of other health professionals and the public. Whereas he was forced to retreat from his territory of practice in one area, the pharmacist expanded it in another. These effects are quite obvious, and so are the reasons for them; pharmacy can not expect these conditions to reverse themselves.

Whereas the aforementioned changes were those brought about by evolution and by external forces, pharmacy is now in the process of bringing about changes of a revolutionary kind, caused by forces within the profession. These internal forces, although inexorable, are not of the same intensity in all quarters, however; in fact, there are factions in pharmacy practice which are satisfied with the evolutionary status quo. But the standard bearers of revolutionary change, for the most part, are coming from the ranks of both practitioners and educators.

If clinical pharmacy is put forward as a new idea, as some believe it is, it is reasonable to expect observers, within the profession as well as outside, to question the motives behind this emphasis. Is pharmacy a failing profession—one which is seizing upon a "new role" to save it from the dimorphous state of business/profession? The business/professional role conflict has received much attention by pharmacy educators in recent years,[12-15] which indicates an increasing concern, on their part, with what is considered to be a dichotomous situation. Not all pharmacists, however, view the entrepreneurial aspects of the profession as detrimental, and some even criticize pharmacy educators for their encouragement of activities which, in their opinion, seem to encroach upon the practice of medicine.[15]

In all fairness, one must at least consider the possibility that the advancement of a "new" concept in a profession might be considered by some professional as well as lay observers to be a *reaction* to the status quo, rather than a *response* to a real need in society. If such an interpretation could arise, it might result in effects truly detrimental to the professional goals of pharmacy.

The response of pharmacy education to the changing nature of the profession cannot be considered in any sense to be *post facto* reaction of recent origin. Changes in, and the lengthening of the program for graduates in pharmacy have been taking place for decades, with an eye towards establishing guidance and new directions for the profession. A convergence of these endeavors occurred when the primary purpose of the practice of pharmacy was recognized in the concept of drug-use control.

Pharmacy education has stated the goals of role expansion in the profession in light of current needs and has been training students to fill these roles. The next requirement, once again the responsibility of educators, is to assess how well these goals have been and are being achieved. Pharmacy educators have continually stressed the need for precise studies of the professional performance of pharmacists in order to expand these services for the purpose of improved health care delivery. During his Remington Honor Medal acceptance address, Parks directed his remarks towards questions of continuing education and competency in pharmacy: "What are the competencies the pharmacist needs and how can they be measured? To my knowledge, no group has addressed this question, and until we have a valid answer to it we will continue to spin our wheels in an aimless manner."[16]

Patient-Oriented Pharmacy Practice

Rather than placing emphasis upon clinical pharmacy as a recent innovation, the profession might well render a more accurate accounting of this ministration by relating the way it has been practiced in the past to the way it is being practiced today. The patient-oriented practice of pharmacy has a rich historical background with a strong European heritage, as well as one dating back to colonial America. Excerpts from hospital procedure manuals in 18th century Italy show that the pharmacist was not only required to accompany the physician during visits to the patient, but visited seriously ill patients independently to examine them and to attend to needs which might suddenly arise.[17] Historical facts such as these should be brought to the attention of health professionals to show the continuity of tradition which is present in today's "new direction" in pharmacy.

Pharmacy educators as well as physicians are not unaware of the plenteous examples of clinical pharmacy that history has to offer. Tyler has referred to patient orientation in the profession as " . . . an avatism, albeit a scientifically oriented one, to the days when pharmacists universally showed a helpful concern for their patients."[18] And Weaver states: "Historically, clinical pharmacy roles could be shown to exist perhaps centuries ago—as with clinical pharmacology."[19] Ebert has observed: "Pharmacy is an old profession and the pharmacist is accepted as a person who has traditionally played a role in the provision of health care. Why not exploit that acceptance and extend the role of the pharmacist rather than create new types of health professionals."[20]

Professionalism

Pharmacy must now, however, rest content with clinical pharmacy as a mere extension of a traditional role, and expect that the impetus of a strong historical background is sufficient to carry it forward to meet the changing needs of society today. It must also measure the contributions of pharmacists *at this time* to reveal the impact of clinical pharmacy. Many of the aspects of pharmacy which are now called clinical are identical to those qualities of practice which are designated to be professional. And although the sociological attitudes concerning professionalism are still in a formative stage, the control of conditions of practice is one of the criteria of a profession.[13] As far as pharmacy is concerned, the subject of control has raised some crucial questions resulting in legal actions. The United States Supreme Court, in 1973, handed down a decision that the majority ownership of North Dakota pharmacies must be in the hands of registered pharmacists in good standing. This decision overrules the Liggett decision of 1928, which held that pharmacy ownership could be controlled by nonpharmacists.[21] The overruling of the Liggett decision restores to the pharmacist some control of conditions of practice, at least by restoring to the individual states the right to decide who shall own pharmacies. In an editorial on this decision, Francke refers to remarks by counsel for the Liggett Company, who argued that: " . . . the doctor and the lawyer performed a *personal* service but the pharmacist did not."[22]

Other aspects of professionalism in which very little research has been done concern the amount of time the pharmacist spends in professional duties as opposed to other tasks, and the determination of the types of individuals with whom the pharmacist interacts during the day. What seems to be required is thorough research into the quality of professional performance of pharmacists. Such research, backed up by the profession's strong historical foundation, will form the baseline from which new directions for an expansion of professionalism in pharmacy can be plotted.

It is quite clear that clinical pharmacy is not new, nor has the concept been invented to save the professional image of pharmacy. Pharmacists have been advising patients and consulting with physicians about drugs, including instructions for their use, warnings concerning their misuse, and recommendations of O.T.C. drugs as a normal activity for generations. Such services are patient oriented, and comprise part of the clinical component of pharmacy practice.

Role in Primary Care

The pharmacist traditionally has provided many elements of primary care although they have not been recognized in the context of the latter. Studies have been made recently which document the fact that pharmacists are participating in the delivery of primary health care in the United States and Canada.[22-25] These studies reflect the attitudes of pharmacists towards providing care of this kind, and also indicate that those pharmacists who have recently entered the profession or have recently taken postgraduate courses express more interest in increasing their professional involvement.

Analyses of recent clinical pharmacy practice, including exhaustive research of case studies in which the activities of pharmacists are examined objectively, will reveal the actual impact of the clinical pharmacy concept on the profession as it exists today. This research will reveal the strengths and weaknesses in pharmacy practice, particularly as they relate to the current needs of society. If compromises must then be made in adjusting an ideal to a realistically achievable goal, the facts will be available upon which one may judge the case. Clinical pharmacy is built upon a strong historical tradition and in its present state of development it is

attempting to respond to the needs of changing social structures.

Comment

The preceding discussion has attempted to show that the changes that are taking place in the name of patient-oriented or clinical pharmacy are probably little more than a modern manifestation of an historic truth. Pharmacy practice from the simplistic times of antiquity to the present day has been devoted to preparing for and distributing medicines to people, a function and a service that by their very nature are patient oriented. This function remains the core of the pharmacist's contribution to society, namely the safe and responsible distribution and use of medicines.

During the intervening centuries many changes have taken place that have influenced this historic relationship, while at the same time the spectrum of the pharmacist's services has expanded and the mode and environment of his practice have changed. The most profound changes that have taken place probably can be attributed to the scientific revolution and the ever expanding body of knowledge and technology that have accompanied it. Social and economic forces and the growth of professionalism have also contributed to the evolutionary changes. One of the characteristics of pharmacy practice that has been eroded by change is the pharmacist-client relationship. This erosion has paralleled the growth of the business-profession dichotomy.

There exists a natural three step sequence that the pharmacist instinctively follows, once he receives a physician's order for a medicine, which focuses *first* on the pharmacist, and the quality of his performance, *second* on the medicine, and the knowledge and skill that its preparation requires, and *third* on the patient, to whom he administers the medicine or to whom he distributes it. This order of events has become distorted. The normal sequence seems to have been interrupted at the second step and the pharmacist's terminal focus has become the medicine, itself, representing as it is, the fruit of his own labors. Interestingly enough, this same analogy can be applied to medical practice and the physician, and the shift of his focus from the patient to the disease itself. Quite likely, this is a universal failure of health care delivery in our times, and appears to be applicable to all health care providers and institutions.

From this perhaps overly simplified explanation, it is easy to interpret what the introduction of the clinical pharmacy concept in these times is doing: it is beginning to realign the historic scope of concern for a client by the pharmacist, again focusing his ultimate concern on the recipient of his service; it is giving a renewed visibility and increasing importance to the third step in the natural sequence. In so doing the pharmacist is not abrogating his responsibilities as a pharmaceutical scientist, because it is his mastery of the body of knowledge, broadly chemical and biomedical, and uniquely pharmaceutical in nature, that justifies his services to society.

Perhaps the most striking influence that the clinical pharmacy concept has had on the pharmacist and the profession is the change that has occurred in the "pharmaceutical attitude" or "outlook." One of the main deficiencies in the existing health care delivery system is its failure to provide the full spectrum of health services for people—not just the special services that each provider is qualified to supply, but other services as well; particularly those that are associated with primary care such as *interventive, enabling* and *formative* services.[26] Society seems to be mandating that each provider assume a responsibility which can be met only if he functions in a dual role, *first*, that of a health

generalist, one who is broadly qualified and motivated to respond to the health problems of society, and *second*, that of a health specialist—physician, pharmacist, nurse—for which each provider is uniquely qualified. It is to this end that the clinical pharmacy concept is directing the profession.

References

1. Parker, P. F.: The Hospital Pharmacist in the Clinical Setting. I., Paper presented at the Second Annual Clinical Midyear Meeting of the American Society of Hospital Pharmacists, Dec. 4, 1967.
2. Francke, Gloria N.: Evolvement of Clinical Pharmacy. *In: Perspectives in Clinical Pharmacy*; ed. by Donald E. Francke and Harvey A. K. Whitney, Jr., Hamilton, Ill.: Drug Intelligence Publications, 1972, pp. 26–36.
3. Rising, L. Wait: Theory and Practice Can be Combined, *Am. J. Pharm. Ed.* 9:557–559 (Oct.) 1945.
4. Youngken, H. W., Jr.: The Washington Experiment—Clinical Pharmacy, *Am. J. Pharm. Ed.* 17:64–70 (Jan.) 1953.
5. Brodie, Donald C.: The Challenge to Pharmacy in Times of Change, Washington, D. C., The Commission on Pharmaceutical Services to Ambulant Patients by Hospitals and Related Facilities, The American Pharmaceutical Association and the American Society of Hospital Pharmacists, 1966, p. 39.
6. *Ibid.*, p. 46.
7. Smith, W. E.: The Future Role of the Hospital Pharmacist in the Patient Care Area, *Am. J. Hosp. Pharm.* 24: 228 (Apr.) 1967.
8. Owyang, Eric, Miller, Robert A. and Brodie, Donald C.: The Pharmacist's New Role in Institutional Patient Care, *Am. J. Hosp. Pharm.* 25:624–630 (Nov.) 1968.
9. Proceedings: *Pharmacy—Medicine—Nursing Conference on Health Education.* Ann Arbor, Mich., February 16–18, 1967.
10. *Ibid.*, p. 42.
11. *Ibid.*, p. 35.
12. Rising, W.: Professional Consulting, a Neglected Function of Pharmacy, *Am. J. Pharm. Ed.* 26:209–216, 1962.
13. Ladinsky, Jack: Research on Pharmacy: Retrospect and Prospect, *Am. J. Pharm. Ed.* 34:550–559 (Nov.) 1970.

14. Avellone, Nick: Trends and Problems in Community Pharmacy Practice, *Am. J. Pharm. Ed. 34*:885–887 (Dec.) 1970.

15. Peterson, Arthur F.: What Differences does it Make? *Am. J. Pharm. Ed. 35*:267–274 (May) 1971.

16. APhA Honors Lloyd Parks with Remington Medal: *APhArmacy Weekly 14*:4 (May 3) 1975.

17. Koup, Jeffrey R.: Letter: Déjà Vu: We have all been here before, *Drug Intell. Clin. Pharm. 7*:191–192 (Apr.) 1973.

18. Tyler, Varro E.: Let's Make Sure They Understand, *Am. J. Pharm. Ed. 35*:131–133 (Feb.) 1971.

19. Weaver, Lawrence C.: Clinical Pharmacy Concerns, Proc. 74th Annual Meeting, Am. Assn. of Colleges of Pharmacy, Scottsdale, Ariz., 1973. *Am. J. Pharm. Ed. 37*:536–538 (Aug.) 1973.

20. Ebert, Robert H.: Changes in the Health System, *J. Am. Pharm. Assoc. NS9*:402–404 (Aug.) 1969.

21. A Landmark Decision: *Drug Intell. Clin. Pharm. 8*:27–31 (Jan.) 1974.

22. Francke, Donald E.: Editorial: The Supreme Court's Reversal of the Liggett Decision, *Drug Intell. Clin. Pharm. 8*: 7 (Jan.) 1974.

23. Linn, Lawrence S. and Davis, Milton S.: Factors Associated with Actual and Preferred Activities of Pharmacists, *J. Am. Pharm. Assoc. NS11*:545–548 (Oct.) 1971.

24. Bass, M.: The Pharmacist as a Provider of Primary Care, *Can. Med. Assoc. J. 112*:60–64 (Jan. 11) 1975.

25. Perry, Paul J. and Hurley, Stephen C.: Activities of the Clinical Pharmacist Practicing in the Office of a Family Practitioner, *Drug Intell. Clin. Pharm. 9*:129–133 (Mar.) 1975.

26. Parker, Alberta W.: The Dimensions of Primary Care: Blueprints for Change. *In: Primary Care: Where Medicine Fails*; ed. by Spyros Andrepoulos, New York: John Wiley & Sons, 1974, pp. 23–26.

19—Levels of Pharmacy Practice

Donald E. Francke

One can identify several levels of practice in pharmacy and one such arbitrary classification is shown in Table 19.1. The criteria I used to judge the five levels of practice was whether 90 percent of one level could perform 90 percent of the responsibilities of the next higher level. If they could not then they are separate levels; if they could, I merged the levels. For example, I believe there is a significant difference between the levels of practice of what the Millis Commission called a generic pharmacist and what I call a clinical pharmacist generalist and that 90 percent of the present generic pharmacists cannot carry out 90 percent of the responsibilities of the clinical pharmacist generalist. In the same way, I believe that 90 percent of the clinical pharmacist generalists cannot carry out the responsibilities of 90 percent of the pharmacotherapeutic specialists or applied pharmacologists. However, until levels of competency are determined and applied, any graduate can continue to claim any level of competency in professional practice he chooses.

At present, an underdeveloped area of pharmacy practice is that performed by the *clinical scientist* who in the words of the Millis Commission is "equally at home at the patient's bedside or in the laboratory."[1] The use

Table 19.1

Levels of Pharmacy Practice

CLINICAL PHARMACISTS
1. Clinical Scientists
2. Clinical Pharmacy Specialists
   a. Pharmacotherapeutic Specialist or Applied Pharmacologist
   b. Clinical Radiopharmacist Specialist
   c. Drug Information Specialist
   d. Pediatric Clinical Pharmacy Specialist
   e. Others
3. Clinical Pharmacy Generalists

GENERIC PHARMACISTS
4. Generic pharmacists involved in a high percentage of professional activities, perform clinical functions and have numerous patient-physician contacts daily.

GENERIC PHARMACISTS—PHARMACY TECHNOLOGISTS
5. Generic pharmacists involved in a low percentage of professional activity, perform little or no clinical functions and have little contact with patients or physicians. Ninety percent of trained pharmacy technologists could perform 90 percent of what these generic pharmacists do.

of the term laboratory has generated a great deal of confusion as to the nature of the clinical scientist and how he will be developed and I am now seeking clarification of this point. However, if we relate the clinical scientist in medicine to the clinical scientist in pharmacy what do we find? First that the large majority of physicians who are clinical scientists possess only their basic professional degree; a few also have a research degree. Second, physicians with this background perform significant research in such fields as lipid research, cancer research, hematology, hypertension and many others. Third, the research team is almost always multidisciplinary and numerous specialists contribute. Fourth, the physician, since he bears the chief responsibility for the patient, is the leader of the research team. It would be my judgment that clinical scientists in pharmacy will develop in somewhat the same manner. A number of those who receive good training in the basic sciences, who have the appropriate motivation, who possess excellent clinical training and who have a proper health care setting for research involvement will become clinical scientists without too much additional formalized effort.

A second level of practice is that which I would call areas of specialization as exemplified by the *Pharmacotherapeutic Specialist* or *Applied Pharmacologist*. In the early days of clinical pharmacy education, I attempted to conceptualize what a clinical pharmacist was and thought of him as an applied pharmacologist. I thought of the clinical pharmacist as being a person who, in addition to his basic pharmacology, had taken courses in pharmacology and therapeutics with medical students, courses in which he would receive a great deal of therapeutics. I thought of him as having graduate level courses in biostatistics, pathophysiology, biopharmaceutics and pharmacokinetics, and the sociology of health care. These courses plus his general educational background in microbiology, pharmaceutics, formulation, etc., plus suitable clinical training such as a residency or clerkship would produce one of the most drug knowledgeable people on the health care team. Some people don't like calling the clinical pharmacist an applied pharmacologist because they think it might antagonize clinical pharmacologists. Thus, I also think of the clinical pharmacist as a pharmacotherapeutic specialist. The important considerations, I believe, are his knowledge of therapeutics and the actions of drugs in humans. In the preface to the first edition of *Applied Pharmacology* which the British physician, A. J. Clark, wrote more than fifty years ago, he said that his objective was "to give an account of the direct scientific evidence for the therapeutic action of the most important drugs, and to demonstrate the importance of this knowledge in the clinical application of drugs."[2] This is essentially the objective of the high level clinical pharmacist whether one calls him a pharmacotherapeutic specialist or an applied pharmacologist.

Of course a number of other specialists may eventually be approved after due consideration by the APhA's Board of Pharmaceutical Specialties.[3] Some of these may be, for example, Clinical Radiopharmacist Specialist, Drug Information Specialist, Pediatric Clinical Pharmacy Specialist, Geriatric Clinical Pharmacist, and perhaps others. However, I would expect that the large umbrella for the areas of specialization would be the Pharmacotherapeutic Specialist or Applied Pharmacologist, or some similar designation. For example, I would expect this person's knowledge and experience would be such that he would be equally at home with patients and physicians in such specialties as medicine, surgery, obstetrics and gynecology, neurology, etc. The principal reason pediatric and geriatric clinical pharmacy may be eventually judged as specialties is because of the differences in metabolism of drugs in the very young and very old. Whether this difference warrants specialization remains to be seen.

A third level of pharmacy practice is exemplified by the *clinical pharmacy generalist.* As this title implies, this person is a generalist with a broad range of knowledge. This person is not as well grounded as the applied pharmacologist in pharmacology, therapeutics, biostatistics or pharmacokinetics and lacks his clinical training and experience. Still he has a sufficient background to be a most valuable member of the health care team.

A fourth level of practice is that exemplified by the hundreds of what the Millis Commission describes as *generic pharmacists* who practice in community and hospital pharmacies. Some of these are involved in a high percentage of professional activities and are engaged in daily patient-physician contacts and perform numerous important clinical services for patients and the health team. In due course, I anticipate that this level will merge with the clinical pharmacy generalist as the colleges improve their educational programs and decrease their student load.

In addition, there is a fifth level of practice carried out by generic pharmacists who are involved in a low percentage of professional activities and perform few if any clinical functions. These are the pharmacists who stand behind a counter all day repetitively filling and labeling prescriptions, turning the filled prescription over to a clerical person to transfer to the patient. In my opinion, this group of generic pharmacists should be merged with trained pharmacy technologists, technicians or dispensing assistants. These technical people could, in my opinion, competently perform 90 percent of what this group of pharmacists do.

I would like to see the profession recognize that it does not require the training a pharmacist receives to carry out the functions now performed by a large number of pharmacists. Once this was accepted, the number of pharmacists enrolled in schools of pharmacy could be greatly decreased. On the other hand, the importance and significance of the pharmacist would be greatly enhanced because they would be trained to perform tasks which are now neglected. Schools of pharmacy would have fewer pharmacy students but they would be superior students trained to an entirely different level than they are at present. The education and training of these students would be such that a professional doctoral degree would be entirely appropriate. Schools of pharmacy would be involved, directly or indirectly, in the training of technical personnel to the level required by the function they will be called upon to perform. I believe that this is the general pattern that will finally emerge and when it does, pharmacy will become a much stronger profession because of it.

References

1. [Millis, John S.]: *Pharmacists For The Future,* Health Administration Press, Ann Arbor, Michigan. 1975.
2. Modell, Walter, et al.: Preface to *Applied*

Pharmacology, American Edition, W. B. Saunders Co. 1976.

3. Board of Pharmaceutical Specialities: Petitioners Guide to Specialty Recognition, 6 page document available from the American Pharmaceutical Association, 2215 Constitution Avenue, Northwest, Washington, D.C. 20037.

20—Roles for Pharmacy Practice

Donald E. Francke

. . . I believe that level 4 of what the Millis Commission called the *generic pharmacist* will merge with the level 3 of what I termed the *clinical pharmacy generalist* as the colleges improve their educational program.[1] In addition, I said that the level 5 *generic pharmacist* who is involved in a low percentage of professional activity should be merged with trained technologists, technicians or dispensing assistants. Now I would like to outline my general concept of the professional role of the *clinical pharmacy generalist* who someday I believe will constitute the large majority of practicing pharmacists. . . .

It is my judgment that all practicing pharmacists should be able to carry out with competence each of the responsibilities for drug related activities as listed in Table 20.1.

I will comment briefly about each of these professional roles.

1. *Drug-Use Control.* Brodie[4] has proposed *drug-use control* as the mainstream function of pharmacy wherever it is practiced. He defines it as "that system of knowledge, understanding, judgments, procedures, skills, controls, and ethics that assures optimal safety in the distribution and use of medication." "This definition," says Brodie,

"relates professional function to patient welfare in the form of drug safety; it is patient oriented. It is the heart of the body of practice . . ." While I agree with Brodie's concept, still I must admit it is as yet an unattained ideal, but certainly one worth striving for. Few pharmacists exercise drug-use control in handling OTC products. Relative to prescription medication, Mickey Smith[5] made what I consider a profound remark when he asked "What is a prescription?" and then answered, "it is a written record of the failure of the pharmacist to gain control of the social object—the drug." Smith was referring to Brodie's concept of drug-use control mentioned above. As Dr. Smith points out, the prescription says, in effect, here are the doctor's orders to the pharmacist and the doctor's orders to the patient. In addition, Smith states, the prescription is too easy a measure of what the pharmacist does and serves as an oversimplified basis for his remuneration.

If the pharmacist is serious about assuming responsibility for the drug and willing to take the necessary steps to accomplish this, then Dr. Smith argues, the prescription should be gradually abolished. This process would be started with the pharmacist maintaining good patient medication profiles

Table 20.1

Roles for Clinical Pharmacy Generalist

RESPONSIBILITY FOR DRUG RELATED ACTIVITIES

1. Supervises all drug distribution activities for drug use control and patient safety.
2. Selects for patients therapeutically effective prescription drug products at reasonable cost.
3. Records patient's medication history of drugs taken and any adverse reactions therefrom.
4. Monitors patient's response to drugs utilizing patient medication profile and other resources.
5. Detects and diagnoses adverse drug reactions and drug interactions.
6. Counsels patients on the use of drugs to assure compliance.
7. Advises patients on selection of OTC drugs.
8. Helps establish dosage regimens for patients.
9. Promotes rational drug therapy by physicians.
10. Integrates the psycho-socio-economic aspects of health care.
11. Prescribes for mild self-limiting diseases.
12. Supervises management of patients with acute and chronic diseases.
13. Detects and overcomes incompatibilities in drug mixtures.
14. Compounds drug preparations to meet specific patient requirements.
15. Supervises the dispensing of prescriptions by dispensing assistants.
16. Has ability to evaluate the drug literature.
17. Performs drug utilization review.
18. Provides health care education to the public.

I am indebted to Dean Goyan[2] and Captain Brands[3] for delineation of several of the roles mentioned in this table.

with increased consultation between physician and pharmacist. As a second step, prescriptions would be written for the drug only while the pharmacist would decide the brand, dosage form and directions for the patient. A third step would occur when the physician provided the diagnosis and decided whether or not drug therapy were necessary and the pharmacist would be completely responsible for the therapy. This plan would take some years to implement and would require a drastic change in the phar-macist's education and training. But it could be done.

2. *Selects drug products.* The pharmacist is well qualified to select drug products and, in fact, must be selective from among reputable sources of supply in the face of extensive product duplication.

3. *Medication history.* The patient's medication history forms an essential part of the data base upon which the pharmacist can make judgments about the patient's response to medication, adverse effects, etc.

4. *Monitors response to drugs.* To accomplish this the pharmacist must establish and maintain suitable records for the purpose of monitoring the drugs prescribed for (or self-selected by) the patient seeking his services. Inherent in this is the responsibility to consult with the prescriber at such time as the record reveals that:

a. The prescribed therapy is inappropriate for this patient due to lack of efficacy, or potential adversities (interactions), or,
b. The patient is not responding to therapy as could be expected, or,
c. The patient is not complying with the recommended regimen, or,
d. The patient has established an abuse pattern for the medication(s) prescribed.

5. *Adverse reactions and interactions.* Pharmacists could easily be trained to diagnose and detect a high percentage of adverse drug reactions and drug interactions which occur as the result of drug therapy.

6. *Assures compliance.* Poor patient compliance with medication regimens is a widespread problem. To assure compliance the pharmacist must consult with every patient receiving a prescription drug to assure that:

a. The patient fully understands the directions for use, and the importance of complying to the regimen,
b. The patient fully understands the intended therapeutic outcome,
c. If a previously prescribed drug, the patient is complying to the directions and regimen intended by the prescriber.

In evaluating compliance there are undoubtedly a number of steps or tests the pharmacists could perform or have performed in order to better evaluate patient compliance. Such steps include taking of blood pressure of hypertensive patients and testing of urine of diabetic patients. A number of protocols to evaluate compliance could be developed cooperatively by physicians and pharmacists.

7. *Selection of OTC drugs.* The pharmacist consults with all patients seeking nonprescription medications to assure that:

a. The patient is not attempting to treat a malady for which OTC medications are not effective, or for which a physician should be seen.
b. The patient will receive the most suitable drug product for the malady for which self-medication is being sought.
c. The patient understands the directions, limitations, possible adversities, and contraindications of the medication being acquired.
d. The medication being sought is not in conflict with other medications the patient may be taking.

In many countries, however, nonprescription drugs are available on open shelves for unsupervised purchase by the public with the pharmacist in no way involved. Observing this, public health authorities may well say "it really doesn't matter who sells the public his OTC medication so long as they are properly packaged and labeled." I believe the pharmacist loses a great deal when he does not accept responsibility to counsel patients relative to their OTC medication. When he fails to do so, it is true that it really doesn't matter where the drugs are sold. When he does perform this function, he becomes an important member of the health care team.

8. *Dosage regimens.* In an institutional setting, the pharmacist often has input into the establishment of dosage regimens before the prescription is written. In community practice this occurs seldom. However, when a prescription is refilled the community pharmacist can note the patient's response to drug therapy and determine if the patient has suffered any untoward effects; whether the patient is obtaining the desired response; should the dose be increased or decreased? Such observations should be discussed with the physician.

9. *Rational drug therapy.* Pellegrino,[6] in discussing rational therapeutics by physicians, states "I do not believe that physicians can meet all other responsibilities being assigned to them and still maintain the kind of detailed information and surveillance of drug use in all their patients. Rather than fearing pharmacists as intruders, they must come to see them as indispensable allies in their attempts to practice the best possible therapeutics."

10. *Psycho-socio-economic aspects.* The affective or emotional aspect of the value of medication is intertwined with the patient-physician relationship, the patient-pharmacist relationship the physician-pharmacist relationship, the placebo effect, the meaning of the prescription to the patient, the condition of illness and other factors such as age, sex, race, etc. These interrelationships are only now being addressed in courses at colleges of pharmacy and the present day pharmacist is ill prepared to cope with these aspects. Some aspects of these problems are discussed by Bush[7] and Francke and Smith.[8]

11. *Prescribes for mild, self-limiting diseases.* One of the proposals the American Pharmaceutical Association has made recently is that an additional class of drugs be created and the pharmacist be authorized to prescribe them for minor, self-limiting illnesses. This proposal is tied in with changes in the education and training of pharmacists and in developing standards of competence for pharmacists so as to minimize dangers of prescribing a drug for conditions the pharmacist may believe to be a minor ailment when it is, in fact, actually serious. It was pointed out that the public now has this possibility of incorrect diagnosis when choosing medication for themselves and that, with

certification, a pharmacist could minimize this. Examples of drugs which the pharmacists might prescribe include pseudoephedrine 60 mg; ephedrine 50 mg; antihistamines such as chlorpheniramine 4 mg, 8 mg and 16 mg; diphenhydramine 25 mg and 50 mg capsules, certain analgesics, etc.

12. *Management of patients.* Pharmacists and physicians working under agreed protocols could greatly expand the effective health care system by having the pharmacist manage the drug-related aspects of therapy as is now done in a few institutions.

13. *Incompatibilities and instabilities.* Detecting and overcoming incompatibilities and instabilities in drug mixtures are traditional roles for the pharmacist.

14. *Compounding of prescriptions.* This is another traditional role which in most countries is performed by pharmacy technicians.

15. *Dispensing of prescriptions.* I recently saw a consumer-oriented TV news sequence of pharmacists dispensing prescriptions in a Washington, D.C. drugstore. It was very revealing. Here the pharmacists were carrying out their dispensing role but neglecting most of their other professional roles. The pharmacists worked behind a prescription counter with no contact with the patient. Still, many believe that dispensing is the principal function of a pharmacist. Brodie has made this comment:[4] "There are those who believe that pharmaceutical dispensing is the mainstream activity of pharmacy service. To those who accept this reasoning, the following statement is pertinent:" continuing he quotes from the *Mirror to Hospital Pharmacy* " . . . the dispensing function of the pharmacist, while important and even vital for patient care, is essentially a superficial practice of the profession which, by itself, does not utilize knowledge or skills sufficiently basic to merit professional recognition to the depth that lies within the grasp of hospital pharmacists."

I am sure the statement applies to all pharmacists. For reasons apparently beyond their control, they have overemphasized their dispensing function and underemphasized those functions which require a knowledge of pharmacotherapeutics, disease states, and the sick patient. I do not deprecate the dispensing function of the pharmacist any more than I would the taking of blood pressure by the physician. Both are essential functions. But the physician can no more practice total medicine by taking blood pressures than can the pharmacist practice total pharmacy by dispensing. Each is but a small part of professional practice. In my view, the dispensing function should be delegated to trained pharmacy technologists, technicians or dispensing assistants and the pharmacist should prepare himself to participate more fully in health care by fulfilling his related functions.

16. *Evaluate literature.* About ten years ago Schor and Karten[9] analyzed articles in ten of the most highly read and prestigious American medical journals and found that the methodology of the studies were acceptable in only 28 percent. Thus, in 72 percent of the articles the conclusions were invalid, or were not supported by the data presented. All pharmacists should have sufficient training in literature evaluation to judge the merits of articles in medical and other professional and scientific journals.

17. *Drug utilization review.* This is usually a function carried out by an interprofessional team at the request of governmental or health insurance agencies or medical societies in which the pharmacist can play an important role.

18. *Health care education.* "A well-informed pharmacist is the best individual to disseminate information about public health" stated Professor Charters of the University of Pittsburgh some years ago. This role is gradually being expanded by pharmacists all over the world according to Griffenhagen[10] who has recently prepared an international summary.

Eventually, I hope that those roles outlined in Table 20.1, and perhaps others, will be commonly performed by all pharmacists. Pharmaceutical education has turned in the direction of preparing pharmacists for these roles, although there still remain many unmet needs.

References

1. Francke, Donald E.: Levels of Pharmacy Practice, *Drug Intell. Clin. Pharm. 10*:534–535 (Sept.) 1976.
2. Goyan, Jere E.: The Professional Responsibility of the Pharmacist, Appendix XV of the Report to the Speaker of the Assembly by the Advisory Committee, California 1973–1974.
3. Brands, Allen J.: Personal communication.
4. Brodie, Donald C.: Drug-Use Control—Keystone to Pharmaceutical Services, *Drug Intell. Clin. Pharm. 1*:63–65 (Feb.) 1967.
5. Smith, Mickey C.: General Practice Pharmacy in the U.K. and the U.S.A.—Some Comparisons and Contrasts, *Pharm. J. 210*:9–12 (Jan. 6) 1973.
6. Pellegrino, Edmund D.: Meddlesome Medicine and Rational Therapeutics, *Drug Intell. Clin. Pharm. 9*:480–484 (Sept.) 1975.
7. Bush, Patricia J.: Psychosocial Aspects of Medicine Use, *In, Perspectives on Medicines in Society*, Wertheimer, Albert I. and Bush, P. J., editors, Drug Intelligence Publications, Hamilton, Illinois 62341, 1976.
8. Francke, D. E. and Smith, Dorothy L.: The Social Psychological Role of the Pharmacist in Drug Usage, *In, Perspectives in Clinical Pharmacy*, Francke, D. E. and Whitney, H. A. K. Jr., editors, Drug Intelligence Publications, Hamilton, Illinois 62341, 1972.
9. Schor, S. S. and Karten, I.: Statistical Evaluation of Medical Journal Manuscripts, *J. Am. Med. Assoc. 195*:1123–1128 (Mar. 28) 1966.
10. Griffenhagen, George B.: The General Practice Pharmacist and Health Education, talk presented at the 26th General Assembly of the International Pharmaceutical Federation, Warsaw, Poland, September, 1976.

Related Readings in This Volume

Readings for a Broader Perspective

1. McLeod, D. C. "Contribution of Clinical Pharmacists to Patient Care," *American Journal of Hospital Pharmacy* 33 (September 1976): 904–11.
2. Kay, B. G., and Adelman, D. N. "How Our Clinical Role Spurs Services in an Ambulatory Care Setting," *Pharmacy Times* 44 (January 1978):48–51.
3. Bellafiore, I. J. "Clinical Pharmacy: Applications to Community Pharmacy," *American Journal of Pharmaceutical Education* 35 (February 1971):85–88.
4. Morris, Lynn "Yes! Clinical Pharmacy in a Retail Pharmacy," *Pharmacy Times* 42 (September 1976):58–60.
5. Francke, D. E., and Whitney, H. A. K. "Patterns of Clinical Pharmacy Education and Practice in the United States," *Drug Intelligence & Clinical Pharmacy* 10 (September 1976): 511–21.
6. Barsness, F. R., and Trinca, C. E. "Activity Analysis and Cost Study of Clinical Pharmacists Practicing in a University Medical Center," *Drug Intelligence & Clinical Pharmacy* 12 (May 1978):284–94.
7. Gong, W. C., Cheung, A., Shrifter, N., and Campa, P. "Primary Care—A Clinical Pharmacist's Role," *California Pharmacist* 23 (June 1976):41–44.

DRUG HISTORY TAKING

21—The Pharmacist-Acquired Medication History

Tim R. Covington and Frederick G. Pfeiffer

The objective of this presentation is to further illustrate how the pharmacist may effectively contribute to patient care by fulfilling certain clinical responsibilities requiring direct patient-pharmacist communication. Although there are several opportunities for direct patient-pharmacist communication, this presentation deals specifically with the pharmacist's role in medication history acquisition and the subsequent need to counsel ambulatory outpatients and patients upon discharge from the hospital regarding proper drug usage.

The Problem

Basic to effective patient interviewing and counseling is the ability to communicate. Effective communication depends largely upon the pharmacist's ability to communicate verbally and interpret nonverbal responses. While it is not within the scope of this paper to enumerate specific communicative techniques, one should not minimize the importance of developing effective communication skills as is revealed in the following nursing service incident-accident report:[2]

Mr. Smith, on April 14, 1966, was given some liquid pHisoHex soap and instructed to take a shower before going to surgery. Instead of taking a shower with pHisoHex he drank it. Because he didn't go to surgery on April 14 Mr. Smith was again given some liquid pHisoHex soap so he could take a shower. Instead, he drank it again. This morning the patient complained to the doctor that the "medicine" made him vomit.

The pharmacist's potential contribution in the acquisition of medication histories is great, but there has been little documentation of his expertise in this area. Physician-acquired medication histories are generally sketchy.[3] Often little effort is made to determine what drugs the patient may have been taking prior to admission. Failure to acquire this information has significant medicolegal implications in that many maintenance drugs should be continued during hospitalization while other drugs having residual effects after discontinuation, such as reserpine or monoamine oxidase inhibitors, may alter the normally predictable response to the treatment regimen. In addition, the physician-acquired medication history is often lacking in information concerning the patient's reliability in taking scheduled doses, frequency with which patients consume other patients' legend drugs, nonprescription drug usage patterns and alcohol consumption patterns. Finally, often the only entry in the physician-acquired medical history concerning medication is the response of the patient when questioned about drug allergies. Even this vital question is not always asked or appropriately documented as was revealed in a study conducted in a university teaching hospital. In this study a retrospective analysis of 270 patient charts revealed that 42 (16%) of the patients were apparently not asked if they had drug allergies, or if they were asked, the response was not recorded.[4] Questions concerning allergies should always be asked and documented lest the patient sustain an unnecessary, expensive and potentially life-threatening allergic reaction.[1]

Methodology

In an effort to demonstrate the pharmacist's ability and expertise in acquiring patient medication histories, 58 inpatients on medicine and surgery units of a 500-bed, municipal, acute care, general hospital were selected at random and interviewed by a pharmacist. Information was recorded on a medication history data sheet. Physician-acquired facts relative to a patient's medication history were transcribed from the chart onto one of these forms and then compared with the data obtained from the same patient by the pharmacist.

Results

Allergies or Hypersensitivities

Perhaps the most surprising finding in this study was the relative infrequency with which physicians documented the patient's history of allergies or hypersensitivities to drugs or other chemicals (see Table 21.1). In only 32 (55%) of the 58 charts was there an entry indicating the physician had asked the patient about prior allergies or hypersensitivities.

While physician-acquired histories noted five patients with prior drug allergies, pharmacist-acquired medication histories revealed 15 prior drug allergies including six to penicillin, two to sulfonamides and one to aspirin. The interviewing pharmacist was careful in assuring that the patient under-

stood the definition of "allergy." In addition, the pharmacist was cautious not to suggest specific allergies that might bias the response. The contrast of reported drug allergies (8.6% of patients according to the physicians and 25.8% of patients according to the pharmacist) speaks well for the pharmacist's communicative skill and ability to extract pertinent information from patients.

The pharmacist also revealed 12 food allergies, three allergies to pets and six allergies to miscellaneous agents which contrasts sharply with physician-acquired data. Finally, in an effort to determine whether there was any familial genetic correlation of allergies or hypersensitivities, it was revealed that 11 of the 15 patients with a history of allergies had at least one member of their immediate family prone toward allergies or hypersensitivities.

Prescription Drug Consumption

Many of the questions asked by the pharmacist are not routine in a physician-acquired medication history but are, nevertheless, essential in maximizing patient safety and rational drug therapy. Regarding prescription drug consumption, the pharmacist documented that the 58 patients sampled were consuming 155 more prescription drugs immediately prior to admission than was revealed in their charts. Physicians documented that 38 prescription drugs were being consumed prior to admission, or 0.65 drugs per patient. The pharmacist determined that 193 prescription drugs were being consumed immediately prior to admission, or 3.2 drugs per patient (see Table 21.1).

Entries in the chart suggested that physicians inquired into prior prescription drug usage only 21 times, although the question may have been asked and not recorded in the chart. At any rate, prior drug usage should be recorded for the benefit of other physicians and health professionals who may become involved with the case.[5]

Table 21.1

**Comparison of Physician-Acquired and Pharmacist-Acquired
Medication Histories for 58 Patients**

Type of Data	Physician Acquired Information	Pharmacist Acquired Information
ALLERGY AND HYPERSENSITIVITY		
Number of times question was asked by physicians as evidenced by entry in chart	32	————
Number of patients with allergies or hypersensitivities to drugs (includes serums and vaccines)	5	15
Number of patients with allergies or hypersensitivities to foods	2	12
Number of patients with allergies or hypersensitivities to pets	1	3
Miscellaneous allergies or hypersensitivities (ragweed, insect bites, dust, etc.)	1	6
Number of individuals whose immediate family had history of allergies or hypersensitivites	0	12
PRESCRIPTION DRUG CONSUMPTION		
Legend drugs consumed immediately prior to admission (number represents prescriptions)	38	193
Number of times above question was asked by physicians as evidenced by entry in the chart	21	————
RELIABILITY OF PRESCRIPTION DRUG CONSUMPTION		
Number of patients with a history of missing doses at home	0	23
CONSUMPTION OF ANOTHER INDIVIDUAL'S PRESCRIPTION DRUGS		
Number of patients with a history of consuming someone else's medication	0	9
NONPRESCRIPTION MEDICATION CONSUMPTION		
Number of nonprescription medications consumed regularly during past year by patients sampled	2	237

Self-Medication Schedules

When asked by the pharmacist if they ever failed to consume prescription drugs as prescribed, 23 patients reported a history of missing doses (see Table 21.1). Comments such as, "Sometimes I forget," "When I run out I usually get a refill in a day or two," "I stop taking them when I start to feel better" or "I cannot afford the medicine" were not uncommon. One female reported she failed to take her oral contraceptive for four days in the midst of the 20 tablet cycle. One study revealed an epileptic patient who did not take his Dilantin and phenobarbital until he "got bad."[5]

Many patients are much too casual about taking drugs. At one extreme are individuals who consume drugs in excess. An example of excessive ingestion was revealed by a 19-year-old, unmarried student nurse presenting with severe iron deficiency anemia, excessive menstrual flow and symptoms of endometrial adenocarcinoma. By chance the physician asked about medication she was consuming and discovered that she had been taking six oral contraceptive tablets per day for three of every four weeks over a period of 20 months. This was done to "guarantee" conception control![6] At the other extreme are patients who abandon their drug therapy regimen for a variety of reasons. Drug defaulting by the drug-consuming public is a tremendous public health problem that has not received the attention it warrants. It is most common for chronically ill patients such as those with rheumatic fever, tuberculosis, diabetes, ulcers, psychiatric disorders, and so forth, to default.[7] It has been estimated that only two-thirds of 6,000 patients on drug therapy and under the care of the Tuberculosis Control Section of the Philadelphia Department of Health take their medication properly.[8] In addition, reports of patients from lower socioeconomic levels selling their drugs or leaving them on buses are not uncommon.[1]

Clearly, there is a great need for some health professional, logically the pharmacist, to vigorously counsel patients on their particular drug therapy regimen, emphasizing the actions of the drugs, why and how the physician's instructions should be carefully followed, and the importance of acquiring refills as prescribed.[9]

Consumption of Another Individual's Prescription Drugs

In this study, nine (15.5%) of the patients interviewed by the pharmacist revealed a history of occasionally taking someone else's prescription drugs. This question was not asked of the patient by any physician as evidenced by no documentation in the charts. Through malinformed self-diagnosis based on symptoms that resembled those under treatment in other individuals, patients have reported the consumption of a friend's or relative's "nerve pills," sedatives, digitalis for lower back pain, pink pain pills for headache, green water pills for fluid, diet pills for

stimulation, and amitriptyline HCl, 10 mg, to make the patient "feel better."[5] Obviously these patients were not aware of the specificity, toxicity and interaction potential of pharmaceuticals. The pharmacist, once again, is the individual best suited by education, training and practice locus to fulfill this public education function. Failure to fulfill this function is a default of professional responsibility.

Nonprescription Medication Consumption

While nonprescription medications are potential sources of drug-drug interactions, adverse drug reactions and iatrogenic disorders, it is significant that only two chart entries concerning prior nonprescription drug usage were recorded by physicians. In sharp contrast, the pharmacist determined that the 58 patients in this study regularly consumed 237 nonprescription drugs during the past year (see Table 21.1). This represents an average regular consumption of 4.1 drugs per patient. One patient consumed 14 nonlegend drugs at regular intervals. Many of these proprietary medications were flagrantly misused and abused, laxatives being the most commonly abused nonprescription drug, followed closely by aspirin. In many instances it was quite obvious that patients do not consider proprietary medications as drugs.

One particular patient, hospitalized with congestive heart failure, correlated his regular ingestion of Alka-seltzer with swelling in his ankles. The interview revealed that his genuine respect for the potency, specificity and toxicity of prescription drugs did not apply to nonprescription medication. As a result, he allowed Alka-seltzer, with a sodium content of 532 mg per tablet, to complicate his primary disease state.

Aspirin was seen to produce varying degrees of nephropathy, complicate a peptic ulcer and prolong bleeding time in patients consuming anticoagulants.

Also of great importance is the fact that

many proprietary products are of questionable efficacy. At the least, they are expensive, but more importantly, their use may delay a person from seeking appropriate medical attention. The consumer is continuously victimized by Madison Avenue marketing practices which extol the virtues of a particular panacea, while never mentioning a word about contraindications or side effects.

The time is long overdue for the pharmacist to project himself into the role of a non-biased health educator-at-large, informing and protecting drug conscious people from their own misinformation relative to non-prescription medications.[1]

Alcohol Consumption

Finally, the pharmacist should inquire into the patient's alcohol consumption pattern as alcohol ingestion and concurrent drug therapy may be the source of significant problems for the patient. Guidelines as to what degree of alcohol consumption constitutes a light, moderate or heavy drinker should be set since arbitrary assignment of these terms is of little use.

Conclusion

Data such as those presented here point out quite vividly the need to acquire a comprehensive medication history and to properly counsel hospitalized patients at discharge and ambulatory outpatients regarding their drug therapy. If the physician does not have the time or inclination to acquire a thorough medication history, he certainly cannot be expected to thoroughly counsel patients regarding proper use of all drugs. The burden, then, is upon the pharmacist to educate and advise the public in drug therapy related matters.

In addition to monitoring drug therapy of inpatients and outpatients via the patient drug profile it is our contention that the

pharmacist should generally make the patient aware of the following points upon dispensing a prescription:[10,11]

1. For whom the medication is intended,
2. The intended therapeutic use of the medication,
3. The name of the medication,
4. How to use the medication,
5. When to use the medication,
6. How long to use the medication,
7. Maximum daily dose,
8. Side effects,
9. What to avoid,
10. Storage, and
11. Miscellaneous auxiliary instructions.

The entire efforts of the health care team become futile if the patient fails to take his medication correctly while at home. The pharmacist, through oral and written communication, can and must do more toward decreasing confusion and increasing the reliability of the self-medicating public. Increased clinical activity by the pharmacist in the acquisition of medication histories and the counseling of patients must occur in order to improve patient care and hasten the evolution of the pharmacist's appropriate professional identity.

References

1. Covington, T. R.: Interviewing and Advising the Patient, ch. 11 *In* Francke, D. E. and Whitney, H. A. K., (eds.): *Perspectives in Clinical Pharmacy*, Hamilton Press, 1st ed., 1972.
2. Zinner, N. R.: Clean Inside and Out (Correspondence), *New Engl. J. Med.* 281:853, 1969.
3. Wilson, R. S. and Kabat, H. F.: Pharmacist Initiated Patient Drug Histories, *Amer. J. Hosp. Pharm.* 28:49–53 (Jan.) 1971.
4. Yim, M. K.: Drug Hypersensitivities of Hospitalized Patients, Thesis for Master of Science in hospital pharmacy at Jefferson Medical College Hospital (May) 1967.
5. Covington, T. R. and Whitney, H. A. K.: Patient Pharmacist Communication Techniques, *Drug Intel. Clin. Pharm.* 5:370–376 (Nov.) 1971.
6. Symmers, W. S.: Curiosa and Exotica—How Many Have You Been Taking?, *Brit. Med. J.* 4:767 (Dec. 26) 1970.

7. Roth, H. P. et al.: Measuring Intake of a Prescribed Medication, *Clin. Pharmacol. Therap.* 11:228–237 (Mar.–Apr.) 1970.
8. Anon.: Deja Vue (Editorial), *Arch. Envir. Health* 20:449 (Apr.) 1970.
9. Anon.: Keep on Taking the Tablets . . . , *Lancet* 2:195–196 (July 25) 1970.
10. Brands, A. J.: Complete Directions for Prescription Medication, *J. Amer. Pharm. Ass. NS* 7:634–635 (Dec.) 1967.
11. Vreugdenhil, P. P.: Patient, Pharmacist, Physician, Prescription. *Can. Pharm. J.* 9:18–21 (Jan.) 1970.

Related Reading in this Volume

Reading for a Broader Perspective

1. Covington, T. R. "Interviewing and Advising the Patient," In Francke, D. E., and Whitney, H. A. K., Jr. *Perspectives in Clinical Pharmacy* (1st ed.). Hamilton, Ill.: Drug Intelligence Publications, 1972. pp. 212–227.

DRUG THERAPY ADVISER

22—How Pharmacists Use their Drug Knowledge to Help Doctors

Your training as a drug expert makes you an invaluable reference source for physicians. But how can you *best* use your knowledge to serve both physicians and their patients? What kinds of drug-related information do physicians most often lack? And what are the circumstances that prompt pharmacists to approach doctors and suggest a change in the prescribed therapy?

These are among the questions that were answered by the pharmacists who responded to a recent national spotcheck conducted by PHARMACY TIMES magazine.

Types of Information

Our respondents indicated that they most often contact physicians to provide information on drug interactions and contraindications, possible alternatives designed to improve therapy, correct dosage instructions, generic drug names, and drug costs.

A physician will sometimes prescribe a drug product for a patient who is allergic to one of the product's ingredients. Or, a physician might not be aware of *all* the drugs (both Rx and OTC) that the patient is taking. Another error involves physicians prescribing a dosage that is much more than the recommended dosage. Pharmacists also noted that doctors often lack knowledge of drug costs.

Specific Examples

In our letter to pharmacists, PHARMACY TIMÉS asked respondents to cite specific examples in which their recommendations convinced physicians to change the prescribed therapy. The following letters are representative of those PHARMACY TIMES received:

"At least once or twice a month, a physician will prescribe medication for a patient on whom we have a patient profile card, and the card will indicate a potential interaction. A frequent example involves tranquilizer medication prescribed for use by diabetics.

"I have repeatedly warned doctors not to give dosage instructions as '1 tablespoon-ful' for medication, such as theophylline. I encourage them to prescribe 15 cc, so that the patient will ask the pharmacist what '15 cc' means. (We provide medication measures with the cc *specifically* indicated for our patrons.)"

RALPH T. MARTINEZ, JR., R.Ph.
Wilshire Apothecary
Tucson, Arizona

"We had a situation where a physician called in for his patient the following prescriptions: Tetracycline and Hycodan syrup.

"Upon checking our profile card for this particular patient, we learned that she was suffering from glaucoma—for which Hycodan is contraindicated.

"We called the physician, of course, and he then ordered Benylin instead of the Hycodan.

"But Benylin is *also* contraindicated for glaucoma patients. So we suggested a product in the Robitussin family to the physician, and he selected Robitussin DM. The physician was grateful to us, and he expressed his thanks accordingly."

A. MICHAELS, R. Ph.
Lexington Apothecary
New York, New York

"I have convinced several physicians to change from prescribing the newer tetracycline analogs back to tetracycline HCl for two reasons—fewer side effects and a lower price to the patient."

PEOPLES PHARMACY
Murfreesborro, Arkansas

"In one case, the prescribing MD was attempting to prescribe generically, but he was confused about the drug's generic name. It was obvious that he had made an error in drug nomenclature, and I was able to tell him the drug's proper name."

APOTHECARY SHOP
Lakeville, Connecticut

"In one instance, a physician prescribed Donnagel-PG for a patient with glaucoma. We phoned the physician and told him that the drug contained belladonna alkaloids, and we reminded him of the patient's glaucoma. He changed the medication for the patient.

"Another physician prescribed Elixophyllin Liquid for a patient on Antabuse. The patient was getting the Antabuse from a local mental health center, and the prescribing physician was not aware of this. When we alerted him to this fact, he switched the prescription to an alcohol-free bronchodilator.

"We have caught many cases of prescriptions for medications which the patient was allergic to. For example, one patient who was allergic to sulfa had a prescription for AVC Vaginal Cream. We called the physician, and he prescribed something else for the patient. The doctor thanked us for the suggestion."

JAMES BENNETT, FACA
James Bennett Apothecary
Corinth, Mississippi

"I suggested to an oral surgeon that he use erythromycin stearate in place of the estolate, because of possible problems.

"In another case, I suggested to a physician that he prescribe colchicine 1/100 every hour until nausea or diarrhea develops, instead of one tablet t.i.d."

DONALD P. REITER, R.Ph.
Joliet Prescription Shops
Joliet, Illinois

"A doctor prescribed Tylenol #3 for a patient who was allergic to codeine. I suggested that the Rx be changed to Dilaudid, and the physician agreed.

"A patient with nocturnal leg cramps claimed little relief from quinine sulfate, so I informed the physician that Benadryl had been reported to help leg cramps."

WASHINGTON CLINIC PHARMACY
Washington, D.C.

"A physician prescribed Naprosyn, 2 tablets t.i.d. When I told him that the recommended dosage was one b.i.d., he changed the prescription to Tolectin, 2 tablets t.i.d.

"Carelessness in prescription writing is increasing—unfortunately."

SADLER APOTHECARY
Clinton, South Carolina

"We are consultants to a nursing home. A patient there was on Mellaril therapy for restlessness. The therapy wasn't completely effective, so the physician changed her to Trilafon—with no improvement. We were asked to suggest an alternative therapy. Upon questioning the nurse, we found that the patient suffered from Parkinsonism. We suggested a phenothiazine and Valium."

BOWMAN PHARMACY
Portland, Oregon

Related Readings in This Volume

25. Clinical Pharmacy on Oncologic Service
33. Pharmacy at the City of Hope
34. Pharmacy in Clinical Community Mental Health Center
41. Retail Pharmacy

45. Standards for Pharmacies in Institutions
48. Geriatric Practice
50. Pharmacies in Rural Areas

Readings for a Broader Perspective

1. Oksas, R. M. "How You Can Consult with Dentists Regarding Prescribing," *Pharmacy Times* 42 (July 1976):46–49.
2. Briggs, G. G., and Smith, W. E. "Pharmacist-Physician Drug Consultations in a Community Hospital," *American Journal of Hospital Pharmacy* 31 (March 1974):247–53.

PATIENT COUNSELING

23—Counseling Encounters, a Facet of 24-Hour Consultation Service by a Community Pharmacist

Max Stollman

"Clinical pharmacy," which might be referred to more appropriately as "patient-oriented pharmacy," is what many community pharmacists practice every day. Some pharmacy schools have oriented students toward the long-term care facility as the place to fulfill the patient/pharmacist relationship. But community pharmacists see their patients over longer periods of time and have far more opportunities to prevent or help mitigate the diseases and illnesses of their patients. The consultation process, enhanced by effective "counseling encounters," is the major ingredient of quality professional care by community pharmacists.

As a community pharmacist, I offer 24-hour emergency consultation. This practice has encouraged patients needing self-care guidance or prescription service to seek me out. Some consultations are complex and place the pharmacist in a counseling posture. The step-by-step progression from customary and usual advice to the counseling encounters which certain situations necessitate, is illustrated by the following hypothetical consultation.

The pharmacist who dispenses a new prescription and tells the patient, "Now be sure to take one tablet daily to control your blood pressure," is not involved in a counseling encounter. But when the pharmacist asks, "How are you about taking medicine? Do you remember to do it as ordered, every day, or do you skip doses?" we have the genesis of a counseling encounter. If the patient replies, "Oh, I'm terrible about taking pills. I always forget," we now have a command performance situation that calls for a counseling encounter. The pharmacist brings out one of those calendar date books that greeting card companies use for promotionals. While the patient looks on, the pharmacist draws a circle around the appropriate day of the week to represent each dose of medicine. The patient is asked to check off each dose as it is taken and to bring the calendar back for inspection when a refill is needed. This is a counseling encounter.

For the purpose of this paper the following definition is offered: A counseling encounter is that aspect of consultation, in the provision of quality professional health care, that requires immediate, energetic, and/or bold activity by the health professional to protect the health of the patient(s) and/or those affected by the patient(s) from significant adverse effect and/or to overcome a deterrent that might otherwise inhibit effective necessary therapy. This definition is applied to the following case histories.

Case Histories

Patient A. Some problems may be solved quite simply. Patient A represented the noncompliant patient pharmacists find out about when they check refill dates against dosage regimen. He was a young man with serious congenital heart disease for which quinidine (Q.I.D.) and digoxin (once daily) were ordered. A personalized checkoff sheet was prepared and given to him. He was instructed to check off each dose and bring the sheet in with each refill. The compliance rate rose with each refill. We both made a game of it, and he reached 95% just before he moved out of state.

Patient B. Pharmacists should be prepared to deal with highly unusual counseling requirements. Patient B was a male-to-female transsexual, approximately 35 years old, who was experiencing both physiological and psychological difficulties. I first met her when she came to my pharmacy with a vaginal dilator prescription. Our counseling encounter disclosed that fear of being rejected as a woman was aggravated by the justifiable concern that her surgically created vaginal orifice was closing.

Although Patient B had received some counseling before and after her operation, she felt that it had been deficient. I gave her the name of a counselor/psychiatrist group that treats homosexuals exclusively. One of the counselors called me to say that she had seen Patient B but could not accept her as a patient because she was not homosexual. She had given Patient B the name of a contact person for a group of transsexuals. Unfortunately, Patient B never consulted with this group.

Our next encounter took place when Patient B dropped by on her way to a doctor who was going to enlarge the vaginal orifice. I had heard of the doctor; it was common knowledge among health care professionals that the man was a charlatan who provided poor cosmetic surgery. I even called the Department of Reconstructive Surgery at the University of California at Los Angeles to prove that the doctor was not qualified. After some discussion I dissuaded Patient B from going to his office.

In the course of our patient/pharmacist relationship I became deeply concerned about Patient B's personal life and continued to urge her to seek professional psychiatric guidance in resolving her conflicts.

Patient C. To be effective, the consultation must be thorough. Solving Patient C's problem required persistence. Patient C was a 69-year-old diabetic with arthritis. She bought regular and NPH insulin from me only sporadically because she could buy it more inexpensively elsewhere. When I asked her how many units of each she used, she complained that the doctor kept changing the doses. I asked her how she gave herself the injections, and she explained that she mixed the two insulins together in one syringe. I was not satisfied with her explanation and asked her to bring all of her supplies to the pharmacy so that I could observe her giving herself the injection. That is how I discovered the reason for her erratic insulin demand.

Her fingers were affected by the arthritis, and she had difficulty in manipulating the syringe. The procedure was complicated: she had to pump air into one vial, draw out insulin, withdraw the syringe, pull the plunger of the syringe to pull in air, put the needle into the second vial, add air, and withdraw the required amount of insulin. But what was really happening was that the contents of the syringe from the first vial were being added to the second vial, and then the total amount of insulin needed was being withdrawn from the second vial, whose potency was compromised with each day's injection.

I called Patient C's physician and told him the problem; he agreed to my preparing a mixture of the two insulins in the proper proportions. I supervised each dose at the pharmacy, and the patient's insulin demand stabilized quickly. Arrangements were then made to have a neighbor give the injections from a bulk mixture that I prepared as needed.

Patient D. Some counseling encounters involve the pharmacist in intimate discussions. The pharmacist should always project a demeanor that does not discourage such consultations.

Patient D had been married at 18 and divorced at 19. At age 22 she decided to "get off the pill" and presented a prescription order for a diaphragm. I showed her the literature that came with the diaphragm kit, went over the details, and answered her questions.

That weekend I attended a 2-day seminar sponsored by the California Pharmaceutical Association (CPhA) on "Human Sexuality, Family Planning, and Venereal Disease." The discussion on diaphragm use included the suggestion that women be encouraged to insert the diaphragm each evening whether or not coitus was contemplated. This routine would help them feel more secure because of the proficiency gained from numerous insertions, and the prior insertion would not detract from the spontaneity of the act of coitus, were it to take place.

A few days later, Patient D was complaining that she was afraid to use the diaphragm because she did not have a regular boyfriend, she "just couldn't stop in the middle of everything" to insert the diaphragm, and she would not insert it correctly because of her nervousness. I told her about the CPhA seminar and suggested regular insertion nightly to help her feel secure and comfortable. She later reported that this was a wonderful suggestion and that she now felt very secure about herself. I now suggest this method of use for every patient who receives a diaphragm for the first time.

Patient E. The pharmacist must always be alert to the possibility of drug misuse or abuse. Patient E called the first time on a holiday when the pharmacy was closed. She had just been released from a small hospital where she had had minor surgery. I called her surgeon, who ordered chloral hydrate elixir and Butisol Sodium (butabarbital sodium) tablets. Delivering the medications to the residence gave me an opportunity to meet the patient. She was 37, lived with her mother in the family mansion, had been divorced three times, and had had a complete hysterectomy (against her better judgment, she claimed) because her ex-husband, a physician, had insisted.

I sensed that the patient had emotional problems she was not handling well. Her conversation drifted back and forth from past to present and back again. I had some doubt about leaving a pint of chloral hydrate and 100 Butisol Sodium tablets.

Two days later, Patient E called for more chloral hydrate. I called the surgeon and attempted a heart-to-heart talk. He said that she was psychotic so he wanted the chloral hydrate diluted in half to be on the safe side. I told him that I could do that, but the patient would probably take twice as much. He wanted it done his way.

A day later the patient called for another pint. I told the surgeon that I wanted to "level" with the patient and establish a controlled situation that would allow a slow, programmed reduction of the chloral hydrate and barbiturate use. The surgeon referred me to the family physician, who agreed to "any program that would help his patient."

I went to see the patient, and we agreed to a psychological game in which I would prepare daily allotments of medications in vials and seal them in small bags. A weekly fee was charged for the service. Under no circumstances was the patient to secure medication from any other source. I also suggested to the patient that she seek professional care about some of her problems, although she never took my advice. With the daily allotment method we were successful in reducing her use of drugs. I kept telling her that I would be pleased when she would no longer need me as her pharmacist. She would joke and say that I was the most expensive pharmacist but the cheapest psychiatrist.

Patient F. Professional courtesy among health care specialists may be instrumental in a successful counseling encounter. Patient F was referred to me by a fellow pharmacist who sensed her need for counseling.

Patient F was a heavy smoker with congestive heart failure, diabetes (requiring insulin), and a "touch" of emphysema. She called from her hospital room to ask me to see her. Her pharmacist had told her about our Succesful Temporary Nonsmoker service. I explained that she would have to secure permission from the hospital and

from her doctor. She did so, and we scheduled a 1-hour visit.

When I arrived, she told me that she had had an insulin reaction the night before but she wanted me to go through with the program. Her physician came in to urge me to stay and help his patient. During the visit I stopped twice because the patient was not feeling well.

In the last part of the program the patient must place the cigarettes in the pharmacist's Successful Temporary Nonsmoker Bank. Patient F put the cigarettes in, but as I was about to leave, she changed her mind. I gave them to her and urged her to think of herself as being a success because she had really tried. I felt that I was the one who had failed, but 2 weeks later when I called her, she claimed that she had gone instantly from her usual three packs per day to one fourth of a pack. Sometimes our success is measurable only by comparison.

Patient G. Occasionally, the pharmacist even loses business when a patient's problem is solved. Patient G was 64; a childhood rheumatic fever attack had left him with a recurring gum infection that manifested itself by an exudate and gave him a "bad taste." For years, his physician had been prescribing antibiotics every time the infection flared up.

Instead of acquiescing to this infection/ antibiotic/infection cycle, I persuaded Patient G to see a periodontist who would treat the source of the infection. The patient's use of antibiotics will lessen, but he will enjoy better health as a result of our encounter.

Counseling Techniques

All these case histories exemplify situations that face many pharmacists. To deal with them successfully, pharmacists must provide a suitable environment and behave in a way that encourages counseling encounters. I have found certain techniques to be effective in patient consultations.

Patient/pharmacist contact. As one of the many pharmacists who practice in an environment that commingles professional services with numerous other nonprofessional business activities, I do not have a private consultation room. I have found that the most effective consultation takes place when I am seated next to or facing the patient, with no desk or table in between. The full view of the patient's body allows better observation of body language and nonverbal communication. Occasionally, for maximum privacy, I request other patients to leave the immediate area until I finish a particular consultation.

To this day I am still trying to improve the skill that enables me to talk to patients about their problems without offending them. This is not always possible. One must be bold when it is necessary, and this involves the calculated risk of offending the patient. More than once I have been discouraged by my inability to find a tactful approach. Naturally, I am encouraged when patients admit that they have a problem and ask for help. But some patients are just as bold about speaking up and in so many words tell me to mind my own business.

Personal commitment. Instead of having members of my staff deal with new patients, I receive new prescription orders directly. During the initial interview I assess the patient's complaint and try to find out whether an immediate dose is needed. I even keep a bottle of milk on hand for medications requiring food or milk. Patients are impressed by a pharmacist who is concerned enough to offer the first dose right away, before the prescription is even filled. Then I personally hand the completed prescription to the patient, review the dosage regimen, and answer questions.

Patient drug file. To keep track of patient medication, I use a folder for storing prescriptions. Each folder receives an account number (I use the patient's address, but any suitable system could be devised). When I explain my filing procedure to patients, they feel that I am concerned about their health.

Professional consultation. While I am consulting with new patients, I try to observe any disease syndromes or problems (twitches, suspicious growths, poorly fitting dentures) or detrimental habits (smoking or nail-biting). I look into their eyes and check clothes, hands, and even purses for clues.

I explain that my 24-hour consultation service means just that: patients may call at any time to discuss medical or health problems. I have a "beeper" that will find me anywhere within a given area. If I am out of town, my answering service refers patients to another pharmacist.

When business is too heavy for a consultation or when I need time to research a problem, I suggest a suitable time (usually in the morning) for the patient to return. Pharmacists should structure their practice to allow for consultation "hours."

Conclusions

I have set forth some of my personal experiences and some of the techniques that I use in dealing with them. Counseling encounters are as much a part of the community pharmacist's business as dispensing medicine. To encourage patients to consult with us, we should emphasize the pharmacist (a person) rather than the pharmacy (an institution). The CPhA is working toward that image by changing its name to the California Pharmacists Association.

Another point that pharmacists as professional health consultants should consider is the financial implication of providing this service. What does it cost to sit with a patient for a 5-minute consultation? Can the prescription fee cover more than a cursory consultation? If quality professional care requires the pharmacist to curtail the sale of other more conventional commodities, is there a subsequent loss of income that must be offset by a consultation fee? Pharmacists have traditionally provided consultation without fee, but are we not ready to re-evaluate this "tradition"? Should we not be paid for the knowledge we possess, for our ability to store and retrieve information, and for our contribution to quality health care provision? Do the questions about economics prompt other questions about moral, ethical, and legal considerations? All of these topics are worthy of consideration for future papers by pharmacists.

24—Compliance and Pharmacists

James M. McKenney

Noncompliance with medical regimens is undoubtedly one of the major unsolved health problems facing pharmacists, physicians and other health care providers today. Regardless of the particular patient group, at least 30 percent and quite often 50 percent or more of patients fail to comply with physicians' orders. This quite naturally has a major impact on health care delivery. It makes little difference how sophisticated or appropriate patient care resources or facilities are, how much expertise physicians put into their diagnosis of a medical problem or how much care pharmacists put into their services if patients do not take the medication as prescribed. This not only deprives the patients of the benefits of therapy, but also may mean that additional medical care will be needed. Thus a further wasteful expenditure of already over-taxed health resources will be required because the medical problem was not solved or adequately controlled.

Why Don't Patients Comply?

At first glance, noncompliance may appear to be a rather simple problem. For example, many practitioners see noncompliance as simply an informational problem; that is, patients do not comply because they have not been given the information about their disease or drug therapy that they need in order to comply. It is true that patients are often deprived of important health information. However, providing it does not necessarily mean that the noncompliance problem will be solved. In this case, knowing does not necessarily mean doing. Many pharmacy students have been given information in the classroom but have failed to correctly use it in a patient care setting. While providing health information is important, it alone is not going to solve the problem.

Some practitioners consider noncompliance to be a phenomenon primarily affecting the poor, indigent and illiterate. However, the rich, healthy and educated are just as likely to be noncompliant. In fact, none of the more than 100 studies on this subject during the past 40 years has been able to clearly establish any consistent socioeconomic, demographic or educational characteristics of noncompliant patients.

To understand noncompliance is to understand patient behavior and that, frankly, is not understood in total by anyone. Why any of us behave the way we do is the result of all the influences in our individual environments. For the noncompliant patient, that environment consists of, among other things, the health care delivery system, health providers, drug regimens, the patient's social and family relationships and the patient's own perceptions and attitudes of illnesses and drugs. No one influencing factor determines compliance; but, to varying degrees, all of them do.

Even though compliant behavior is complex, it is also learned. No patient comes to the health provider with experience in taking potent drugs for unfamiliar medical problems according to a rigid schedule that interferes with a normal daily life style; and, not infrequently, produces adverse effects. This behavior must be learned and that is where the health care provider can make a contribution.

An approach that has the best chance of solving the noncompliance problem involves addressing those factors in the patient's environment that make it difficult to comply and thereby creating a new environment in which the patient will be more willing or able to learn to follow drug use directions approximately. With this approach, health professionals are obligated, at least professionally if not ethically and morally, to examine those services within their sphere of responsibility to insure that patients are given the best possible chance of complying and thereby receiving the maximal benefit from therapy. For the pharmacist, this does not necessarily mean that specific services need to be pulled from a "bag of tricks" when a noncompliant patient is detected. Instead, experience strongly suggests that certain basic services considered a minimal part of any good pharmacy practice can have a dramatic impact on the noncompliance problem and should be offered routinely. Some of these services are considered below.

How Can the Pharmacist Measure Compliance?

Before any services designed to improve patient compliance can be offered, it is important that we be able to detect the noncompliant patient. Since pharmacists often have more frequent contact with patients returning for prescription refills than do other health care providers, they are in a unique position to measure patient compliance. In addition, pharmacists have at their disposal several specific, readily accessible, non-invasive methods of measurement which are of sufficient sensitivity to identify most noncompliances. Two of these measures are the drug history and the patient medication profile.

Pharmacists should, as a routine part of their practice, inquire about the drug use patterns of patients. Part of this inquiry should deal with the patient's compliance. This is accomplished best not by direct questions such as, "Have you taken your medication as you were directed?" but by indirect questioning such as: "Tell me exactly how you took X medication yesterday," or "During the past three days, how many doses of X medication have you taken?" or "What do you do when you miss a dose?"

Unfortunately, when compared with pill counts or blood levels of drugs, this method of estimating patient compliance is one of the least accurate. However, the quality of the inquiry should significantly improve the accuracy of the measurement. Also, studies have shown that when patients do admit noncompliance, you can be reasonably certain that this is accurate (Pack, L. C. and Lipman, R. S.: "A comparison of patient dosage deviation reports with pill counts," *Psychopharmacologia*, 6:299–302, 1964).

Pharmacists should also routinely review the patient's medication profile for compliance. With the basic information contained in this profile, the pharmacist can use the prescribed dosing schedule and quantity dispensed to the patient to project when patients should return for a prescription refill or compare the quantity of drugs dispensed with what should have been consumed, thereby estimating compliance. This method of measuring compliance is readily accessible, inexpensive and more accurate than the drug history. It is also particularly valuable for measuring compliance of chronically ill patients who return routinely for prescription refills.

How Can the Pharmacist Improve Compliance?

As the provider of the product for which compliance is such a problem, the pharmacist is in a unique position to provide services to improve compliance. This doesn't mean that the problem rests with the pharmacist alone. Rather, it recognizes that only at this one point in the normal delivery of care in the community will the patient, the product and the professional come together when services to improve compliance can be offered. These services, as mentioned previously, should be routine among pharmacists.

Drug Regimen

The pharmacist should discourage the use of unnecessary nonprescription drugs and encourage simple drug regimens. It is clear that the greater the number of doses per day or total number of drugs in the regimen, the less likely patients are to comply. While pharmacists are not responsible for prescribing drugs, they are often consulted on the use of nonprescription drugs. They can encourage compliance by discouraging the use of unnecessary agents. Because pharmacists maintain patient medication profiles, they are often the only health professionals aware of patients' total drug regimens. With this

perspective, pharmacists consult with prescribers when drug regimen problems are uncovered.

Practice Setting

The pharmacist should improve the image of the practice setting in order to change the patient's expectations and improve compliance. It is very difficult to determine just what influence the image of pharmacists and their environment has on the way patients comply with medications. However, at least one recent study (Ludy, A. J.; Gagnon, J. P.; and Caiola, S. M.: "The patient-pharmacist interaction in two ambulatory settings," *Drug Intell Clin Pharm*, 11:81–89, 1977) strongly suggests that providing patient-oriented pharmacy services in a private consultation room instead of through an open window can have a significant impact on patient satisfaction with services and on compliant behavior.

Time

The pharmacist should organize a dispensing procedure that is time-efficient. Even the hardiest of patients may be discouraged from having their prescriptions filled initially or returning as needed for prescription refills if they are required to wait an inordinate amount of time for these services. To lessen this problem, it is important that a well-organized dispensing system and the proper use of technical assistants be developed and maintained.

Costs

The pharmacist should help keep drug costs down. Drug costs are clearly a barrier to some patients and interfere with compliance to some extent in many patients. Unfortunately, many of the determinants of drug costs are beyond pharmacist control. However, encouraging generic prescribing, when appropriate, and knowing community resources that may aid patients unable to afford prescriptions are certainly possible pharmacist actions.

Prescription Labels

The pharmacist should provide a prescription label with explicit instructions including a clear administration schedule and indication.

Far too often the prescription label is incomplete and is the immediate source of misunderstanding by the patient as to how the medication is to be taken. Unfortunately, the prescription label is often a function of the written prescription, which is also incomplete. As a part of their professional responsibility, pharmacists should assure that prescription label directions are clear, complete and as explicit as possible.

Patient Education

The pharmacist should supply patients with information on which to form correct beliefs. Behavioral scientists have suggested that certain health beliefs affect patient compliance. Their health belief model, simply defined, suggests that patients will be more willing to comply if:

* they perceive a susceptibility to the disease;
* they perceive a threat from the disease; and
* they perceive a benefit from prescribed therapy that outweighs any perceived or actual barriers (i.e., drug costs, side effects and complex regimen).

Pharmacists should address each of these precepts in the instructional process and provide the reinforcement needed for patients to adopt correct beliefs.

Pharmacists should also supply explicit information to patients regarding drug regimens so patients clearly understand what is expected and what to expect. Even though compliance is a learned behavior, it begins with a cognitive (informational) stage. Patients must first be taught how to take medications correctly and why taking them as directed is important. This information should be explicit and relate to the precise information patients need to take their medications. The following items, for example, should be reviewed with patients when applicable:

* Drug name.
* Intended use and expected action.
* Route, dosage form, dosage and administration schedule.
* Special directions for preparation.
* Special directions for administration.
* Precautions to be observed during administration.
* Common side effects—their avoidance and action required if they occur.
* Techniques of self-monitoring.
* Proper storage.
* Potential drug-drug/food interactions.
* Prescription refill information.
* Action to be taken in the event of a missed dose.
* Information peculiar to a specific patient or drug.

This information should be given verbally and, when possible, reinforced with written instructions or audiovisual programs.

The pharmacist should learn to be an effective communicator. Not only is the particular message content important. A good counsellor uses effective communication to establish a relationship with the patient that engenders trust and confidence and that ultimately fosters patient compliance. The counsellor specifically avoids confrontation, tension, attempts to "control" the patient or other factors known to impair the relationship with the patient. Communication should be clear, explicit, reinforcing and two-way; the basic attitude is one of concern and compassion, freely providing feedback to the patient after information has been solicited.

The pharmacist should consistently communicate to each patient: friendliness, authority, and responsiveness to patient compliance or admissions of noncompliance. The pharmacist should give justification or rationale for medication taking with an emphasis on what is expected from taking medication, while trying to learn the patient's medication-taking habits. In a recent study (Svarstad, B. L.: "Physician-patient communication and patient conformity with medical advice," in *The Growth of Bureaucratic Medicines: An Inquiry Into the Dynamic of Patient Behavior and the Organization of Medical Care*, Edited by D. Mechanic, pp. 220–238, John Wiley & Sons, New York, 1976), each of these elements of communication was associated with improved compliance. All of them, when provided with explicit instruction, were present when the vast majority of patients were compliant. This evidence strongly suggests that, in terms of patient compliance, how we communicate is as important as what we communicate.

Monitoring

The pharmacist should solicit feedback from patients on response, compliance, side effects and drug use problems and provide methods for patients to adapt to these findings through tailoring, goal setting, explanation, recommendation and/or referral. Compliance is improved if practitioners solicit (as well as allow) patient descriptions of their drug therapy problems and concerns during each return visit. This not only uncovers bar-

riers to full compliance but demonstrates interest and concern on the part of the health providers. Once this information has been uncovered, it is vitally important to continued compliance for the practitioner to offer ways patients may deal with these problems. Some ways to respond to these problems may be to:

- develop a specific dosing schedule tailored to daily activities (i.e. brushing teeth) for patients with complex regimens;
- select a goal patients can follow routinely to demonstrate drug benefit;
- explain the origins or characteristics of the problem;
- clarify misconceptions;
- provide reassurance of the benign or self-limiting nature of a side effect;
- recommend ways to specifically correct detected problems; or
- refer the patient to the physician for diagnosis and management.

Even if the above services are made routinely available by pharmacists, there will remain a group of patients of undeterminable—but probably small—size who will continue to be noncompliant with prescribed regimens. The reasons for this noncompliance will vary from forgetfulness to deliberate rejection of the therapy. For these problems, some of the following special services tailored to meet the individual patient's needs may be offered.

Patients who are noncompliant because they dislike taking medications, fear their consequences or are not convinced of their efficacy may benefit from routine interaction with a group of patients with similar diagnosis or drug therapy where peer support and encouragement may be provided. Groups are more likely to succeed if:

- there is a common ground for participation;

- there are officers, scheduled meetings and programmed activities, similar to other organizations;
- meetings are held in a group member's home; and
- health providers participate only as advisors to the group.

There are patients who are noncompliant because they have a pessimistic outlook on their prognosis or the efficacy of their therapy. These "Tarzan-types" who ignore their own vulnerability to their disease or deny therapy to punish themselves or gain attention may benefit from the support or supervision of family members. Pharmacists can describe to family members the nature of the medical problem and what precise steps should be taken by the patient in order to prevent problems.

Noncompliance is a complex behavioral problem that is at least strongly influenced, if not caused by, a complicated, sometimes unresponsive, impersonal and busy health care delivery system. However, it is likewise a function of the regimen, the patient and the illness. Thus, the solution of the noncompliance problem does not rest in changing any one of these factors. Rather, the solution requires a mutual recognition of and response to the problem by all health providers, each of whom is sensitive to the needs of patients and makes a concerted effort to routinely offer quality services. For pharmacists, this means routinely:

- providing verbal and written explicit instructions on how medications are to be taken;

- measuring patient compliance;
- reinforcing explicit instructions and motivation to comply;
- soliciting feedback on problems and providing appropriate solutions; and
- showing interest and concern.

Related Readings in This Volume

1. Comprehensive Pharmacy Services
7. Pharmacist and Family Planning
12. Pharmacist and Preventive Medicine
15. Self-Medication
16. Over-the-Counter Medications
32. Pharmacist and Hyperalimentation Programs
34. Pharmacy in Clinical Community Mental Health
41. Retail Pharmacy
50. Pharmacies in Rural Areas

Readings for a Broader Perspective

1. Hood, R. L. "Why There Are Many Different Facets to Counseling Patients," *Pharmacy Times* 43 (November 1977):41–45.
2. O'Hara, G. L., and Sperandio, G. J. "Patient Education for Better Compliance," *The Apothecary* 89 (May/June 1977):18–21, 62.
3. Coutts, K. W. "How We Promote Patient Compliance with Drug Therapy," *Pharmacy Times* 43 (November 1977):66–74.
4. Conte, R. "Provider's Prescription, Patient's Problem," *California Pharmacist* 25 (June 1978):18–21.
5. Hussar, D. A. "Optimizing Drug Therapy—The Patient's Need to Know," *American Journal of Pharmacy* 149 (May/June 1977): 65–74.
6. Covington, T. R., and Whitney, H. A. K. "Patient-Pharmacist Communication Techniques," *Drug Intelligence & Clinical Pharmacy* 5 (November 1971):370–76.

THERAPEUTIC MONITORING

25—Prescription 'Errors' Should Not Occur

Khairy W. Malek

According to a survey published in *The New York Times*,* "30,000 Americans accept the drugs prescribed for them and die as a direct result. Perhaps 10 times as many patients suffer life-threatening and sometimes permanent side effects such as kidney failure, mental depression, internal bleeding, and loss of hearing or vision. These figures are among the more conservative to be found in studies of the prescription drug problem by the medical profession itself."

There are many reasons for these frightening data, reasons which impose a heavy responsibility on health professionals to find a means of minimizing patient injuries. Some of the factors contributing to prescription errors are:

• The vast number of drugs on the market—most have potential side effects and drug interactions with which not all physicians are familiar;

• Errors in interpretation of physician's orders and dispensing of drugs by nonpharmacists in many hospitals;

• Defensive medicine and overprescribing of drugs;

• Failure on the part of some pharmacists to keep up with the scientific literature;

The pharmacy profession can do much more than it is doing now to alleviate the problem. Some suggestions are:

• The present pharmacy curriculum should be increased from five to six years nationwide. Greater emphasis should be placed on pharmacology, drug interactions and side effects. In addition, some basic medical science courses, such as physiology, microbiology and pathology, should be expanded. Such courses would also give the pharmacist a greater understanding of package inserts and medical literature. This expanded education is particularly recommended for hospital pharmacists because of the nature of their work. Also, "for every 18 prescriptions written in a hospital, one adverse reaction occurs. Ten percent of the reactions are major and 1.2 percent are fatal," according to the *Times* survey.

• Continuous up-to-date education must be a condition for renewal of pharmacy licenses.

• There should be greater cooperation between the American Medical Association (AMA) and the American Pharmaceutical Association (APhA) in disseminating drug information to physicians and pharmacists.

Some articles have been written concerning prescription errors by nurses in interpreting physicians' orders when they recopy the

---

* "Thousands a Year Killed by Faulty Prescriptions," *The New York Times*, January 28, 1976.

orders and forward them to the hospital pharmacy. Most of the blame should be placed on hospitals which still follow this procedure, since nurses are not pharmacists.

Other errors were also attributed in part to failure by some pharmacists to take notice of obvious prescription errors before the medicine reached the patient.

Physician Prescription Errors

In this article, I shall concentrate on physicians' prescription errors. These were found relative to dose, route of administration, wrong combination of drugs, pharmacological action, or unwarranted use of certain drugs.

During my work as a hospital pharmacist, I encountered hundreds of prescription errors. Some were made by residents, but others were made by attending physicians and specialists. Although many of the errors were minor, others were major, and a few may have been fatal. All errors are documented. Since human lives and health are very precious, and since to err is human, I believe strongly in a useful role which a well-prepared pharmacist can assume as the last check before the medicine is dispensed. This can be done by rendering intelligent advice, and wise discussion with the prescriber after first consulting all references at hand so as to avoid disturbing him or her for imaginary mistakes.

Sample Errors

The following are some of the errors encountered:

• Order for Pro-Banthine, Maalox and Indocin capsules. The combination of Pro-Banthine and Maalox made me suspect a peptic ulcer. By checking the diagnosis, it was found to be a duodenal ulcer. The pre-scriber was contacted and advised about the dangerous possibility of massive hemorrhage with Indocin for peptic ulcer patients. He was very grateful and canceled the Indocin immediately.

• Order for Chloromycetin suspension for a two-month-old child. I informed the physician about the possibility of a fatal "grey syndrome" from Chloromycetin at this age. She said the child had diarrhea and changed the order to Kaopectate.

• Order for acetic acid solution 10 percent for wound irrigation. I informed the doctor that this concentration is very irritating and that the strength usually used for this purpose is ½–1 percent. He changed the order to a one percent solution.

• Order for Kantrex injections, ½ g every six hours. The doctor was informed that the maximum dose is 1½ g daily and should not be exceeded specifically for this drug. He reduced the dose from 2 to 1 g daily.

• Order for Kantrex capsules 500 mg, four times daily. I knew that the patient had burns and asked the nurse to check if the patient had any intestinal problems. The answer was negative; consequently, I informed the physician that Kantrex cannot be used as a systemic antibiotic orally since it is not absorbed from the intestines and its effect there is local. He asked me to cancel the order.

• A nurse from the intensive care unit came to the pharmacy asking for 6 g neomycin for daily intramuscular injections (1 g every four hours). I told her that neomycin is very rarely given by injection and if so the maximum dose would be 1½ g. I also advised her that 6 g daily could be fatal. She advised that she had been at the pharmacy the day before and had asked another pharmacist for the drug. This pharmacist also thought the dose was high and called the patient's physician, who insisted on the dose as ordered.

The pharmacist dispensed the neomycin injections to the nurse, who then gave the patient 1 g every four hours intramuscularly. From the combination of drugs ordered, I understood that the patient probably had cirrhosis of the liver. This condition was confirmed by checking the file. I phoned the physician, who said that he was following the treatment ordered by an internist.

In checking the chart, it was found that the internist had written "neomycin 1 g every four hours" without specifying the route of administration. I informed the internist that it was my understanding that in a case of cirrhosis of the liver neomycin is prescribed *orally* to reduce ammonia formation in the intestine, and he said "That is obvious." I also advised him that the patient's family physician had ordered it as an injection and that it had been administered to the patient for 24 hours before I refused to dispense it. He asked me if the patient was "still alive" and thanked me for saving the man's life.

• Order for Kantrex and Loridine injections together for the same patient. I advised the physician that it is not recommended that these two drugs be given at the same time since they are both nephrotoxic (the patient was 70 years old). The physician asked me to cancel the Loridine.

• Prescription for Cafergot tablets. On the prescription order form the blood pressure of the patient was recorded as 240/130. I called the resident who had written the prescription and informed him that it was dangerous and contraindicated to give Cafergot to a patient with such high blood pressure and that the patient's headache could be due to the elevated pressure. The resident said he appreciated the fact that I was aware of the contraindication, and asked me to change the order to Darvon Compound 65.

Later, a nurse came back to the pharmacy with the Darvon Compound. Since the attending physician had originally prescribed the Cafergot, she had called him about the change in order. The attending physician refused the Darvon Compound and insisted on the Cafergot. I asked the nurse to have

him phone me since I would not dispense the Cafergot to the patient under any condition. She returned to advise that the doctor had changed the order from Cafergot to "Serpasil ampule."

From these examples of prescription errors it is clear that pharmacists must take an active role in preventing the kinds of problems cited here. Patient welfare depends on the utmost skill and up-to-date continuing education when it comes to the best drug therapy.

Related Readings in This Volume

1. Comprehensive Pharmacy Services
6. Adverse Reactions
8. Monitoring Diabetic Patients
12. Pharmacist and Preventive Medicine
14. Hypertension Patients in a Community Pharmacy
24. Compliance
26. Management of Ambulatory patients
33. Clinical Pharmacy on Oncological Service
34. Pharmacy in Clinical Community Mental Health
45. Standards for Pharmacies in Institutions
46. Comprehensive Hospital Pharmacy Services
48. Geriatric Practice
49. Pharmacy Service for the Elderly

Readings for a Broader Perspective

1. Wernik, D. J. "Patient Profiles: 19 Examples of Their Value in a 7–Day Period," *Pharmacy Times* 44 (May 1978):68–72.
2. Sax, M. J., Cheung, A., Brinkman, J., and Brady, E. S. "A Systematic Approach to Drug Therapy Monitoring," *Hospital Pharmacy* 12 (April 1977):155–62.
3. O'Hara, G. L. "Patient Medication Profile Monitoring," *J. Am. Pharm. Assoc.* NS 16 (May 1976):248–49, 270.
4. McCarron, M. M. "A System of Inpatient Drug Monitoring," *Drug Intelligence & Clinical Pharmacy* 9 (February 1975):80–85.
5. Doering, P. L., and Stewart, R. B. "The Extent and Character of Drug Consumption During Pregnancy," *Journal of the American Medical Association* 239 (February 27, 1978): 843–46.

6. Solomon, D. K., Baumgartner, R. P., Glascock, L. M., Glascock, S. A., Briscoe, M. E., and Billup, N. F. "Use of Medication Profiles to Detect Potential Therapeutic Problems in Ambulatory Patients," *American Journal of Hospital Pharmacy* 31 (April 1974): 348–54.

7. Stewart, R. B., Cluff, L. E., and Philp, J. R. (eds.) *Drug Monitoring: A Requirement for Responsible Drug Use.* Baltimore: The Williams and Wilkins Co., 1977. 309 pp.

THERAPEUTIC MANAGEMENT

26—Pharmacist Management of Ambulatory Patients Using Formalized Standards of Care

Philip O. Anderson and David A. Taryle

The Indian Health Service (IHS) of the U.S. Public Health Service has been likened to a system of prototype health maintenance organizations (HMO's) in which a number of innovative services have been implemented.[1] Several pharmacy services have been developed in the IHS which may have application in other organized health care settings.

It is the purpose of this paper to discuss one of the direct patient care services provided to selected ambulatory patients by the pharmacist at the IHS hospital in Clinton, Oklahoma, from April 1972 to July 1973.

The Maintenance Care Program

The Clinton Indian Hospital is a 26-bed inpatient facility offering general medical, obstetrical and pediatric care to approximately 4,000 Cheyenne-Arapaho Indians in western Oklahoma.

During the period covered by this report, the Clinton medical staff of four physicians also maintained six smaller field clinics in addition to the inpatient and outpatient facilities at Clinton. Generally, only two physicians were at Clinton at any time during the four hours of each weekday that the outpatient clinic was open. The pharmacy was staffed by one pharmacist with part-time help provided by a pharmacy student intern. Over 10,000 patient visits per year were made to the hospital's outpatient department.

All outpatient prescriptions were dispensed directly from the patient's medical record which was organized in the problem-oriented format. The advantages of the problem-oriented record to the pharmacist and patient are many and have been discussed previously.[2]

To better serve patients with medical problems requiring the chronic use of medications, the pharmacist and physicians developed a program whereby the pharmacist may assume responsibility for the management of such patients. The medical problems included in the program are congestive heart failure, epilepsy, estrogen replacement, essential hypertension, isoniazid preventive therapy, oral contraception and thyroid replacement.

Methods of Pharmacy Involvement

There are two distinct methods by which to implement a program of maintenance care by the pharmacist. The first could be described as a "dependent" method in which the pharmacist interviews the patient, evaluates his health status and then decides to either refill the patient's medication or refer the patient to a physician. The physician must countersign the pharmacist's chart entries for legal purposes and thereby assumes responsibility for the pharmacist's actions. This system, analogous to the functioning of a medical student or a physician's assistant under the preceptorship of a physician, was used at Clinton both prior to the development of the formalized program and to some extent afterwards. Other pharmacists have successfully functioned in this manner also.[3-5]

The logistics of this method can be cumbersome in a busy outpatient clinic, however. The pharmacist must repeatedly contact the physician throughout the day for approval and countersignature of his actions, and the routine of both practitioners may become disrupted.

The second method involves delegated responsibility to the pharmacist via a set of specified protocols previously agreed upon by both physician and pharmacist. This method is analogous to the use of "standing orders" under which a nurse is allowed to perform treatment in the absence of a physician. From April 1972 to July 1973, a similar method was employed at the Clinton Indian Hospital whereby the pharmacist followed selected patients with stabilized, chronic medical problems. The patients were selected by the medical staff and assigned to the program with the patient's consent. A total of about 50 stabilized patients were assigned to the maintenance program utilizing these protocols during the period covered by this report. Examples of two of the protocols are provided in Figure 26.1.

On each pharmacy visit, the pharmacist interviews the patient, requests laboratory and clinical measurements as specified in the protocols, evaluates the data and decides whether to refill the patient's medications. Should the condition of the patient appear unstable, the pharmacist will consult a physician and a joint decision is made on the appropriate action to be taken.

The chart of each patient followed by the pharmacist is supplied with a flow sheet on which are recorded specific parameters and the patient's medications. The flow sheet, patterned after those described by Schulman and Wood,[6] is valuable in summarizing and correlating patient data, drug regimen and patient response.

Conceptually, the protocols may be considered to be the minimum standards of care which are applied to patients with certain chronic medical problems. Once the standards have been agreed upon, it remains only to be decided which providers of care are best suited to carry out the indicated functions. At our facility, the authority for actions and decisions regarding the monitoring of a patient's condition between physician visits was delegated to the pharmacist. It should be emphasized that for any particular patient, the physician may decide that the pharmacist should acquire additional data to adequately monitor the patient's status.

Furthermore, the standards of care are necessarily limited by practical considera-

Figure 26.1

Sample protocols which delineate the minimum standards applied to outpatients; time intervals for specific patients are determined by the physician and baseline data are collected by the physician at the designated intervals; monitoring data are collected on each patient visit unless otherwise stated; clinical data are obtained through the patient interview by either the physician or the pharmacist.

Definitions of Terms

Baseline Data: Information that will be collected by the physician before the patient is assigned to the protocol and as indicated on the particular protocol. The baseline data relate only to the monitoring of chronic drug therapy and does *not* attempt to define standards for any part of the patient's initial work-up.

Monitoring Data: Information that will be collected on each visit or at the specified interval by the pharmacist or physician.

Clinical Data: The pertinent clinical information which should be obtained on each visit by the physician or pharmacist through interview or observation of the patient.

PHARMACY CHRONIC CARE MONITORING
PROTOCOL—ORAL CONTRACEPTION

Physician evaluation: Every 6 to 12 months.
Pharmacist evaluation: Every 3 months.

A. Drugs possible:
   norethindrone 1 mg and mestranol 80 μg.
   norethindrone 1 mg and mestranol 50 μg.
B. Baseline data:
   Breast exam, pelvic exam and Pap smear:
      Women 35 years or under: every 12 months.
      Women over 35 years: every 6 months.
C. Monitoring data:
   1) Blood pressure.
   2) Weight.
D. Clinical data:
   1) Compliance with regimen.
   2) Breakthrough bleeding, vaginal discharges.
   3) Leg aches, calf pain, chest pain.
   4) Breast tenderness, lumps or discharge.
   5) Fluid retention or swelling.
   6) Headaches.
   7) Mood changes.
   8) Observe for jaundice.

PHARMACY CHRONIC CARE MONITORING
PROTOCOL—CONGESTIVE HEART FAILURE

Physician evaluation: Every 3 to 6 months.
Pharmacist evaluation: Every 1 to 2 months.

A. Drugs possible:
   digoxin, digitoxin, hydrochlorothiazide,
   furosemide, spironolactone, potassium chloride
   solution.
B. Baseline data:
   1) EKG, chest X-ray every year.
   2) Serum creatinine every 6 months.
C. Monitoring data:
   1) Blood pressure.
   2) Weight.
   3) Pulse and regularity.
   4) BUN every 3 months.
   5) Urinalysis every 3 months.
   6) Serum potassium every 3 months unless
      unstable; then, every month.
   7) CBC every 6 months.
   8) FBS every 6 months if on hydrochlorothiazide.
D. Clinical data:
   1) Palpitations, arrhythmias.
   2) SOB, DOE, PND, orthopnea.
   3) Nocturia.
   4) Anorexia, nausea, vomiting, diarrhea.
   5) Visual abnormalities.
   6) Muscle weakness.

tions such as laboratory capability and availability of specialized diagnostic equipment. For example, renal function is monitored via blood urea nitrogen (BUN) values with the realization that the serum creatinine level is a better index of renal function. However, in our laboratory it took the technologist about ten minutes to determine the BUN value versus about 40 minutes for the creatinine.

The protocols are quite like the minimum care criteria described by Kessner et al.,[7] except that ours are designed primarily for the application to maintenance care, whereas Kessner's are used in the initial workup and stabilization of a patient. Our experience was similar to that described by the above authors in regard to the need for flexibility, periodic revision and limitations dictated by practicality.

The use of formalized protocols by the pharmacist in the management of patients receiving long-term drug therapy was first developed in the IHS by Streit at the Cass Lake, Minnesota Indian Hospital in 1970.[8] Since then, this system has become widespread in the IHS and has been the subject of another report in the *Am. J. Hosp. Pharm.*[9] Pharmacists outside the IHS have also described similar programs utilizing formalized protocols.[10]

Although no review procedures were employed by us in conjunction with the maintenance care program at the Clinton Indian Hospital, the establishment of minimum care standards for both initial workup and maintenance care is appropriate for use with data obtained through a professional standards review organization (PSRO). Data collected by the PSRO serves as a feedback to aid in the refinement and periodic revision of the standards to insure that the standards are suited to the population being served.[7,11] Cooperative physician-pharmacist ventures in professional standards review have been undertaken elsewhere with good results.[12-15]

Success of the Program

Patients at the Clinton Indian Hospital readily accepted the pharmacist as a primary provider of health care and to our knowledge did not question his competency in this role. This acceptance was due in part to the explanation of the program to each patient when he was assigned to it. We believe that the further activities of the pharmacist are viewed by patients as a logical extension of the expanded role already played by the pharmacist in the Indian Health Service. The acceptance of a practitioner by a patient seems to be based more on the competency demonstrated by the practitioner than on the professional category into which he falls.

Acceptance of the program by physicians has been especially good. They feel that the protocols have been followed well and that the pharmacist is better utilizing his knowledge with the result that there is more rational drug use. There has been no question of the pharmacist assuming responsibility beyond that agreed upon, nor do the physicians feel in any way threatened or that their "power" is being usurped. To the contrary, it is felt that more patients could be handled in this fashion. Indeed, the concept of the pharmacist managing chronic care patients has been given approval and support by the Senior Clinician of the Indian Health Service. A three-year study is presently being performed at the Cass Lake Indian Hospital to attempt to determine the effectiveness of the pharmacist in the management of ambulatory patients using formalized protocols.

General Applicability of the Role and Implications

The role that we have outlined for the pharmacist as a provider of maintenance care is but one of many roles which a clinically-trained pharmacist is capable of performing.[16] The role would be most suitably performed in a group medical practice, HMO, rural health care delivery system or satellite facility such as a neighborhood health center. This view is consistent with the role of the pharmacist in the primary care setting of the emerging health care system as outlined by Dr. Edmund Pellegrino who sees the pharmacist as the person most responsible for proper drug therapy on a team of diverse health professionals.[17]

With the pharmacist assuming increasing responsibility for direct patient care, the question arises as to the type of practitioner that will assume the traditional drug distribution functions. In our experience at Clinton, the limiting factor in the utilization of the pharmacist in direct patient care was the pharmacist's involvement in drug distribution which was, by necessity, his top priority. We suspect that a conflict in priorities for the pharmacist's time will frequently exist when he must perform both drug distribution and direct patient care roles. Although subprofessionals can be used effectively to perform many tasks in the drug distribution process, the necessity of having a professional responsible for drug procurement, storage and distribution is undeniable. In order to use pharmacy manpower most efficiently, one is led to the conclusion that two types of pharmacy practitioners must be formally recognized by the profession. Two recent dissertations have acknowledged this necessity and have related it to a perceived need for two distinct courses of study in pharmacy: a doctoral program emphasizing the clinical use of drugs and a baccalaureate program, perhaps of less than five years, emphasizing drug distribution.[16,18]

Conclusion

As the delivery of ambulatory care becomes more organized through the formation of HMO's and similar systems, the delivery of health care through a team approach draws closer to becoming a reality. The clinically-trained pharmacist promises to make a unique contribution to patient care as a drug therapy expert. A role for the pharmacist as a provider of maintenance care to ambulatory patients is presently being developed in several settings. By establishing and applying standards of care, not only can more uniform care be provided, but

a medium is created through which the pharmacist can be integrated into the health care system and participate readily in peer review procedures.

From our experience at the Clinton Indian Hospital, we believe that a role for the pharmacist as a manager of chronic drug therapy is a viable one with considerable potential.

References

1. Johnson, E. A.: Government's Role in Hospital-Based Health Care Delivery Systems, presented at the Seventh Annual ASHP Midyear Clinical Meeting, Las Vegas, Nevada, Dec. 3–7, 1972.
2. Borgsdorf, L. R. and Mosser, R. S.: The Problem-Oriented Medical Record: An Ideal System for Pharmacist Involvement in Comprehensive Patient Care, *Amer. J. Hosp. Pharm. 30*:904–907 (Oct.) 1973.
3. Dunphy, T. W.: The Pharmacist in the Management of Chronic Disease, presented at the 119th Annual Meeting of the American Pharmaceutical Association, Houston, Texas, Apr. 22–28, 1972.
4. Miller, W. A. and Corcella, J.: New Member on the Team, *Ment. Hyg. 56*:57–61 (Spring) 1972.
5. Coleman, J. H., Evans, R. L. and Rosenbluth, S. A.: Extended Clinical Roles for the Pharmacist in Psychiatric Care, *Amer. J. Hosp. Pharm. 30*:1143–1146 (Dec.) 1973.
6. Schulman, J., Jr. and Wood, C.: Flow Sheets for Charts of Ambulatory Patients. *J. Amer. Med. Ass. 217*:933–937 (Aug. 16) 1971.
7. Kessner, D. M., Kalk, C. E. and Singer, J.: Assessing Health Quality—The Case for Tracers. *N. Engl. J. Med. 288*:189–194 (Jan. 25) 1973.
8. Streit, R. J.: Long-Term Drug Therapy—A Program Expanding the Pharmacist's Role, *J. Amer. Pharm. Ass. NS13*:434–443 (Aug.) 1973.
9. Ellinoy, B. J. et al.: A Pharmacy Outpatient Monitoring Program Providing Primary Medical Care to Selected Patients, *Amer. J. Hosp. Pharm. 30*:593–598 (July) 1973.
10. Mattei, T. J. et al.: Hypertension: A Model for Pharmacy Involvement, *Amer. J. Hosp. Pharm. 30*:683–686 (Aug.) 1973.
11. Sanazaro, P. J., Goldstein, R. L. and Roberts, J. S.: Research and Development in Quality Assurance: The Experimental Medical Care Review Organization Program, *N. Engl. J. Med. 287*:1125–1131 (Nov. 30) 1972.

12. Ellinoy, B. J., Schuster, J. S. and Yatsco, J. C.: Pharmacy Audit of Patient Health Records—Feasibility and Usefulness of a Drug Surveillance System, *Amer. J. Hosp. Pharm. 29:*749–754 (Sept.) 1972.

13. Kunin, C. M. and Dierks, J. W.: A Physician-Pharmacist Voluntary Program to Improve Prescription Practices, *N. Engl. J. Med. 280:*1442–1446 (June 26) 1969.

14. Laventurier, M. F.: A Prototype Pharmacy Foundation Peer Review Program, *Calif. Pharm. 19:*36–38 (May) 1972.

15. Laventurier, M. F. and Talley, R. B.: The Incidence of Drug-Drug Interactions in a Medi-Cal Population, *Calif. Pharm. 20:*18–22 (Nov.) 1972.

16. Brodie, D. C., Knoben, J. E. and Wertheimer, A. I.: Expanded Roles for Pharmacists, *Amer. J. Pharm. Educ. 37:*591–600 (Nov.) 1973.

17. Pellegrino, E. D.: Relationship of Medical and Pharmacy Education, Proceedings, Conference on Challenge to Pharmacy in the 70's, University of California School of Pharmacy, 1970, United States Department of Health, Education and Welfare, National Center for Health Services Research and Development, Rockville, Maryland [DHEW Publication No. (HSM) 72-3000], p. 83–91.

18. Goyan, J. E.: Pharmaceutical Education: A Ticket to Professional Survival or Extinction, The T. Edward Hicks Lecture, State University of New York at Buffalo, School of Pharmacy, Mar. 7, 1972.

Related Readings in This Volume

Reading for a Broader Perspective

1. Kradjan, W. A. "A Pharmacist's Experience in a Teaching Program for Patients on Anticoagulant Medication," *Hospital Pharmacy* 11 (July 1976):257–58, 262–64, 270.

Clinical Pharmacokinetics

27—An Orientation to Clinical Pharmacokinetics

Gerhard Levy

Background

The development of the new discipline of clinical pharmacokinetics is the culmination and logical outcome of recent advances in the areas of pharmacokinetics, clinical pharmacology, analytical chemistry, and biopharmaceutics, among others. Sensitive and specific methods are now available to determine the concentration of many drugs and their metabolites in biologic fluids and tissues; a therapeutic plasma concentration range has been identified for a number of widely used drugs; pharmacokinetic theory has been developed for almost all major types of biologic systems and dosage regimens; computer methodology for descriptive and at least tentatively predictive purposes in pharmacokinetics is well established; the pharmacokinetic characteristics of many important drugs have been determined; at least a beginning has been made in rigorously correlating the time course of action of some drugs with the time course of their concentrations in plasma, plasma water, or in certain extravascular tissues.

With the aid of these capabilities it has been determined that there are pronounced inter-subject variations in the elimination kinetics of certain drugs; that the absorption, distribution, and elimination of one drug may be influenced by another drug or by the environment; that a substantial number of patients do not take their medication in accordance with the physician's directions; that drug absorption from some pharmaceutical products may be erratic and incomplete; that age and disease may modify not only the absorption, distribution, and elimination of a drug but that these two variables may also affect the relationship between drug concentration in plasma and intensity of pharmacologic effects.

Because of many of these factors, it has been found that there is usually a considerably better correlation between plasma concentration and pharmacologic response than between the prescribed dose and the pharmacologic response. For the same reasons it has been necessary to individualize the dosage of many drugs. While in the ideal case such individualization of dosage regimens should be based on the therapeutic response (and in some instances on the occurrence and intensity of adverse effects), this is usually not feasible. In fact, most types of thera-

peutic response are difficult to quantitate (the best available data are usually obtained by averaging results from many subjects) and the onset of response is often delayed. Some drugs are intended primarily for prophylactic purposes (anti-epileptics, anti-asthmatics) and it would not be in a patient's interest to use exacerbations or acute attacks of the disease as an index of adequate drug dosage. Similarly, it is unwise to wait until an overdose or a drug interaction results in acute manifestation of drug intoxication (hemorrhage produced by anticoagulants, hypoglycemia from tolbutamide) rather than to adopt measures to prevent such incidents.

Consequently, it is now preferred in many cases to individualize drug dosage regimens on the basis of a targeted range of plasma concentrations known to produce the desired therapeutic response in most patients, taking into consideration the variables which are known to affect the relationship between dose and plasma concentration and utilizing feedback information from drug concentration monitoring to make subsequent adjustments of dosage as required. It is understood that these efforts should constitute an important part of the input for decision-making in the therapeutic management of the patient, but that they should never take the place of proper clinical observation and assessment by the attending physician who must ultimately be responsible for the proper care of the patient and whose judgment should be based on all pertinent considerations in addition to the pharmacokinetic aspects of the case.

Definitions and Functions of Clinical Pharmacokinetics

Simply stated, clinical pharmacokinetics is a health sciences discipline which deals with the application of pharmacokinetics to the safe and effective therapeutic management of the individual patient. Its functions include the following:

a. Initial design of drug dosage regimens (dose, dosing interval, route, dosage form) for individual patients upon request of the attending physician, based upon the generally available knowledge of the pharmacokinetics of the drug, the intended purpose of the medication, the disease(s) or tentative diagnosis and such variables as age, sex, body weight or surface area (or lean body mass), race or other indicator of possible pharmacogenetic influence (family history, tests of acetylator status, etc.), renal function, plasma albumin concentration, hemotocrit, preceding and/or concomitant use of other drugs, urine pH, and blood electrolytes, where applicable.

b. Refinement and re-adjustment of dosage regimens, where necessary, based usually on serial monitoring of drug concentrations in plasma or other fluids but sometimes on direct assessment of clinical response or on indirect assessment of response, for example, on the basis of changes in certain biochemical parameters.

c. Pharmacokinetic diagnostic work-ups to help determine the reasons for a quantitatively unusual response (usually lack of therapeutic effect or pronounced adverse effects) to a drug. Such diagnostic work-up, if carried out properly by a qualified individual, should lead to the detection of lack of compliance by the patient, bioavailability problems, medication errors, drug interactions, unusual distribution and elimination kinetics, or certain pharmacogenetic effects including unusual receptor site sensitivity.

d. Consultation with necessary follow-up in special situations such as assessment of need for intermittent dosage adjustment for patients on hemodialysis or peritoneal dialysis, and the management of acute drug intoxications.

e. Retrospective assessment of potential or suspected therapeutic mishaps or mis-

management (clinical conferences, post-mortems).

f. Educational activities (directed to physicians, pharmacists, nurses, and under certain circumstances to individual patients) to help assure that drugs are used safely and effectively.

g. Research, including an assessment of cost-benefit aspects of clinical pharmacokinetic services for individual drugs under various conditions, discovery of bioavailability problems and as yet unrecognized drug interactions, pharmacokinetic measurements to enlarge the data base (half-life, renal clearance, apparent volume of distribution, etc.) for a particular drug, and definition of parameters which may be useful in the design of individualized dosage regimens.

The General Approach

Since clinical pharmacokinetics focuses on the individual patient, the approach to problem solving must be individualized in accordance with the specific situation presented by any one patient. It may be helpful, however, to outline a general approach which, appropriately modified for individual needs, can be useful in many instances. The clinical pharmacokineticist will usually become involved with a particular patient problem in response to one of three types of requests from the attending physician: (a) a request to recommend a dosage regimen for the initiation of therapy or a modification of an ongoing dosage regimen which does not seem to be satisfactory; (b) a request for information or consultation involving a complicated problem in therapeutics which may have a pharmacokinetic basis; and (c) a request for a "blood level".

Requests of type (c) may originate from physicians with little or no orientation in pharmacokinetics who have, through casual reading of the literature, become aware of the fact that there is an established, generally safe and effective therapeutic plasma concentration range for such drugs as digoxin and diphenylhydantoin for the average patient. The type (c) request should be recognized as an opportunity to inform the physician of the proper role and capabilities of the clinical pharmacokineticist. The specific response to the request must be based on the reasons which motivated the physician to make it: a real patient problem, a self-protective measure, or simply "because this service is available."

Requests of type (a) and (b) usually come from physicians who have an adequate awareness of the kinds of services which the clinical pharmacokineticist can provide. These requests for consultation are usually responded to in the following manner: First, a clear statement of the problem as he sees it is elicited from the physician. An appropriate history, embodying the kind of information outlined in paragraph (a) of the preceding section, is gathered from the attending physician, the patient's chart, and if necessary, from interviews with the patient and such other individuals as the situation may dictate: nurses, residents, clinical pharmacists, consulting physicians, etc. Time and conditions of drug administration, possible use by the patient of non-charted drugs or home remedies and other such information may have to be obtained. If it is decided that certain additional blood chemistries or other biochemical tests are necessary and if determinations of drug concentrations in plasma or other fluids are indicated, then the types and timing of sample collections must be established and these collections must be ordered. For example, the timing of consecutive plasma samples (such as for the control of dosage by constant rate intravenous infusion) must be based on the rate of accumulation of the drug (which is a function of its biologic half-life), the therapeutic index, and the turn-around time of the assay procedure. The number and timing of blood, urine, or saliva samples during a dosing interval at the steady state produced by regular administration of maintenance doses (tablets, capsules, etc.) must be determined on the basis of the characteristics and expected magnitude of drug concentration fluctuations during the dosing interval. The analytical procedure must be decided upon; the concurrent use of two distinctly different types of analytical procedures (for example, radio-immunoassay and gas chromatography) may be indicated if the patient has received other drugs which might interfere with the assay.

It is essential to clearly define the line of communication between the clinical pharmacokineticist and the physician responsible for the individual patient. Upon pharmacokinetic assessment of the case, recommendations and/or comments will be communicated to the physician. The factual basis and rationale for any recommendations, the assumptions on which they are based and the uncertainties involved should be explained clearly but succinctly. Upon adoption by the physician of any recommendations concerning the drug dosage regimen for a particular patient, a subsequent verification or assessment of the patient's status should be arranged. This will usually take the form of follow-up determinations of drug concentrations or of the patient's response (such as frequency of seizures, blood clotting time, etc.). The results of the follow-up will be used as feedback information for further adjustment of drug dosage, if necessary. These various inputs to decision making, and the position of clinical pharmacokinetics in this process are outlined schematically in Figure 27.1.

Last but not least, a final conference or communication between physician and clinical pharmacokineticist should be devoted to an assessment, on as objective a basis as possible (the physician's assessment may be overly generous as a matter of courtesy!), of the contribution of the clinical pharmacokinetics consultation to the management of the

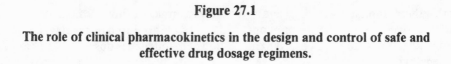

Figure 27.1

The role of clinical pharmacokinetics in the design and control of safe and effective drug dosage regimens.

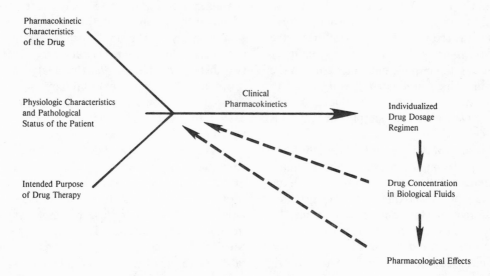

particular patient. Since such consultations may be costly and the number of competent clinical pharmacokineticists is (and will for some time) be limited, regular collection of data for the determination of cost-benefit ratios is important.

Hopefully, this exposition of a general approach to a problem in clinical pharmacokinetics has also served to indicate clearly what this discipline is not. It must be more than a service for supplying "blood levels," i.e., a laboratory which accepts vials of plasma, blood (usually hemolyzed), serum, urine or other fluids taken at random from patients who are described only by name or case number and which then generates a number (i.e., the drug concentration) that at best may be meaningless and at worst is misleading. While these requests for "blood levels" may be annoying, they should be received with understanding. Most of the usual biochemical tests (BUN, creatinine, serum bilirubin, etc.) do not require strict temporal control because these "levels" are indeed relatively level; they do not fluctuate

as much as do drug concentrations produced by repetitive dosings. Also, the physician is trained to utilize the "raw" biochemical data while the interpretive and consultative role of the clinical pharmacokineticist is more comparable to that of the pathologist or radiologist.

The Physical Setting of the Clinical Pharmacokinetics Laboratory

While the contribution of a clinical pharmacokinetics service to the quality of patient care (and the cost of such service) remains to be established in detail, it is already apparent that this service can contribute significantly in certain areas (such as therapy with cardioactive and antiepileptic agents). A clinical pharmacokinetics service should therefore be available directly in every major hospital. Ideally, this should consist of a properly qualified clinical pharmacokineticist and technical personnel to carry out drug analyses. It should have available adequate resources for standard analytical procedures (at least spectrophotometry, fluorometry, gas chromatography, and radioimmunoassay), access to a digital computer and to a good drug information center, and established relationships with consultants in such disciplines as clinical pharmacology, analytical chemistry and pharmacokinetics.

Smaller hospitals should have some sort of arrangement to utilize the clinical pharmacokinetics service of larger institutions, at least for emergencies and unusual problems in patient management. Such hospitals would benefit greatly by having on their pharmacy staff a clinical pharmacist who has received some training in clinical pharmacokinetics. It will probably be found advantageous in the future to centralize certain analytical services for specific drugs within a region (for example, all digoxin assays for ten hospitals in a large city may be carried out in one location); this is likely to improve quality and provide greater economy. Such an arrangement is not usually suitable for drugs for which rapid feedback information is required (such as lidocaine in an acute cardiac care center). It may also be feasible for several hospitals to "share" a clinical pharmacokineticist, such as is done in the case of certain other specialists. The clinical pharmacokinetics service should also be available to outpatients seen in clinics or by private physicians, but an adequate model for such a service has yet to be evolved.

Educational Requirements and Training Facilities

The clinical pharmacokineticist requires formal training in pharmacology, pharmacokinetics, biopharmaceutics and drug analysis at an advanced level. Consequently, he (or she) will have taken course work covering the prerequisites for these several types of courses: physiology, biochemistry, (ideally) pathology, biostatistics, calculus, basic pharmaceutics, basic chemical analysis, and medicinal chemistry. This type of course work is uniquely and characteristically offered in the better schools of pharmacy, and particularly as part of the graduate program of certain departments of pharmaceutics.

In addition to this formal training, the student in clinical pharmacokinetics requires extensive practical experience in a clinical pharmacokinetics laboratory which is located in a high quality and very active clinical setting. He should have the opportunity to become involved in a wide variety of consultations (thus the need for training in a general hospital or for rotation in various specialty hospitals such as a pediatric hospital, a chronic disease hospital, and an outpatient facility). He should gain experience in the de-bugging and trouble-shooting of analytical procedures. He must learn to relate to other professionals in the sociologically complex setting of a hospital. In particular, he must learn to communicate effectively with his physician-clients and he must have full appreciation for and an understanding of the role of other medical service groups such as clinical chemistry, pathology and toxicology. Ideally, there should be a fully operative drug information center, usually functioning in association with a school of pharmacy and staffed by clinical pharmacists with specialty training in drug information. The teaching faculty in clinical pharmacokinetics must include a "critical mass" of individuals who are actively engaged in this activity (this should never be a one man operation!) as well as professorial staff in basic pharmacokinetics, drug analysis, and clinical pharmacology. There is a danger that the current great interest in, and the glamor of clinical pharmacokinetics may cause some institutions to intitiate a formal training program without having the staff or facilities to do so properly. This must be discouraged because it is the patient who ultimately will suffer the consequences of such lack of responsibility.

Relationship with Other Disciplines and Professions

The clinical pharmacokineticist is likely to have essential and therefore strongly developed relationships with two types of disciplines and professionals: those who, in the immediate sense, are served by the clinical pharmacokineticist, and those who provide the body of knowledge and techniques upon which clinical pharmacokinetics is based. In the former group is primarily the physician directly involved in patient care, be he specialist or general practitioner. The diagnostic and therapeutic (in the broadest sense) skills of the physician, his ability to assess the therapeutic response, his understanding of the disease state and of the phenomena associated with it, together with the ability of the clinical pharmacokineticist to design and modify drug dosage regimens on a rigorous and objective basis, his inclination for and training in quantitation, his analytical capabilities, and his special knowledge of drug absorption, distribution, elimination and of drug interactions, invest in this combination of two professionals a capability for the safe and effective use of drugs which simply cannot be embodied in any one individual.

Grouped together with the practicing physician must be the clinical pharmacist, who like the clinical pharmacokineticist is part of a newly evolving discipline. Properly trained clinical pharmacists, particularly graduates of Doctor of Pharmacy programs, are able to serve as drug consultants to physicians and in many institutions accompany physicians on rounds, take drug histories, monitor adverse effects, and maintain medication records. Requests for clinical pharmacokinetics consultation may often be initiated upon their recommendation, and they can "translate" and expand upon the results of such consultation, particularly for the benefit of the young and relatively inexperienced physician. They can also consolidate and organize for transmittal to the clinical pharmacokineticist the patient information required for the consultation.

In the second group of disciplines and professions, i.e., those who provide basic knowledge and techniques utilized by clinical pharmacokineticists, the clinical pharmacologist plays a very important and prominent role. Since the aim of pharmacotherapy is to elicit a desired therapeutic response (rather than a defined "blood level"), there must be available adequate information concerning the relationship between drug concentration and pharmacologic effect. The clinical pharmacologist is uniquely trained to determine this relationship. If (as is the case) there is very limited concentration-effect information for many drugs, it is due to the unfortunately small number of clinical pharmacologists, their lack (until recently) of adequate resources and support from other medical disciplines, and perhaps their occasional preoccupation with areas of research not central to their primary function or training (for example, studies of the fate and disposition of drugs with no reference to the temporal, concentration, and disease related aspects of drug action). There must be strong bonds of collegiality between clinical pharmacokineticists and clinical pharmacologists, particularly in those few institutions (usually university health sciences centers) which can afford and obtain the services of both of these professionals.

The average, non-university related hospital will not be able to obtain the services of a clinical pharmacologist in the forseeable future in view of the many demands for these individuals by industry (for new drug trials), by universities (for teaching and research) and by government (for regulatory activities). Nor is it likely that a strong case can be made for the effective utilization of this type of physician in the average hospital. On the other hand, there is a vast amount of knowledge yet to be acquired concerning the relationship between drug concentration in biologic fluids and the intensity of drug action, and the effect of disease on this relationship. There is also a tremendous need for more definitive studies of drug efficacy. We depend greatly upon clinical pharmacologists to acquire these kinds of information and clinical pharmacokineticists therefore have a strong commitment to support and cooperate with their colleagues in clinical pharmacology.

Clinical pharmacokineticists must also have well developed working relationships with basic pharmacokineticists, analytical chemists concerned with drug analysis, and other kind of pharmaceutical scientists. These individuals will constitute the support base for dealing with special problems arising from the operation of the clinical pharmacokinetics laboratory such as the development of new analytical methods, automation and quality control of such methods, development of computer methodology for pharmacokinetic guidance and consultation, etc. The basic pharmacokineticist in particular will generate the fundamental information concerning the absorption, distribution, and elimination of a drug without which the clinical pharmacokineticist cannot function.

The Future

Future developments in clinical pharmacokinetics will depend considerably on: a) the availability of sensitive, specific, rapid, and economical assays for many more drugs; b) progress in clinical pharmacology particularly as it pertains to the capability of assessing drug efficacy and pharmacologic response; and c) the results of ongoing and future studies concerning the cost-benefit aspects of a clinical pharmacokinetic service. The experience to date with such drugs as digoxin, diphenylhydantoin, and theophyl-

line is very encouraging. Efforts must now be extended to other drugs.

The recent development of non-invasive, indirect methods of plasma concentration monitoring by determining drug concentrations in saliva is very exciting and at least preliminary evidence of the usefulness of this approach is available with respect to theophylline, diphenylhydantoin, and a number of other anti-epileptics, digoxin, lithium, and certain sulfonamides. Indications are that it may be advantageous or is necessary to measure the free rather than total concentration of certain highly protein bound drugs and it will be important to develop rapid, accurate, and economical means for making these measurements. There is need for microanalytical methods for use in pediatrics and particularly in neonatology; this need may be served largely by the increasing variety of radio-immunoassay procedures. Computer-aided drug therapy, based on multiple correlations with certain patient characteristics and incorporating continuous feedback capability, may be found useful. The clinical pharmacokineticist may in the future be concerned with the proper utilization and verification of the performance of sophisticated programmed drug delivery systems. Thus there are many exciting opportunities for research and service in our new discipline and there will be the satisfaction of being able to contribute measurably to the improvement of patient care. . . .

Readings for a Broader Perspective

1. Gibaldi, M., and Levy, G. "Pharmacokinetics in Clinical Practice: I. Concepts," *Journal of the American Medical Association* 235 (April 26, 1976):1864–67.
2. Gibaldi, M., and Levy, G. "Pharmacokinetics in Clinical Practice: II. Applications," *Journal of the American Medical Association* 235 (May 3, 1976):1987–92.
3. Levy, G. "A Training Program in Clinical Pharmacokinetics," *Drug Intelligence & Clinical Pharmacy* 12 (April 1978):204–09.

Critical Care

28—The Clinical Pharmacist in Emergency Medicine

Robert M. Elenbaas, Joseph F. Waeckerle and W. Kendall McNabney

The recent pharmacy literature has contained many papers describing the activities of pharmacists in a variety of health care settings. Hypertensive clinics,[1,2] chronic care facilities,[3,4] primary health care programs[2,5] and total parenteral nutrition programs[6] (to name only a few) have been the subject of previous reports. It is evident that pharmacists are becoming involved as active components in virtually all aspects of medical care where drugs are used. Papers have appeared which describe the drug distribution procedures in emergency rooms,[7] content of emergency drug boxes[8] and activities of pharmacists on a cardiorespiratory resuscitation team.[8,9] However, little has been written describing the activities of a pharmacist in emergency medicine. It is the purpose of this paper to describe the role of a pharmacist within the specialty of emergency medicine and to present an evaluation of physician and nurse attitudes toward this role.

The Department of Emergency Health Services is an independent department of Truman Medical Center (formerly Kansas City General Hospital), the primary teaching hospital of the University of Missouri-Kansas City, Schools of Medicine and Pharmacy. Over 30,000 patients currently are seen annually in either the emergency room or the initial care clinic; Table 28.1 indicates the general types of problems treated by the Department of Emergency Health Services. Professional personnel consists of four attending physicians (surgeon, internist and two emergency medicine specialists), 18 emergency medicine residents, the nursing staff, a paramedic coordinator and the phar-

Table 28.1

Representative Patient Care Statistics for the Department of Emergency Health Services (Fiscal Year 1975–1976)

Category	No.
Patient encounters	
Major medical-surgical	2,706
Minor medical-surgical	10,006
Coronary disease	340
Drug overdose	520
Major trauma	1,600
Minor trauma	6,416
Psychiatric problem	1,236
Obstetrical	239
Gynecological	1,747
Hospital admissions via emergency department	
Major medical	1,267
Coronary	212
Major surgical	509
Minor trauma	1,474
Ob/Gyn	308

macist. Residents from other departments and hospitals, pharmacy residents, and medical and doctor of pharmacy students rotate to the emergency room for a four- to six-week experience.

The pharmacist (RME) joined the Department of Emergency Health Services in July 1974; his salary is supported jointly by the department and the School of Pharmacy of the University of Missouri-Kansas City. The pharmacy program at Truman Medical Center and the University of Missouri-Kansas City has been described previously[10]; the docent teams provide the focus for health care delivery and education. Although a formal docent team, as such, does not exist within the Department of Emergency Health Services, the concept of team delivery of health care prevails.

Description of the Role

As can be seen in Table 28.1, a large number of patients seen in the emergency department have problems which require drug therapy. Although not all of these represent immediate life-threatening emergencies, the prehospitalization care administered to medical or surgical admissions, or the emergency room care given to ambulatory patients, would be expected to greatly affect their outcome. It is, therefore, the general responsibility of the pharmacist to promote and assure rational pharmacotherapeutics within all aspects of health care offered by the Department of Emergency Health Services. To fulfill this responsibility the activities of the pharmacist can be conveniently divided into the three classic areas of clinical practice, education and research. A brief description of each of these activities follows.

Clinical Practice. Clinical activities primarily include:

1. Physician-nurse consultation—pharmacotherapeutic and pharmaceutic consultation to design, implement and monitor a patient-specific therapeutic plan using the most efficacious, least toxic and most economical drugs available;

2. Patient education—directed toward increasing patient understanding and appreciation of medication use to assure minimal therapeutic failure, toxicity or noncompliance;

3. Medication use—assists in maintaining emergency department compliance with pharmacy procedures and assists in developing and maintaining an appropriate formulary of medications in the emergency room (although drug distribution functions are not a part of this activity);

4. Drug therapy management—directly initiates and continues the drug therapy of selected patients within the emergency department (i.e., drug overdoses, asthma, seizures, etc.); and

5. Committee service—the pharmacist is active on both hospital and community agency committees concerned with emergency drug use. The Mid-America Regional Council for Emergency Rescue (a community agency coordinating prehospital emergency health care) has been developing policies regulating infield, paramedic drug administration, and the pharmacist has served as a consultant to this agency in developing these and other policies.

To be readily available for consultation when most needed, the pharmacist is "on duty" in the emergency department primarily in the afternoon and evening. Because all departmental attending staff have their offices located within the emergency room the pharmacist is easily accessible during other times of the day and can easily monitor E.R. activities. Residents in clinical pharmacy also assist in providing evening and night coverage while on rotation to the department.

Education. The pharmacist is involved in a variety of formal and informal educational programs. It is virtually impossible to offer a pharmacotherapeutic consultation without the experience also being an educational session for one or both parties. Formal educational activities include instruction to:

1. Medical staff and residents—in addition to daily informal educational encounters, the department has a structured conference program for its members and students, which the pharmacist regularly participates in and conducts;

2. Nursing staff—scheduled inservice programs are offered for the nursing personnel;

3. Medical students—through the design of the University of Missouri-Kansas City, School of Medicine, the clinical pharmacy faculty are largely responsible for medical student education in pharmacology and therapeutics,[10] and the pharmacist holds a joint faculty appointment in the schools of pharmacy and medicine;

4. Emergency medical technicians (paramedics)—the Department of Emergency Health Services conducts a 500-hour paramedic training program, and the pharmacist is responsible for the pharmacology portion of the curriculum;

5. Continuing education—extramural physicians and nurses may participate in organized continuing education programs in emergency medicine offered through the department; and

6. Pharmacy students (B.S. and Pharm. D.) and pharmacy residents—activities of the pharmacist in the educational programs of pharmacy students and residents have been extensively described elsewhere.[10]

University faculty appointment, of course, carries the usual amount of administrative and committee responsibilities.

Research. There exists a striking need for well conducted research in clinical pharmacy[11] and emergency medicine.[12] All attending staff of the Department of Emergency Health Services, therefore, are pursuing research interests; the pharmacist is par-

ticularly involved in projects relating to drug use in emergency medicine.

Evaluation

A questionnaire was developed in an attempt to determine physicians' and nurses' attitudes toward the pharmacist and clinical pharmacy services in emergency medicine. The authors developed a rough draft of the questionnaire which was then reviewed by two individuals not associated with the Department of Emergency Health Services, but with knowledge of questionnaire design. The questionnaire was subsequently pretested on a small number of individuals to identify weaknesses in the design of the survey questions. The evaluation was distributed in June 1976. A total of 54 questionnaires were distributed: 17 to physicians (resident and attending staff) of the Department of Emergency Health Services (EHS), 20 to all residents from other departments or hospitals who had spent at least a one-month rotation within the E.R. during the preceding year (non-EHS), and 17 to all nursing staff of the department. Specifically excluded from the survey were medical students in rotation to the emergency room and the nonprofessional personnel of the department.

Thirty-nine of 54 (72%) of questionnaires were completed and returned: 17/17 by physicians of the department, 9/20 by nondepartmental residents and 13/17 by nursing personnel. The results are shown in Table 28.2. Statistical analysis was performed using either Chi-square or The Exact Test as appropriate.

Discussion

Results of the questionnaire indicate that the pharmacist is a well accepted and recognized component of emergency medicine practice at Truman Medical Center and is

Table 28.2

Physicians' and Nurses' Evaluation of Clinical Pharmacy Services in the Department of Emergency Health Services

Question and Response	No.		Question and Response	No.	
	M.D.s	R.N.s		M.D.s	R.N.s
Interpretation of pharmacist's role:			Background of literature and basic sciences or literature		
Patient care					
Primary	1	7	background	26	10
Secondary	18	2	Primary clinical experience with either basic science or		
Tertiary	3	3	literature background	0	0
Teaching			Unable to evaluate	0	3
Primary	21	5			
Secondary	1	7	Consultation recommendations followed:		
Tertiary	0	0			
Research			Always	3	7
Primary	0	0	Most of the time	23	3
Secondary	3	3	About half of the time	0	0
Tertiary	19	9	Never	0	0
Not ranked	4	1	Unable to evaluate	0	3
Benefit to patient care:			The pharmacist is available for		
Yes	26	12	consultation when needed:		
No	0	0	Yes	26	10
Unable to evaluate	0	1	No	0	1
Benefit to educational activities:			Unable to evaluate	0	2
Yes	26	13	Capable of offering primary care to		
No	0	0	selected patients:		
Unable to evaluate	0	0	Yes	21	11
Benefit to research activities:			No	3	0
Yes	16	7	Unable to evaluate	2	2
No	1	0			
Unable to evaluate	9	6	Role transferrable to other emergency departments:		
A necessary component of			Yes	22	10
department:			Only to university setting	6	2
Essential	10[a]	10	To any E.R.	16	8
Useful but not essential	16[b]	2	No	1	0
Unessential	0	0	Unable to evaluate	3	3
Unable to evaluate	0	1			
Knowledge and recommendations are based upon:			Willing to have patients pay for clinical pharmacy services (asked of physician only):		
Only textbook and literature information but little clinical			Yes	19	—
			No	4	—
experience	0	0	Unable to evaluate	3	—

[a] EHS physicians: 9; non-EHS physicians: 1.

[b] EHS physicians: 8; non-EHS physicians: 8.

considered a benefit to the patient care, educational and research activities of the department. Reasons listed by physician responders for their beliefs included statements like: "supplying information concerning therapy, particularly designed to include physiological reasoning along with drug properties"; "quality control and counsel on what otherwise would have been an arbitrary and unscientific administration of drugs and dosage regimens."

Although "teaching" is considered by physicians to be the pharmacist's primary activity, it is interesting to note that most physicians also feel the role to be transferrable to emergency departments not necessarily having training programs. This apparent discrepancy probably arises for several reasons and is not difficult to explain. Is a consultation given regarding the treatment of a specific patient a "patient care" or a "teaching" activity? Undoubtedly both, since the patient receives appropriate drug therapy and the "student" has gained information and expertise in dealing with a given problem. In a university environment where the consultation often is given to a resident or student it will probably be interpreted as a teaching function, while in a nonuniversity setting the same activity may well be judged a patient care act. The significant difference ($p < 0.002$) between physician and nurse interpretation of the pharmacist's primary and secondary roles also tends to reinforce the concept that the same act may be interpreted as two different functions by various individuals. It appears that the "student attitude" of resident or academically-based physicians causes them to see the pharmacist as a teacher, while the "service attitude" of the nurse causes them to see him more as a provider of patient care. Regardless, when one considers the need for continual education among health care practitioners, the "teaching" role of the pharmacist would seem vital.

It is interesting to note that although all questionnaire responses indicate the pharmacist to be an important component of the Department of Emergency Health Services, the strength of this attitude among physicians may differ between those who are members of the department and those who only spend a relatively short rotation within the emergency room. Even though no statistically significant difference existed between the reported attitudes of EHS and non-EHS physicians concerning this point, the relatively low return of questionnaires (9/20) from non-EHS physicians as compared to EHS physicians (17/17) may have biased the results. It is probable that if a larger percentage of non-EHS physicians had returned the questionnaires a difference would have existed between EHS and non-EHS physicians. This is not unlikely since those individuals who did not bother to complete and return the questionnaire would not be expected to consider the pharmacist an "essential" component of the department. The possible difference could represent the relative amounts of contact the two groups of individuals have with the pharmacist and the degree of appreciation they can gain for his capabilities during this time.

The pharmacist is actively recognized and used as an information source. His consultative recommendations are interpreted as being based upon an appropriate blend of "literature and textbook" information supported by clinical experience and almost always are followed by both physicians and nurses. Although not the primary responsibility of the pharmacist, almost all physicians and nurses feel that he is capable of delivering "primary care" to certain patients once the diagnosis has been made by a physician. Examples of patients identified were those with asthma, COPD, hypertension and arrhythmias. This role has been well developed elsewhere [1,2,5] and appears to be a well accepted component of the pharmacist's activities within this department as well. Of interest in this case, however, is that the pharmacist may be responsible for the management of a variety of acute medical problems instead of the chronic, insidious disease processes described in other reports.[1,2]

Of importance are the observations that almost all physicians and nurses feel the role of the pharmacist to be transferable to other emergency departments, both university- and nonuniversity-affiliated, and that the physicians surveyed appeared to support a fee-for-service charge mechanism for clinical pharmacy services. If clinical pharmacy services are to transfer to the private sector of health care or truly thrive in the university environment, such a fee mechanism would seem mandatory.

Conclusion

The results of this survey indicate that the pharmacist has been successful in establishing a unique practice within the specialty of emergency medicine. As this medical specialty gains further recognition and physicians graduate from our residency program, we hope to establish other clinical pharmacy role models in emergency medicine.

References

1. McKenney, J. M., Slining, J. M., Hendersen, H. R. et al: The effect of clinical pharmacy services on patients with essential hypertension, *Circulation 47*:1104–1111 (Nov) 1973.
2. Reinders, T. P., Rush, D. R., Baumgartner, R. P., Jr. et al: Pharmacist's role in management of hypertensive patients in an ambulatory clinic, *Am J Hosp Pharm 32*:590–594 (Jun) 1975.
3. Mattei, T. J.: Clinical involvement for the pharmacist in chronic care, *Am J Hosp Pharm 31*:1053–1056 (Nov) 1974.
4. Hamilton, S. F.: Therapeutic problems in nursing home patients, *Drug Intell Clin Pharm 10*:703–707 (Dec) 1976.
5. Johnson, R. E. and Tuchler, R. J.: Role of the pharmacist in primary health care, *Am J Hosp Pharm 32*:162–164 (Feb) 1975.
6. Skoutakis, V. A., Martinez, D. R., Miller, W. A. et al: Team approach to total parenteral nutrition, *Am J Hosp Pharm 32*:693–697 (Jul) 1975.
7. Mar, D., Hanan, Z. and LaFontaine, R.: A data process assisted, single unit packaged emergency room medication system, presented at the 11th Annual ASHP Midyear Clinical Meeting, Anaheim, California, December 7, 1976.
8. Schwerman, E., Schwartau, N., Thompson, C. O. et al: The pharmacist as a member of the cardiopulmonary resuscitation team, *Drug Intell Clin Pharm 7*:299–308 (Jul) 1973.
9. Elenbaas, R.: Pharmacist on resuscitation team, *N Engl J Med 287*:151 (Jul 20) 1972.
10. Anon: Clinical role models for service and education, clinical pharmacy program, University of Missouri-Kansas City School of Pharmacy, Kansas City, Missouri, 1976.
11. Romankiewicz, J. A.: Spanning the gap—clinical research, *Drug Intell Clin Pharm 9*:324 (Jun) 1975.
12. Sims, J. K.: Plea for research in emergency medicine, *J Am Coll Emerg Phys 5*:994 (Dec) 1976.

Related Reading in This Volume

Readings for a Broader Perspective

1. Stollman, M. "They Call 'Em Urgency Exits," *California Pharmacist* 24 (October 1977): 28–33.
2. Woolley, B. H. "Practical Pharmacology During Cardiopulmonary Resuscitation," *The Apothecary* 90 (September/October 1978): 34–37.

Drug Information

29—Drug Information: An Overview and Prospect for the Future

James R. Ruger and Sr. Jane M. Durgin

Introduction

The years following World War II were witness to a proliferation of printed material that was unprecedented in the history of civilization.[1,2] Technical and military documents confiscated from the conquered nations Germany and Japan gave early evidence and, in some cases, laid the foundations of future developments. Soon after, an "information explosion" of scientific and technical research became visible. This phenomenon has continued until today.[3] Vinken[4] cites that the major cause of the exponential growth of literature is a "twigging effect," that is, a greater trend towards professional specialization. The capabilities of information manipulation have gained momentum during recent years and it is speculated that the changes to come within the next ten years will far surpass those of the last fifty.[5] These changes will be the result of factors such as new and improved automated systems, high-speed facsimile capabilities, micrographics, library-information center networks, and space satellite telecommunications.

The idea of processing, controlling and disseminating drug information developed practically parallel to the concept of clinical pharmacy. One of the first drug information centers originated in 1959 at the Los Angeles County/U.S.C. Medical Center.[6] The services provided included question answering, adverse drug reaction reporting and the production of a monthly news bulletin. However, the center was staffed exclusively by physicians and was not placed under the directorship of a pharmacist until June, 1973. The first fully operational drug information center under the auspices of a pharmacist originated in 1962 at the University of Kentucky.[7] Data concerning medications used in all areas of medical practice were collected, classified, cataloged, stored, evaluated and disseminated. This center has served as the prototype for many later organizations.[8]

This article proposes to discuss levels of drug information services, to describe the functions and to help delineate some of the competencies that need to be developed in the education and training of future drug information practitioners.

The Need and Demand for Drug Information Services

McCarron[9] describes five factors which cause significant drug therapy problems in the hospital: (1) poor systems of drug distribution, administration and record keeping; (2) improper application of product information to the preparation and administration of drugs; (3) inadequate drug information on the part of prescribers; (4) lack of knowledge of the pharmacokinetics of the products used and (5) a lack of concern by hospitals and physicians towards recognizing and reporting adverse drug effects. Problems two to five are basically due to inadequate knowledge, information, or the generation of data concerning drug entities. A drug information service attempts to increase the prescriber's awareness of drug entities and their proper use, thereby decreasing the frequency of drug therapy problems.

The desire for improved adverse drug reaction recognition and reporting techniques has been stressed by the American Pharmaceutical Association,[10] the American Medical Association,[11,12] and the Federal Government.[13,14] However, as Wintrobe points out,[15] physicians and hospitals continually fail to meet these needs. The identification of adverse drug reactions is a primary objective of the clinical pharmacist, but in many hospitals clinical pharmacy practice is nonexistent or in an early developmental stage. The result is an estimated 60,000 to 140,000 deaths per year due to adverse drug reactions[16] and the relinquishing of drug surveillance responsibilities to other health professionals.[17] Affiliation with an existing drug information center, or formation of regional services can facilitate the collection and dissemination of drug data as well as aid in decreasing drug therapy problems in hospitals where expanded clinical services are unavailable.

In the introduction to *Meyler's Side Effects of Drugs*, volume eight, Dukes writes, "Information on the undesirable effects of medicines is increasing so fast, and that information needs differ so widely . . . (that) it will be a long time before every drug prescriber has ready access to a computer terminal and even longer until such channels

provide him with all the detailed and often conflicting material he may need to form his own judgment. That is the basic problem with drug information: the most important material is often that relating to matters which are still nascent, disputed, or poorly quantified."[18] It is estimated that over 100,000 biomedical publications are produced annually[19] and access to this material varies from manual indices to satellite-computer telecommunication networks.[20] Furthermore, it has been observed[21] and demonstrated[22] that a great many pharmacy school seniors and recent graduates are unfamiliar with even the basic professional literature. Without guidance, many of these "future pharmacists" may never read more than a package insert for a particular drug. The task of developing improved, evaluative retrieval systems and of educating practitioners as to the importance of drug information lies with the drug information specialist.

A survey by Rosenberg et al.[23] reveals that the majority of hospital affiliated drug information practitioners function in a part-time capacity (128 part-time; 78 full-time). Although a part-time service is a great asset,[24] it cannot hope to access and manipulate all the medicinal data presently available. Therefore, the responsibility of providing smaller services with essential information that is not easily obtained may be handled through the formation of drug information networks. The network concept originated with the proposed "Voice of Peace" in 1964.[25] This United Nations Agency was "to act as a world source of knowledge and references for the collection, communication, and dissemination of all types of information useful for peaceful purposes throughout the world." The need for a centralized drug information clearinghouse which would collect, evaluate and disseminate medical information on a national level was recognized by Senator Hubert Humphrey in his address to the D.I.A./F.D.A./ N.L.M. symposium on unusual and underutilized drug information resources.[26] Until such a national service is a reality, communications between existing centers can be improved. Cooperative networks, depending upon input from all their members, may be formed. These can improve the quality of information access and expand the data base of all the participants.

A recent study, sponsored by the American Association of Colleges of Pharmacy, identified a primary deficiency in health care as a lack of available drug information and the failure of the present system of pharmacy to develop, organize, and distribute knowledge and information about drugs.[27] The problem is not the unavailability of drug information, but rather its access. The clinician requires information to practice effectively, it is demanded by the public, and it is intrinsic to improved health care. Knowledge is gained through information and only with improved systems can the drug data base be expanded and better manipulated. The need and demand, to be answered by future drug information specialists, is the development of more efficient, clinical systems, thereby improving the transfer of knowledge and patient care.

Specialized Knowledge Useful to the Operation of a Drug Information Service

Communication is the major method by which information is transferred. Communication can be verbal, written or observed, therefore, one of the most important behavioral skills to drug information transfer is the ability to recognize relevant data and transmit it effectively. The clinician compiles much patient data from the patient interview. Not only is pertinent information concerning medical, familial and personal histories obtained, but judgements regarding patient attitudes and drug compliance can be

formed. Thus, the interview often provides the basis of therapeutic management. A drug information specialist may provide consultations to patients on the proper administration and use of their medications. This service requires an individualized knowledge of the patient and his or her disease state. The patient interview can enhance the drug information specialist's insight into the patient's characteristics, thereby enabling him to evaluate the quantity of information to be transmitted to that patient. In addition to interviewing the patient, the drug information practitioner needs to be adept at conducting another form of interview which is inherent to the concept of question negotiating. This communication technique is called the reference interview.

The reference interview attempts to uncover any "hidden" information needs which are not specifically stated by the inquirer.[28] Fosket[29] points out that the question is a basic unit with which information science deals and it is one of the first steps taken in solving a problem. Fosket further adds, "When a research worker begins to make a search, he has become aware of a gap in his knowledge that he wants to fill, but he cannot know the extent of his ignorance." The enquirer may then overelaborate or oversimplify his request in a nebulous way. This nebulous area requires clarification, which is accomplished through a stepwise, systematic approach termed the reference interview. Figure 29.1 charts the reference interview process. As Taylor observed, "An inquiry is merely a microevent in a shifting non-linear adaptive mechanism . . . the question is open-ended, negotiable and dynamic."[30] This concept is the underlying principle to be kept in mind as the drug information specialist obtains requests for data from users of the drug information service.

The ability to write effectively and to accurately analyze written documents are two essential processes in the communication of knowledge with which the drug

Figure 29–1

Flow chart of the reference interview.

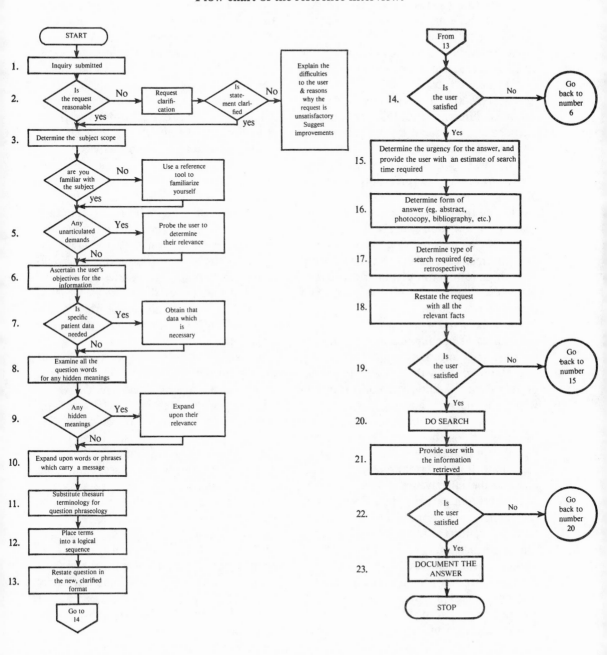

*Based on the concept of body language.
+Based on thesauri or other form of term control used by the particular center.

information specialist is concerned. Answers to questions, reports and articles must be composed in a clear, concise manner. Abstract writing, a major device for information storage, retrieval and transfer, demands careful preparation. The abstracter must be sensitive to the needs of the abstract readers. For example, an abstract which serves a current awareness function may have to be written in a different style than an abstract intended for permanent storage and use as a retrospective searching device. The preparation of these terse literature surrogates requires an accurate interpretation of the document's contents, as well as a keen sense for identifying and eliminating superfluous language from a written concept. The abstract must fulfill its mission: to give its readers a fast, informative account of an article's content. Often formal training in abstract writing and evaluation can greatly improve an abstract writer's ability.

The spoken and written word are not the only forms of communication which concern the drug information specialist. Drug information deals with the communication of knowledge. Additional modes through which this may be accomplished are the media (e.g., telecommunications), signal transmission (e.g., body language) and automated data processing systems. To be successful, a drug information system must increase the effectiveness with which the communication of drug data occurs. The transmission of information is only successful when it effects a change in the receiver of that information. The relevance of the change is a measure of the effectiveness. To illustrate: an adverse drug reaction is discovered by a clinical pharmacist who then gathers documentation to substantiate his find. The information is effectively communicated to the physician who discontinues the drug. The pharmacist then suggests alternative therapy which is accepted and implemented. Thus, the information, having been effectively communicated, resulted in a relevant therapeutic change.

All forms of communication are prone to three levels of problems: 1) technical e.g., proper grammar in speech and writing; 2) semantic e.g., interpretation of concepts; 3) behavioral e.g., trying to increase a patient's compliance. Hence, a situation occurs where a technical error could lead to a semantic difficulty and both could form the basis of a behavioral perplexity. A simple illustration is the pharmacist who incorrectly copies the directions for a medicine's use onto the label. As a result, the patient experiences side effects to the medicine and develops an innate distrust of all pharmacists from then on. Information science attempts to rectify all three levels of problems, for it is concerned with the effective transfer of *knowledge*.[31] *Drug information* tries to improve the transmission of drug knowledge and, therefore, tries to eliminate the errors which occur in McCarron's previously mentioned drug therapy problems.

In 1967, Walton[32] described two types of drug information specialist: 1) The drug literature specialist or documentalist who is concerned with increasing the efficiency and usefulness of document retrieval and 2) The clinical drug information specialist who is concerned with increasing the efficacy of patient care by providing close, continuing support to the clinician.

Today we are faced with a situation where information output and technology are progressing so rapidly that, in order to be effective, the clinical drug information practitioner can no longer neglect the function of documentalist. He must become intricately involved with systems use, theory and design. Likewise, the documentalist cannot be effective if he is not clinically involved.[33] Drug information practice is evolving to the point where Walton's two concepts are beginning to merge. When the merger is complete, the result will be a highly trained specialist capable of designing and applying clinically oriented drug information systems which possess a high degree of relevance.

A recent survey[34] regarding the adequacy of physicians' and pharmacists' sources of drug information revealed that both professional groups regarded themselves as inadequate (or non-relevant). These physicians and pharmacists stated that they would prefer written documentation, as could be provided by a drug information center, over many other sources of information.

Without knowledge of information science concepts, systems theory and methods of data manipulation, the effective transmission of knowledge is limited and the dissemination of information becomes a purely technical and mechanical process. An untrained information dispenser, for example, may be satisfied with supplying a quester with a terse, one-line response to a question. He may not have recognized unstated information needs, for he was unfamiliar with the concept of body language. The failure to properly state a request while using an online retrieval system is another way that a lack of systems theory may generate erroneous data, as well as waste time and money. Finally, inadequate knowledge of a system's purpose and design may complicate a search process. For discussion purposes, let us assume that a person unfamiliar with the format of the de Haen *Drugs In Use* system, improperly files away the cards. The result is that the indices are now rendered useless and time is lost as a searcher must read all the cards on a drug entity in order to find his desired information.

The concept of "peripheral data" plays an important part in the amount of information to be given to a user. If unaware of this concept, an information disseminator may be prone to supplying too little or too much data. This can result in unfulfilled information needs on the part of the quester, or wasted time and effort by the disseminator.

A simple guide is: If 95 percent of the information provided is acceptable to the enquirer, the search may have been too narrow. If less than 80 percent of the information furnished is acceptable, the search was too wide. An 85–90 percent acceptance of information by the quester assures with a fair amount of certainty that any peripheral needs were met and that extraneous data was minimal.[35]

The relevance of the data collected and disseminated relies upon a keen sense of pharmaceutical and medical knowledge. Without the subject speciality, evaluative analysis of literature sources, patient information and the relation of retrieved data to the clinical environment is extremely difficult, if not impossible. Laboratory data, patient progress notes, nursing notes and medication sheets all reveal specific clues concerning a patient's status. The patient-oriented drug information specialist needs to be able to recognize and interpret any problem signs appearing in these sources.

The "invisible college," or more explicitly colleague consultation, has been a major mode of information transmission to physicians for many years.[36,37,38] In order to provide efficacious drug consultation services, the clinically-oriented drug information practitioner must communicate on a peer basis with physicians. A lack of competence in the pharmaceutical sciences not only prevents intellectual peer status but also increases the chance for erroneous literature analysis. In the hospital environment this can be disastrous.

Several surveys, [39,40,41] as well as statements by the American Medical Association[42,43] have disclosed that many physicians are reluctant to allow pharmacists to practice clinically and use them sparingly as a source of drug information. To reverse this sentiment the pharmacist must demonstrate his clinical proficiency. The drug information specialist attempts to make health professionals aware that the pharmacist is an essential source of drug information.

Drug Information Functions and Services

Francke[44] sketches the function of the pharmacotherapeutic specialist, or applied pharmacologist, as an educator possessing expertise in pharmacology, therapeutics, pharmacokinetics and biostatistics. The drug information specialist provides these practitioners with relevant data and thus enables them to perform more effectively. Information science therefore deals with relevance.[45] The separation of the pertinent from the irrelevant is what detaches the true information scientist from "wholesale information disseminators." Confronted by an enormous body of literature, the drug information specialist is particularly concerned with relevance. It is his task to isolate those documents that are vital to improving health care and to relate their importance to the clinician.

The success or failure of an organization is greatly dependent upon its guidelines and objectives.[46] Before specialized services can be offered, general activities must be outlined. Table 29.1 lists the general activities of three different systems: a special library, an information center and an information analysis center. If the objectives of an organization are unclear, the services offered may not fulfill their desired purpose. In order to provide an effective drug information service, the information needs of the user community must be identified. The functions the center should perform can then be delineated and the proper services implemented. It is unrealistic to assume that all drug information centers can perform each of the activities listed in Table 29.1. Manpower with the ability to adequately staff drug information centers, is scarce and funds are difficult to obtain. In addition, many institu-

tions do not need some of the listed functions, especially the highly individualized services, such as the selective dissemination of information. One method by which a wide variety of services can be offered at moderate cost is through the formation of drug information networks. Each participating center could fulfill certain specific functions, thereby augmenting the services offered by the entire system.

The development and construction of a center's data base is a vital function. Again, relevance is central. The users' present and future needs must be recognized and satisfied. If the user can obtain more relevant material elsewhere, the center will fail. The drug information specialist must know where and how to obtain pertinent, new material. Books, though forming the literature core, are a small part of a drug information collection. Pamphlets, journals, monographs, reprints, government documents, technical reports, patents, indices, abstracts, file-card systems and micrographics comprise the congregate mass. Training beyond a basic pharmaceutical education is desired if such materials are to be properly accessed.

Automation further compounds the problem of data collection. System compatibilities, flexibility of soft and hardware, processing language, choice of retrieval packages and costs must be analyzed. This is a highly specialized function and extremely important if finance is a factor.

The processing of materials is a technical activity. Works are prepared and stored in a prearranged manner. Documents can be extracted or abstracted, photo-copied, vital information can be "torn out," converted to microfilm, placed in a computer system or stored in the original form. Data are classified and indexed or cataloged, according to the terminology utilized by the center. Therefore, subject headings or thesauri must be adopted and then adapted to satisfy the center's needs. An aptly designed retrieval system greatly facilitates data access.

Table 29.1

**General Activities of a Special Library,
Information Center and
Information Analysis Center**

Activity	Special Library	Information Center	Information Analysis Center
A. *Collection*			
1. Documents*	M	M	M
2. Data*	r	M	M
B. *Storage in Original Form*	M	m	m
C. *Materials Processing*			
1. Documents	m–M	M	M
2. Data	O	M	M
D. *Analysis*	r	M	M
E. *Retrieval Forms*			
1. Entire Document	M	m	m
2. Fact of Information	m	M	M
F. *Services Offered*			
1. Bibliographic Searches	M	M	m
2. Automatic Dissemination	m	M	m
3. Selective Dissemination	r	M	M
4. Current Awareness	m	M	m
5. Automated Data Bases	M	M	M
6. Thesauri Design	m	M	M
7. Systems Design	r	M	M

M = major activity; m = minor; r = rare; O = no activity

* Document is any printed matter; data are any bit of information, not necessarily printed

The evaluation and analysis of information sources is focal to the concept of relevance. The foundation of this function was formed in pharmacy school and completed during graduate education. Pharmacology, pharmacokinetics, pharmaceutics, therapeutics, toxicology, and biostatistics are all pertinent to determining the relevance of given information. The interpretation of information is of great consequence, especially when contradictory data are retrieved.

Individualized, special services are paramount to information centers, and few place limits upon them.[47] Drug information should not be an exception. If qualified personnel and systems are both available, such services may lend more support to a center than the question and answer service. Current awareness is a basic responsibility of a drug information service. This is accomplished via lectures, written articles and news bulletins. A more individualized service which is not offered by many centers, is selective dissemination of information (SDI). User profiles are prepared and some form of alerting device is employed to keep the user abreast of developments in a pre-specified subject field. Alerting mechanisms range from bibliographies to photo-copied articles.

The design of new, evaluative retrieval systems is a specialized function. Presently, drug interactions,[48] laboratory test interferences,[49] patient profiles,[50,51] and on-line retrieval systems (i.e. Medline) are accessible by computer. However, the clinical aspects of all these can be beneficially improved.[52]

Training the drug information specialist in computer programming and systems design can facilitate such improvements.

The drug information center may also function as a source of legal information to pharmacists, physicians and nurses. If the center is to function in this capacity it needs to collect legal documents and be adept at acquiring current data concerning laws. Drug information is not only subject to health regulations, but also to the Freedom of Information Act (PL89–487),[53,54] the Privacy Act (PL93–579), [55,56] and the Copyright Revision Act (PL94–553).[57] Developments concerning computer thefts[58] and conclusions by the National Commission on New Technological Use[59] will influence information storage and transfer. The Freedom of Information Act has increased the importance of government documents. The Food and Drug Administration, for example, which once withheld 90 percent of its information from the public will now make 90 percent available.[60]

Administration and public relations are general, yet important necessities. The preparation of objectives, guidelines, budgets, reports and manuals are responsibilities that must not be neglected. The services provided need to be promulgated and evaluated. Guidance to students of drug information is an educative activity and participation in hospital conferences is essential.

Services that are presently available from many drug information centers include: patient, physician, pharmacist and nursing drug consultation services; educational lectures; question and answer services; interviewing, reviewing, and disseminating pharmaceutical manufacturer representatives' information; adverse drug reaction reporting; patient drug monitoring; investigational drug data; literature searches; and publication of newsletters. A poison control information service must take priority over less important duties. The center may also act as a clearinghouse for research conducted with-

in the parent institution. Benefits derived from this function include a reduction in the duplication of experimental efforts and savings in time and funds.

The needs of an organization may be determined only through careful analysis. One may then decide which services to offer and which functions to fulfill. The drug information specialist needs to be a learned judge of human nature, knowledgeable in pharmacy and astute in information science to be able to break through long-existing professional barriers.

Education

The preceding discussion has produced evidence for the necessity of providing the drug information practitioner with a distinct form of education. The concept of training the drug information specialist in library and information science originated in the mid–1960's.[61,62] The first formal graduate degree in drug information, offered through a school of library and information science, was announced in October, 1973 by Case Western Reserve University.[63] The program was open to registered pharmacists who desired to expand their professional expertise. Individuals wishing to further their medical knowledge were permitted to elect courses from Case Western [Reserve's] Medical School. The degree program consisted of thirty-six semester hours leading to a Master of Science in Library Science with a certificate of specialization in drug information.

The Arnold and Marie Schwartz College of Pharmacy and Health Sciences of Long Island University (formerly Brooklyn College of Pharmacy) offers a thirty-six semester credit program leading to a Master of Science in Drug Information.[64] In contrast to the Case Western [Reserve] degree, this program is directed through a college of pharmacy. Most of the courses are pharmaceutically-oriented, with several informa-

Table 29.2

Drug Information Courses Offered Through Colleges of Pharmacy*

College	Course Title	Drug Information Degree
Arkansas, Univ. of	Scientific Literature Retrieval	No
Arnold and Marie Schwartz College of Pharmacy	36 credit M.S. Degree	Yes
Auburn University	Pharmaceutical Literature	No
Connecticut, Univ. of	Drug Information Services	No
Duquesne University	Pharmaceutical Literature	No
Florida, Univ. of	Drug Information	No
Iowa, Univ. of	Drug Lit. Retrieval and Eval.	No
Kentucky, Univ. of	Poison Information and Control	No
Missouri, Univ. of	Research Literature	No
North Carolina, Univ. of	Drug Information Analysis and Retrieval	No
Oklahoma, Univ. of**	Intro. To Pharm. Lit. (U.G.) Pharmacy Literature (Grad.) Drug Interactions and Lit. Eval. Readings in Pharm. Sciences	No
Ohio State University	Pharm. Record Keeping and Information Systems	No
Oregon State University	Drug Information Services	No
Philadelphia College of Pharmacy	Electronic Data Processing	No
Purdue University	Drug Information Services	No
St. John's University	57 Credit Dual Master's Degree	Yes
Utah, Univ. of	Drug Information Retrieval; Clerkship in Drug Information and Poison Control	No
Washington, Univ. of	45 Credit M.S. Degree	Yes
Also: Case Western Reserve Library School	36 Credit M.S. L.S. Degree	Yes

* Information obtained from 1975–76 college bulletins and brochures.

** U.G. with U. of Oklahoma means undergraduate course.

tion science courses offered as electives.

St. John's University, New York, realizing the necessity for both forms of education, has taken advantage of two of its resources.[65] A program where the applicant receives a Master of Science in Pharmacology and a Master of Library and Information Science has been implemented as of January, 1977. The program consists of fifty-seven credits, twenty-seven in library and information science and twenty-four in pharmacology together with six elective credits. Applicants must be graduates of an accredited college of pharmacy.

Table 29.2 lists eighteen colleges of pharmacy which offer courses in drug information. Many hospital residency programs provide drug information experience[66] and Masters' degrees are being offered by other Universities (i.e., the University of Washington). Specialized education combined with practical experience will enable the drug information practitioner to better accomplish the task of improving information access, storage, manipulation, and dissemination techniques.

Conclusion

The need and demand for drug information has been a topic in the literature for nearly twenty years. The distribution of drug information is a function of pharmacy which will continue to increase in importance as time passes. Neglecting this service not only ignores the pharmacist's professional responsibility but also opens the way for other health professions to incorporate this function into their own areas of practice.

The problems of identifying and reporting adverse drug reactions, collecting and disseminating drug data and accessing the immense body of biomedical literature must be approached in a scientific manner. This great, new responsibility must be faced by highly trained individuals capable of meeting the demands of this emerging pharmaceutical specialty.

References

1. Fairthorne, R. A.: The Information Revolution—A Britisher's Perspective, *Bull. Am. Soc. Info. Sci. 2*:11–13 (Sept.-Oct.) 1975.
2. Werdel, J. A. and Adams, S.: U.S. Participation in World Information Activities, *Bull. Am. Soc. Info. Sci. 2*:44–48 (Mar.) 1976.
3. Burchinal, L. G.: Recent Trends in Communication of STI, *Bull. Am. Soc. Info. Sci. 2*:9 (Sept.–Oct.) 1975.
4. Vinken, P. J.: Developments in Scientific Documentation in the Long Term, *J. Am. Soc. Info, Sci. 25*:109–112 (Mar.–Apr.) 1974.
5. Baker, D. B.: Information in Revolutionary Times, *Bull. Am. Soc. Info. Sci. 2*:3–4 (Sept.–Oct.) 1975.
6. McCarron, M. M. and Thompson, G. A.: Drug Information, *Principles of Clinical Pharmacy Illustrated by Clinical Case Studies*. McCarron, M. M. (Ed.), Drug Intelligence Publications, Inc., Hamilton, Ill., p. 12, 1974.
7. Hirschman, J. L.: Building a Clinically-Oriented Drug Information Service, *Perspectives in Clinical Pharmacy*, Francke, D. E. and Whitney, H. A. K. Jr., (Eds.), Drug Intelligence Publications, Inc., Hamilton, Ill., p. 151, 1972.
8. Burkholder, D.: Some Experiences in the Establishment and Operation of a Drug Information Center, *Am. J. Hosp. Pharm. 20*: 506–513 (Oct.) 1963.
9. McCarron, M. M.: Inpatient Drug Monitoring, *Drug Intell. Clin. Pharm. 9*:80–85 (Feb.) 1975.
10. Bender, J. J., McKenzie, M. W. and Stewart, R. B.: Defining the Adverse Drug Reaction Sequence, *J. Am. Pharm. Assoc. NS 16*:244–247 (May) 1976.
11. Ballin, J. C.: The ADR Numbers Game Revisited, *J. Am. Med. Assoc. 234*:1257 (22 Dec.) 1975.
12. Karch, F. E. and Lasagna, L.: Adverse Drug Reactions: A Critical Review, *J. Am. Med. Assoc. 234*:1236–1241 (22 Dec.) 1975.
13. American Pharmaceutical Assoc.: A.Ph.A. Reps. Bacon, Wolf Named to New Commission to Monitor Utilization, ADRs, *Pharm. Weekly 15*:1 (4 Dec.) 1976.
14. Martin, E. W., (Ed.): Request for Adverse Drug Reaction Reports: Gratifying Response from Professionals, *FDA Drug Bulletin 6*:34 (Aug.–Oct.) 1976.
15. Wintrobe, M. M.: The Problem of Adverse Drug Reactions, *J. Am. Med. Assoc. 196*:118 (2 May) 1968.
16. Shimomura, S. K. and Watanabe, A. S.: Adverse Drug Reactions: Illustrated by Clinical Case Studies, *Drug Intell. Clin. Pharm. 9*: 190–197 (Apr.) 1975.
17. Johns, M. P.: The Nurse and Drug Surveillance, *Drug Inf. J.*:75–77 (Apr.–Sept.) 1976.
18. Dukes, M. N. G. (Ed.): How to Use This Book, *Meyler's Side Effects of Drugs: A Survey of Unwanted Effects of Drugs Reported in 1972–1975*, Vol. VIII, Excerpta Medica, Amsterdam. Elsevier Pub. Co., Inc., New York, pp. viii–ix, 1975.
19. Wilk, C. K.: Computer Telecommunications Policies: Critical Crossroads, *Drug Inf. J.*:66–70 (Apr.–Sept.) 1976.
20. NASA—Lewis Research Center: *Communications Technology Satellite*, Lister Hill National Center for Biomedical Communications (Nov.) 1975.
21. Porter, L. K.: The Literature and the Pharmacist, *Drug Intell. Clin. Pharm. 9*:513–514 (Sept.) 1975.
22. Herman, C. M., Rodowskas, C. A. Jr. and McGhan, W. F.: Examining the Use of Sources of Drug Information, *J. Am. Pharm. Assoc. NS 16*:239–241 (May) 1976.
23. Rosenberg, J. M., Guzzetti, P. J. and Zupko, A. G.: Pharmacist-Manned Drug Information Centers are Increasing, *Pharm. Times 40*:43–53 (June) 1974.
24. DiPirro, M. N., Kelly, W. N. and Miller, D. E.: Developing a Clinically Oriented Drug Information Service in a Community Hospital, *Lipp. Hosp. Pharm. 10*:434–440 (Oct.) 1975.
25. Aines, A. A.: Infoscope: Opportunities Missed?, *Bull. Am. Soc. Info. Sci. 2*:7–8 (Nov.) 1974.
26. Howard, F. H.: Message to the Symposium

from Senator Hubert H. Humphrey, *Drug Inf. J.*:98–99 (May–Sept.) 1975.

27. American Assoc. of Colleges: *Pharmacists for the Future: The Report of the Study Commission on Pharmacy*, Health Administration Press, Univ. of Michigan, Ann Arbor, Mi., 1975.

28. Katz, W. A.: *Introduction to Reference Work: Vol. II.* Second edition. McGraw-Hill Book Co., New York, pp. 69–97, 1974.

29. Fosket, D. J.: *Information Service in Libraries*, Philosophical Library, New York, p. 75, 1961.

30. Taylor, R. S.: Question-Negotiation and Information Seeking in Libraries, *Coll. Res. Libs. 29*:178–194 (May) 1968.

31. Saracevic, T.: Relevance: A Review of and a Framework for the Thinking on the Notion in Information Science, *J. Am. Soc. Info. Sci. 26*: 321–343 (Nov.–Dec.) 1975.

32. Walton, C. A.: Education and Training of the Drug Information Specialist, *Drug Intell. 1*: 133–137 (Apr.) 1967.

33. Johnston, P. M., Harelik, J. H. and Ryan, M. R.: The Adequacy of Physicians' and Pharmacists' Sources of Drug Information, *Drug Inf. J.*:16–19 (Jan.–Mar.) 1976.

34. Hirschman, J. L.: Building a Clinically-Oriented Drug Information Service. op. cit. p. 152.

35. Beltran, A. A.: The Craft of Literature Searching, *S.L.A. Sci. Tech. News 25*:113–116 (Winter) 1971.

36. Miller, R. R.: Prescribing Habits of Physicians: A Review of the Studies on Prescribing of Drugs, *Drug Intell. Clin. Pharm. 7*:492–500 (Nov.) 1973.

37. Smith, G. H., Sorby, D. L. and Sharp, L. J.: Physician Attitudes Toward Drug Information Resources, *Am. J. Hosp. Pharm. 32*:19–25 (Jan.) 1975.

38. Czapek, E. E.: What the Physician Learns From His Colleagues, *Drug Inf. J.*:47–49 (Jan.–Apr.) 1975.

39. Norwood, G. J., Seibert, J. J. and Gagnon, J. P.: Attitudes of Rural Consumers and Physicians Toward Expanded Roles for Pharmacists, *J. Am. Pharm. Assoc. NS 16*:551–554 (Oct.) 1976.

40. Hodapp, W. J.: Forces Affecting Drug Information Delivery in the Physicians Future, *Drug Inf. J.*:18–26 (Jan.–Apr.) 1975.

41. Miller, R. R.: Prescribing Habits of Physicians: A Review of Studies on the Prescribing of Drugs, *Drug Intell. Clin. Pharm. 7*:81–92 (Feb.) 1974.

42. American Pharmaceutical Association: In

Brief: AMA Resolution Critical of Profession, *Pharm. Weekly 15*:2 (4 Dec.) 1976.

43. American Pharmaceutical Association: AMA Again Opposes DPS, but Agrees to Resolution that Recognizes Substitution, *Pharm. Weekly 15*:3 (18 Dec.) 1976.

44. Francke, D. E. (Editorial): Roles for the Pharmacotherapeutic Specialist, *Drug Intell. Clin. Pharm. 10*:651–652 (Nov.) 1976.

45. Schultz, A.: *Reflections on the Problem of Relevance*, Yale University Press, New Haven, Conn. 1970.

46. Strauss, L. J. et al.: *Scientific and Technical Libraries: Their Organization and Administration*, Becker and Hayes, N.Y. 1972.

47. American Society for Information Science: Information Brokers: Who, What, Why, How, *Bull. Am. Soc. Info. Sci. 2*:11–20 (Feb.) 1976.

48. Tataro, D. S., Briggs, R. L., Chavez-Pardo, R., Feinberg, L. S., Hannigan, J. F., Moore, T. N. and Cohen, S. N.: Detection and Prevention of Drug Interactions Utilizing an On-Line Computer System, *Drug Inf. J.*:10–17 (Jan.–Apr.) 1975.

49. Young, D. S., Pestaner, L. C. and Friedmon, R. B.: Laboratory Oriented Computerized Drug Information System, *Drug Inf. J.*:182–189 (May–Sept.) 1975.

50. Knight, J. R. and Conrad, W. F.: Review of Computer Application in Hospital Pharmacy Practice, *Am. J. Hosp. Pharm. 32*:165–173 (Feb.) 1975.

51. Crootof, L. M., Veal, J. H. and Brunjes, S. D.: Pharmacy Information System for a Health Maintenance Organization, *Am. J. Hosp. Pharm. 32*:1058–1062 (Oct.) 1975.

52. McEvilla, J. D. and Lewis, M. C. G.: The Use of Computers in Pharmacy in the Year 2000, *Drug Intell. Clin. Pharm. 9*:439–446 (Aug.) 1975.

53. Belair, R. R.: Inadequate Privacy Protection in FOIA and the Privacy Act, *Bull. Am. Soc. Info. Sci. 3*:13–16 (Oct.) 1976.

54. Fisher, P. L.: The Freedom of Information Center, *Bull. Am. Soc. Info. Sci. 3*:18–19 (Oct.) 1976.

55. Neir, A.: The Freedom of Information Act, the Privacy Act and You, *Bull. Am. Soc. Info. Sci. 3*:20–21 (Oct.) 1976.

56. Medow, C. T.: On Privacy—A Discourse With Myself, *Bull. Am. Soc. Info. Sci. 3*:22–23 (Oct.) 1976.

57. American Library Association, *Washington Newsletter 28*:1–10, 1–38 (15 Nov.) 1976.

58. Lowe, T. C.: Computer Security Safeguards for Privacy: The Technical Role of NBS, *Bull. Am. Soc. Info. Sci. 3*:16–18 (Oct.) 1976.

59. American Library Association, *Washington Newsletter* 28:3–4 (8 Sept.) 1976.
60. Wenninger, J. A.: FDA's Cosmetic Data Information System: The Program, Design and Public Access to Data, *Drug Inf. J.*: 60–65 (Apr.–Sept.) 1976.
61. Henley, S., Tester, W. H. and Knapp, R.: Dissemination of Drug Information, *J. Am. Hosp. Assoc.* 42:99–102 (16 June) 1968.
62. Burkholder, D. F.: Establishing a Drug Literature Evaluation Program, *Am. J. Pharm. Ed.* 32:871–875, 1968.
63. Worthen, D. B.: Development of a Professional Degree Program in Drug Information, *Drug Inf. J.*:43–46 (Jan.–Apr.) 1975.
64. The Arnold and Marie Schwartz College of Pharmacy (Pamphlet): *Graduate Pharmacy Programs, 1976*, Long Island University, Brooklyn Center, New York.
65. St. John's University: *Proposed and Approved Program for Dual Master's Degree in Pharmacology/Library and Information Science, 1977*, St. John's University College of Pharmacy and Allied Health Professions and Division of Library and Information Science, Jamaica, New York.
66. Francke, D. E. and Whitney, H. A. K. Jr.: Patterns of Clinical Pharmacy Education and Practice in the United States, *Drug Intell. Clin. Pharm.* 10:511–521 (Sept.) 1976.

Related Readings in This Volume

Readings for a Broader Perspective

1. Watanbe, A. S., et al. "Systematic Approach to Drug Information Requests," *American Journal of Hospital Pharmacy* 32 (December 1975):1282–85.
2. Rosenberg, J. M., and Kirschenbaum, H. "How Pharmacy's Drug Information Centers are Enhancing Safe and Efficacious Therapy," *Pharmacy Times* 42 (January 1976):66–72.
3. Zellmer, W. A. "The 'New Pharmacist' and the Pharmaceutical Writer," *Medical Marketing and Media* 10 (August 1975):25–27, 30.
4. Green, L. W., and Fedder, D. O. "Drug Information, the Pharmacist, and the Community," *American Journal of Pharmaceutical Education* 41 (December 1977):444–48.
5. Sewell, W. *Guide to Drug Information*. Hamilton, Ill.: Drug Intelligence Publications, 1976. 218 pp.
6. Collins, G. E., and Lazarus, H. L. *Drug Information Services Handbook*. Acton, Massachusetts: Publishing Science Group, 1975. 180 pp.
7. *Drug Information Journal*. Published by the Drug Information Association. A. D. Berton, editor. Medical Documentation Service, 19 So. 22nd St., Philadelphia, Pennsylvania, 19103.

Geriatrics

30—The Senescent Drug "Abuser": A New Sociologic Problem

Allen Morgan Kratz

We are witnessing a time where combinations of sociologic, ecologic, and economic phenomena are resulting in serious new problems. The Toflerian need to design new solutions to unthought of problems can best be witnessed in the field of gerontology. One hundred years ago there were 1.2 million elderly persons in the United States. Today there are 25 million. Life-expectancy in the U.S. has risen from 49 years in 1900 to 73 today. During the same time period, the proportion of elderly has gone from 4 to 11% of the population. The "young-old," newly retired, often to active retirement communities, have little in common with the "old-old" who are usually infirm or house-bound. This is the generation that has lived through the technological revolution—the discovery of the airplane, psychotherapy, the atomic bomb, and now, space travel. They have also benefited from tremendous advances in medicine, with more yet to come. Every day 4000 more Americans join the 65–plus generation while 3000 older persons die. In 25 years the proportion of elderly over 85 will more than double.

At the same time, it is in the past half century that we have made miraculous discoveries in the medical field, particularly in the development of drug therapy which have made such an enormous impact on demographic life-expectancy factors. This article will comment on the interface between these medications and the demographic results of longer life in the larger proportion of elderly in our society. It will also look at some of the philosophical changes that have taken place in our senescent populus through their lifespans—changes that range from the days of wearing garlic around their necks to today's full acceptance of the American credo, "Better living through chemistry." In describing the problem, Dr. Wendell R. Lipscomb commented about the iatrogenic "spaced-out" grandma syndrome:[1]

> This syndrome is a collection of signs and symptoms one might expect in the youthful hippie drug experimenter. But I have increasingly been called on to consult about the ancient chemical hippies who owe their spaced-out status to the good intentions of their family doctors. What has happened is that a woman, usually in her 70's has been overtreated for multiple conditions—arthritis, hypertension, periodic headaches, occasional sleeplessness, and mood swings. Each complaint is dealt with on a pragmatic basis of one symptom, one drug. Somehow the total effect of the therapeutic cocktail is never considered.

In reviewing the literature, it is unfair to pin the blame of drug "abuse" in the elderly solely on iatrogenesis—a physician induced ailment. The etiology of the problem stems from a synergistic interface between three poorly informed, and often noncommunicative, components of the gerontologic health care system: the physician, the pharmacist, and last, but not least, the patient.

Measuring the severity of the drug "abuse," or misuse, problem in the elderly is most difficult. Research now being undertaken is looking at the medication usage patterns of senescent persons in the Miami area. Anecdotal data tell a very sad story. Virtually everyone interviewed was on three or more medications. The record holder is an 81-year-old lady who was taking a total of 28 medications. In South Miami Beach, one observes what can be defined as the "chemical dresser" syndrome. This is an old piece of furniture usually about 42 inches high, the top of which is covered with a variety of vials and liquid medicine bottles in numbers which could easily stock a pharmacy shelf. Many of these containers are empty. Many are better than 10 years old. Yet they sit in a special place of pride along with family pictures and other memorabilia relating to the life of this senescent individual.

This individual is often suffering from some degree of an organic brain syndrome which in itself can cause confusion and often lead to overmedication or actual unintentional overdosing. A classic paper providing basic source data on elderly persons who were treated for nonfatal, but acute, drug reactions in a hospital emergency room is one published by Drs. David Petersen and Charles Thomas. They collected data from all 1128 persons treated for acute drug reactions at Jackson Memorial Hospital in Miami during 1972. Looking at the group 50 and over, they discovered that this age group accounted for 5.4% of all admissions. The drug emergencies in this group were, however, significantly different. All admissions of the elderly involved the use of a legend drug as opposed to an illicit one. Of these, 80.9% involved the misuse of a psychotropic

drug and 10.6% were related to an overdose of a nonnarcotic analgesic. The most frequently implicated drugs were *Valium, Tuinal*, phenobarbital, and *Darvon*.[2]

In a British study which reviewed 5 years of admissions to three general hospitals, 46% of self-poisoning admissions were accidental as opposed to intentional. It is interesting to note that in those admissions over the age of 75, the accidental self-poisoning rate had actually gone down to 36%. There were no significant differences between the number of drugs taken in accidental overdoses and in true suicide attempts. Sedatives and hypnotics comprised the largest group. Of the 291 accidental deaths during this period, 33 emanated from self-poisoning.[3]

Of course, the degree of severity of the drug problem should not be based on the known statistics from these or other studies, but rather, from the unknown. Since severe illness and death in the elderly is so much an *expectation*, objective, detailed investigation is the exception rather than the rule. There is no way of knowing how many cases of chronic organic brain syndrome wasting away in nursing homes were originally precipitated by acute drug reactions. It is also not known how many hip fractures emanated from falls unnecessarily caused by a drug-induced vertigo or visual misperception. There is no way of knowing how many unautopsied deaths of an elderly person in his or her sleep were in fact caused by an acute drug reaction or interaction. Just as gerontologic suicide is undercounted, the dimensions of drug-related illness and death are grossly underestimated.

Looking at the three interactive agents that have caused this drug misuse problem, the physician must shoulder a large portion of the blame. Medical training all but ignores the senescent patient. No medical school in the country has developed a geriatric specialty to this date. Too often, the medical ego, ubiquitously seeking cures, cannot tolerate the chronic degenerative processes that are seen in many of our elderly. Often the elderly patient is a burden to the physician's practice. The combination of Medicare and other third-party billing paperwork along with the additional time it may take to properly treat an elder results in many physicians discouraging that aspect of their caseload.

What are some of the specific problems created by the physician in the area of gerontologic drug "abuse"? Oftentimes the physician does not take the time and make the effort to appropriately titrate medication dosage to the individual patient. The dosage prescribed may be well suited to the imaginary 28-year-old, 70-kg male that pharmaceutical companies use as their test model but not for the frail 70-year-old. Secondly, the physician often does not appreciate the common interactions that exist among medications. This is especially serious in the elderly who suffer from a multiplicity of problems and are often receiving a variety of drugs related to each of these conditions, many times prescribed by a variety of physicians as well. The physician does not realize that drug therapy in the elderly has special hazards because of the anatomic, physiologic, and biochemical changes that accompany aging.[4,5] Physicians generally do not take the time to monitor medications once they have been prescribed. Often adjusting the dosage will make the difference between therapeutic failure and success with a given medication. Relying on the pharmacist as an aid in monitoring patient response to medication seems a logical solution to this problem. Too many physicians treating the elderly are quick to want to satisfy their client. Physicians must share frustrations over the elder who comes into the office and is extremely disappointed if no prescription is written. How many mild tranquilizer prescriptions are written simply to meet the predetermined expectation of the patient? Many of these physicians do not take the time to educate their patients towards the realities of the aging process and the limita-

tions of medications towards treating some of the chronic illnesses from which they suffer.

The pharmacist is the second aspect of this "Bermuda triangle." Remember the days when the pharmacist represented the neighborhood physician-extender? Generally, the pharmacist was intimately involved with each and every patron, trying to be helpful, knowing the neighborhood physicians as well as the products that were sold without a prescription. He was also intimately involved in the preparation of the prescribed medication, with the mortar and pestle or the graduate. Unfortunately, today, most of this intimacy has been lost as has the professionalism in the practice of community pharmacy. Yet, the potential for this professionalism does exist in the form of a subtle record-keeping program known as the patient medication profile. Many pharmacies have adapted this technique or system and in some states it has been mandated as a public health safeguard. The pharmacist maintains a master record for each patient which includes information on each prescription dispensed as well as pertinent data such as drug allergies, medical history, and previous treatments. The pharmacist can serve as a quality control check on the prescribing physician and appropriately question a given prescription in light of knowledge he maintains about other medications previously prescribed or purchased over-the-counter by the patient. This profile is also used to screen for possible drug-drug, drug-food, and drug-laboratory test interactions. The pharmacist can also detect when a patient is visiting more than one physician for the same symptoms or complaints as some of our elderly often do. It is not unusual to find a little old lady taking three different medications from three different physicians all for the same indication or malady. Computer systems are now available and utilized by some progressive pharmacists that are programmed to scan for possible contraindications, allergies, and interactions. They alert pharmacist and physician to possible situations of inappropriate medication, potential interactions, or possible counter-prescribing by two or more physicians. If a prescription ordered does not fit the profile of that patient, the computer will reject the order and indicate to the pharmacist the reason for rejection. If appropriate, the pharmacist would contact the prescribing physician and explain the problem, hoping to arrive at a logical alternative or solution to the problem. This profile system can be maintained by a concerned and well-trained pharmacist using a simple index card or a sophisticated computer. The present day pharmacist, clinically trained, is probably the most overeducated and underutilized member of the health care team.

The pharmacist also sees the massive utilization of over-the-counter medications that are often useless, and occasionally dangerous to the elderly person who seeks relief from discomfort by doing what his/her television directs. Whether curing headaches, arthritis, or constipation, the uninformed consumer may well create a complicating drug reaction based on responding to a televised suggestion. A favorite story is that of the 76-year-old man who took *Ex-Lax* every morning and *Kaopectate* every evening for years.

The pharmacist and his supplier, the pharmaceutical company, can do a great deal more in the area of packaging medications for the elderly. Clever birth control pill packaging has helped many women achieve the therapeutic benefits for which the pill was designed. It seems incomprehensible that the same packaging and marketing efforts cannot be made for commonly prescribed medications for the elderly. "Child-proof" containers as we came to find out are in actuality "aged-proof" as well. Many elderly and their families have developed adaptations because of sensory and memory deficits ranging from commercially obtainable daily pill boxes to the clever adaptation of a fishing tackle box using colors, num-

bers, and large painted letters to assist an elderly grandfather with appropriate utilization of his medication. It should be noted that some companies are, in fact, looking at packaging alternatives to better serve the aged population. However, the industry as a whole has not been profoundly responsive to the overall problem.

Let us look at the third component and perhaps the most significant: the patient. Who is the drug-abused geriatric patient? First, organic brain changes often make this person forgetful. "Did I take that pill an hour ago? Well, I better take one now." One must remember that organic brain changes can create a level of forgetfulness that totally eradicates all new learning input. The organic brain syndrome patient, who, one half hour after eating, complains about not having eaten simply because he has forgotten, is the classic example of this all too common situation.

We also see a philosophy among many of our elders that is based on some logical assumption that "if one pill will get me better, two pills will get me better twice as fast." Lack of understanding about the side effects and contraindications of medications is a serious problem. This also manifests itself in the popular pill swapping game that is observed throughout areas where the elderly congregate. "Oh, your doctor gave you a blue pill to help your stomach. My doctor didn't give me anything for my stomach. I'll give you my red arthritis pill if you give me your blue stomach pill." It happens and continues to happen without regard to the potentially harmful effects of such transactions. As mentioned previously, the philosophy that underlies the entire aspect of this problem is that of better living through chemistry. A belief that medication can cure often incurable, degenerative problems of the senescent.

Medicare as a medical insurance program has helped the elderly in many ways. However, inexpensive physician care has led to a doctor "shopping" epidemic. Often, when a physician does not prescribe a medication, or enough medications, the elderly patient takes off the next day to visit another physician who hopefully will serve as a more adroit supplier. Accidentally or purposefully, the patient often neglects to tell one physician what another has prescribed. Sometimes, even the well-intentioned elder forgets what they take for occasional aches and pains in their back, or their lumbago, or headache, or the medication they take on a second day without a bowel movement. Also many elderly are afraid that they would insult their physician if they told him about the other doctor or two they are seeing. So they fail to mention the other physicians, and prescriptions involved in their care. If the elder had all his prescriptions filled and obtained all his health needs solely from a single source—one pharmacy with a patient profile system—this problem could be alleviated.

Finally, we do know that the elderly suffer a variety of sensory deficits. The two that impact on this problem are decreased vision and hearing. Younger people often have a difficult time reading the dosage instructions on prescription containers. For the elder, this can become an impossible act. The pharmacist should be asked to type the instructions in capital letters. Likewise bottle and dosage form color discrimination is a difficult task due to reduced visual acuity and color perception. Listening to the physician's and/or pharmacist's verbal instructions may also be a futile effort on the part of the hearing-impaired elderly person. Yet, as with other minorities, the senescent suffers from the psychological "native" syndrome in a land of colonials. They are often frightened to speak up about their deficits, their concerns, their needs, and their questions.

Before looking for some potential solutions, some attention should be given to those 5% of the elderly that are in nursing homes or long-term care facilities. Even though a relatively small percentage, they represent a major area of concern. In 1973,

there were about 21,800 nursing homes in the United States, containing almost 1.3 million beds and providing care to about 1.2 million residents. Of all nursing homes 77% were proprietary; 17% were nonprofit homes, while about 6% were government sponsored. During fiscal year 1975, nursing home expenditures in the United States reached 9.0 billion dollars or 7.6% of the total expenditures for health services and supplies.[6]

Dr. Sidney Cohen, former director of the National Institute of Mental Health Division of Narcotic Addiction and Drug Abuse and Clinical Professor of Psychiatry at the University of California at Los Angeles Neuropsychiatric Institute, recently wrote:[1]

> Oversedation of many nursing home members is part of a general picture of overmedication. In part, this results from piling on drug orders without a periodic review of the chart to eliminate the unnecessary but long forgotten items. Furthermore, eccentricity, nonconformity, even irascibility are not indications for sedation. Our problem is that we have pills easily capable of making the crotchety complaint-free, the demanding dulled, and the surly sedated. Why should the staff put up with any disrupting influences whatsoever? One answer is that we don't want to chemically obliterate all personality features, however obstreperous. Another answer is that these drugs have side effects that require other drugs that have side effects. Since the source of geriatric sedative abuse is, almost invariably, the physician's order or prescription, more enlightened prescribing practices could do a good deal to solve the problem.

In a study of 91 nursing homes by Raymond Glasscote of the Joint Information Service, one conclusion read:[7]

> It is easy to conclude that primary care physicians widely prescribe small doses of major tranquilizers in a routine and "precautionary" way, since older patients with neurological damage are likely to be restless, irritable and uncomfortable. Whether nearly so large a percentage of patients

need even a small routine dose of a major tranquilizer certainly might be questioned.

The consultant pharmacist responsible to the skilled nursing facility has been given the specific task of reviewing patient medications on a monthly basis in hopes of preventing this type of overutilization. An effective drug utilization review will also reduce the overall costs by reducing the amount of unnecessary medications prescribed for these long-term care patients. Again, effective use of the clinically trained pharmacist as a member of the gerontologic health care team will pay dividends to all concerned.

For the institutional elderly, greater supervision by the regulatory agencies will also help to eliminate much of the problem. In institutions, one need not worry about many of the community elderly drug abuse concerns, since medications are handled by the nursing staff, recorded, and administrations are generally supervised with professional care. It is interesting to note the emergence of safer unit-dose systems designed for the long-term care environment similar to systems employed in hospitals. Considering the differences in personnel administering medications in the long-term facility as compared to the acute care facility a safer drug distribution system should be a prerequisite in nursing homes.

With regard to problems in the community, one must look at all components of the triad for potential solutions. Education is the key for the physician, pharmacist, and patient. One recent article emphasized that health education designed to meet the consumer's need for health care information in simple, direct terms was a viable means for coping with this problem.[8] Unfortunately, our communities have not as yet adequately responded to this need. Yet, the combined resources of the health and mental health systems, colleges and universities, the public schools, and indigenous senior citizens organizations could well together provide adequate input to make a significant inroad on the problem of drug "abuse" in the elderly.

Drug "abuse" in the senescent is a much easier problem to solve than illicit drug use in the young. The solution requires a significant amount of public attention, combined efforts at education to all concerned, and finally, where indicated, increased governmental regulatory controls of an already legally sanctioned system of drug advertising and distribution. The informed 82-year-old "abusers" will not hit the streets looking for a *Valium* connection . . . or will they??

This is one opportunity for those concerned with the health and welfare of our senescent populace without some new bureaucracy to find solutions to a problem without creating new problems as a result of these solutions.

References

1. Geriatric drug abuse said virtually ignored problem. *Psychiatric News*, April 1976.
2. Petersen, D. M., Thomas, C.: Acute drug reactions among the elderly. *J. Gerontal 30*:552, 1975.
3. Bean, P.: Accidental and intentional self-poisoning in the over 60 age group. *Gerontol Clin 15*:259, 1973.
4. Aadaargard, G.: Drug therapy in the aged. *Postgrad Med 52*: 115, 1972.
5. Wynne, R. D., Heller, F.: Drug overdose among the elderly: a growing problem. *Perspectives on Aging 2*: March–April 15, 1973.
6. U.S. House of Representatives Subcommittee on Oversight and Investigations, Committee on Interstate and Foreign Commerce: "Fraud and Abuse in Nursing Homes: Pharmaceutical Kickback Arrangements," April 1977.
7. Glasscote, R.: *Old Folks at Homes*, Joint Information Service, Washington, D.C., 1976, 74.
8. Plant, J.: Educating the elderly in safe medication use. *Hospitals 51*: April 16, 1977.

Related Readings in This Volume

Readings for a Broader Perspective

1. Lesko, L. J. "Biopharmaceutical Aspects of Geriatric Pharmacy," *The Apothecary* 89 (March/April 1977):21–26.

2. Kluza, R. B. "Monitoring of Geriatric Drug Therapy," *The Apothecary* 89 (March/April 1977):27–31.
3. "Elderly Targeted for Medication Education," *NARD Journal* 100 (December 1978):24–25.

Intravenous Drug Therapy

31—Justification for a Pharmacy-Coordinated I.V. Therapy Team

Daniel L. Kopp and Richard J. Hammel

Intravenous therapy and the administration of medications by the intravenous route has become an integral part of patient care. Over one-fourth of hospitalized patients receive intravenous infusions.[1] This results in at least 8 million patients who receive I.V. therapy each year.[2] The modern era of I.V. therapy dates back to 1923 and the discovery of pyrogenic substances by Siebert.[3] Significant developments since 1923 include the introduction of the plastic catheter in 1945,[4] the use of total parenteral nutrition,[5] development of complex infusion systems, and a proliferation of I.V. medications. The increased usage of I.V. therapy, the addition of multiple medications to I.V. fluids, and the availability of the laminar flow I.V. hood led to the development of centralized pharmacy I.V. additive services in the late 1960's.[6-8] The concept of a pharmacy-coordinated I.V. admixture and administration service (I.V. team) also developed in the late 1960's.[9] The benefits of a centralized pharmacy I.V. additive service have been documented[6-10] and

will not be discussed further. The concept of the pharmacy-coordinated I.V. administration service or I.V. team is being promoted more frequently. This article will attempt to provide the hospital with the procedures and justification necessary for approval of a pharmacy-coordinated I.V. therapy team.

The I.V. Therapy Team

The I.V. therapy team is a multidisciplinary team responsible for the proper initiation, maintenance, and monitoring of I.V. therapy. Primary therapy is performed by the I.V. team nurse or I.V. therapist under the direction of the I.V. Committee or other authorized hospital department. The I.V. team should be able to draw on the expertise of the pharmacy, nursing and medical staff. The concept of an I.V. therapy team can develop in numerous ways. The idea may develop from one person (nurse, pharmacist, physician) or may result from discussions or evaluations of current I.V. therapy. Once the idea has been born, the "team dream" to be successful and viable must seek a broad base of support.[11]

The increased technology and sophistication in medical care is forcing the physician to shift perspectives concerning paraprofessionals. The physician has become increasingly dependent on paraprofessional teams.[12] The paraprofessional team must develop a sense of teamwork. Webster defines teamwork as "joint action by a group of people, in which each person subordinates his individual interests and opinions to the unity and efficiency of the group; coordinated effort."[13] This definition of teamwork indicates that each member of the team be utilized to his highest level of competence and that no member would have an absolute role. Teamwork must be an integral force in the development, initiation, and success of an I.V. therapy team. If adequate support and teamwork are present, the team approach to I.V. therapy merits consideration. If strong opposition is encountered from administration, physicians, nurses, or pharmacists, the program will stand little chance of approval or success. If enthusiastic support or support to further evaluate the idea is received, the team concept can proceed through more specific and formal channels of approval.

I.V. Team Proposal

The formal channels of approval for the I.V. team will vary from hospital to hospital. The most common hospital committee to develop an I.V. team proposal is a joint pharmacy and nursing committee.[9,14,15,16] The pharmacy and therapeutic committee,[17] infection control committee, patient care committee, and the hospital administration must all be actively involved in developing guidelines and policies and procedures for the I.V. team. Communication is imperative. It may be advisable to form an *ad hoc* committee representing the medical, nursing, pharmacy, laboratory and dietary staff. This committee would be responsible for establishing the scope and objectives of the I.V. team, develop guidelines and policies, and justify the need and expense of an I.V. team.

The proposal should begin with a statement of the scope and objectives of the I.V. therapy team. These should be statements upon which justification for the program can be developed (Table 31.1).

Table 31.1

Beginning of Proposal for I.V. Therapy Team[18]

Scope
1. To provide adequate trained personnel proficient in mixing additives to I.V. fluids and in making venipunctures.
2. To establish centralized accountability of the use and charging of I.V. fluids.
3. To provide a central point of information concerning I.V. fluids.

Objectives
1. To maintain a department having an adequate understanding of the principles and techniques which intravenous therapy demands.
2. To provide for the efficient administration of intravenous fluids, medication, blood and blood derivatives.
3. To maintain a department skilled in the venipuncture procedure to provide greater patient comfort.
4. To minimize the physiological effect on the patient receiving intravenous therapy.
5. To provide an additional check and control for greater patient safety by reducing medication errors.
6. To keep accurate records of the types of fluid and medications given and of any reaction to either.
7. To provide a central point of information on intravenous fluids.
8. To shift compounding duties from nursing units to pharmacy guidance where it belongs.
9. To reduce waste and provide proper labeling.
10. To save nursing time.
11. To provide accurate charging of intravenous fluids.

The second step for the I.V. team committee is to define the responsibilities of the various team members and develop standard policies and procedures. In defining these responsibilities, I would like to describe a system which can accomplish most of the potential benefits of an I.V. team and can be adapted into most hospitals without excessive increases in staff or expense.

The physician's responsibilities are to advise the team concerning proper procedures, new techniques, and to evaluate the functioning of the team. The physician should also play an active and vital role in education of the team.

In a pharmacy-coordinated I.V. team, the pharmacist would have numerous responsibilities (Table 31.2).

Nursing responsibilities can be divided into two areas, the I.V. team nurse and/or I.V. therapist and the unit nursing staff. The I.V. team nurse and/or I.V. therapist (trained LPN or I.V. technician) and unit staff nurses' responsibilities are listed in Table 31.3.

The third step for the I.V. team committee

Table 31.2

Pharmacist's Responsibilities of Pharmacy-Coordinated I.V. Team

1. To ensure proper functioning and coordination of team activities.
2. To provide financial management and budgeting of team activities.
3. To maintain I.V. additive services.
4. To provide a source of I.V. information.
5. To educate and train I.V. team members.
6. To maintain workload and team statistics.
7. To maintain adequate supplies.
8. To establish a quality control program.
9. To maintain close communication with nursing, medical and administrative personnel.

is to justify the need and forecast the expense of the I.V. team. The I.V. team committee must document the need for an I.V. team and present a review of the literature. To document the need, a number of studies might be considered. These studies might include the savings in total personnel time, equipment required, additional staff requirements, usage of I.V. therapy, and an evaluation of current I.V. therapy. These studies would then be utilized to document the need

Table 31.3

Responsibilities of I.V. Team and Unit Staff Nurses

The responsibilities of the I.V. team nurse and/or I.V. therapist:
1. To perform the initial venipuncture and restarts.
2. To monitor flow rates at least each shift.
3. To change and date I.V. sets every 24 hours.
4. To change dressings at appropriate intervals.
5. To survey for phlebitis, infiltration or hematoma at least once per shift.
6. To coordinate the administration of drugs with the I.V. additive service.
7. To administer blood and blood products.
8. To maintain heparin wells and locks.
9. To assist with subclavian catheterization, dressing changes three times per week, and monitor total parenteral nutrition and enteral alimentation therapy.
10. To monitor and report infection control data.
11. To maintain appropriate workload statistics.
12. To insure accurate charging of I.V. fluids.

The responsibilities of the unit staff nurse:
1. To monitor flow rate of the I.V. at least every hour.
2. To provide additional fluids as ordered and administer intermittent medication via piggyback.
3. To check for phlebitis, infiltration and hematoma.
4. To monitor input and output data.
5. To page I.V. team nurse for restarts or problems.

for the I.V. team to the hospital administration, executive board, and the board of trustees. A thorough literature search will also provide a firm basis for approval of an I.V. therapy team. The remainder of this article will deal with the justification of the I.V. therapy team on the basis of the literature.

Justification for an I.V. therapy team can be divided into the advantages for the patient, the hospital, and the financial implications which result.

Patient Care

Patient care is becoming more complex in all areas and I.V. therapy is no exception. The proliferation of potent I.V. medication, complex delivery systems, total parenteral nutrition (TPN), cardiac catheterization and other advances have made I.V. therapy a specialty.[19] The general unit nurse, who is responsible for all aspects of patient care, can no longer be expected to provide optimal care and knowledge of I.V. therapy. The unit nurse, however, should not be relieved completely of I.V. responsibilities. This division of responsibilities insures the patient of optimal care by the I.V. team and allows the unit nurse more time to administer other therapy. The I.V. team nurse can expand her knowledge, expertise, and experience in providing comprehensive I.V. therapy. The American Association of I.V. Therapists, the National I.V. Therapy Association, and the I.V. Therapists Association of Greater New York have been established to promote the education and utilization of I.V. therapists.[20] The American Journal of I.V. Therapy is published bimonthly to aid the I.V. therapist. The I.V. therapist also promotes improved patient care by strictly adhering to policies and procedures developed by the hospital I.V. committee. It has been shown that proper attention to established protocols will decrease I.V. complications and improve patient care.[21,22] The traditional

system with the feeling that "anyone can handle I.V. therapy" is not consistent with optimal patient care.

Complications resulting from I.V. therapy can pose serious threats to the well-being of hospitalized patients. The most serious threat is I.V.-related sepsis. Numerous investigations have shown varying positive catheter culture and sepsis rates. Positive cultures of I.V. catheters range from 3.8% to 57% with associated sepsis rates ranging from zero to 8%.[23] Bentley's study indicated that the specially trained transfusion therapy service maintained 90% of all catheters, but resulted in only 11% of the catheter-related septicimias. House physicians maintained the remaining 10% of catheters but were responsible for 89% of the related septicemias.[24] Their conclusion stated, "the skill and experience in inserting catheters atraumatically was undoubtedly one of the factors for the transfusion therapy services low complication rate. The second, and perhaps the most important reason, was the daily and sometimes twice daily observation of the catheter site." This study, however, was retrospective and uncontrolled. Fuchs reported a very low colonization rate (3.8%) of indwelling catheters and attributed this low value in part to the hospital's population and in part to the hospital team of specially trained "I.V." nurses for insertion and maintenance care of I.V. catheters.[25]

Many other articles have recommended I.V. therapy teams as the most efficient and effective system for minimizing I.V. complications.[23,26,27,28,29] The case for the I.V. therapy team is also strongly supported by the U.S. Center for Disease Control in Atlanta. In its *Recommendations for the Prevention of I.V. Associated Infections*, in 1973, the Center for Disease Control (CDC) points out that "experience has indicated that proper maintenance of intravenous fluid systems is most efficiently and effectively carried out if intravenous "teams" are responsible for intravenous therapy throughout the hospital. Heterogenous groups of individuals, such as house officers, staff doctors, and nurses, have been much less successful in methodically and meticulously following the above recommendations."[30]

The importance of adequate care is even more difficult to achieve when special procedures such as hyperalimentation are considered. Kaminski and Stolar demonstrated that there were significant deficiencies between the actual practices and the proposed guidelines for the administration of total parenteral nutrition.[31] These deficiencies led to a series of recommendations which include a multidisciplinary hyperalimentation team. In another study, metabolic complications of total parenteral nutrition utilizing a team approach resulted in 2.7% electrolyte aberrations and 5% for significant glycosuria.[32] This compares with 28.1% electrolyte imbalances and 27.4% glycosuria reported by Kaminski and Stoler.[31] The maintenance of total parenteral nutrition and other specialized I.V. procedures by an I.V. team will promote patient care.

It has also been reported that I.V. teams have reduced the incidence of phlebitis. Multiple factors appear to predispose the patient to the development of phlebitis. These include: 1) the anatomic location of the vein-cannulated legs is more vulnerable; 2) position of the cannula tip-short plastic catheters terminating in extremity veins is more irritating than central venous catheters; 3) duration of cannulation-phlebitis increases with time; 4) type of cannula-steel needles causes less phlebitis than plastic catheters, probably due to smaller bore size, ease of insertion, and relatively nonthrombotic surface; 5) size and length of catheter; 6) type of infusion–acidic, hypertonic; 7) intravenous medications such as cephalosporins and cytotoxic medications irritate veins.[33] Considering these predisposing factors, the I.V. therapy nurse could effectively reduce phlebitis complications by proper selection of vein, proper selection of needle or catheter, proper

insertion techniques, and frequent surveillance. To evaluate I.V. complications and phlebitis, a study at Hamot Medical Center from July 1974 to August 1975 showed phlebitis complications of 18.5% non-team to 10.0% for the I.V. team. The total amount of I.V. related trouble was 41.7% non-team versus 23.3% for the I.V. team[17] (Table 31.4).

Table 31.4

Results of I.V. Therapy Team (July 1974–August 1975)[17]

I.V.'s started or DC'd because of	Number of Venipunctures	
	Non-Team (2757)	Team (7376)
Phlebitis	18.5%	10.1%
Infiltration	15.5%	9.8%
Pain, sore or tender	6.4%	3.4%
Poor sites	1.3%	0 %
Total amount of trouble	41.7%	23.3%

Another important consideration of proper patient care is the avoidance, recognition, or prompt discontinuation of incompatible or unstable medications. The majority of I.V. incompatibilities can be averted through a centralized pharmacy I.V. additive program. It is imperative, however, that the I.V. therapist be aware of common I.V. incompatabilities and adverse reactions. This awareness can be provided through an adequate training program.

Training of I.V. Therapists

Last and not least, patient and staff education about I.V. therapy will improve understanding, cooperation, and patient care. An important component of existing I.V. teams is their emphasis on education and training of I.V. therapists.[11,15,17] The training of I.V. therapists should be handled as a joint responsibility of the nursing, anesthesiology, and pharmacy departments. The curriculum should include the areas listed in Table 31.5. In addition, the I.V. therapist must be monitored periodically to ensure proper techniques. Quality control measures should include a review of the venipuncture records of each I.V. therapist. Once a baseline is established for each therapist, breakage in techniques or performance can be easily spotted.

Table 31.5

Curriculum for I.V. Therapists[17]

1. Fluid and electrolyte balance.
2. Aseptic techniques.
3. Emotional aspects of I.V. therapy.
4. Familiarization with I.V. sets and filters.
5. The difference between extracaths, intracaths, and needles, and their appropriate use.
6. Familiarization with I.V. fluids.
7. Familiarization with I.V. incompatabilities.
8. The use of I.V. controllers and pumps.
9. Relationship of I.V.'s to laboratory tests.
10. Techniques of venipuncture.
11. Methods to retard phlebitis.
12. Administration of blood and blood products.
13. Subclavian catheter care.
14. Enteralimentation/hyperalimentation.
15. Intradermal skin testing.

Patient Education

Education of the patient has resulted in a better understanding and acceptance of I.V. therapy. The I.V. therapist can explain the reasons for I.V. therapy, what will happen to the patient, and how the patient can help assure successful I.V. therapy. Because of the time involved and a desire to provide written material to the patient, some hospitals have developed an I.V. handbook for patients to supplement the therapists' discussion. For example, the handbook at Northside Hospital in Atlanta, Georgia contains sections on I.V. admixtures, indications for I.V. therapy, how the nurse selects a suitable vein, patient responsibilities, and warning signs. The section on warning signs states, "You should call the nurse if any of the following situations become apparent

during the course of your I.V. therapy: 1) your arm becomes swollen and/or red around the needle site; 2) you feel soreness or a burning sensation around the needle site (this is sometimes due to drugs you are receiving in the I.V. bottle); 3) the I.V. stops dripping or is running excessively fast; 4) the I.V. bottle is empty; 5) fluid is leaking somewhere from the I.V. system."[34] Although the handbook and education will not benefit all patients, the idea that patients become participants in their care can produce marked improvement in cooperation, understanding, and overall care for many patients.

Pharmacy Coordination and Control

The I.V. therapy team must also be justified on its advantage to the hospital. One of the first questions is, under which department should the I.V. therapy team function? I.V. teams have been placed under anesthesiology, nursing, and pharmacy departments. The department of anesthesiology in most hospitals is removed from the day-to-day operation of patient care. The opportunities for the I.V. team to grow and expand its functions are limited. The anesthesiology department, however, is an excellent area for the training and education of I.V. therapists. If nursing service is selected, a communication problem may exist between the pharmacy centralized I.V. additive service and the nursing I.V. therapy team. Combining the I.V. additive service and the I.V. team under the pharmacy department will provide advantages for the I.V. therapist, the pharmacy, and the hospital.[35]

Advantages to the hospital will include a much closer working relationship between departments, especially pharmacy and nursing. The pharmacy department will become increasingly involved in patient care areas. The I.V. therapist is a vital communication link between pharmacy and nursing and can promote pharmacy involvement. Through the I.V. therapist, the pharmacy may better realize and identify areas of additional pharmacy services. The I.V. therapist will have prompt access to the pharmacists' knowledge of I.V. incompatibilities, recommended dosages, and administration methods. The I.V. fluid will be prepared aseptically, reviewed by a pharmacist, and be ready for the I.V. therapist to administer when needed. This synergistic relationship of pharmacy and nursing would increase efficiency in the delivery of I.V. therapy.[36]

The management of the I.V. additive and I.V. team would also be more effective if budgeting, control, and procedures were delegated to the pharmacy department. Because of improved communication, the accountability and waste associated with many I.V. additive programs would be minimized. Budgeting and workload statistics could be correlated and an equitable I.V. charge could be computed. The standardization and evaluation of I.V. equipment may result in reduced inventory and increased efficiency.

Developmental and Operational Costs

The greatest advantage to the hospital and the hospital's ultimate goal is to improve patient care. A pharmacy-coordinated I.V. team can improve patient care and decrease the hospital's liability against improper I.V. care.

The cost of developing an I.V. team will vary considerably depending on the level of service the hospital provides. The best method to determine costs is to perform several studies to determine nursing time saved, staffing patterns, and personnel needs. In justifying the nine positions at St. Francis Hospital in Cincinnati, Ohio, Wuest demonstrated that the cost of seven I.V. therapist positions would come from unfilled nursing positions, one from reduced need of a house physician, and one additional hospital bud-

geted position.[16] The cost of the I.V. team also depends on the I.V. team personnel. Will the team consist of one or two registered nurses plus LPN and I.V. technician therapists or will the team consist of registered nurses only? This decision may be regulated by the law in each individual state.

Costs may be reduced through standardization of equipment, decreased inventory, and decreased wastage due to improper selection or unsuccessful venipuncture. Substantial savings might also be generated if I.V.-related items, which were improperly or not charged under the traditional system, were now being charged by the I.V. team.

Staffing the I.V. team will vary from hospital to hospital as will the range of services provided. A study should be undertaken to determine the usage and staffing pattern required.[37] The time required to start an adult I.V. has been estimated at 15 minutes, 15 to 30 minutes for pediatric I.V.'s and 20 minutes per liter of hyperalimentation. Provision must be made for restarts, dressing changes, surveillance, and complications.[38]

Equipment requirements will be minimal if a centralized I.V. additive program is in operation. The only other equipment required might include a small office, some additional storage space, a file cabinet, and a desk.

Conclusion

In conclusion, the I.V. therapy team is an extension of today's complex medical system. Advances in I.V. therapy, I.V. medications, and the proliferation of knowledge has made I.V. therapy a specialty similar to the operating room nurse, pediatric nurse, emergency room nurse, pediatric nurse, emergency room nurse, or intensive care unit nurse. The team approach permits the most knowledgeable, motivated, and best trained people to manage I.V. therapy.

The organization of the I.V. team should be under the direction of the pharmacy department. A pharmacy-coordinated program produces a good marriage between the I.V. additive services and the I.V. therapy team. Communication, understanding, and efficiency are maximized when the management and day-to-day operation of the team is placed under the pharmacy department. The development of the I.V. team must be carried out by a multidisciplinary committee responsible for justification, developing policy and procedures, and evaluation. The justification can be divided into the benefits to the patient, the hospital, and the financial alternatives.

The benefit to the patient is significant. The major benefits result from improved nursing care. The I.V. therapist's primary responsibility is the proper insertion, care, and maintenance of I.V. therapy. With a relatively small staff, the I.V. therapists are able to adhere to and practice standard policy and procedures established by the hospital. This adherence to standard protocols can reduce the infection complications associated with I.V. therapy. The quality of venipuncture is largely a matter of practice, expertise, and specialized care. Nurses who rarely initiate I.V. therapy are at a definite disadvantage, as is the patient. The therapist is also trained on selection of catheter site and maintenance of catheters. The I.V. therapist provides closer surveillance of the patient than ward personnel, and is a valuable link to the pharmacy department. The I.V. team concept controls and centralizes the reporting of infections and the reporting of appropriate statistical records. Education of the patient plays a critical role in eliciting cooperation, understanding, and a feeling of participation in the patient's therapy.

Benefits to the hospital include increased efficiency in the delivery of I.V. therapy, improved communication, decreased liability, and improved patient care. The cost, personnel needs, and staffing will depend on the individual hospital. A portion of the cost may be offset by a transfer of nursing positions, decreased inventory, greater account-ability, decreased waste, and accurate charging of I.V. solutions and equipment. The hospital I.V. committee through the documentation from various studies must be able to establish a need for the I.V. team and the cost of providing that service.

References

1. Francke, D. E. (Editor), *Handbook of I.V. Additive Reviews*. Hamilton, Illinois, Hamilton Press, 1970, p. 18.
2. Anon., The Nation's Hospitals: A Statistical Profile. *Hospitals* 45:447, 1971.
3. Siebert, F. B., Fever-producing substance found in some distilled waters. *Amer J. Physiol.* 67:90–104, 1923.
4. Meyers, L., Intravenous catheterization. *Am. J. Nursing* 45:930–931, 1945.
5. Dudrick, S. J., Wilmore, D. W., Vars, H. M., and Rhoads, J. E., Long-term total parenteral nutrition with growth, development, and positive nitrogen balance. *Surgery* 64:134–142, 1968.
6. Meisler, J. M., and Skolaut, M. W., Extemporaneous sterile compounding of intravenous additives. *Am. J. Hosp. Pharm.* 23:557–562 (Oct) 1966.
7. Ravin, R. L., "Steps in starting an I.V. additive program. *Drug Intell. Clin. Pharm.* 4:13–14 (Jan) 1970.
8. Ragland, J. G., and Knoll, K. R., Pharmacists and nurses benefit from I.V. additive programs. *Hospitals* 42:136–140 (Aug 16) 1968.
9. Pulliam, C. C. and Upton, J. H., A pharmacy coordinated intravenous admixture and administration service. *Amer. J. Hosp. Pharm.* 28:92–101 (Feb) 1971.
10. Skolaut, M. W., Long-term benefits of a centralized I.V. additive service. *Am. J. Hosp. Pharm.* 25:536–537 (Sept) 1968.
11. Kimmel, R. A., Dream to working reality: how to start an I.V. team. *Am. J. I.V. Therapy* 4(2)39–45 (1977).
12. Cain, R. M., and Kahn, J. S. The pharmacist as a member of the health team. *Am. J. Publ. Health* 61(11)2223–2228 (Nov) 1971.
13. *Webster's New World Dictionary*, College Edition, 1957, p. 1495.
14. Willett, R. D., Developing an I.V. therapy team in a small hospital. *Am. J. I.V. Therapy* 3(5) 18–20 (Aug–Sept) 1976.
15. Paoloni, C. V., Procedure for handling intravenous additives: the nursing team approach. *Hosp. Management* (Sept) 1969, pp. 12–22.

16. Wuest, R. J., Justifying an I.V. additive program. *Drug Intell. Clin. Pharm.* 4:125–126 (May) 1970.

17. Kelly, W. N., and Miller, D. E., Initiating and justifying an I.V. team. *Am. J. I.V. Therapy* (Oct–Nov) 1975, pp. 34–38.

18. Wuest, R. J., Initiating an I.V. additive service: 3. Development of policies and procedures. *Drug Intell. Clin. Pharm.* 4:183–185 (July) 1970.

19. Geri, D. M., Is I.V. therapy a specialty for you? *Nursing* 5:81–86, 1975.

20. Isler, C., The hidden danger of I.V. therapy. *RN* (Oct) 1973, pp. 23–31.

21. Corso, J. A., Agontinelli, R., and Brandriss, M. W., Maintenance of venous polyethylene catheters to reduce risk of infection. *J.A.M.A.* 210:2075–2077, 1969.

22. Ryan, J. A., Abel, R. M., Abbott, W. M., et al., Catheter complications in total parenteral nutrition. *N. Engl. J. Med.* 290(14)757–761 (Apr) 1974.

23. Maki, D. G., Goldmann, D. A., and Rhame, F. S., Infection control in intravenous therapy. *Ann. Intern. Med.* 79:867–887, 1973.

24. Bentley, D. W., and Lepper, M. H., Septicemia related to indwelling venous catheter. *J.A.M.A.* 206(8)1749–1752 (Nov) 1968.

25. Fuchs, P. C., Indwelling intravenous polyethylene catheters. *J.A.M.A.* 216(9) 1447–1450 (May) 1971.

26. Goldmann, D. A., Maki, D. G., Rhame, F. S., et al., Guidelines for infection control in intravenous therapy. *Ann. Intern. Med.* 79:848–850, 1973.

27. Maki, D. G., Infection control and the I.V. therapist. *Am. J. I.V. Therapy* (June–July), 1975, pp. 23–27.

28. Steere, A. C., How to avoid bacterial contamination of I.V. catheters and solutions. *Am. J. I.V. Therapy* (June–July) 1975, pp. 31–34.

29. Bergman, H. D., Incompatibilities in large volume parenterals. *Drug Intell. and Clin. Pharm.* 11:345–360 (June) 1977.

30. U.S. Center for Disease Control, *Recommendations for the prevention of I.V. associated infections* (Aug) 1973.

31. Kaminski, M. V., and Stolar, M. H., Parenteral hyperalimentation—a quality of care survey and review. *Am. J. Hosp. Pharm.* 31:228–235 (Mar) 1974.

32. Skoutakis, V. A., and Martinez, D. R., Miller, W. A., and Dobbie, R. P., Team approach to total parenteral nutrition. *Am. J. Hosp. Pharm.* 32:693–697 (July) 1975.

33. Wilson, J. A., Infection control in intravenous therapy. *Heart and Lung* 5(3) (May–June) 1976, pp. 430–436.

34. Lee, G., and Walker, T. R., A handbook for I.V. therapy patients. *Am. J. I.V. Therapy* 4(2)17–20 (Mar) 1977.

35. Spoon, J., The I.V. team in the pharmacy. *Supervisor Nurse* 4:48–54 (1973).

36. White, S. J., Pharmacist and I.V. therapist: synergistic interaction. *Am. J. I.V. Therapy* 3(6)17–22 (Oct–Nov) 1976.

37. Wuest, R. J., Staffing an I.V. additive service. *Drug Intel. and Clin. Pharm.* 4:153–154 (June) 1970.

38. Godfrey, D., How to set up an I.V. team. *Handbook*, Abbott Seminar, 1976.

32—The Pharmacist's Role in Inpatient and Home Care Hyperalimentation Programs

Philip Schneider

Hyperalimentation or total parenteral nutrition (TPN) is a development in patient care which can create many opportunities for the clinical pharmacist. It can be a means to interdisciplinary involvement for pharmacy in your hospital. In this paper I will review the hyperalimentation therapy process and emphasize ways in which pharmacists have an opportunity to contribute.

Solution Preparation

The most obvious area for pharmacist involvement is the preparation or compounding of the hyperalimentation solution. This is a task for which the pharmacist is legally responsible and has unique expertise. The pharmacist is knowledgeable about chemical incompatibilities, sterile technique, and is able to perform the dosage calculations required for proper preparation of the solution.

In the medical literature the pharmacist has been recognized as the person who should take responsibility for preparing TPN solutions.[1,2] Pharmacists in institutions without IV admixture programs have used this opportunity to begin involvement in preparing parenteral solutions for the hospital. Physicians look to the pharmacy for expertise in qualitative and quantitative preparation of hyperalimentation solutions. The medical literature can go a long way toward justifying equipment, space and personnel required to begin an IV admixture program. There is no excuse for use of hyperalimentation solutions which have not been prepared by a pharmacist.

Policy Formulation

Pharmacists who are active in policymaking bodies such as the Pharmacy and Therapeutics Committee or Infection Committee can become involved in policy formulation regarding use of hyperalimentation solutions. Because of the critical nature of hyperalimentation use and the difficulty in training hospital physicians and personnel in proper procedure, formulation and implementation of proper procedures are impor-

tant. Elements of hyperalimentation use which must be addressed are:

1. Use of proper antiseptic on dressings.
2. Use of final filters in administering hyperalimentation solutions.[3]
3. Infection control guidelines
   a. Preparation and storage of solutions
   b. Insertion of catheter
   c. Changing IV sets.[4]
4. Developing protocols or hyperalimentation team.[5]
5. Training patients to self-administer solutions at home.[6-8]

The first step in establishing guidelines for use should be obtaining and reviewing the document from the Center for Disease Control "Infection Control Guidelines for Total Parenteral Nutrition Programs."[4] Pertinent points in this document for pharmacists include:

1. The team approach, in which a pharmacist is a member of the team, is recommended.
2. Protocol for hyperalimentation solution preparation, distribution and use should be approved by necessary committees, including "pharmacy standards" committee.
3. Solution components must be mixed by a "trained member of the hospital staff" using a laminar flow hood.
4. The catheter site should be disinfected with iodine 1% and 70% alcohol.
5. Use of antimicrobial dressing is recommended.
6. Filters are discussed but not recommended for routine use.

In preparing guidelines, initial efforts should be directed toward formulating policies which effect preparation and use of hyperalimentation solutions rather than their prescription. Necessary policy decisions include:

1. Who should make the solution.
2. How solutions are stored.
3. How IV sites are maintained (use of iodophor ointment).
4. Use of final filters.
5. Equipment and drugs on hyperalimentation "tray" used for catheter insertion.

More comprehensive planning should include protocols for hyperalimentation solutions used in the hospital. Even though this therapy is indicated and used for a variety of conditions, many physicians are unfamiliar with its use. The pharmacist should meet with a knowledgeable and interested physician to develop such a protocol.

Standard III in the Joint Commission on Accreditation of Hospitals also points out the need for pharmacists to work closely with physicians in developing comprehensive hospital policies of hyperalimentation solution use. Interpretation of this standard states: "In the interest of safety of preparation and administration and effective nutritional content, overall directions shall be provided by a qualified physician when total parenteral nutrition products (hyperalimentation) are required."[9]

Part of an IV admixture program and TPN preparation procedure in the pharmacy must include the development of a document which records hyperalimentation formulas used for each patient. These flow sheets allow the pharmacist to follow changes in additives and identify potential errors and incompatibilities. Physicians may elect to use this form for comprehensive review of a patient's ongoing formulas.[3]

Hyperalimentation use is safer when a team is developed; such a team should include a pharmacist. The team described by Skoutakis et al.[3] takes entire responsibility for hyperalimentation use in the hospital, performing its service after consultation. The team usually performs its service by using a protocol. Pharmacist responsibilities can include:

1. Monitoring patient therapy using hyperalimentation metabolic charts,
2. Keeping and storing all records of use,
3. Compounding and dispensing solutions,
4. Recommending solutions and additive of choice and changes in therapy based on monitoring the patient,
5. Maintaining and servicing equipment (pumps, filters),
6. Teaching pharmacy students.

The value of this team was measured by Skoutakis et al. by determining the incidence of hyperalimentation-related sepsis. An incidence of 1% is significantly lower than that published in other studies, indicating the positive effects of the service.

Further, the 2.7% incidence of electrolyte disturbances and 5% significant glycosuria found in patients whose solutions were prepared by the team compares favorably to the 28.1 and 27.4% cited by Kaminski and Stolar.[3]

Home Care Hyperalimentation

A final step in providing care to patients is training them to administer their own hyperalimentation solutions at home. Development of this technique was begun in 1970 by Belding Scribner[10] and by Maurice Shils.[11] Two reports of pharmacist involvement in training patients for hyperalimentation self-administration have subsequently been published.

Tsallas et al. report an outpatient who self-administered three liters of solution daily at home.[12] The pharmacist's role in this program included bulk sterile compounding of the solutions. The patient received 84 liters of hyperalimentation fluid from the pharmacy every month when she came to the hospital for follow-up visits. In addition, pharmacy supplied the patient with vitamin additives, in-line filters, administration sets and catheter care items such as disinfectants and antibiotic dressings. The program resulted in a weekly savings of about $600 when costs of home care hyperalimentation were compared with those of hospitalization.

More recently, Ivey et al. reported pharmacist involvement in training a patient to self-administer hyperalimentation solutions at home.[8] This report includes expanded roles for the pharmacist in training the patient to prepare these solutions daily at home.

Training by the pharmacist involves general orientation on the IV therapy system, care of the catheter, preparing the solutions, changing tubing, starting and stopping infusions, maintenance, trouble shooting and management of complications. Training lasts from 10 days to two weeks. The authors report that 40 patients have been successfully trained.

Home care programs offer pharmacists an excellent opportunity to cost-justify a clinical program. Significant savings result when patients are able to avoid hospitalization and administer their own solutions at home. These savings are of interest to third-party agencies who wish to see reduction in hospital costs.

Some pharmacists have been successful in obtaining authorization from Blue Cross and other agencies for this type of pharmacy service.[13] At current hospital costs, patients save about $1400 per week through training given at Ohio State University to self-administer these solutions at home. Blue Cross reimburses pharmacists $70 for each patient they instruct. To this date four such patients have been trained.

Research Involvement

Research efforts should evolve from pharmacist involvement with hyperalimentation use. Research should be directed toward:

1. Documenting and quantitating problems of procedure (utilization review).
2. Measuring effectiveness of various programs on problems which currently exist (role effectiveness review).
3. Cost-justifying pharmacist involvement in hyperalimentation use in hospital (cost effectiveness review).

Some documentation of problems has already been done. Kaminski and Stolar[3]

conducted a survey to document the quality of hyperalimentation care. Significant discrepancies were found between recommended standards and actual practices. An unacceptably high incidence of avoidable complications was found as well. Studies by Ryan et al.[2] document the nature and the incidence of catheter-related complications in patients receiving total parenteral nutrition. This study documents a reduction in sepsis rate from 11% to 3% when proper catheter care procedures were used. Studies which need to be performed in this area are:

1. Incidence of contamination of hyperalimentation solutions prepared outside the laminar flow hood.
2. Utilization review study to evaluate the prescribing habits of physicians.

If pharmacists aid in implementing hospital policies and programs to improve hyperalimentation use, the effectiveness of these changes should be measured. The impact of policies related to hyperalimentation prescribing and to use must be assessed. Effectiveness of protocols and teams which are implemented must also be evaluated. Studies such as those of Ryan et al.[2] and Skoutakis et al.[3] include such data and provide support to justify a policy or service.

Cost justification is the final step. Savings resulting from home care programs are obvious; more data need to be published. The more challenging job of cost justifying these teams and pharmacist involvement on such teams has yet to be done.

TPN use can indeed be a "doorway" to interdisciplinary involvement for pharmacists. This paper has discussed some of the problems to which pharmacists can address themselves. Pharmacists can be involved in establishing programs to help solve these serious problems. Interested individuals should not miss the opportunities to get involved in hyperalimentation therapy, to help improve patient care through safe and rational drug therapy and elevate the level of pharmacy practice in the hospital.

References

1. Myers, R. N., Smink, R. D., and Goldstein, F.: Parenteral hyperalimentation: Five years clinical experience. *Am. J. Gastroenterol.* 62:313–324 (Oct) 1974.
2. Ryan, J. A., Abel, R. M., Abbott, W., Hopkins, C., Chesney, T. M., Colley, R., Phillips, K., and Fischer, J.: Catheter complications in total parenteral nutrition. *N. Engl. J. Med.* 290:757–761, 1974.
3. Skoutakis, V. A., Martinez, D. R., Miller, W. A., and Dobbie, R. P.: Team approach to total parenteral nutrition. *Am. J. Hosp. Pharm.* 32:693–697 (Jul) 1975.
4. Goldman, D. A., and Maki, D. G.: Infection controls in total parenteral nutrition. *JAMA* 223:1360–1364, 1973.
5. White, P. L., Nagy, M. E., and Fletcher, D. C.: Total Parenteral Nutrition, Acton, Mass., Publishing Sciences Group, Inc., 1974, pp. 329–347.
6. Shils, M. E.: A program for total parenteral nutrition at home. *Am. J. Clin. Nutrition* 28:1429–1435 (Dec) 1975.
7. Jeejeebhoy, K. N., Zohrab, W. J., Langer, B., Phillips, M. J., Kuksis, A., and Anderson, G.: Total parenteral nutrition at home for 23 months, without complications and with good rehabilitation. *Gastroenterology* 65:811–820 (Nov) 1973.
8. Ivey, M., Riella, M., Mueller, W., and Scribner, B.: Long-term parenteral nutrition in the home. *Am. J. Hosp. Pharm.* 32:1032–1036 (Oct) 1975.
9. Tousignant, D. R.: Joint Commission on Accreditation of Hospitals 1977 Standards for Pharmaceutical Services. *Am. J. Hosp. Pharm.* 34:948 (Sept) 1977.
10. Scribner, B. H., Cole, J. J., and Christopher, T. G.: Long-term total parenteral nutrition: The concept of an artificial gut. *JAMA* 212: 457, 1970.
11. Shils, M. E., Wright, W. L., Turnbull, A., and Brescia, F.: Long-term parenteral nutrition through an external arteriovenous shunt. *N. Engl. J. Med.* 238:341–344, 1970.
12. Tsallas, G., and Baum, D.: Home care parenteral alimentation. *Am. J. Hosp. Pharm.* 29:840–846 (Oct) 1973.
13. Fudge, R. P., and Latiolais, C. J.: Blue Cross pays for clinical pharmacist services in training hemophiliacs for home care self-therapy. *Pharmacy Times* 42:36–41 (Jan) 1976.

Related Reading in This Volume

46. Comprehensive Hospital Pharmacy Services

Readings for a Broader Perspective

1. Muraida, R. M. "Pharmacy-Nursing Communications in an Intravenous Admixture Program," *American Journal of Hospital Pharmacy* 32 (September 1975):889–91.
2. Powell, J. R., and Cupit, G. C. "Developing the Pharmacist's Role in Monitoring Total Parenteral Nutrition," *Drug Intelligence & Clinical Pharmacy* 8 (October 1974):576–80.

Medical Oncology

33—Clinical Pharmacy Activities on a General and Oncologic Surgical Service

LeRoy S. Ezaki and Marshall Gilston

The City of Hope Medical Center, located in Duarte, California, is a treatment and research institution for catastrophic disease, with a primary emphasis on cancer. As a means of better patient care, a satellite pharmacy was opened in late 1969 on the general and oncologic surgery service. A medication room of about 150 square feet was converted into the satellite pharmacy.

With this satellite pharmacy, located immediately adjacent to the nursing station, 35 private and semiprivate beds are served in addition to four intensive care beds. A complete unit dose drug distribution system is provided from the satellite, with two medication carts and exchange cassettes used.

The satellite pharmacy is staffed by one full-time clinical pharmacist and a technician who assists in filling medication orders and preparing intravenous solutions. During evenings and weekends, additional pharmacists and technicians are available to process the medication orders.

The surgery service is staffed by four full-time permanent physicians. However, almost all of the medication orders are written by third- and fourth-year surgical residents who are affiliated with the City of Hope for periods of four to 12 months for training in oncology.

The role of the clinical pharmacist at the City of Hope has expanded and evolved over a period of several years. This role expansion was made possible because of the close rapport which has developed between the clinical pharmacist and the physicians. When a physician sees the same pharmacist on a daily basis, it seems to promote more reliance and trust in the professional judgement of that pharmacist. We will discuss the principal activities of the clinical pharmacist at our institution.

Pharmacist Functions

Cancer Protocols

The pharmacist is actively involved with physicians in preparing cancer therapy protocols. His involvement includes researching data, establishing administration guidelines, gathering data on results and writing the chemotherapy orders in the patient's chart (according to the established protocols). All orders written by a pharmacist on a patient's chart must be countersigned by the physician at his earliest convenience (usually within 48 hours).

The pharmacist may assist the physician by monitoring and following the progress of patients on various protocols. For example, while an inpatient is receiving chemotherapy, the clinical pharmacist checks the hematology results each day and authorizes the giving of that day's dose if the laboratory results meet the requirements of the protocol.

Patient Consultations

When a patient is admitted, the clinical pharmacist takes a medication history. The pharmacist also advises the patient before discharge on self-medication procedures to be followed when the patient is at home.

Conference Attendance

The pharmacist is invited and expected to attend all surgical service conferences. In addition, he frequently attends x-ray, tumor board and resident's disease and treatment presentations.

Monitoring

The clinical pharmacist monitors the drug regimens for all inpatients on his unit. The monitoring of drug therapy is not productive unless it leads, when necessary, to appropriate corrective action. Whenever any difficulties or potential medication problems are noted, the patient's physician is contacted.

During teaching and working rounds, the objective of the clinical pharmacist is to interact directly with the physician to improve drug therapy. Success depends upon freedom of communication in which suggestions can be candidly evaluated.

Writing Medication Orders with Prior Approval

Once the clinical pharmacist on the unit is accepted as a member of the health care team, he can expand his role by seeking additional responsibilities. At the City of Hope, this led to the utilization of "verbal authorization forms" (Fig. 33.1). During the first month of his affiliation at the City of Hope,

each surgical resident is asked if he would authorize the clinical pharmacist on his unit to write medications from the "approved list" as verbal orders. The physician must countersign the pharmacist's orders at his earliest convenience.

The authorization form was presented to 11 resident physicians during their last year; no resident was selectively omitted. The responses are seen in Figure 33.1. Signed forms were kept on file by the clinical pharmacist. Drugs listed on the final approved list include laxatives, antacids, antinauseants, hypnotic-sedatives and anti-anxiety agents.

The physician could also indicate his willingness to allow the pharmacist to renew outdated medication orders, convert the route of pain medication(s) and order a specific laboratory test to evaluate and monitor possible drug toxicity.

Evaluation

The clinical pharmacist on the oncologic surgery service prepared an evaluation form to be completed and signed by each surgical resident at the conclusion of his affiliation with the City of Hope. These evaluations were collected over a three-year period from January, 1973 to January, 1976.

This sample population included all the residents (except one who left the program early and did not complete an evaluation) who were affiliated with the City of Hope surgery service during the time of the study. Each resident completed the evaluation and returned it to the pharmacist (Fig. 33.2). At the end of the study period there were 28 completed evaluations. Due to the small sample size, statistical analysis was not used.

Following each question was space for comments by the physicians. The comments seen on Figure 33.2 are direct quotes from the evaluations and are representative. Almost all the comments were included in this report and no attempts were made to influ-

Figure 33.1

**Verbal authorization form and physician's response to it. The formal authorization
for pharmacists to carry out the indicated activities is shown,
as are the responses of the last 11 residents completing the form.**

City of Hope Medical Center
Duarte, California

To _____   Date _____

From ___Lee Ezaki, W-6 pharmacist___   Subject _____

With your approval, the Clinical Pharmacist on Wing 6 may write as verbal orders the following which must be counter-signed by the physician at the earliest convenience:

		Yes	No
1.	Renew outdated medication orders (outdated one or more days). (The pharmacist will inform the respective physician regarding the renewal of antibiotics and steroids.)	(10)	(1)
2.	Order, on request by RN or patient, or as needed:	(11)	(0)
	a. Laxatives Colace MOM Dulcolax, suppository/tablet		
	b. Antacids Maalox Mylanta Amphogel	(11)	(0)
	c. Antinauseants Compazine Tigan	(10)	(1)
	d. Hypnotic-sedatives Dalmane	(11)	(0)
	e. Antianxiety agent Only Valium or Librium	(6)	(5)
3.	Convert route of pain medication(s) from IM to PO, or vice versa, as when postop patient is placed on liquid diet. Convert Demerol Injection to Tylenol #3 Convert Tylenol #3 to Darvon	(11)	(0)
4.	Order a specific lab test to evaluate and monitor possible drug toxicity, as creatinine for genta-micin, kanamycin, etc.	(10)	(1)

ence the results. It should be pointed out that only a few residents volunteered comments, while most merely answered the questions.

Conclusion

This retrospective study seems to indicate that the physicians were willing to authorize and delegate to the clinical pharmacist re-sponsibilities traditionally restricted to phy-sicians. The authors believe that the major factors influencing these results were the institutional setting and the ability of the clinical pharmacist to communicate effec-tively. Many physicians requested that the authorization to write verbal orders be re-stricted to the clinical pharmacist perma-nently assigned to the unit.

Physicians were generally in favor of

Figure 33.2

Evaluation questionnaire for surgery residents.

1. Has the ordering of laxatives, antacids, hypnotics, etc., by the pharmacist caused any problems?

   Yes   0   0%
   No   28   100%

   Comments: "Great help."

2. Evaluate the activities of the pharmacist regarding renewing and ordering new medications (laxatives, antacids, antinauseants, etc.)

   Favorable   27   96.4%
   Neutral   0   0
   Unfavorable   1   3.6%

   Comments: Very favorable.

3. Do you feel that the pharmacist has infringed too far into the area of the physician?

   Yes   0   0%
   No   28   100%

4. Did you feel comfortable knowing that the pharmacist was ordering drugs from the "approved list" for your patients?

   Yes   25   89%
   No   3   11%

   Comments: "The rapport with the pharmacist was excellent and all the drugs ordered by him had been discussed previously." "Has saved much time and numerous nuisance calls."

5. Would you allow the pharmacist to order Valium or Librium for nervousness?

   Yes   16   57%
   No   12   43%

   Comments: "Probably this should be evaluated by the physician as nervousness; may be a sign of some more significant disorder." "Yes, in small doses." "No, nervousness sometimes presages catastrophic complications."

6. Would you allow the pharmacist to order specific lab tests to evaluate specific drug toxicity (i.e. creatinine)?

   Yes   26   93%
   No   2   7%

   Comment: "Should be discussed with physician as routine drug orders are discussed;" "Yes, if for his own interest but not for patient management;" "Yes, for special cases like IV methotrexate therapy;" "Certainly;" "Yes, as long as discussed with physician."

7. Do you approve the practice of letting the pharmacist taper dose of analgesics (converting patient from IM narcotic to oral agent such as Tylenol #3)?

   Yes   22   79%
   No   6   21%

   Comments: "Yes, only if patient contact and interaction maintained;" "Yes, if both previously ordered."

8. Any further suggestions concerning pharmacy activities?

   Comments: "Well done job;" "Good work and thank you;" "Keep it up;" "Help in developing and monitoring chemotherapy orders, useful liaison."

   "It has been both a pleasant and educational experience to have someone readily available to discuss problems with. I also think it serves the patient's best interests."

allowing the pharmacist to renew outdated medication orders, and to order new medications such as laxatives, antacids and antinauseants. One exception was the ordering of antianxiety agents by the pharmacists. About one-half of the residents believed that the need for such drugs should be evaluated by the physician. Most physicians indicated they would let the pharmacist order laboratory tests to evaluate specific drug toxicity. In performing these duties, the residents did not feel that the pharmacist had infringed too far upon the traditional role of the physician. These conclusions must be qualified since they were obtained in a unique environment and are certainly not representative of hospital pharmacy as a whole.

The results of the clinical pharmacy program at the City of Hope Medical Center can be summarized by paraphrasing a comment from one of the former residents. He thought that the City of Hope policy for pharmacist participation in the ordering of drugs was excellent. It allowed the physician to spend valuable time on other needed tasks. He said, "I found the pharmacists pleasant, cooperative, informed members of the health care team who welcomed questions about drugs, routes of administration, dosages and side effects.

Readings for a Broader Perspective

1. Morris, C. R., and Hickman, M. J. "Medical Oncology Pharmacy: A New Role for the Clinical Pharmacist," *American Journal of Pharmaceutical Education* 41 (August 1977): 278–80.

Mental Illness

34—Clinical Pharmacy Practice in a Community Mental Health Center

Glen L. Stimmel

Introduction

New roles and role models for pharmacists in patient care responsibility are slowly but steadily growing in number. Pharmacists have become actively involved in many aspects of medical care involving drug therapy. Examples include extended care facilities, rural health care, obstetrics, general medicine and mental health facilities.[1-4] Expanded roles for pharmacists continue to be discussed as part of the expected future trends in pharmacy practice.[5] Schools of pharmacy are giving increased attention to clinical training of pharmacy students.[6] A crucial question is if these new roles for clinically trained pharmacists allow justification of the schools' effort, time and money to provide clinical training of the current magnitude. A perceptive criticism of many pharmacy students, as well as pharmacists in practice today, is that most clinical pharmacy roles exist only within the academic institution and have no relation to possible pharmacy practice outside the institution. Thus, there exists a clear need to document viable community-based clinical pharmacist roles. It is the purpose of this article to describe one such role.

In March 1973, the city and county of San Francisco funded and hired a full-time clinical pharmacist for District V Mental Health Center. This position represents a true community-based clinical pharmacy practice and has definite implications for increasing clinical pharmacy involvement within community mental health centers.

Origins

In 1971 the director of District V Day Treatment Center invited pharmacy student participation to monitor patients' drug therapy and assist in drug distribution. Two students began a three-month clerkship at the Day Treatment Center in September 1971. The clerkship training program that emerged from this beginning has been previously described.[7] From this student experience at the Day Treatment Center, it became clear that a clinically trained pharmacist could provide a valuable service as part of the mental health center staff. A proposal detailing the duties of a clinical pharmacist in a mental health facility was drawn up, and in March 1972 was presented to the director of the District V Mental Health Center. With his support and that of the Citizens' Advisory Board, the proposal was submitted as part of the budget, and was approved and funded by the City and County of San Francisco.

Description of Facility

Community mental health is a relatively new concept for mental health care delivery. Prior to the 1950s, the public had not begun to accept the idea that a mentally ill person could be treated and his illness controlled outside a mental hospital. Public attitudes began to change in the 1950s as the mass media publicized the potential of psychoactive drugs and improved treatment techniques. The public responded with interest, then hope, and then a growing demand for additional public funds to provide better treatment for the mentally ill. With strong support from President Kennedy, the Community Mental Health Centers Act was adopted in October 1963. The statute reflected the progress in treatment and the attendant shifting in public attitudes by establishing the location of the new mental health centers within the communities where patients and their families lived.[8]

Each community mental health center has responsibility for providing mental health care to a specified number of people residing in a geographic area known as the "catchment area." District V Mental Health Center is one of five community mental health centers serving the City and County of San Francisco. Mental health services are many and varied, including—inpatient crisis intervention, geriatric day treatment, adult day treatment, adolescent day treatment, three outpatient clinics, home visiting team, social skills program, board and care home enrichment program and a halfway house.

As the clinical pharmacist for the entire district, involvement with most of the units mentioned above is primarily consultative. Direct patient care responsibility involves only the adult day treatment center and two of the outpatient clinics. These three areas were chosen based on where it was felt drug monitoring and information would best be directed. The day treatment center was chosen because patients at the center are most often just recently discharged from an inpatient service, their acute psychotic, depressive or suicidal episode not yet resolved, and their medication at large doses and causing significant adverse effects. Managing psychotropic medication at this stage is the most difficult and challenging since the goal is to lower medication to maintenance levels, treat and prevent adverse effects, and still maintain therapeutic efficacy. Clinical pharmacy input at this point seemed to be most appropriate. Outpatient clinics were chosen as a second area of direct patient care involvement since outpatients often present with problems of noncompliance, persistent adverse effects necessitating drug therapy modification and other medical illnesses being treated by other prescribing physicians.

Role of the Clinical Pharmacist

Perhaps no other specialty of medicine has better accepted a team approach to health care delivery as has psychiatry. Community mental health has widely accepted a team approach—with mental health care responsibility shared among psychiatrists, psychologists, psychiatric nurses, psychiatric social workers and community workers. For this reason it was easier to discuss with mental health administrators the need for clinical pharmacy involvement. To propose that an additional discipline be added to an already multidisciplinary team could sound unnecessary. What had to be documented was that the role of a clinical pharmacist in community mental health is unique and is not a duplication of existing roles. In addition to the unique contributions clinical pharmacy can make, the following description of duties demonstrates the blurring of his own role to make him an active member of the staff. Some duties in fact are not directly related to drug therapy. There must be a willingness to participate as an active

member in mental health care delivery, which includes, but is not limited to, clinical pharmacy-related activities.

Adult Day Treatment Center

The primary function is to monitor patients' total drug therapy. The clinical pharmacist has his own group of patients to follow weekly for medication evaluation and adjustment. Assessment of drug therapy response and adverse effects is made, and appropriate drug or dosage changes are made. Consultation with a psychiatrist is available for questions or problems. Close contact is maintained with each patient's primary therapist for additional information regarding the patient's progress that should be reflected in medication needs. Medication prescribed by physicians for other medical illnesses as well as use of non-prescription drugs is monitored to insure prevention of potential adverse effects or interactions.

Some new patients also are assigned to the clinical pharmacist for medication needs. This can involve initiating drug therapy as well as changing drug or dosage. In addition to his own patients, the clinical pharmacist is responsible for the monitoring of drug therapy of patients who are interviewed and followed by pharmacy students.

A second major function is consultation with other staff members regarding specific drug therapy problems or questions. This includes not only psychiatrists but also other staff members whose patients are on medication. Responding to these questions requires a fair knowledge of the patient, his particular symptoms and past history, so that the response is clinically relevant and applicable to the patient. Within a year it became easier to become acquainted with most of the 120 patients and their particular medication-related problems.

A third major function is as a primary therapist for patients. The clinical pharmacist carries a small caseload of patients for whom he is primary therapist. He sees most of his patients individually for psychotherapy sessions, with a few assigned to small group therapy. The role of primary therapist denotes much more than doing psychotherapy, however. As a primary therapist, the clinical pharmacist does initial intake interviews, may meet with the family of the patient, makes referrals to other programs such as vocational rehabilitation, helps the patient to plan living and financial arrangements, arranges for hospitalization of his patients if necessary, and arranges for follow-up treatment when patients are discharged from the Day Treatment Center. Obviously there is much sharing among staff in making many such decisions, but the responsibility for these duties lies with the individual primary therapist.

This aspect of the clinical pharmacist's duties is essential for his involvement as part of the staff, and equally as important, helps to place the use of drugs into a proper perspective as one of many treatment methods for psychiatric disorders. Being totally involved in patient care allows a proper evaluation of various treatment methods and their respective roles in a total treatment plan for patients.

A fourth responsibility is supervision of pharmacy students and administration of their psychiatric clerkship program. The clinical pharmacist teaches pharmacy students in an elective community psychiatry clerkship offered by the University of California school of pharmacy, San Francisco. The clinical pharmacist supervises students as they monitor patient drug therapy at the Center, and teaches a weekly conference on psychiatric disorders and drug treatment.

A last responsibility at the Day Treatment Center is participation on various committees. The clinical pharmacist, with the director, initiated a psychiatric library for staff use. A library committee was formed and a half-time librarian named to continue improvement and expansion of the library. Other committees are the trainee committee and medical records committee.

Outpatient Clinics

The major function of the clinical pharmacist in the outpatient clinics is participation on a regular basis in several medication groups. The psychiatrist and clinical pharmacist see patients together for medication evaluation and renewal. Advice regarding appropriate drug therapy and adverse effects is given as necessary, and drug therapy is mostly a mutual decision.

Direct involvement with the outpatient clinic medication groups has varied depending on the psychiatrist involved and available time. Earlier, three different psychiatrists' medication groups were regularly attended by the clinical pharmacist, but turnover in psychiatrists and increasing patient care responsibility at the Center has resulted in a continuation of involvement in one outpatient medication group weekly with about 25 patients.

The other major responsibility in the outpatient clinics is consultation regarding drug-related problems or questions. Telephoned consultations are frequent from psychiatrists in the various outpatient clinics as well as from other staff members. Most of the consults are in regard to drug therapy questions or problems with individual patients. Response is thus directed to being specific and relevant to the particular patient involved. Drug information given most often is reflected in the patient's prescriptions.

District-Wide Responsibility

District-wide responsibility essentially involves scheduled lectures and discussions regarding some aspect of drug therapy. Initially, this function developed slowly, but has escalated markedly to the point where now one or two lectures per week is average. Lectures first were given to staff of the outpatient clinics and the Center. Because of the large number of mental health services provided by District V, there are many more units who work with patients on psychotropic drugs, and these units requested inservice education by the clinical pharmacist. Such talks have included the staff of the halfway house, social skills program, and the board and care home enrichment program. Talks regarding psychotropic medication also have been given to the various trainees in the District, including psychology, nursing, social work and pharmacy students.

A specific scheduled inservice series is held for the psychiatrists employed by District V Mental Health. These sessions are held every other month, and topics include specific issues of recent concern or new literature information on specific topics. The format consists of the clinical pharmacist presenting information, followed by discussion among the group, often comparing literature information with clinical experiences and impressions. These conferences are an excellent vehicle for the clinical pharmacist to bring new information to all the prescribing psychiatrists in the District, as well as discuss problems observed by the clinical pharmacist as reflected by prescribing habits. Specific topics have included—indications for tricyclic antidepressants, rational use of antiparkinson agents, fluphenazine enanthate versus fluphenazine decanoate, sedative-hypnotics versus sedating phenothiazines for insomnia, and limitations of antianxiety agents in psychiatry.

The second major responsibility of the clinical pharmacist for the District is supervision and administration of the drug distribution system. Since there had not been pharmacy involvement in this community mental health district before, the drug distribution system was in definite need of improvement. Prescription medications and stock drugs were still being sent back and

forth from the county hospital (across town) to the various clinics through messenger. Lag time between prescription order writing and the patient receiving the medication was about one week. Thus the primary task of the clinical pharmacist upon arrival was development of a drug distribution system for the District. Contracts were established between community pharmacies located near each clinic and the City and County of San Francisco. Patients now are seen for medication evaluation and renewal, and are given prescription orders to take to a pharmacy within walking distance of the clinic. Details and results of this distribution system are still being evaluated and will be published at a later date.

City-Wide Responsibility

Several invitations were extended by other groups involved in mental health care for lectures and discussions regarding psychotropic medication. A series of three sessions was given to city psychologists, and several lectures given to board and care operators in the city. One other community mental health district also requested several inservice education sessions for their staff.

Results

As mentioned earlier, new roles for clinically trained pharmacists have appeared in the literature. Many consist of a proposal, others an established role within an academic institution. An important feature of the role described in this article is that it is in actual practice, is totally supported and funded by a community mental health district and is separate from any pharmacy institution. The merits of clinical pharmacy practice are recognized and supported by a community mental health center. Because the role as presented was not designed as a structured research project but rather evolved as a true clinical pharmacy practice position, there are no documented statistical results to present. A study comparing mental health facilities with and without a clinical pharmacist has begun and will allow presentation of such data. But several observations deserve mention at this point based upon 16 months of experience.

The most significant area of influence is in education regarding medication. Individual consultation by psychiatrists regarding drug information is directly reflected in the prescription orders written in the majority of cases. The regular discussions with the District psychiatrists focus on specific clinical drug issues, and changes in prescribing habits are readily observed in the weeks following the meeting. Examples include a definite switch from fluphenazine enanthate to fluphenazine decanoate, and definite decrease in the use of antiparkinson agents prophylactically. A third area is in other staff members' ability and comfort in working with their patients who experience adverse drug effects. Their increased understanding of adverse effects, and the efforts made to minimize, but not always eliminate adverse effects, results in increased ability to work with their patients and this problem.

A final observation is the total incorporation of the clinical pharmacist as an integral part of the staff. Many duties do not directly involve drugs and drug therapy, but rather involve a close working relationship with patients and staff. Identity as a pharmacist is almost lost and is replaced by a feeling of being an integral member of the mental health staff with drug information a specific area of expertise.

Conclusion

Because our schools of pharmacy have made a major commitment to teaching clinically oriented pharmacy, it is essential that roles develop that will utilize this training.

Funding of clinical pharmacy roles by non-pharmacy sources is a major step in the development of viable clinical pharmacy practice. A role model for clinical pharmacy practice, funded by the City and County of San Francisco through District V Mental Health Center, has been described. Efforts must be made to continue documentation and development of new roles, both by educating pharmacists as well as other professionals of the present and potential state of clinical pharmacy practice.

References

1. Letourneau, K. N., "Drug Utilization Review in an Extended Care Facility," *Drug Intell. and Clinical Pharm.*, 8, 108 (March 1974)
2. Baumgartner, R. P., Land, M. J., and Hauser, L. D., "Rural Health Care—Opportunity for Innovative Pharmacy Service," *Amer. J. Hosp. Pharm.*, 29 (5) 394 (1972)
3. Anon., "The Clinical Pharmacist in Obstetrics," *Contemp. Ob/Gyn.*, 4, 40 (July 1974)
4. Miller, W. A., and Corcella, J., "Professional Pharmacy Functions in Community Mental Health Centers," *JAPhA*, NS 12 (2) 68 (1973)
5. Brodie, D. C., Knoben, J. E., and Wertheimer, A. I., "Expanded Roles for Pharmacists," *Amer. J. Pharm. Educ.*, 37, 591 (Nov. 1973)
6. Skinner, W. J., "Report on the Current Status of Clinical Pharmacy Programs," *Amer. J. Pharm. Educ.*, 36, 403 (Aug. 1972)
7. Stimmel, G. L., Katcher, B. S., and Levin, R. H., "The Emerging Role and Training Program of Clinical Pharmacy in Psychiatry," *Amer. J. Pharm. Educ.*, 38, 179 (May 1974)
8. Yolles, S. F., "Past, Present and 1980—Trend Projections," in *Progress in Community Mental Health*, Vol. 1. L. Bellak and H. H. Barten, eds., Grune and Stratton, New York, 10 (1969)

Readings for a Broader Perspective

1. Dugas, J. E., and Brown, S. "Community Mental Health Centers: A Milieu for Expansion of Pharmacy Services," *Hospital Pharmacy* 13 (February 1978):78, 81–82, 84, 86–87.
2. Evans, R. L., Kirk, R. F., Walker, P. W., Rosenbluth, S. A., and McDonald, J. "Medication Maintenance of Mentally Ill Patients by

a Pharmacist in a Community Setting," *American Journal of Hospital Pharmacy* 33 (July 1976):635–38.

3. Sax, M. J., Chow, C., Namikas, E., Wilson, C.

L., and Cheung, A. "Improving Psychotropic Drug Utilization," *California Pharmacist* 24 (April 1977):40–43.

Nuclear Pharmacy

35—An Introduction to Nuclear Pharmacy

Harriet L. Behm and Rodney D. Ice

A new specialty of pharmacy practice is nuclear pharmacy. Nuclear pharmacy deals with radioactive drugs (also commonly called radiopharmaceuticals) used in the practice of medicine. Because these drugs are radioactive, the sites where they localize in the body can be visualized externally, thus providing a noninvasive technique for the evaluation of body function and anatomy.

Being drugs, the properties of the radiopharmaceuticals are the same as those of nonradioactive drugs; however, additional properties, arising from the fact that the drug is radioactive and is not administered in pharmacologically significant doses, must be considered. Instead, the mass of the drug is purposely reduced to minimize noticeable pharmacological effects. At the same time, the quantity of radioactivity is optimized to permit the radiopharmaceutical to be used in diagnosis and, on occasion, for radiation therapy.

Radiopharmaceutics is the science of nuclear pharmacy and radiopharmaceuticals. Radiopharmaceutics deals with traditional pharmacy, such as pharmacology, biophar-

maceutics, pharmaceutics, calculus, medicinal chemistry, dispensing, and clinical pharmacy. In addition, it includes radiation physics, radiation biology, radiation dosimetry, nuclear medicine, nuclear instrumentation, and the practice of nuclear pharmacy.

Types of Nuclear Pharmacies

The first nuclear pharmacies were associated with nuclear medicine departments of large institutions. In recent years, some of the institutionalized nuclear pharmacies have branched out to service surrounding hospitals and clinics in their geographical area and thus are now called central nuclear pharmacies. Another developing area of nuclear pharmacy is that of private practice, which operates independently of the hospitals. Community nuclear pharmacies generally serve a number of hospitals and clinics in nearby locations with radiopharmaceuticals.

A nuclear pharmacy can have various functions and can be of different sizes, depending on the health needs of the community. In small hospitals where the nuclear pharmacy is located within the pharmacy, the pharmacist may only be responsible for formulation and quality control of radiopharmaceuticals. . . . After the products are prepared, they are dispensed on a unit-dose basis, precalibrated for radioactive decay to the time of dose administration. The prepared radiopharmaceuticals are then delivered to the nuclear medicine unit where the physician injects the drug into the patients. A small nuclear medicine unit that has a qualified nuclear pharmacist on the hospital staff could easily be serviced in this manner.

Pharmacists in larger hospital-based nuclear pharmacies are responsible for compounding, product formulation, quality control, and dispensing. In most hospitals the nuclear pharmacist also serves as a consultant to physicians on drug interactions, regulatory aspects and use of radiopharmaceuticals. In university nuclear pharmacies, teaching and research duties are involved as well as new product development. University-based nuclear pharmacies are usually affiliated with colleges of pharmacy and/or medical schools.

The newest type of practice is the community nuclear pharmacy. These operations are owned by pharmacists (or other interested persons) and supply a complete inventory of radiopharmaceuticals to hospitals located within their trading area on a daily basis. A unit dose system is used by some community nuclear pharmacies, in which radiopharmaceuticals are requested on individual patient prescriptions. Other community nuclear pharmacies dispense the radiopharmaceuticals in multidose vials. . . . Patient doses are drawn from these vials in the nuclear medicine units just prior to the time a patient is injected. Standing orders, sent out daily by the nuclear medicine units, are dispensed by the community nuclear pharmacy, as well as call-in orders for pharmaceuticals which can be used in emergencies or for studies not performed on a routine basis. Community nuclear pharmacies that dispense radiopharmaceuticals in the final injectable form relieve the nuclear medicine unit of radiopharmaceutical formulation, quality control, and dose calibrating responsibilities.

The Nuclear Pharmacist

A special committee on radiopharmaceuticals of the American Association of Colleges of Pharmacy has listed seven minimal professional responsibilities of a nuclear pharmacist.[1] They are:

1. to prepare, procure, store, compound, and dispense radiopharmaceuticals
2. to provide radiopharmaceutical quality control
3. to develop and maintain control procedures and records
4. to identify drug interactions
5. to carry out clinical consultation with patient and physician
6. to conduct routine health physics procedures
7. to fulfill requirements of regulations and licensure.

The ability to perform these duties requires special training that is not generally offered in the traditional program of study in pharmacy. Additional courses must also cover subjects involved in the general field of radiopharmaceutics.

Nuclear pharmacy education in the nation's colleges of pharmacy has increased greatly in the last few years. The American Association of Colleges of Pharmacy conducted a survey and found that 48 schools offered some form of education in the nuclear pharmacy area.[2] These programs ranged from a non-credit course for continuing education credit to a Ph.D. degree with specialization in nuclear pharmacy.

A B.S. pharmacist with training in nuclear

pharmacy is capable of performing routine dispensing, compounding and quality control procedures. The M.S. or Pharm.D. pharmacist, who receives advanced training in the specialty, is capable of handling a larger and more complex operation. The master's degree emphasizes research, whereas the Pharm.D. degree is clinically oriented. Persons trained at the Ph.D. level perform basic research, direct programs in nuclear pharmacy, teach, and also provide nuclear pharmacy services.

Nuclear pharmacy assistant programs have been developed to train technicians to assist in the dispensing of radiopharmaceuticals. These programs are approximately of one year duration and are oriented towards persons with one year of college credit in the sciences.[3]

In addition to the pharmacist there are three other types of nuclear medicine personnel involved with radiopharmaceuticals, i.e. the physician, technologist, and health physicist. The physician, as head of a nuclear medicine department, oversees the entire clinical operation. The physician's primary clinical function is the interpretation of the nuclear medicine diagnostic procedures (both scans and function tests) and the determination of the radiation treatment levels for therapeutic procedures. Technologists properly position the patients and obtain the diagnostic nuclear medicine images using radiation scanners and cameras sensitive to the ionization radiation emitted by the radiopharmaceutical. Health physicists are concerned with the radiological protection of personnel and patients. The health physicist also handles the regulatory requirements associated with the receiving, handling decontamination, and disposal of radiopharmaceuticals.

A 1972 survey of nuclear medicine physicians[4] indicates that there are 7,000 physicians actively involved in the practice of nuclear medicine. This survey also showed that nuclear medicine physicians associated with medical centers averaged over two thousand nuclear medicine procedures each year. Thus a conservative estimate of the number of radiopharmaceutical doses to patients in 1972 would be greater than 10 million, compared to a 1967 figure of 4 million doses to patients. The total sales of radiopharmaceuticals in the United States are estimated to be about $40–$45 million per year.[5]

There are about 400 pharmacists in the United States actively practicing nuclear pharmacy today. There is an obvious need for increased participation by the pharmaceutical profession. With the advent of new radiopharmaceuticals, and greater utilization by smaller hospitals, pharmacists both in hospital and community practice must become aware of this particular area of pharmacy practice.

Nuclear Pharmacy Operation

Generator systems have provided a convenient and simple means for obtaining short-lived isotopes on a daily basis. With generators, a short-lived daughter radiopharmaceutical can be easily obtained from a parent radionuclide that has a much longer half-life. . . . Radiopharmaceuticals or radionuclide generator systems can be purchased from companies such as Abbott, Mallinckrodt, New England Nuclear, Squibb, and Union Carbide. These companies also supply "kits" which are themselves not radioactive, but with the addition of the proper radionuclide, obtained from a generator system, can be used to make a radiopharmaceutical suitable for imaging a particular organ or measuring organ function.

Using the radionuclide generator systems and the "kits", pharmacists compound the radiopharmaceuticals. Each manufacturer, as well as the pharmacist, may prepare kits using different formulations. Thus the pharmacist must evaluate the formulations, do the necessary quality control, and select the best product to meet patient needs.

Quality Control

Quality control is a major function in the practice of nuclear pharmacy. Radiopharmaceutical quality control includes the testing and interpretation of data resulting from chemical, biological, and physical tests on radioactive drugs to determine their suitability for use in humans or animals, including internal test assessment and authentication of product history. Quality control includes a large number of tests, e.g. radionuclidic, radiochemical, chemical purity, as well as radioassay.

Radionuclidic purity is the proportion of the total radioactivity which is the stated radionuclide, such as the amount of ^{131}I in a radiopharmaceutical as compared to the total amount of radioactive iodine (i.e. [125]I, ^{123}I). This property can be measured using a multichannel analyzer or a spectrum scanner on a single channel analyzer. Both of these instruments have the ability to distinguish the energies of photons emitted from individual radionuclides.

Radiochemical purity is the proportion of total radioactivity which is present as the stated chemical form, i.e. the percent of labeled ^{131}I-iodocholesterol present in the radiopharmaceuticals.

The radiochemical purity of the product can be measured by thin layer chromatography, thus enabling the pharmacist to assess product stability and expiration dates (or hours).

Chemical purity is the proportion of the chemical form of the drug which is in the desired chemical state, for example, the percent of L-selenomethionine in a mixture of L-selenomethionine and D-selenomethionine.[6] Chemical purity can be assayed using spectrophotometric procedures or thin layer chromatography.

Radioassay is the quantitative determination of the amount of radioactivity present. The amount present must be within 10% of the amount calculated by the pharmacist. A dose calibrator, an instrument that can detect the quantity of emitted radiation, is used for radioassay [. . . .]

Over 80% of the radiopharmaceuticals used today are administered intravenously. All intravenous drugs must be checked for sterility and pyrogenic contamination. U.S.P. sterility and pyrogen tests are not applicable to products that must be used within twelve hours after preparation. A six-hour bacterial contamination test has been developed in which the radiopharmaceutical is added to a culture media containing ^{14}C-labeled glucose.[7] Any bacterial utilization of this glucose results in the emission of $^{14}CO_2$, which can be detected by radiation monitors. The Limulus test is an *in vitro* pyrogen test that takes one hour to perform. The test involves the incubation of the radiopharmaceutical with limulus amebocyte lysate, which is made from the circulating blood cells of the *Limulus Polyphemus*, or horseshoe crab.[8] After incubation, the formation of an opaque gel indicates pyrogenic contamination.

Because of the very short physical half-life of radiopharmaceuticals, some products must be used immediately after their preparation. Thus, there is a large responsibility on the pharmacist to have an established, proven technique that maintains product integrity. The technique of the pharmacist must be regularly tested [. . . .]

Dispensing and Record Keeping

Accurate records must be kept concerning the receipt, transfer, and disposal of all radioactive drugs. A nuclear pharmacy must be able to account for all radiopharmaceuticals, from the time of receipt, to their use in humans or until their disposal.

The unit dose system is often used for radiopharmaceuticals. A dose is based on the patient's body surface area, calculated on height and weight of the patient. The product is compounded in a multidose vial and the proper unit dose is withdrawn, precalibrated to the time of injection based upon the radioactive decay law: $A = A_o e - \lambda t$, where A is amount of radioactivity at time t, the time elapsed since the original calibration; A_o is the amount of radioactivity at the initial calibration; λ is the decay constant characteristic of each radionuclide equal to 0.693 divided by the physical half life. Syringe shields are used when transporting the radiopharmaceutical to the place of injection. [. . . .] This system enables the pharmacy to control the dose given to the patient and to assure the quality of the product until the time of injection. Accurate records must be kept of all radiopharmaceuticals compounded and dispensed.

In a multidose system the radiopharmaceutical is delivered to the nuclear medicine unit in a single vial. Patient doses are withdrawn at the nuclear medicine unit by the physician or technologist. This system allows a larger number of nuclear medicine facilities to be serviced with minimum nuclear pharmacy personnel.

The nuclear pharmacy must record all compounding procedures as well as quality control results. The nuclear medicine unit maintains records on doses administered to patients.

- patient's name;
- prescriber's name;
- prescription number;
- date dispensed;
- name of the institution or pharmacy;
- pharmacist's signature or initials;
- name of the radionuclide;
- chemical state of its complex;
- lot number;
- amount of radioactivity present at a specific calibration time;
- nuclear medicine procedure to be performed. In addition, a magenta-yellow radiation control label must be affixed to the containers.

Equipment

The capital outlay for the opening of a nuclear pharmacy involves approximately $20,000–$30,000. Essential equipment includes: the fume hood, for volatile radiopharmaceuticals; laminar flow hood, for aseptic procedures; dose calibrator, for radioassay; prescription balance; refrigerator; scintillation counter, for the assay of radionuclides; incubator, for sterility testing; hot air oven and autoclave, for depyrogenation and sterilization of equipment; microscope; a portable radiation detector for detecting loose radioactivity; adequate supplies (glassware, utensils, chromatography apparatus, gloves, shields, standards, remote handling devices); typewriter; and record-keeping supplies.

Extra equipment varies according to the scope of the nuclear pharmacy operation. Examples include a liquid scintillation system for radiopharmaceuticals which emit beta particles, syringe shields for unit dose distribution, and a multichannel analyzer for evaluating radionuclide purity.

Regulations

Radiopharmaceuticals, which are classified as drugs, are subject to all rules and regulations of the Food and Drug Administration (FDA) and the state Boards of Pharmacy. These pharmaceuticals, because of their radioactivity, are also regulated by the Nuclear Regulatory Commission (NRC) and/or state agencies responsible for radiological health.

The NRC regulates byproduct material. Byproduct material includes those radionuclides produced in the process of nuclear activation in a nuclear reactor, the process by which a majority of the radiopharmaceuticals are made. The FDA has the authority to govern the quality, the labeling, and advertising of radioactive drugs. The function of the Boards of Pharmacy is to regulate nuclear pharmacy practice within the state.

To date, only the Boards of Pharmacy in Arizona and California have adopted rules and regulations pertaining to the practice of nuclear pharmacy. Other states are recognizing the practice of nuclear pharmacy and are in the process of promulgating regulations.

References

1. Ice, R. D., Keesee, R. E., Shaw, S. M., Wolf, W., "Final Report of the Special Committee on Radiopharmacy," *Amer. J. of Pharmaceutical Education*, 39, 492 (1975).
2. Nuclear Pharmacy Educational Program, Survey of Colleges of Pharmacy, American Association of Colleges of Pharmacy, Bethesda, Maryland (1974).
3. *Programs in Radiopharmacy*, University of Southern California, School of Pharmacy, Los Angeles, California 90007, Walter Wolf, Director (1974).
4. McAfee, J. G., Powell, M. R., O'Mara, R. E., Friedman, B. I., Holmes, R. A., and Nelp, W. B., "Survey of Academic Divisions of Nuclear Medicine in the U.S. Medical Schools", April, 1972, Conducted by the officers of the Academic Council of the Society of Nuclear Medicine, and presented before the Council July 12, 1972.
5. "The Nuclear Industry," U.S. Atomic Energy Commission, Washington, D.C., 119 (1971).
6. Lathrop, K. A., Johnston, R. E., Blau, M., Rothschild, E. O., "Radiation Dose to Humans from 75-Se-L-Selenomethionine," *J. Nucl. Med.*, Suppl. (6) MIRD Pamphlet No. 9, 7–30 (1972).
7. DeLand, F., Wagner, H. N., "Automated Radiometric Detection of Bacterial Growth in Blood Cultures," *J. Lab. Clin. Med.*, 75 (3) 529 (1970).
8. Cooper, J. F., "Principles and Applications of the Limulus Test for Pyrogen in Parenteral Drugs," *Bulletin of the Parenteral Drug Association*, 29, 122 (1975).

Readings for a Broader Perspective

1. Porter, W. C., Ice, R. D., and Hetzel, K. R. "Establishment of a Nuclear Pharmacy," *American Journal of Hospital Pharmacy* 32 (October 1975):1023–27.
2. Rhodes, B. A., and Friedman, B. "Why Nuclear Medicine Spurs the Need for More Radiopharmacists," *Pharmacy Times* 44 (April 1978):94–96.
3. *American Pharmacy* NS 19 (June 1979):20–26.
4. Pollock, M. L., Strane, T. R., Brown, G. J., and McNeil, K. F. "Nuclear Pharmacy: A Student's Perspective," *Contemporary Pharmacy Practice* 2 (Fall 1979):190–94.
5. Wolf, W. "Chair Report for the Special Committee on Radiopharmacy," *American Journal of Pharmaceutical Education* 39 (May 1975): 151–52.
6. Rhodes, B. A., and Croft, B. Y. *Basics of Radiopharmacy*. Saint Louis, Missouri: The C. V. Mosby Company, 1978. 195 pp.

Pediatrics

36—Pediatric Dosing—The Pharmacist's Dilemma

Paul J. Munzenberger and Patrick McKercher

The medical treatment of pediatric patients frequently confronts health care providers with significant problems related to appropriate medication dosing. Children may suffer from diseases primarily restricted to their age group. Also, clinical drug trials generally are conducted on adult populations providing little experience and knowledge regarding the metabolism of the drug in the pediatric patient. When compared to adults, the drugs used to treat pediatric diseases may react differently in children. Therefore, determining the correct drug dose may prove difficult.

Methods for determining pediatric drug doses have been the subject of a number of published articles. In 1961, Glazko[1] described a procedure for calculating drug doses in infants and children using a slide rule specifically designed for this purpose. In 1965, Shirkey[2] published a review of a number of methods for determining pediatric dosage. In 1974, Habersang and Kauffman[3] reviewed the basic pharmacokinetic principles affecting pediatric dosing. More recently, Gill and Ueda[4] described a unique method of determining pediatric dosage based on differences in body water between children and adults.

Certainly one of the most well-known methods for determining pediatric doses is the use of mathematical rules. These rules usually are based on the child's age, weight, or surface area and have been published in medical and pharmacy reference books and as journal articles. "Remington's Pharmaceutical Sciences"[5] and "Perspectives in Clinical Pharmacy"[6] both contain one or more of these rules and Vaughan has referred to Clark's rule in his "Textbook of Pediatrics"[7]. Additional references to rules are found in other published articles.[8,9]

Although these rules have received considerable attention, little proof exists documenting their usefulness. This study was undertaken to compare the possible dosage variation which might be observed in the application of these rules.

Methodology

This study was conducted at a 310-bed, pediatric hospital located in Detroit, Mich. This hospital is a teaching hospital associated with Wayne State University. The data for this study were collected from patient charts for a 3-month period. All patients, 3–14 years of age, admitted to the medical units, and receiving one or more drugs, were candidates for inclusion.

Data collected included patients' age, weight, height, (if available), diagnosis, drug administered along with administration route, and the actual initial dose. From these data the patient's surface area was derived using a West nomogram. Additionally, the actual initial 24-hour dose was computed for each drug prescribed for the study patients. Using Clark's weight rule, Clark's surface area rule, Young's age rule, and Shirkey's dosing recommendations,[10] initial 24-hour doses also were computed for each prescribed drug. These rules are as follows:

Clark's weight rule–

$$\frac{Wt\ (lbs.)}{150} \times Adult\ Dose = Child\ Dose$$

Clark's surface area rule–

$$\frac{SA}{1.73} \times Adult\ Dose = Child\ Dose$$

Young's age rule–

$$\frac{Age\ (Years)}{Age + 12} \times Adult\ Dose = Child\ Dose$$

The adult dose appearing in each of these rules was derived from the drug product's package insert with appropriate consideration of the patient's diagnosis and disease severity. Similar considerations were applied using Shirkey's dosing recommendations.

The actual initial 24-hour dose was then compared to those calculated using each of the four previously described methods. A *t* test analysis was done comparing the actual initial dose with the doses calculated by each of the four methods.

Results

During the collection period the data for 159 patients were collected. Of this total, 82 (52%) drugs were ordered by the intravenous route, 71 (45%) orally, five (3%) by intramuscular injection, and only one was ordered as a rectal suppository. The oral and intravenous routes represent 96.2% of the total sample number.

Intravenous aminophylline represents 35 samples (22%) while oral acetaminophen represents 34 samples (21%). The third most frequently encountered drug administration route was intravenous ampicillin with 13 samples (8.2 percent). Antibiotics as a class of drugs represented 36.5 percent of all drugs and analgesic antipyretics represented 31 percent. A total of 29 drug administration route entities was identified.

A total of 25 different clinical conditions was identified; asthma represented the most frequently encountered diagnosis (29 percent). Patients with infectious diseases, either alone or in combination with another condition, represent the most frequently encountered type of diagnosis. This explains why antibiotics were the most frequently prescribed drug class. There were 85 patients (53 percent) diagnosed as having some type of infectious process.

Statistical Analysis

Independent Variable. Qualitative, categorical variables—age, drug, and administration route—were selected as independent variables. Patients 3–5 years old were assigned to the first age category and each subsequent 3-year ages were similarly assigned. The distribution of the resulting four categories is cross-tabulated with administration route in Table 36.1. The relative infrequency of some drugs necessitated the

Table 36.1

Cross-Tabulation of Age Categories by Route of Administration[a]

Age Category	Route of Administration		
	Oral	i.m.	i.v.
3–5 years	14	1	27
6–8 years	28	1	29
9–11 years	15	4	15
12–14 years	13	0	11

[a]$x^2 = 11.2$, $df = 6$, not significant.

assignment of drugs to an antibiotic or non-antibiotic category.

Dependent Variable. The criterion or dependent variable was the deviation of doses from the administered dose using four dosing methods: Shirkey's dosing recommendations; Clark's weight rule; Young's age rule; and Clark's surface area rule. The ranges of dose deviation are given in Table 36.2.

Table 36.2

Ranges of Dose Deviation Calculated versus Administered Dose

Method or Rule	Administered Dose with Range of Deviations for Calculated Doses
Shirkey	(−7,930 mg)|—•—|(3,750 mg)
Clark's weight rule	(−6,800 mg) (10,200 mg)
Young's age rule	(−4,800 mg) (10,100 mg)
Clark's surface area rule	(−12,300 mg) (9,410 mg)

Analysis. Paired comparison *t* tests were applied to the administered and calculated doses. The summary statistics of this analysis are shown in Table 36.3. Clark's surface area rule did not differ significantly from the administered dose. However, the dosing deviation range from administered dose was the greatest for this rule. Apparently, unusually high doses are counterbalanced by unusually low doses resulting in average group doses similar to the administered dose.

Discussion

Appropriate dosing of the pediatric patient involves more than pediatric textbook mathematical rules. Comparison of the actual dose administered with doses calculated using the four published methods yielded a large variation. Much of this variation is in error or within group variance which should be expected considering the variety of disease conditions.

Shirkey's recommendations yielded a range of dose deviations between calculated and administered dose which was about one-half the range observed with Clark's surface area rule (see Table 36.2). Shirkey's dosing recommendations are more consistent with observed dosing practices and analysis of these data suggests some modification for age categories and administration route may

Table 36.3

Comparison of Administered Dose in Milligrams with Dose Calculated by Dosing Rules

Dosing	Number of Cases	Mean	SD	Mean Difference	SD of Difference	t	2-Tail Probability
Shirkey's	159	1801 1486	2338 2349	314.6	1237	3.21	0.002
Clark's weight rule	159	1801 1179	2338 2604	622.2	1817	4.32	0.001
Young's age rule	159	1801 1129	2338 2306	672.5	1558	5.44	0.001
Clark's surface area	159	1801 1683	2338 3491	117.7	2345	0.63	0.528

be the standard practice. Shirkey's recommended dose for children 3–5 years old averaged only 96 mg. greater than administered dose. The overall dose deviation for all drug administration route categories averaged 304 mg. The average deviation from the administered dose within categories for Shirkey's recommendations is less than the deviation observed with the other dosing rules.

Finally, the variations resulting from the use of these methods indicate that considerable caution should be exercised with their use. Furthermore, Shirkey's recommendations provide the most reasonable approach to pediatric dosing. However, pharmacists should monitor these patients carefully and recommend dosage adjustments whenever necessary. Monitoring is essential if serious adverse reactions, toxicities, and subtherapeutic doses are to be avoided.

References

1. A. J. Glazko, Simplified procedures for calculating drug dosage from body weight in infancy and childhood, *Pediatrics*, 27, 503 (1961).
2. H. C. Shirkey, Drug dosage for infants and children, *J. Am. Med. Assoc.*, 193, 443 (1965).
3. R. Habersang and R. E. Kauffman, Drug doses for children, *J. Kans. Med. Soc.*, 75, 98 (1974).
4. M. A. Gill and C. T. Ueda, Novel method for the determination of pediatric dosages, *Am. J. Hosp. Pharm.*, 33, 389 (1976).
5. "Remington's Pharmaceutical Sciences," A. Osol and J. E. Hoover, Eds., Mack, Easton, Pa., 1975.
6. D. E. Francke and H. K. Whitney, "Perspectives in Clinical Pharmacy," Drug Intelligence, Hamilton, Ill., 1972.
7. V. C. Vaughan, R. J. McKay, and W. E. Nelson, "Textbook of Pediatrics," W. B. Saunders, Philadelphia, Pa., 1975.
8. M. J. Reilly, Pediatric drug dosage, *Am. J. Hosp. Pharm.*, 29, 699 (1972).
9. I. Libert, Modifying therapy for the young, *Drug Ther.*, 1 (4), 6 (1976).
10. H. C. Shirkey, "Pediatric Therapy," C. V. Mosby, St. Louis, Mo., 1975.

Readings for a Broader Perspective

1. Masaki, B. W. "O-t-c Drugs and the Pediatric Patient," *J. Am. Pharm. Assoc.* NS 15 (May 1975):239–46.
2. Ericson, A. J. "The Fetus: Conception to Birth," *The Apothecary* 90 (January/February 1978):27–32.
3. Lesko, L. J. "Pharmacokinetics of Drugs in the Neonate," *The Apothecary* 90 (January/February 1978):33–38.
4. Hays, D. P. "Drug Use in the Infant, Toddler, and Small Child," *The Apothecary* 90 (March/April 1978):33–38.
5. Munzenberger, P. J. "The Pharmacist as a Consultant to Children with Chronic Disease," *J. Am. Pharm. Assoc.* NS 16 (October 1976): 560–61.

Poisoning

37—The Pharmacist and Poisoning

William G. Troutman

As a compounder and dispenser of drugs, the pharmacist has always had a natural interest in the toxic effects of drugs, particularly when they are taken in accidental or intentional overdose. Coupling this natural interest with the pharmacist's ever increasing ability to utilize his knowledge of drug actions, uses, side effects and kinetics to improve patient care, the result is a health care practitioner who can make a significant contribution to the care of the poisoned patient. The role of the pharmacist in poisoning was reviewed by Kinnard in 1971,[1] but there have been some substantial changes in that role in recent years.

It has been impressive to watch, in the past few years, the growth of pharmacist-dominated regional poison information centers, both in numbers and in stature. While the growing trend toward regionalization of poison information activities will sound the death knell for many of the nation's nearly 600 small poison control centers, increased pharmacist involvement in regional programs will assure the profession a continued position of prominence in this field. Pharmacists practicing in regional poison information centers are involved in many thousands of poisoning cases each year and, most often, they are the first health professional contacted by the patient. Their position is that of a triage officer: determining the potential toxicity of the poison, recommending first aid procedures to be carried out, and determining the level of definitive care needed by the patient. Should the patient require an emergency room visit or hospitalization, the poison information center pharmacist is capable of advising the physician of the most appropriate treatment plan to follow. The skills required by pharmacists trained in drug information retrieval and analysis can be directly applied to the selection of correct therapy for the poisoned patient.

Another area in which pharmacists have increased their direct participation in the health care process is the emergency service of major hospitals. The pharmacist is rapidly gaining recognition as a valuable source of information and advice for a busy emergency department.[2] These pharmacists are capable of directly affecting the care of hundreds of poisoned patients each year, providing advice on treatment protocols and monitoring the progress of the patient toward recovery. The combination of the information resources of a regional poison information center and the direct on-site involvement of the emergency service pharmacist can produce a powerful joining of knowledge and talent, all directed toward improved patient care.

The vast majority of pharmacy practitioners are neither working in a regional poison information center nor assigned to the emergency department of their hospital, yet they are capable of making a substantial contribution to the care of the poisoned patient. The pharmacist should be a member of the hospital's poison response team. His familiarity with the appearance and ingredients of drug products can be of great value in the correct identification of the ingested product, an important first step in the management of poisonings. The pharmacist should also accept the responsibility for maintaining an adequate supply of "antidotal" drugs in both the emergency department and in the pharmacy. For the emergency department, this may be accomplished through the development of a special drug tray or cabinet to be used only for poisonings. The contents of this supply can be determined through consultation with a regional poison information center.

Poisonings are often preventable emergencies and all pharmacists, regardless of practice, have an obligation to participate in poison prevention activities. This is particularly true today when the public often views the pharmacist's sole contribution in this area to be the use of child-resistant (and sometimes adult-resistant) containers. Pharmacists can promote poison prevention through the distribution of public education materials, the preparation of mass media materials and by talking to school and civic groups about poisons and poisoning. This activity must go on all year, not just during Poison Prevention Week.

The pharmacist cannot help but be exposed to poisonings, and it is important that he be prepared to make a valuable contribution to the prevention and management of this widespread problem.

References

1. Kinnard, W. J. Jr.: The role of the pharmacist in the control of acute poisoning, *Clin Toxicol* 4:659–663 (4) 1971.
2. Elenbaas, R. M., Waeckerle, J. F. and McNabney, W. K.: The clinical pharmacist in emergency medicine, *Am J Hosp Pharm* 34:843–846 (Aug.) 1977.

Readings for a Broader Perspective

1. Bates, L. S. "Poison Control Today," *The Apothecary* 90 (September/October 1978): 14–15, 61–62.
2. Manoguerra, A. "Poison Prevention Month," *California Pharmacist* 25 (March 1978):18–19.
3. Schwartzmyer, P. R. "Techniques in the Management of Acute Poisoning: Part 1," *Hospital Pharmacy* 12 (September 1977):432–34.
4. Schwartzmyer, P. R. "Techniques in the Management of Acute Poisoning: Part 2," *Hospital Pharmacy* 12 (October 1977):501–04.
5. *American Pharmacy* NS 19 (February 1979):21–24.

PRIMARY CARE

38—Primary Care by a Pharmacist in an Outpatient Clinic

Steven H. Erickson

The Indian Health Service (IHS) has long been recognized for its progressive practice of pharmacy. Some pharmacists in the IHS have provided primary care for ambulatory patients with acute and chronic illnesses by protocol.[1-3] The following is a report of the data and experiences of a pharmacist providing primary care at an outpatient clinic and his impact on the delivery of health care services.

The Lummi Indian Health Center is an outpatient clinic located about 10 miles northwest of Bellingham, Washington. The clinic serves about 2,500 Lummi and Nooksack Indians. Two small hospitals in Bellingham provide inpatient facilities for those patients requiring hospital services. The Lummi Indian Reservation, located in Whatcom County, is not in a medically indigent area. The county population of 85,000 is served by over 100 physicians. The clinic staff at the time these data were collected included a physician, nurse, pharmacist, pediatric nurse practitioner, dentist, psychologist, public health nurse and supportive personnel.

Pharmacy Responsibilities

The clinic has always provided free medications, but it was without the services of a pharmacist until 1974. Prior to that time, drug ordering and dispensing responsibilities were shared by the nurse, physician and pediatric nurse practitioner. In July 1974, a pharmacist was added to the staff. Pharmacy functions included dispensing prescriptions, drug monitoring, patient counseling, ordering and maintaining drug supplies, and serving as the drug consultant for the health care team. Because this was a small clinic and funding did not permit a full-time pharmacist and laboratory technician, the pharmacist also provided limited laboratory services. As there was only one physician—who was overworked—primary care responsibilities were made a part of the pharmacist's job description.

The pharmacist was trained to perform many routine laboratory tests. A list of these tests can be found in Appendix A. The pharmacist also drew all blood specimens required for serology, chemistry and other blood tests. Training in laboratory procedures was received in Gallup, New Mexico, where the pharmacist spent several weeks in the medical laboratory of the Gallup Indian Hospital in a structured course. Prior to the pharmacist's arrival at this clinic, laboratory work was done by the physician and nurse. The pharmacy and laboratory were physically combined in one room. An aide worked in the pharmacy/laboratory to assist in the laboratory work.

Primary Care

Primary care responsibilities of the pharmacist included the diagnosis and treatment of certain acute illnesses and the management of selected chronic disease patients. The pharmacist learned diagnostic clinical skills while serving at another IHS facility in the Southwest. Protocols were written by the pharmacist and physician to cover 31 acute illnesses (Appendix B) and seven chronic conditions (Appendix C). Several other chronic diseases were followed without protocols, but in close cooperation with the physician.

The pharmacist invested much time searching for appropriate protocols, modifying existing protocols and writing new ones. . . . The style and format of Runyan[4] were used in developing these protocols with changes made to tailor the protocols to the clinical skills of the pharmacist. . . . [The] form of the oral contraceptive protocol [was] adopted from the pharmacy department of the Phoenix Indian Medical Center.[5]

A patient coming to the Lummi Clinic for health care was first screened by the receptionist. Depending on the reason for the visit, the patient was assigned to see the physician, nurse or pharmacist. The receptionist referred patients to the pharmacist for medication refills, chronic disease monitoring and acute complaints that could be managed

by the pharmacist. The receptionist kept a list of chief complaints that were to be referred to the pharmacist. Cough, sore throat, diarrhea, earache and minor skin sores were symptoms that the receptionist would routinely refer to the pharmacist. All patients requesting to see the physician were referred to the physician. Patients who were referred to the pharmacist were made aware that they were to be seen by a pharmacist. Some chronic disease patients also had pharmacy appointments for medication monitoring and refills. Most pharmacy appointments were made for the early morning, as the afternoon clinics were normally very busy with a large number of unscheduled patients. The medical charts of pharmacy patients were placed in a rack inside the pharmacy by the receptionist. All clinic and pharmacy patients waited in a common room. Patients were called to the pharmacy by the pharmacist when they were to be seen.

The pharmacy, measuring 6 m by 6 m, was equipped with a small table, two chairs and an examination table. A door to the waiting room could be closed so that privacy could be maintained. Diagnostic equipment such as an otoscope, stethoscope and blood pressure cuff were also in the pharmacy along with drugs and laboratory apparatus.

For each patient seen, the pharmacist obtained subjective and objective data, made assessments and carried out a plan as per protocol. The type of objective data collected depended on the nature of the pharmacy visit. When appropriate, the pharmacist took a blood pressure reading, examined the ears, nose and throat, auscultated the chest, or palpated the abdomen. The pharmacist wrote a problem-oriented note and dispensed any medication that he prescribed. Each patient was appropriately counseled as to the use, storage, benefits and expected side effects for the prescribed medication.

Duration of pharmacy visits varied depending on the nature of the visit. For example, a weekly disulfiram refill may only require five or 10 minutes, an acute otitis media visit about 15 minutes, and a patient with hypertension, diabetes, and congestive heart failure may require 20 to 30 minutes for monitoring and refills.

Complications not covered by protocols could be managed by one of three methods. The pharmacist could consult the physician, refer the patient immediately to the physician or have the patient see the physician at a later time if the problem was not an emergency.

Pharmacy Visits

Pharmacy visits accounted for almost a third of the clinic visits in 1975 (Table 38.1).

Table 38.1

Number of Clinic Visits in 1975

Primary Care Provider[a]	Clinic Visits	
	Number	Percent
Physician	5,800	48.8
Pharmacist	3,729	31.4
Nurse	1,633	13.7
Others	730	6.1
Total	11,892	100.0

[a] Only one primary care provider per patient visit.

For each clinic visit only one provider was credited as being the primary care provider. For example, if a patient came to the clinic with an earache and saw the physician who made a diagnosis of otitis media and wrote a prescription for ampicillin that was dispensed by the pharmacist, then the physician was designated as the primary care provider. If, however, this patient with an earache did not see the physician but was referred to the pharmacist who diagnosed and treated this otitis media, then the pharmacist was the primary care provider.

The diagnosis and treatment of the 10 most common acute illnesses made up over

Table 38.2

Ten Most Common Acute Illnesses Seen by the Pharmacist in 1975

Illness	Number	% Total Pharmacy Visits
Upper respiratory infection	679	17.9
Pharyngitis—tonsillitis	227	6.0
Gastritis—gastroenteritis	117	3.1
Otitis	115	3.0
Skin infections	108	2.9
Urinary tract infections	96	2.5
Oral	56	1.5
Iron deficiency anemia	39	1.0
Ectoparasitic	38	1.0
Conjunctivitis	27	0.7
Total	1,502	[39.6]

40% of these pharmacy visits (Table 38.2). Upper respiratory infections and pharyngitis-tonsillitis accounted for over half of these acute visits. Most patients presenting with a sore throat or cold symptoms could be examined by obtaining subjective data and a quick examination of the ears, nose and throat. In those patients giving a history of a productive cough, the pharmacist auscultated the chest. In diagnosing gastroenteritis and gastritis, the pharmacist took a careful history to rule out other causes of abdominal pain. Eight percent of the pharmacy visits were for common pediatric problems such as otitis media, skin infections (mostly impetigo) and ectoparasitic infestations (nits, lice, scabies and pinworms). The 96 visits for urinary tract infections were mostly follow-up visits. Usually the physician diagnosed the infection, and the patient reported to the pharmacist in several days for follow-up. The pharmacist checked the culture and sensitivity reports, questioned the patient about symptoms, changed antibiotic therapy if indicated and ordered a repeat culture after termination of therapy. Oral illnesses included the diagnosis and treatment of thrush and mouth sores, and the prescribing of pain medication for dental pain when the dentist was out of town.

The 10 most common chronic conditions monitored by the pharmacist accounted for another 40% of the pharmacy visits (Table 38.3). The chronic management of hypertension and other cardiovascular problems (rheumatic heart disease prophylaxis, angina, arrythmias) constituted the largest group of patients. The relatively large percentages of visits for anxiety and depression reflect the clinic policy of dispensing only small quantities of the benzodiazepines. Most of these visits were for refills of antianxiety or antidepressant drugs. The pharmacist maintained a close alliance with the physician and the psychologist in the management of these patients. Patients on oral contraceptives were seen every three to six months, and blood pressure changes and side effects were checked for on each visit.

The pharmacist also dispensed prescriptions written by the physician, dentist and nurse practitioner. Prescriptions were ordered in the patient's chart, and each patient was appropriately counseled about his medication. In 1975, the pharmacist dispensed 4,723 new prescriptions, monitored and refilled 2,479 prescriptions, and prescribed and dispensed 2,933 additional prescriptions. He provided clinical counseling services on 7,205 occasions.

Conclusion

Both the patients and clinic staff accepted this expanded role of the pharmacist. Some patients felt less threatened by the pharmacist and preferred seeing the pharmacist for minor acute problems or chronic medication monitoring. Also, the pharmacist was generally more accessible than the physician, who usually had a full appointment schedule. The pharmacist was able to provide patient monitoring between visits to the physician and extend the interval between such visits. The pharmacist was able to diagnose and treat a large number of acute illnesses that otherwise would have required physician visits.

In fiscal year 1974, prior to the arrival of the pharmacist, there were 9,500 outpatient visits at the clinic. In 1975 there were 11,892 outpatient visits. Because there were only part-time pediatric nurse practitioner services provided in 1975 and full-time services in 1974, the pharmacist's impact was actually greater than the 2,500 difference in total patient visits.

These data suggest that pharmacists, with some additional training, can take care of a large variety and volume of acute and chronic diseases in an outpatient clinic.

Table 38.3

Ten Most Common Chronic Conditions Followed by the Pharmacist in 1975

Condition	Number	% Total Pharmacy Visits
Hypertension and cardiovascular	284	7.5
Anxiety—depression	202	5.3
Family planning	184	4.9
Eczema—urticaria	155	4.1
Arthritis	145	3.8
Chronic respiratory disease	138	3.7
Diabetes	101	2.7
Alcoholism	83	2.2
Gastrointestinal disease	61	1.6
Epilepsy	60	1.6
Total	1,413	37.4

Appendix A

Laboratory Tests Performed by Pharmacist

Hematocrit
White blood cell count
Erythrocyte sedimentation rate
Throat culture
Urine culture
Gynecologic culture
Wound culture
Sensitivities
Pregnancy test
Urine analysis with microscopic examination
Potassium hydroxide preparations
Saline preparations
Gram stain
Blood sugar

Appendix B

Acute Illnesses Diagnosed and Treated by the Pharmacist

Pharyngitis
Tonsillitis
Acute bronchitis
Upper respiratory
  infection
Sinusitis
Gastritis
Gastroenteritis
Cholelithiasis
Menstrual cramps
Eustachian tube
  dysfunction
Acute otitis media
Chronic otitis media
Otitis externa
Cerumen
Serous otitis media
Impetigo
Superficial abrasions
Cellulitis-minor
Urinary tract infections
Teething
Herpes stomatitis-
  aphthous ulcers
Dental pain
Eye irritation
Allergic conjunctivitis
Conjuctivitis—bacterial
  vs. viral
Sty
Foreign body in eye
Pregnancy
  Morning sickness
  Esophagitis
  Iron and vitamin
    therapy
Anemia—iron deficiency

Appendix C

Chronic Conditions or Medications Handled by the Pharmacist

Arthritis
Epilepsy
Rheumatic fever prophylaxis
Oral contraceptive refill
High blood pressure
Congestive heart failure
Diabetes
Thyroid replacement
Isoniazid prophylaxis
Disulfiram therapy for alcoholism
Chronic obstructive pulmonary disease

[Appendix D and E omitted]

References

1. Ellinoy, B. J., Mays, J. F., McSherry, P. V., et al.: A pharmacy outpatient monitoring program providing primary medical care to selected patients, *Am J Hosp Pharm 30*:593–598 (Jul) 1973.
2. Anderson, P. O. and Taryle, D. A.: Pharmacist management of ambulatory patients using formalized standards of care, *Am J Hosp Pharm 31*:254–257 (Mar) 1974.
3. Streit, R. J.: A program expanding the pharmacist's role, *J Am Pharm Assoc NS13*:434–443 (Aug) 1973.
4. Runyan, J. W.: Primary care guide, Harper and Row, Hagerstown, Maryland, 1975, p. 10–15.
5. Anon: Oral contraceptive refill protocol, prepared by the Pharmacy Department, Phoenix Indian Medical Center, January 1974.

Related Readings in This Volume

8. Monitoring Diabetic Patients
12. Pharmacist and Preventive Medicine
14. Hypertension Patients in Community Pharmacy
26. Management of Ambulatory Patients
28. Clinical Pharmacy in Emergency Medicine

Readings for a Broader Perspective

1. Dolan, M. "Emil Baker Emphasizes Services Instead of Salesmanship," *American Pharmacy* NS 18 (May 1978):22–26, 41.
2. Brands, A. J. "How Primary Care Training Enhances the Pharmacist's Health Role," *Pharmacy Times* 44 (October 1978):50–53.
3. Eshelman, F. N., and Campagna, K. D. "Pharmaceutical Services for the Primary Care Health Team," *Hospital Pharmacy* 11 (August 1976):295–300.
4. Longe, R. L., and Calvert, J. C. "Physical Assessment and the Clinical Pharmacist," *Drug Intelligence & Clinical Pharmacy* 11 (April 1977):200–03.
5. Johnson, R. E., and Tuchler, R. J. "Role of the Pharmacist in Primary Health Care," *American Journal of Hospital Pharmacy* 32 (February 1975):162–64.

COMMUNITY PHARMACY

39—From Drug Store to Apothecary Shop

Ira Wellins

There may be more involved in converting from a conventional drug store to an apothecary shop than remodeling the physical plant and eliminating cigarettes, newspapers, school supplies, greeting cards and hair coloring. In some cases an attitudinal change may also be required.

The paramount question that kept me from converting over the years was, "Will it succeed?" There never had been anything like it in my area; and I felt people might resent being forced to go elsewhere for the stamps, newspapers, cigarettes and shampoos which they were accustomed to having available at the drug store. I could fill up this magazine with the excuses I gave myself for not converting.

I hesitated to leave the seeming safety and security of the successful conventional drug store, even though the pressures for change were mounting rapidly. The soda fountain had become a hang-out detrimental to the rest of the store. Increasing prescription volume was straining the cramped quarters of the back room. The layout was not conducive to giving necessary information to the patient.

These problems were solved in 1968 by a major remodeling, which for me was a daring departure from the norm. The fountain, magazines and some minor sundries were eliminated, and a greatly enlarged prescription department was placed right in the center of the store. It was a raised island with a wide aisle surrounding it. I now could talk with patients without raising my voice. It physically placed the one department unique to pharmacy where I thought it belonged, right in the heart of things.

The new layout worked too well. Within four years my prescription volume had grown by 60 percent, and again we were cramped. I had underestimated the stimulating effect of a more professional looking store.

The fact that my prescription department now could sustain my entire operation was brought home forcefully when the adjoining hardware store caught fire and the entire building was gutted. I was able to save the patient profiles and prescription files, however, and with those records we did business from a 60 by 12 foot rented trailer in the parking lot during the eight months it took to rebuild. Even though space limitations restricted us to prescriptions and a very few over-the-counter drug items, we only lost slightly over 11 percent of our gross volume, and our net profit actually increased. This proved to me that my remaining sundries, greeting cards, school supplies, beauty aids, post office, hosiery and so forth, were not only detracting from the professional appeal of the store but also were draining the business financially.

I have tried often to analyze the reason for our sustained growth despite location in a heavily competitive area, which has larger and better merchandised stores within a two-mile radius. The only conclusion I could draw was that our concentration on clinical and people-oriented services had a growing market in our area.

What can you do to get into this market?

Keeping thorough patient profiles and using them to maximum patient advantage are essential. A thorough patient profile not only lists the patient's name, address, and prescriptions filled, with quantity, name, and strength of drug, but also notes pertinent medication information such as reactions and allergies to drugs, chronic and present ailments, and any special diets or lab tests.

Since the purpose of a patient profile is to protect the patient as much as possible, it must be consulted before a new prescription is filled, and entry of the prescription on it should occur before dispensing. Waiting for a slow period to do entries is too risky, in my experience; too many patients come in with prescriptions from different doctors twice in one day. It is not rare for a general practitioner to prescribe penicillin for a strep throat in a teen-ager, while two hours later the dermatologist orders tetracycline for acne. I might add that I have actually seen this combination prescribed on a single prescription blank.

If you are thinking, "This is all fine, but how much will this add to the cost of filling each prescription?" my reply is this: the only part of this procedure which must be done by a professional is the review before filling, which averages under ten seconds. Nonprofessional or pharmacy technician time for pulling the profile, entering the prescription, and refiling is about thirty seconds. In my area, this costs approximately two cents of pharmacist and three cents of technician

time, plus about two cents' worth of paper forms. However, the use of the profile will necessitate an increase in time spent communicating with patients, physicians, and other health professionals. I cannot estimate the cost of this, except to state that no advertising campaign of equal cost will do so much to increase your prescription business and your professional status in the community, and to elevate pharmacy itself.

Since the assistance of technicians is necessary to implement successful patient profiles and other clinical services, we must look at the main objections to their use.

Technicians are illegal. In most states, the law does not define exactly what constitutes filling a prescription. Typing the label, getting the correct bottle off the shelf, counting or pouring the correct amount, putting it into a bottle, and affixing the label are all tasks most technicians can do under the immediate supervision of the pharmacist. This applies to technicians who are formally trained and those who are trained by you. Check with your state pharmaceutical association as to what is allowed in your state. I might add that hiring pharmacy students not only gives you a super-technician, but also helps you keep up-to-date.

Pharmacists will lose jobs. Did the advent of the nurse in the doctor's office put any physicians out of practice? Did the plumber's helper cause hardship among plumbers? Of course not! They contributed to efficiency by freeing the physician and plumber from routine jobs that did not require a person of their qualifications, and so increased the time they could spend using their full training. If we do not use technicians to free us from the routine tasks for which we are overqualified, we will not have the time to communicate our drug knowledge for the patients' benefit. As a result, pharmacy's image will continue its downward spiral, and we eventually will be replaced by dispensing machines already being used in certain hospitals. That is what will cause pharmacists to lose jobs.

There are so many areas where a great need exists for pharmacists to involve themselves in drug usage and monitoring, and so much has been written, that I will mention briefly only a few.

Scheduling the drug regimen for the patient, if the physician has not done so. B.I.D., T.I.D., and similar terms may be translated into specific times, taking into account the illness, mealtimes, and rising and sleeping times.

Monitoring for compliance, and explaining the risks of noncompliance as well as the benefits expected: in short, the "why" of taking the drug in question.

Information stickers are good: "Don't take with milk, after, or before meals," and so on. But stickers plus the pharmacist's reinforcement, explaining why, are more effective than stickers alone.

Counseling on over-the-counter products. People always ask for "the best" cough medicine or laxative. The pharmacist could explain that the "best" varies with the condition being treated. He could determine the cause of the cough and its type by questioning the patient. It might be helpful to explain the difference between expectorants and cough suppressants, between stool softeners, bulk formers, irritants, and the saline cathartics. Sometimes a few questions to elicit the reason the patient is taking medication can give you an inkling of a more serious underlying condition. For example, not all "indigestion" is treatable with antacids. Some patients with this complaint really may be suffering from a heart attack.

Warnings about potential drug side-effects and symptoms, so that patients will recognize these effects and call their doctor if they occur. Of course, this must be done carefully lest the patient be scared into not starting needed drug therapy.

These are but a few of the possible areas of clinical involvement open to you. With thought and imagination you can determine the specific needs of the patients in your community, and devise methods of meeting those needs. Pharmacy technicians give you the time to do this, and doing it increases your prescription volume. When prescription volume and sickroom and convalescent supplies become the major part of your practice, all that is needed is to remodel the place where you practice to reflect what you are doing.

However, a sudden, untested changeover from conventional drug store to apothecary shop seems unnecessarily risky to me. It seems sensible first to change methods and attitudes before changing the physical plant—to become knowledgeable through study and to apply that knowledge through patient-oriented services; namely, the patient profile and the communication of information on drugs. If a resultant rise in prescriptions creates an increasing need for space, it then seems logical to begin dropping sundry departments one at a time (hardware, magazines or school supplies, for instance). This gradual process minimizes risk, because you are dropping small percentages of your sundry volume only as your pharmaceutical volume warrants it.

Throughout this article I have been alluding directly or indirectly to the necessity of keeping up-to-date through continuing education. Pharmacy is a broad field, so each pharmacist must decide which method would be best, whether it be correspondence courses, extension courses, audio tapes, journals, manufacturers' literature, or homework in his own library.

I am not the person to recommend any particular set of titles for your library, as that is not my field. Your needs will vary according to how long you have been out of school, what you have done since, and what goals you wish to set for yourself. For my purposes these are the works I most often consult:

Hansten's *Drug Interactions*
Goodman & Gilman's *Pharmacologic Basis of Therapeutics*
Manual of Medical Therapeutics
Physicians' Desk Reference
Dorland's Medical Dictionary

Drug company hand-outs (some with cassette tapes) on specific disease states and the drugs used in treatment

Case studies in clinical pharmacy (from *Drug Intelligence*).

I also find two journals especially valuable:

Drug Intelligence and Clinical Pharmacy
APhA Journal

Perhaps reading about the numerous factors involved in moving toward a more professional practice makes it seem more difficult than it is. There are only two requirements that must be met in my experience—resolving to continue your education on a regular basis, which may mean setting a goal of one hour a day for study; and examining your own motives when a patient requests your advice. Does a product really suit the patient's need? Talking people out of buying anything at all when they really need no drugs is one of the best ways to earn their respect and confidence.

These two factors, education and attitude, are the heart of an apothecary shop.

40—Patient End Results of Community Pharmacy Service

Mickey C. Smith

One could quote scores of references to the workings of the "health care team." Within the literature of pharmacy scores of additional references concerning the role of the pharmacist in general, the role of the pharmacist on the "team" and the "clinical" role of the pharmacist have appeared. Although a rather tentative classification scheme describing the clinical role of the pharmacist has appeared,[1] the elements of this scheme remain largely undocumented in any quantitative fashion. Further, such reports as have appeared describing incidents or groups of incidents which involve the pharmacist and which might clearly fall under the umbrella of a "clinical" designation, have been largely anecdotal. Relation of such incidents to the broad medical care system or to similar incidents in medical

practice are generally lacking but certainly needed.

The important work which served to prompt the study reported here was that of Sanazaro and Williamson.[2,3] The research technique employed was a modification of the critical incident method.[4] This useful research tool has been employed successfully in studies in dentistry[5] and nursing.[6]

Methodology

The critical incidents gathered in this study were obtained by a mail survey of pharmacists previously identified by faculty members of schools of pharmacy as practicing a "high level" of community pharmacy. These pharmacists were asked to provide written reports of at least one positive and one negative incident from their practices. The wording of the respondent's instructions asked that he "describe an incident which caused you to gain or retain a patient or which was for some reason a source of professional satisfaction to you," for a positive incident. A negative incident was one "which may have caused the loss of a patient or which you would handle differently if faced with the situation or problem again." Examples of critical incidents from the dentistry study were provided for guidance.

Because of the nature of the sample and the type of information requested the results of this survey should be regarded as descriptive only. No claim is made that they are representative of community pharmacy nationally. Nevertheless, we feel they are of considerable value in illustrating episodes of community pharmacy practice which have important beneficial and sometimes deleterious effects on the health, function and attitudes of the consuming public.

Results

One-hundred and ninety-two pharmacists provided accounts of episodes of care. A total of 424 incidents, 192 negative and 235 positive, were received. Twenty-two incidents were judged as "paradoxical" in that they had both positive and negative results. Each incident was further analyzed to determine specific outcomes resulting from it. This analysis yielded a total of 665 end results of which 428 were positive and 237 were negative. These end results were categorized using an adaptation of the work of Sanazaro and Williamson in their study of physicians. . . . [2,3]

Discussion

More than four of five of the end results in this study were "process outcomes." Further, the attitude of patient and physician toward the pharmacist involved one of three positive and six of ten negative results. This finding may be the result of several factors, but two suggest themselves strongly. The first is the current involvement of pharmacy in the professionalization process,[7] which normally results in a high level of concern with prestige and status. The second is the effect of attitudes on number of clientele. It is still much easier to change pharmacists than it is to change physicians. That this may be a factor is borne out by pharmacist assessments of what constitutes a "critical" incident. Sixty positive incidents (25.5 percent) were explicitly identified with gaining a client, while 94 negative incidents (49 percent) were similarly involved with the loss of a client.

Also interesting is the relatively high proportion of pharmacy incidents involved with causing or preventing risks, particularly the latter. The majority of these incidents involved drug incompatibilities. While it is not the purpose of this paper to discuss the contribution of pharmacy to medical care, some of the incidents described were quite dramatic. . . .

We were interested in two types of "end results" in this study. The data reported are divided into these two major categories. "Patient end results" are those in which the patient, his physical condition or disease undergo some change—hopefully for the better, but not always so. "Process outcomes" are end results observable as a result of contact with the health care system and only occurring when such contact is made. The implicit assumption is that a favorable "process outcome" will result in a favorable "patient end result." This is neither necessarily so, nor always possible to determine. Neither in this study were both types of end results observed and/or reported.

It should be emphasized that some of the differences in the general distribution of results between "process outcomes" and "patient end results" must come from inability of the pharmacist to determine (or at any rate to report) the ultimate outcome of an incident in terms of its physiological or psychological effects. Thus, while it might (perhaps justifiably) be assumed that warning the patient against taking antacids and tetracycline together would both assure proper drug use and result in relief of physical abnormalities, the assumption of the latter was not made unless specifically reported. Certainly this must account for a major portion of the difference between the proportions identified for pharmacy and those reported for medicine in the medical study cited earlier.

In spite of the foregoing the critical incidents supplied suggest the possibility of a much deeper involvement by pharmacists in patient outcomes than the simple dispensing of a prescription. Indeed the correct or incorrect technical manipulation of the prescription order was rarely involved in a reported critical incident. An examination of a few of the critical incidents received will illustrate this.

What follows are actual critical incidents of the positive, negative and paradoxical types as submitted by the pharmacist respondents. With the exception of minor editing, they are presented in the words of the respondents themselves.

Positive Incidents

1. A patient presented a prescription for Aralen from a noted dermatologist. The patient had a scalp condition that might be simple dandruff or psoriasis. Aralen is contraindicated in psoriasis so I questioned the patient. He said "my regular physician is treating me for psoriasis." I called this dermatologist on a special phone and talked to him about the patient's condition. He told me to dispense the drug. By this time the patient suspected something was wrong. I told him of the situation and also that as his pharmacist I would not dispense the drug.

The patient was happy, returned to the physician and secured another prescription for his problem, which we dispensed.

2. A man about 65 years of age came into our pharmacy at about 5:15 p.m. He asked me if we had anything that would give quicker relief for "stomach pains" than Tums. I discussed his problem for several minutes and learned that he was in deep distress. After several minutes I got him to take a seat in our waiting room, learned his name and that of his doctor. I called the doctor and told him my thinking about his patient. He came to the pharmacy within 10 minutes and took the patient to the hospital in his car. The hospital is two blocks from our pharmacy. The patient suffered a massive coronary within minutes after his arrival at the hospital.

3. I dispensed a prescription for Indocin 25 mg capsules, No. 30, take one tablet twice a day. Upon presenting this prescription to the patient (who happened to be my former grammar school principal) I asked if the doctor had told him to take this medication with food or milk. He said yes, the doctor had told him this and proceeded to ask why he should take the medicine in this manner. I said I had checked because taking the drug on an empty stomach could possibly cause stomach irritation. Therefore, taking it with food or milk would lessen the chance of this occurring. I found out later that the patient had spoken to my parents (my father is also a pharmacist) and told them that he was impressed with my evident knowledge about this drug and its proper administration.

4. Late one evening an elderly gentleman came in and asked if I had any Vicks cough syrup. In looking at him I noticed that he had beads of perspiration on his upper lip. I thought this rather odd for such a cold evening so I asked him how he knew he needed cough syrup. His reply was that he had a pain in his chest and guessed he must have "Hong Kong flu." I asked him if his left arm hurt and he replied that it did, especially at the elbow. I asked him if he would have a

seat and let me call his doctor, that he just might be having a heart attack. He didn't have a doctor and asked me to pick one. I called one who happened to be at the hospital. I described the symptoms and he asked me to give the patient 1/150 of nitroglycerine under the tongue and then bring him to the hospital. Before I had gone a block, the old man doubled over and I thought he was a "goner." However, after a few more blocks he straightened up and said "I am OK now." I told him that inasmuch as this doctor was looking for him, we had better go on and get him checked out. He agreed to this and after he was admitted I waited around for a while. The doctor came out and told me that the old man had had a massive heart attack. He was in the hospital for about 30 days but he came out of it. The doctor told me something amusing about it. He said he asked the old man if he had ever had a pain like that before and he replied "Not since I had the flu." The doctor asked him when that was and the old man said "In 1918." Anyway I had a patient and in addition a great deal of satisfaction because the physician told me that there was no doubt that I had saved his life and that if I had just sold him the bottle of cough syrup he had asked for, he probably would never have made it through the night. I have always wondered what would have happened if he had gone to a grocery store or supermarket and asked for the cough syrup.

5. A hypertensive patient complained of insomnia and asked for an over-the-counter sleeping tablet. I recommended calling the doctor to see if he agreed that the patient should be taken off Reserpine due to the possibility that it is causing "depressive insomnia." The doctor agreed and changed the patient to Valium and increased his diuretic dosage. Result—the patient's insomnia gradually disappeared and his blood pressure was adequately controlled by the new regimen.

6. This incident concerns a patient who had suffered from a severe rash in the mouth for several months. She had visited several physicians and had been treated with every known ulcer medication—Gentian Violet, Mycostatin, smallpox vaccine and many others. After one of her many visits to another "specialist," we noticed that along with her prescription she purchased a well-known brand of laxative containing phenolphthalein. I passed this information along to the patient's local physician who had referred the patient to the "oral specialist." The physician in turn called the patient and told her to change laxatives, which she did, and the mouth rash cleared up. In this case we did not make many points with the patient as we had only discussed the problem with the physician. But the physician appreciated our interest and has so demonstrated on several occasions since that day. Anyway, the patient was relieved of a most uncomfortable mouth rash, started eating again, regained her health and this is just what our profession is all about anyway.

7. Noticing on subsequent visits that an apparent fever blister was not appearing to heal, I inquired of a patient about the age of the ulceration and what he had been doing for treatment. The treatment period had extended far too long for not having obtained more positive results from the usual home remedy. I suggested the application of one of a triple antibiotic combinations with the admonition that, if some positive progress toward healing was not noted in a couple of days, he should consult his family physician and have him rule out the possibility of a skin cancer. Several weeks later the patient reappeared with his repaired lip and a "sincere" thanks for having guided him to the proper treatment before more radical surgery would have been required.

8. Because of the actual physical layout of our pharmacy in a medical center, communication between pharmacist and physicians is quite complete. One of the doctors was talking to me one day about a patient he knew that I knew. This patient was not a prescription patient of mine but is a very good customer otherwise. The doctor told

me that he had overlooked the fact that she was taking an anticoagulant and had prescribed Atromid-S for her. These prescriptions were filled at a "cut-rate drugstore" which did not keep patient profile cards so no warning was given to the patient. The patient ended up in the hospital. The same patient also ended up in the hospital while taking aspirin for pain relief with the anticoagulant. Knowing about these things, I was alerted when she came in one day with a prescription from a dentist for Phenaphen No. 3. I didn't want to alarm her but called her doctor instead. He was out of the office that day but I finally got hold of him the next day. He said he would call her and tell her not to take them but if I saw her first to tell her to have her Darvon refilled. Fortunately she came by a few hours later and I was able to give her the message without alarming her.

At that time she had a prescription from an oral surgeon for tetracycline. The next morning she was also in the pharmacy and happened to tell me that the tetracycline had upset her GI tract. She had called the oral surgeon who had told her to take the medication with an antacid. I called the dentist and reminded him of the effects antacids have upon the availability of tetracycline. He had not read this information and was grateful to get it. He changed the prescription to another antibiotic. That afternoon the patient was in after the oral surgery with a prescription for Tylenol with codeine. I had just finished reading about a survey done on the effects of acetaminophen on anticoagulants. While this survey was done on a very small number of people, I felt it might be significant in this patient. I talked to her doctor and we both concurred that no chance should be taken. We told her to simply use Darvon as necessary.

9. Recently an elderly lady (approximately 75 years) entered our pharmacy and wanted to purchase an over-the-counter sleeping medication (highly advertised) con-taining a scopolamine alkaloid. She had had cataract and glaucoma surgery within the prior three to four months. Knowing her and her medical background, we suggested she contact her ophthalmologist first before using this type of medication. Upon hearing from this patient the physician was most positive about her not using this type of remedy for sleeplessness and prescribed chloral hydrate. We also received a thank you note from him which was much appreciated.

10. Mrs. X is going to two different physicians who have both prescribed for her hypertension. On receiving a prescription order from Doctor A for a medication which would have doubled the diuretic action of Doctor B's prescription, I consulted with the patient and explained to her the necessity of keeping all of her physicians aware of what she was taking and who she was seeing. She then explained that Doctor B had referred her to Doctor A and she thought that Doctor A knew all the medication she was receiving. I phoned Doctor A and informed him of the situation explaining that according to the medication record she was taking two prescriptions from Doctor B. He expressed appreciation and interest for the keeping of family records. I then phoned Doctor B to let him know what was going on (he thought the patient would tell Doctor A what she was taking). He also thanked me for the call and interest. The result was that Doctor A had Mrs. X discontinue one prescription from Doctor B and begin a third prescription. Both physicians and the patient were pleased.

Negative Incidents

1. A geriatric patient entered the pharmacy with a prescription for sodium salicylate. In trying to save time I did not fill the prescription as such but gave her a bottle over the counter. The physician called a few

days later and was very upset over my action. It seemed the patient complained of pain and the physician wanted this as a placebo prescription to prevent giving her a stronger analgesic which he felt she did not need. Consequently, good relations were lost between physician and patient.

2. On a busy day in my pharmacy I received a new prescription for Thorazine concentrate for a boarding home patient from one of our state mental hospitals. I dispensed it as usual but failed to instruct the nursing personnel as to the need for diluting the medication in another vehicle. About a week later one of the workers at the home told me that they had nearly fought with the patient for two days trying to get him to take the prescribed dose directly into his mouth from the dropper. They had finally read the manufacturer's label (which I had covered with my pharmacy label) and put the medication in juice. The patient was now doing fine. I did not lose the boarding home business but they were quite put out at me for not making them aware of the situation.

3. When I was a student in college, a man came in and asked for a laxative. I asked him whether he wanted something that would work immediately or after a night's rest and he said he wanted something to work immediately. I asked no more questions. He went over to the soda fountain, took the medication and left (citrate of magnesia). In about 10 minutes he was back and wanted to use our bathroom. I let him. After about 30 minutes I had to go downstairs for something else and I could hear someone moaning in the bathroom. I checked and it was him. I called an ambulance and got him comfortable in the truss room and also called a doctor. The doctor got there first but suspected that maybe the man was faking to begin with. They took him in an ambulance to the hospital and did some testing and finally put him into surgery about one hour after admission. Ruptured appendix was the problem. There were also peritoneal ulcers

and the one ulcer was almost paper thin. He lived and all came out fine but the one dose of that purgative could have almost been the cause of death.

4. A lady hypochondriac patron was taking Seconal placebos. We were making the placebos by emptying the active ingredient and replacing it with lactose. This lady was paranoid, and one day she suspected what we were doing. She opened a capsule and tasted the powder and then called the pharmacist and confronted him with her suspicions. He admitted that we were doing just what she suspected. Needless to say, she quit patronizing me and even threatened to sue. She blamed us for all her problems, even though the physician had prescribed the placebo. This incident could have been prevented by good common sense judgement on the part of the pharmacist. He should have known the instability of the woman and could have tactfully reassured her that she was getting just what the doctor ordered.

5. This incident involves a patient who had frequent dizzy spells accompanied with severe headaches. She often watched television promotions of headache medication and felt that there was no need to see a doctor. Therefore she came in for something for her headache. Having several prescriptions to dispense with no time to secure previous conditions and activities that led up to her complaint, she was sold Empirin Compound tablets. After a few days information came to us that she had had a slight stroke which probably could have been prevented with proper advice and treatment in the early days of the symptoms.

6. A lady with an earache went to an ear-nose-throat doctor and received two prescriptions. One was for an antibiotic capsule and the other for Nilstat suspension with the directions 1 cc three times a day. On the next afternoon after the prescriptions were dispensed, the lady called the pharmacy wondering if the Nilstat was to be placed in the ear as she was currently doing. Because of

the way Nilstat looks she wasn't sure if it was an eardrop or not. It was explained to her over the phone that it was to be taken orally and not to be used in the ear. In a couple of hours the daughter of the lady came into the pharmacy and said they had called the physician and he told them that we should have placed on the label "for the throat." The prescription was shown to the daughter along with an explanation that it was labeled as the doctor had specified on the prescription. The daughter was very upset and left the pharmacy in a very disgusted mood.

7. This incident concerns a prescription I misread as 25 mg which was actually 2.5 mg. It could have had serious results but fortunately things worked out satisfactorily. It was a prescription for Coumadin and the doctor indicated the strength as /0025. At the time I dispensed the prescription I commented to the daughter of the patient that it was somewhat unusual to be using a dose that high. The patient and daughter went to see the doctor a couple of days later and the daughter happened to mention to a nurse that it apparently was a high dose. The nurse checked the situation, reported to the doctor and it was necessary to restabilize the patient. The patient reported the mistake to me and I discussed the problem with the doctor. I did not lose the patient as a patron but it certainly affected our relationship.

8. This incident concerns a new patient of the pharmacy expecting her first child. Her obstetrician had given her a prescription for prenatal vitamins. The directions to the patient were poorly written and the pharmacist hastily interpreted them as saying one capsule twice a day instead of one capsule once a day. After the first supply was used the patient returned with another new prescription for the same vitamin. This time the prescription was dispensed correctly. Upon examining the second prescription label the patient called the pharmacy and asked why the directions were different. She became alarmed when it was explained to her that an error had been made. Fearful of any damage to her unborn baby, the pharmacist informed the physician of his error. The physician assured him that there was nothing to fear in this case. The pharmacist called the patient and explained that he had conferred with the physician and that no harm had been done. Perhaps this was not enough because the patient never returned to the pharmacy.

9. I make it a habit to explain directions for new prescriptions to caution my clientele about any obvious side effects. A new patron came into my pharmacy one day with a prescription for Declomycin. I cautioned her about prolonged exposure to the sun with this drug. Unbeknownst to me, this particular patient was very much an alarmist about drugs and interpreted the caution to mean that this drug was very dangerous and potent. She immediately called the doctor and asked him why he gave her such a potent drug and that she wasn't going to take it under any circumstances. Naturally he called me and expressed his feelings about the situation (which were highly negative). I still feel it is necessary for the pharmacist to give this information to the patients, and I still do. However, I also feel it is necessary to know your customer first and use the correct approach in explaining these things.

Paradoxical Incidents

1. A patient had been seeing both a psychiatrist and a general practitioner on a regular basis and was receiving medication from both. On one occasion the general practitioner telephoned a prescription to our pharmacy which would have conflicted with the medication prescribed by the psychiatrist. I advised the general practitioner of this conflict at which time he inquired of all the prescriptions this patient was receiving from other doctors and said that he would consult with the patient. The next contact was the

patient's husband calling me to complain that the general practitioner should not have been advised of the other medications as he was treating a completely different problem. I attempted to explain to him that while the problems were different the patient was the same and conflicts can arise in medication, as medications do not act only on the problem but also affect the rest of the body. This was my last contact with the patient or her husband over two years ago.

2. Last week one of our adult female patients called to have her prescription for 60 Percodan tablets refilled for her pain resulting from back surgery. She also asked us to call another local pharmacy for a copy of another unrelated prescription for thyroid. Upon comparing notes with the other pharmacist, we discovered she had been receiving Percodan from another physician in the community. We then called for renewal authorization of the two medications (Percodan and thyroid) and informed the MD of the duplication of Percodan prescriptions. What happened is predictable. The physician "scolded" the lady for taking too much Percodan and we lost a patron. We feel remorse for losing her as a patient but would still have it no other way.

3. This concerned a physician with whom we were checking a drug interaction. We had three prescriptions for this particular patient and two of the prescriptions contained 5 grains of aspirin, each with other ingredients, while the third was for 5 mg of Coumadin, a direct incompatibility due to increased activity in Coumadin when combined with aspirin. My associate called the doctor's office and related the problem to the office girl as we most often have to do and the office girl said that she would call us right back. She later called us and said that the patient would only be using the aspirin products whenever needed so that the interaction would be alright to dispense. I questioned this in my own mind since if they were used as needed then a stabilized prothrom-

bin time would not be probable and the chance for hemorrhage would still be present.

I called the physician's office once again and just to clarify the problem to satisfy my second thoughts, the girl informed me that she would put the doctor on the line right away. When he came on the line he asked "Just what is this all about anyway?" I related my story again calmly underlining my thoughts on a disruptive prothrombin time. He informed me that he had been aware of this interaction for a long time and wanted to know if I asked my patrons on "thinners" to be in for regular pro times each week and if I did this, this was enough. I answered that we did do this and were merely trying to clarify the information that the office girl had told me. He then told me to send the prescriptions back to him if I was so concerned and he would direct the lady to have them dispensed elsewhere. I assured him that I was not trying to usurp his right to prescribe but just to complete our responsibility to him and his patient to warn of interactions whereupon he stated that this was "his responsibility and not mine" and to "please just send the prescriptions back and he would have them filled elsewhere." Again I assured him that we would be happy to take care of the patient.

Now we will probably lose his prescription patients for some time, even though I wrote him a follow-up letter reiterating the fact that we were only trying to help and asking him if he had any suggestions as to how we might better serve him and his patients. We were just trying but we found out that apparently we were trying to this particular doctor and will probably suffer since he felt that we overstepped our boundary. However, I can sleep tonight.

The above incidents and the hundreds of others provided striking evidence that the pharmacist plays a vital role in the medical care system. His services and the effectiveness with which he provides them, *do* make a difference in the outcome of medical care.

Examination of all the incidents received shows the possibility of using such data for justifying further family record systems, for improving communications skills and for expansion of undergraduate and continuing education programs in the areas of patient behavior, consumer economics and drug interactions to name a few.

Theorizing is a poor substitute for an analysis of what is actually going on in the pharmacy. Much more research in the community practice of pharmacy is vitally needed.

Conclusion

I have noted elsewhere that the prescription is "too easy a measure of what the pharmacist does."[8] Inadequate attention has been given to research documentation of the total potential for medical good and harm

from all of the pharmacist's health-related activities.

This study has provided anecdotal and partially quantified evidence that the pharmacist's impact on the outcome of medical care may extend well beyond the proper or improper execution of a prescription order. Extensive, controlled studies in this area are vitally needed as documentation for the frequent references to the vital role of the pharmacist in the health care system.

References

1. Task force on the Pharmacist's Clinical Role, "Report," HSRD Briefs, Washington (1971)
2. Sanazaro, P. J., and Williamson, J. W., "End Results of Patient Care: A Provisional Classification Based on Reports by Internists," *Med. Care*, 6, 123 (1968). . . .
8. Smith, M. C., "General Practice Pharmacy in the United Kingdom and the United States of America: Some Comparisons and Contrasts," *The Pharmaceutical Journal*, 210, 9 (Jan. 6, 1973)

41—How the Retail Pharmacist Quietly Serves Physicians and Patients

Howard L. Wood

Over the years, I have had my professional pharmacy training, knowledge, and expertise "tapped" many times—both by patient-customers and by members of the medical profession.

I was an independent pharmacy owner for 21 years, and am presently a chain store manager for Achter's Key Drug of Rochester, New York. In the quarter century I have

practiced retail pharmacy, I have heard our profession praised and criticized—both by fellow professionals and by laymen.

But our profession can be no more than we make of it; and I can attest that Pharmacy has offered me endless opportunities to participate in life-saving decisions. I would like to cite a few examples.

The most recent instance occurred when I

learned that a woman patient was taking Coumadin and Nembutal capsules, simultaneously. This combination could result in decreased prothrombin time-response and could, of course, be injurious to the patient. A call to her physician stopped the Nembutal—and earned the physician's deep gratitude.

Once I received a prescription for Tincture of Belladonna for an infant. As written, it called for a teaspoon dose. A phone call to the physician—who had to be tracked to Boston—resulted in a corrected dosage, and the thanks of a very grateful man.

In a similar incident, a sulfa drug prescription—calling for a dosage of one tablespoon—was written for an infant. Again, a phone call to the physician resulted in a corrected, smaller dosage and avoided trouble, all around—a happy ending.

Panicky Parents

Over the years, I've received numerous phone calls from panicky parents whose children have taken some of the parents' prescription medicine. The pharmacist asks a few calm questions; and, with his knowledge of pharmacology, dosage, and side effects, he is able to advise what should be done. This kind of service never fails to earn undying gratitude from frightened parents.

It is not unusual for mothers to come into the pharmacy, asking about which medication should be given to a baby with a fever and/or diarrhea. A few questions are asked, and it is discovered that the child is an infant—only a few weeks old. The mother is urged to consult her physician at once. No sale is made—but a responsible medical referral has been made.

As a consultant to a nursing home, it is my responsibility to review patients' drug charts, check for proper drug storage, etc. On a recent occasion, I discovered a patient was on tetracycline and was also taking massive doses of an antacid which cancels the effec-

tiveness of the antibiotic. The situation was corrected at once.

Another nursing home patient was being continued on a medication beyond the prescription period. That medication, too, was stopped, as soon as the situation was discovered. We also learned that some elderly patients were on medications which had to be crushed, because of the patient's inability to swallow solids. The nurse in charge was advised to consult with the doctor and ask him to order that same medication in liquid form—which we knew to be available.

On a personal note—how many times have I, and other local pharmacists, been called out in the middle of the night to fill an emergency Rx for a very grateful patient and his family?

During one of the bad winter storms of 1977 in New York State, a 6-year-old boy was brought into my pharmacy with 8 of his fingers frozen solid. With my pharmacist's training, I was able to give him proper emergency treatment, before having him transferred to the local hospital. The boy's parents were very grateful for this unexpected service from a pharmacist.

In another case, a father came into the pharmacy and asked for an OTC medication for his 6-year-old daughter who had been nauseated and vomiting for 3 days! The father was told that this could be a serious situation, and he was urged to call his doctor at once.

Physicians often call pharmacists to ask what they may prescribe in order to obtain a specific combination of drugs; and we, the pharmacists, quickly inform them.

Not infrequently—and because we remain watchful for such things—we discover patients who are receiving controlled drugs from different doctors, for the same therapy. A few discreet phone calls to the doctors involved are sufficient to alert them to the situation and resolve the problem, saving a patient from potential addiction.

A fellow pharmacist questioned a physician's prescription order for phenobarbital—

1½ grains, 3 times a day, for a 4-year-old child. Upon calling and questioning the physician, he learned that the physician had intended to prescribe ¼ grain, 3 times a day.

How many times has the pharmacist been asked by a patient-customer to prescribe something for a child's earache? Too many times to count, I'm sure. But after asking a few questions, it is usually discovered that the child also has a sore throat and/or fever. The wise pharmacist will not sell an OTC ear medication, but will, instead, advise the parent to consult the child's physician.

Not too long ago, a young mother came into our pharmacy to purchase a bottle of Robitussin DM. Asked if the medication was for an adult, we learned it was intended for her 4-month-old infant. The mother said her doctor had advised her to buy the medicine, and that she was instructed to give the child a teaspoonful 3 times a day. We informed the mother that it was quite a strong medication, and we questioned the size of the dosage for so small an infant. We then called her physician for clarification. It turned out that he had instructed the mother to get Robitussin *plain*, and give ¼ teaspoonful per dose. He expressed his gratitude for our concern, and for our being alert to a potential problem.

People frequently ask pharmacists to recommend a proper OTC cough syrup for use by diabetics. In such cases, we are able to recommend a sugar-free product—available for this very purpose.

To maintain his awareness of drug inter-actions, a pharmacist must continually rely on his knowledge of pharmacology. It is his primary responsibility to educate customer-patients about the proper use of their medi-cations—and the pharmacist's instructions must go beyond the directions issued by physicians.

Ordinarily, patients are advised to take prescription drugs 3 or 4 times a day. But a conscientious pharmacist will not stop with those limited instructions. His education of the patient will also include:

• Informing him as to whether or not the medication should be taken before meals or after meals;
• Cautioning him to avoid taking antac-ids with tetracyclines;
• Advising him to take his medication *with* food or milk—if the drug is an irritant;
• Alerting him when a certain drug may cause his urine to turn red in color, etc.

While these are only a few instances which attest to the pharmacist's professional and educational role, I have no doubt that other practicing pharmacists can furnish many more successful examples.

In any event, there seems little doubt that the pharmacist who uses his training effec-tively makes a *most valuable contribution* to the public, the community, and to his fellow professionals in the medical field. With that thought in mind, we believe that when a pharmacist is asked what he does for a living—he should respond with justifiable pride: "*I am a pharmacist!*"

42—The Bottom Line is Fairly High

The phone rings in Royce Friesen's paneled office, interrupting his study of a thick print-out. He fiddles with his pen as he listens, then says, "If we don't need someone at that hour, we don't want them around. You've got to keep your expenses down."

The call is from one of his store managers, who wants advice on juggling some hours for one of her employees.

"He's worked here a long time and I'm usually willing to go along," he says to the caller, "but we don't want people standing around just to make up some hours. You've got to keep expenses down because it all comes out in the percentages, Connie, and the percentages are what *you* get." Pause. "Well, whatever it takes for a business to run smoothly."

That routine little exchange fairly well typifies the way Friesen oversees his five Northern California pharmacies, a successful, medically-oriented operation whose annual gross sales hover around the $2 million mark. First is his desire to be fair in the strictest sense—to himself as well as to others. He *is* usually willing to go along, but no nonsense. He doesn't have a lot of rules and regulations for his employees, just a few simple ones that everyone lives with. Whatever it takes.

Then there's the percentages. The bottom line. The final score. The thing about the percentages is that Friesen's managers share in the profits and, thus, have a direct interest in how well they run their store. What's good for business is good for them.

So successful is his business that he is frequently called on to show others how he does it. He has been asked to speak at a number of CPhA's pharmacy management C.E. seminars, including one this fall . . . and he was a member of a five-man panel speaking on future employment conditions during CPhA's Annual Meeting this past April. He was one of the original directors of the Academy of Pharmacy Management, after serving four years as the District 1 representative to the CPhA Board of Trustees, and he is beginning his second consecutive year as chairman of the academy board.

The nail on which Friesen hangs his finan-cial philosophy is expressed in his oft-repeated creed, "Expenses. You've got to know what they are; you've got to keep them down."

"Most pharmacies judge their success by the number of prescriptions they fill. But that's the worst way. You've got to know what your expenses are."

As a part-owner of his first pharmacy in Redding in the mid-60s, he recalls, "Four chains opened up and five independents had to close. We had to figure out how to compete with the chains or else we'd be working for them. Later, when I got four stores, I knew that if we didn't set up a corporate structure, we'd get eaten alive."

So, rather than trying all by himself to run his pharmacies as one business, Friesen set up a system where he is the president of a pharmacy management service as well as a partner or full owner of each pharmacy. The management service—called Apothe-Care, Inc.—handles much of the pharmacies' paperwork chores. For this and other services, each pharmacy—four Owen's Pharmacies in Redding and Ehorn's Pharmacy in Red Bluff—pays a percentage of its gross sales to Apothe-Care. Each store is an individual corporation, and each has its own profit/loss statements.

"Apothe-Care does all the payrolls, banking, negotiations on insurance, and the like," he explains. "But we don't centralize our stock just to increase purchase discounts, because then you have too much inventory lying around and you have to hire an extra man just to deliver it."

While the stock is not centralized, the ordering is. "We use a computer print-out and we have an on-line link with Fresno. The terminal looks just like a hand calculator, only bigger. Every night we just flip a switch and punch in a six-digit number for every order. We tried inventory sheets, but we didn't like them. This is the best way.

"We probably buy better than the average chain, even though we buy in smaller quantities and our per-unit cost is higher. The chains are so far apart, they can't receive, say, a shipment of 12 in Redding, then ship six to Sacramento or Chico. It costs them too much. But we have five stores within a 30-mile radius, and our regular delivery people can distribute them."

Friesen's lieutenants are his five store managers, with whom most of the responsibility for day-to-day operations rests. "After they're with me about three years, and if we get along and it looks like they want to stay with the organization, I start selling them stock. We start a little at a time, but eventually they can buy up to a full 50%. I don't insist on owning the majority interest, because that stigma of 49%–51% can do more harm than good.

"I pay my managers a salary plus a percentage of the net profit on his own store. If I gave them a percentage of the gross profit, then they wouldn't be as cost-conscious. Chain employees earn a lot, but that salary is all they've got. They get burned out by the time they're 50, and that's too young to quit. But my managers have a real interest in our success. They're involved."

Says Jack Schalo, a 50% owner of Owen's No. 1 and vice president of Apothe-Care, "Each manager sets up his own store, and we know what Royce wants. He doesn't come around and lean on anybody. It's up to each manager to run his own staff."

"My managers have come along," Friesen says. "You give me a top pharmacist and it will take me three years to turn him into a top manager. Jack Schalo is an old schoolmate of mine. I hired people who want to get out and talk to people. I want our patients to feel that our pharmacists are *their* pharmacists. Our system allows our pharmacists to spend 95% of their time being pharmacists. Instead of writing checks in their free time, they're out talking to patients."

Which is another Friesen creed. Lest anyone think that he is obsessed with the percentages to the extent that he locks himself in a

room full of receipts and adding machines, he has de-emphasized front-end merchandising and concentrates on health care and consultation.

"Seventy percent of our business is prescription. People have got to know about the drugs they're taking—what to avoid, what to expect. And if you identify with a patient and call him by name, sure, he'll drive across town to see you, as long as your prices aren't out of line."

Friesen himself fills prescriptions—"works the plank" as they say in Redding—three days a week. While he's not a glad-hander or back-slapper, his pharmacies stress service. Their waiting areas offer easy chairs, recent magazines, and free coffee. Patients apparently like it that way.

"We don't have to advertise much," he says, "maybe once a week just to keep our name visible. We never advertise prescription prices, because then the discount becomes the standard price. We advertise our service, and we sponsor a Little League team, but our best advertising is word of mouth. We'd rather spend our money on service."

Friesen, 39, has between 30 and 35 employees spread throughout his five stores and the Apothe-Care headquarters. "I let my employees know how much it costs me to hire them—their salaries, payroll taxes, fringes, etc. I have seven full-time pharmacists, and I pay for their C.E. courses and their CPhA membership because I want them involved. I don't want to pay the lowest wages, because then you can't keep good people. But I don't pay the highest, either. I want my employees to be motivated, not complacent."

To that end, he holds frequent meetings with his managers. "Once a week if we can. Because of expenses, inflation, and salary raises [he has a low employee turnover] we've got to get 8% more this year just to stay where we are. But I don't sit down and tell them what to do. We have what we call 'input management.' I would rather be an advisor than go in and make a decision that my manager may not agree with but would have to live with. I leave as many decisions as I can up to them. Again, this way they have more incentive and more going for them."

With an outlook like that, no wonder the percentages are with them.

Related Readings in This Volume

1. Comprehensive Pharmacy Services
2. Serving the Woodstock Nation
4. Office Practice of Pharmacy
5. Uniform Cost Accounting
6. Adverse Reactions
7. Pharmacist and Family Planning
10. Drug Abuse Education
12. Pharmacist and Preventive Medicine
14. Hypertension Patients in Community Pharmacy

15. Self-Medication
16. Over-the-Counter Medications
23. Counseling
24. Compliance
50. Pharmacies in Rural Areas
54. Capability to do More
60. Third-Party Prescription Programs
62. Independent Pharmacist as Buyer

Readings for a Broader Perspective

1. "The Word's Go, The Way's Up for Today's Store Managers," *Chain Store Age-Drug Edition* 54 (November 1978):22.
2. Hackney, E. "How We Provide Pharmaceutical Services to a Cancer Hospital," *Pharmacy Times* 44 (July 1978):68.
3. Libby, G. N., and Kirk, K. W. "Are Chain Pharmacists Happy or Unhappy?" *Pharmacy Times* 42 (February 1976):68–72.
4. *American Pharmacy* NS 19 (March 1979): 12–17.

FEDERAL FACILITY

43—Pharmacists in the Veterans Administration

Professional Pharmacists in VA's Modern Hospitals and Clinics

Over 1,400 licensed pharmacists staff more than 200 pharmacies serving VA hospitals and outpatient clinics located throughout the United States. The Veterans Administration offers pharmacists a challenging and varied program in areas of pharmacy administration, clinical pharmacy, inpatient and outpatient dispensing, medication systems, bulk compounding and formula development, and research in professional and administrative problems.

- You have the personal and professional satisfaction of working with other members of the health team in planning and executing pharmacy's contribution to the health and welfare of patients.
- You practice pharmacy in modern hospitals and clinics provided with specialized equipment for pharmaceutical compounding and dispensing.
- You are provided a well-balanced pharmaceutical library which maintains current texts and periodicals on related professional and scientific subjects.
- As a member of the health care team, you participate in programs directed toward patient recovery. You contribute to education and training by preparing lectures

and demonstrations for the medical staff, nurses, residents and interns, and provide professional data to the medical, dental, and nursing staffs.

The Qualifications

For the GS–9 grade entrance position, applicants normally must meet *all* of these requirements: (1) Bachelor's degree in Pharmacy through a 5-year course in an approved school; (2) 1-year internship; and (3) current license in a State or Territory of the U.S. or in the District of Columbia.

Various degrees of additional professional education, training or experience are required for grades GS–11 and above. (Over 80% of VA's Pharmacists are in grades GS–11 through GS–14.)

Plan Your Professional Career

If you are still in high school or have just entered college, consider the advantages of a professional career in Pharmacy and plan your curriculum so that you may meet the educational requirements to qualify for this rewarding health profession. . . .

For complete details about VA employment we encourage you to visit, write, or call one of the VA hospitals or clinics. . . . Personnel or Pharmacy officials will be glad to tell you about the Pharmacy program.

VA Pamphlet 10–62 (Revised August 1977), Veterans Administration, Washington, D.C.

Features of Employment as a VA Pharmacist

Comparable Pay

Salary rates for the various Federal Civil Service "GS" grades are revised periodically to insure comparability with private enterprise. For specific information on current salary rates, consult the bulletin boards at U. S. Civil Service Commission offices, College Placement Offices, or the Personnel Officer at VA. . . .

Training and Development Program

A career development program to assist individual pharmacists to advance on the professional career ladder to the highest level consistent with their interest and ability.

Continuing education and inservice training—on-the-job and at educational institutions, while earning regular salary.

Other Top Flight Benefits

Annual leave for vacation and other personal business. Those with less than 3 years of service earn 13 workdays a year; 3 to 15 years, 20 workdays; 15 years or more, 26 workdays.

Sick leave for illness. Thirteen workdays a year. No maximum accumulation.

Holidays—Nine paid each year.

Military leave for reservists. Fifteen days with pay each year when ordered to active duty or training.

Liberal retirement available with full annuities at age 62 with 5 years of service; age 60 with 20 years; or age 55 with 30 years. VA "matches" employee's contribution to the retirement fund.

Hospital and medical insurance. Choice of group plans with reasonable rates and excellent protection. No medical exams or waiting periods. VA shares the cost.

Term life insurance with double indemnity for accidental death. VA shares cost.

Scheduled salary increases within each GS grade. Additional increases for superior job performance.

Cash for suggestions or outstanding job performance.

Compensation for loss of pay due to job-connected injury or illness.

Moving expenses involved in transferring from one VA station to another (subsistence and transportation of self and family, mileage, expenses of selling and buying home, and other miscellaneous expenses).

Uniforms—Special allowance provided.

Application Procedures

These positions are in the Federal Civil Service. No written test is required; however, you must have your qualifications evaluated by the U.S. Civil Service Commission on the basis of education, experience and training. For specific application instructions, contact a Civil Service Commission "Federal Job Information Center." These Centers are located in most major cities. Consult any Federal agency or the white pages of your telephone directory for the Center nearest you.

If you have already received an eligibility rating from the Civil Service Commission, you may wish to inquire directly to VA Hospitals about immediate job vacancies.

Special Postgraduate Training Programs

Pharmacy Intern Training

This one-year non-academic training program in hospital pharmacy provides pharmacy school graduates with pre-licensure experience necessary for registration by

State Boards of Pharmacy. Practicing pharmacists desiring specialized clinical experience in hospital pharmacy are also accepted for internships. Graduation from an accredited school of pharmacy is required.

The primary objective of this program is to develop well-qualified staff pharmacist practitioners who are prepared to perform well in all professional and administrative areas of VA Pharmacy Service.

Interns serve 39 hours per week at the proportionate part of the full-time annual salary for GS–7.

Residency in Hospital Pharmacy

This 24-month University-VA program offers qualified practicing pharmacists specialized clinical training in pharmacy concurrent with postgraduate academic education leading to the Doctor of Pharmacy or Master of Science degree in Pharmacy. Qualifications include graduation from an accredited school of pharmacy, current state license, and acceptance for admission to the graduate school.

The primary objective of this program is to develop well-trained and competent potential Chiefs of Pharmacy Service who are prepared to provide professional leadership to pharmacy-related health care programs of the Veterans Administration.

Residents serve about 28 hours per week at the proportionate part of the full-time annual salary for GS–9. (Financial assistance authorized by the VA under laws pertaining to educational benefits for veterans is also available to those who qualify.)

And When You Finish. . . .

. . . . Excellent opportunities exist after completion of internship or residency for appointment to career positions in the VA. Moving expenses are normally paid by VA when transfer to another location is involved.

[Note: Comparable job opportunities and benefits are available in other federal agencies such as the Department of Defense and the U.S. Public Health Service.]

Readings for a Broader Perspective

1. Donehew, G. R. "The Career and Training of an Army Pharmacy Officer," *J. Am. Pharm. Assoc.* NS 14 (December 1974):679–81.
2. "Pharmacists in the Wide Wide World of PHS," *Tomorrow's Pharmacist* 2 (January 1980):4–7.

GROUP MEDICAL CLINIC

44—Pharmacy and Family Practice

Robert E. Davis, William H. Crigler and
Henry Martin, Jr.

Introduction

In recent years the practice of medicine has seen the development of a new concept, that of a team approach to the care of the entire family. Medicine is becoming too complex and the bureaucracy of health care delivery too intricate for individual professionals to perform efficiently and effectively alone. Teams of health professionals are now emerging, who coordinate their efforts towards delivery of the best quality of care possible to individuals and their families. The general practitioner has now specialized in family practice, the nurse is able to obtain additional training as a family nurse specialist or practioner and the pharmacist is able to obtain advanced academic and clinical training specializing in family practice. . . .

This team, encompassing three professions, provides a cooperative approach to the delivery of health care. Each professional's role is quite clear in such a family practice center. The physician, as the team captain, acquires a data base, assesses the problems and initiates a treatment plan. The nurse is involved in direct patient care by aiding the physician, screening patient problems, follow-up, and dissemination of patient education materials. The pharmacist works on patient education, acute and chronic therapy compliance, monitoring chronic patients, calculating dosage and screening for adverse reactions and drug interactions. This type of role model has been discussed in other published papers.[1-4]

The Model Plan and Concept Origination

Lexington Family Practice is located in a rural-suburban area on the perimeter of Lexington, South Carolina. The center is unique in that it is a totally privately financed ambulatory health care center practicing a team approach to health care. It is also unique in that a fee is paid by the patient to the pharmacist for his consultation services.

The concept of this program originated during the authors' training with the Department of Family Practice at the Medical University of South Carolina. Physicians had daily exposure to, and contact with, the services offered by the pharmacy in the training program. The physicians became aware of the time the pharmacist could save them by counseling the patient on medication and of the safeguard of having the pharmacist screen for drug reactions and interactions. The pharmacist developed an appreciation for the concept of family practice and for the intensive training and background that these physicians have. While at the University, the authors decided that upon graduation they would initiate the concept on a private basis without any public funding or university assistance.

The building consists of 4,300 square feet, with medical, pharmacy, laboratory and business office components located under one roof. . . .

The practice opened in August 1976. Since then it has been developing rapidly and at present the authors are looking for additional personnel to participate in the practice concept. The center currently employs two family practice physicians, two registered nurses, a clinical pharmacist, a prescription-oriented pharmacist, a pharmacy technician and a part-time clinical psychologist.

Acceptance by the community has been excellent. Many physicians have contacted the authors with questions about the concepts involved and the services provided. The center's functions were explained to physicians in the area and the feedback was very good. Patients have been quick to come to the facility and to utilize all of its services. The best indicator of the center's value, however, has come in the form of patient referrals, telephone conversations with the patient and from direct patient feedback.

Model Flow

The routine procedure for a patient's visit can be outlined as follows. . . . The patient checks in with the receptionist and is given forms to fill out concerning past medical and family history. After these are completed, the receptionist notifies the nurse, who ushers the patient to the examination room, records the vital signs and obtains the chief complaint.

The physician then reviews the past medical and family history and the nurse's notes, interviews and examines the patient and notes his findings. After the diagnosis is made, the physician decides on a plan of therapy, writes a prescription when this is warranted and dictates the problem-oriented medical record. The nurse gives the patient further instructions about the disease or disease process if this is required, e.g. diabetic education, and takes specimens for any lab work that is necessary.

The patient is then shown to the pharmacy consultation room. The clinical pharmacist is given the patient's record and the prescriptions written by the physician. From the patient's record, the pharmacist can obtain all the information collected on the patient. This information is vital to the concept of the practice and enables the pharmacist to discuss the use and indications of the medications with the patient. In essence, the pharmacist knows how to tailor his presentation to, and conversation with, the patient.

If the patient is new, a drug history is taken. This begins the patient's profile card which will always remain as a part of the patient's medical record, so that the physician, the nurse and the pharmacist can have access to it. The prescription is next reviewed by the pharmacist with the patient and questions are answered on any information important to the treatment.

The patient then has the choice of having his medications filled in the center or of taking them to another pharmacy. If the patient chooses to have the prescriptions filled at the center, the technician prepares the medications and the prescription-oriented pharmacist dispenses it. Finally, the patient pays for the entire service, including the physician's visit, lab fees, pharmacy charges and miscellaneous charges, by making one payment to the receptionist before leaving.

The Pharmacy

The pharmacy has four basic components: the consultation room, the dispensing area, the waiting room and the clinical pharmacist's office. . . . The consultation room is used to greet the patient and to provide clinical services. The dispensing area resembles the professional pharmacy in which the medications are stored and prepared for dispensing. The waiting area is a sub-area of the medical waiting room which allows the pharmacist's patients to be isolated in another part of the waiting room but still within the center. The fourth component is the clinical pharmacist's office which is used for business operations and includes the pharmacy library and a storage area for the material required by federal law. The entire pharmacy area consists of about 600 square feet, of which 50 percent belongs to the pharmacy dispensing and storage areas.

The Pharmacist's Duties

The clinical pharmacist has a responsibility to both the patient and to the physician. He tries to improve the delivery of health care to the patient and aids the physician in his continuing education and with the plan of therapy.

In the flow pattern discussed previously, a drug history is taken when the patient arrives at the pharmacy consultation room. This history begins the patient's profile card which always remains a part of the patient's medical record and includes current medications, allergies, idiosyncrasies and chronic diseases.

After the history is taken, the prescription is reviewed by the pharmacist who calculates the correct dose, the quantity required for treatment and the brand of product to be used. The prescription is compared to the patient's profile card and screened for allergies, idiosyncrasies and drug interactions.

Next, the prescription is reviewed with the patient. The patient is informed of the name and strength of the medication, the proper time of administration, the use and care of any special devices for its administration, products to avoid while on the medication, significant side effects, the length of time before results can be expected and the total length of treatment required.

After this, the patient is given any printed information that is available to aid him or her in understanding the diagnosis and the use of the medication. These aids are designed to improve patient compliance. Finally, questions are answered on the above information or any other information important to the treatment.

It is therefore clearly defined that in the consultation the pharmacist is involved with the education of the patient. The pharmacist also has responsibilities to the physician. These responsibilities include drug and poison information, dosage calculations, product evaluation, product identification, the monitoring of hypertensive patients through monthly blood pressure checks and checks on compliance, the follow-up on acutely ill patients and the follow-up on physician interpretation of cultures, to insure the patient was maintained on the proper medication as the cultures and sensitivities indicated.

To enable the pharmacist to provide these services, a library of pharmacy and medical text books is located in the center. If information cannot be found from these sources, a cooperative program with an area hospital and the Medical University in Charleston can be utilized to obtain information through literature searches.

The pharmacist manages two patient follow-up programs for compliance. The chronically ill patient is requested by the physician to return to the pharmacy consultation room on a monthly basis. At this time, the patient's compliance is monitored and side effects are reviewed to make sure the patient is experiencing no adverse effects which could cause him or her to stop taking the medication. In the follow-up of the acutely ill, a call is usually made after three to five days of therapy. This is to check on the improvement of the patient and to remind him or her of the regimen he had been placed on. This improves the patient's compliance and confidence in the pharmacist. It also decreases the need for return visits by the patient to the center, thus enabling the physicians to see more acutely ill patients.

After the physician interprets the results of cultures and sensitivities, the pharmacist compares these with the patient's medical record, making sure proper treatment was administered. The patient is called after the results of the culture are received in order to reinforce the needs for him or her to continue the therapy and to check on compliance. If the initial therapy chosen was inadequate, then, with the physician's approval, the patient is notified and the proper treatment is started immediately. Such action is recorded in the medical record by the pharmacist and indicates that the proper treatment was instituted.

Two dentists have recently moved into the area and occasionally require consultations on patients who are seen in their offices and who are on several medications. For the dentists, these consultations are a precaution, to make sure that they are not giving medications which could create drug interactions. They also consult on the proper choice of antibiotics and the dose required.

The time spent in consultation with the patient varies from as little as 30 seconds to as long as ten minutes. The consultation with a new patient requires an average of four minutes, in which the history is taken and the procedures and protocol for our center are explained. After an initial history has been taken from the patient, it takes on average approximately one to one and one-half minutes to discuss the prescription with the

patient. The time taken varies with each patient and with each prescription. For example, it may take as long as ten minutes for an explanation of medications and the establishment of a dosage schedule for a chronically ill patient taking multiple medications on his first visit. In future visits, it may take as little as one to two minutes to make sure the patient is not experiencing any side effects or adverse reactions.

For a return patient with a new or acute problem, the explanation usually takes from one to one and one-half minutes. On a follow-up visit from an acute illness, the time may be as short as 15 to 30 seconds.

During consultation, consideration must be given to the time required to fill the prescription. At this center there is very little difference in the time required to fill the prescription as compared to any other pharmacy; although, there is a certain amount of paperwork done to update profile cards and compliance charts to make sure that all the information is in the patient's record. On average, it takes about one and one-half minutes to fill the prescription and to update the profile card and the patient's record. This time must be multiplied by each prescription filled.

In summary, each visit by a new patient would take eight to nine minutes for a history, consultation and for the filling of the prescription. For a return visit, the time required varies from four to five minutes.

Dispensing of Medications

It is believed that dispensing a patient's medication from the center is to the patient's advantage and this was therefore initiated at our center. Some of the advantages that we felt to be very important are as follows:

1. Convenience to the patient. It offers a convenient system which allows parents of ill children, people with very busy schedules or the elderly to have their medications filled immediately after receiving the physician's services.

2. Savings to the patient. The physicians follow a formulary which allows the pharmacy to purchase on contract various pharmaceuticals in large volumes, thus obtaining discounts which are passed along to the patient. Also, all medications are dispensed at the cost of medication plus a professional fee.

3. Improvement in compliance. The patient has a very good understanding of why he or she is taking the medication and what is expected of him or her from the physician and the pharmacist; the patient is more apt to follow any directions fully, thereby improving compliance. Also, in an acute illness, a follow-up call is made by the pharmacist to make sure that instructions have been followed and to see how the patient is progressing. To improve patient compliance in chronic illness, refills are monitored and the need to take the medication regularly is verbally reinforced during the patient's monthly visits to the pharmacist.

4. Assurance of a quality product. Each product selected for our formulary is reviewed by the pharmacist for problems in bioavailability and for acceptance by the patient. The cost, dosage form and schedule are considered in the assessment of patient acceptance.

Fee System

Income is derived directly from patient receipts. Few transactions occur with third party payments. For each visit the patient is charged a center fee. In this fee the patient is paying for the physician's services, the nursing services and the pharmacist's consultation. The pharmacist receives a set fee from each patient for having his pharmaceutical consultation services available. The fee is charged to every patient, whether or not any prescriptions are filled at the pharmacy. This fee was initiated because of the strong feeling of the authors that the availability of a pharmacist's time for consultation and for answering the patient's questions was not only important but valuable. It also prevented any conflict of interest with other pharmacists in the area on the subject of prescriptions being filled within the center. The consultation fee for the pharmacist's services enables the pharmacist's salary to be based on his availbility to the patient and the physician, and not on how many prescriptions are filled.

To further supplement the clinical pharmacist's salary, he receives money from the dispensing component of the pharmacy. The average fee is $2.15 for each prescription filled. This fee pays for the overhead of the pharmacy and includes income to serve in the dispensing component function. The physicians receive no income from the pharmacy or from pharmacy consultation.

Educational Role Model

There are few role models currently available to the pharmacy student to enable him to develop skills and gain training in Family Practice Pharmacy. Therefore, Lexington Family Practice, in cooperation with the College of Pharmacy and the Department of Family Practice at the Medical University of South Carolina, is initiating a training program of this type. . . .

The center provides an experience to the student which is not available at any other site. The student gains training not only in the day-to-day aspects of a dispensing pharmacy and business management, but also in the consultation and provision of drug information and chronic patient observation. The student also maintains daily contact with residents and physicians at the site, thereby increasing his or her knowledge of diagnosis and treatment while learning the technique of professional interaction. This program was established at the request of the authors and is thought to be an asset to the patient.

Summary

This paper has described the concept, the establishment, the practice model procedure, the patient flow, the pharmacist's roles, the time involved for consultation and the fees charged for a pharmaceutical component within the Family Practice Center. This setting allows the physician, the nurse and the pharmacist to interact in the treatment program of the patient. It allows the pharmacist and nurse to become integral parts of the health care team. The physician, amidst the complexities of therapeutics, has a close-working ally in the pharmacist. The uniqueness of the system allows the pharmacist to concentrate on drug education and consultation, and rewards him for time spent which is not directly related to the dispensing activity. The program has been well-received by the community, both the professional and the private sector; this is evident from the growth of the practice since its opening in August of 1976. In the future, the center will be expanding its services to include more physicians, nurses and additional ancillary personnel.

References

1. Maudlin, R.: The Clinical Pharmacist and the Family Physician, *J. Fam. Pract.* 3:667–668 (June) 1976.
2. Juhl, R. et. al.: The Family Practitioner-Clinical Pharmacist Group Practice, *Drug Intell. Clin. Pharm.* 8:572–575 (Oct.) 1974.
3. Perry, P. and Hurley, S.: Activities of the Clinical Pharmacist Practicing in the Office of a

Family Practitioner, *Drug. Intell. Clin. Pharm.* 9:129–133 (Mar.) 1975.
4. Leedy, J. and Schlager, C.: A Unique Alliance of Medical and Pharmaceutical Skills, *J. Am. Pharm. Assoc. NS* 16:460–462 (Aug.) 1976.

Related Readings in This Volume

Readings for a Broader Perspective

1. "What It's Like to Operate an In-House HMO Pharmacy," *American Druggist* 178 (September 1978):88–89.
2. Gardner, M. E., and Trinca, C. E. "The Pharmacy Clinic: A New Approach to Ambulatory Care," *American Journal of Hospital Pharmacy* 35 (April 1978):429–31.
3. Roberts, R. W., Stewart, R. B., Doering, P. L., and Yost, R. L. "Contributions of a Clinical Pharmacist in a Private Group Practice of Physicians," *Drug Intelligence & Clinical Pharmacy* 12 (April 1978):210–13.
4. Perry, P. J., and Hurley, S. C. "Activities of the Clinical Pharmacist Practicing in the Office of a Family Practitioner," *Drug Intelligence & Clinical Pharmacy* 9 (March 1975):129–33.
5. Juhl, R. P., Perry, P. J., Norwood, G. J., and Martin, L. R. "The Family Practioner-Clinical Pharmacist Group Practice—A Model Clinic," *Drug Intelligence & Clinical Pharmacy* 8 (October 1974):572–75.
6. Lofholm, P. W. "The Clinical Pharmacist in an Interprofessional Group Practice." In Francke, D. E., and Whitney, H. A. K., Jr. *Perspectives in Clinical Pharmacy.* (1st ed.) Hamilton, Illinois: Drug Intelligence Publications, 1972. pp. 270–85.
7. Dolan, M. "Family Practice: A New Approach in the New South," *American Pharmacy NS* 18 (August 1978):25–29.

HOSPITAL

45—Minimum Standard for Pharmacies in Institutions

Introduction

Pharmaceutical services[a] in institutions have numerous components, the most prominent being: (1) the procurement, distribution and control of all pharmaceuticals used within the facility, (2) the evaluation and dissemination of comprehensive information about drugs and their use to the institution's staff and patients, (3) the monitoring and assurance of the quality of drug use. These functions, and other professional activities (e.g., patient drug counseling, primary care responsibilities, drug blood-level monitoring), are carried out in cooperation with other institutional departments and programs.

The primary function of this document is to serve as a guide for the development and provision of pharmaceutical services in institutions. It will also be useful in evaluating the scope and quality of these services. It does not, however, provide detailed instructions for operating a pharmacy—other Society publications serve this function.

Standard I: Administration

The pharmaceutical service shall[b] be directed by a professionally competent, legally qualified pharmacist. He or she must be on the same level within the institution's administrative structure as directors of other clinical services (e.g., surgery, pediatrics, nursing). The director of pharmaceutical services[c] is responsible for: (1) setting the long- and short-range goals of the pharmacy based on developments and trends in health care and institutional pharmacy practice and the specific needs of the institution; (2) developing a plan and schedule for achieving these goals; (3) supervising the implementation of the plan and the day-to-day activities associated with it; (4) determining if the goals and schedule are being met and instituting corrective actions when necessary.

[a] The terms "pharmaceutical services" and "pharmacy" as used in this document are synonymous. The term "pharmacist" is used in the collective sense, referring to the pharmacy staff.

[b] The terms "shall" and "must" are used to indicate a mandatory statement. The term "should" reflects the commonly accepted or recommended method; it permits the use of equally effective alternatives.

[c] The title "director of pharmaceutical services" or a similar title is preferred over "chief pharmacist" or "consultant pharmacist."

The director of pharmaceutical services, in carrying out these tasks, shall employ an adequate number of competent and qualified personnel.

- The director of pharmaceutical services must be thoroughly knowledgeable about hospital pharmacy practice and, preferably, have completed a pharmacy residency in an institution accredited by the American Society of Hospital Pharmacists.
- sufficient supportive personnel (technical, clerical, secretarial) shall be available in order to minimize the use of pharmacists in nonjudgmental tasks. Appropriate supervisory controls[d] for supportive personnel must be maintained.
- The director of pharmaceutical services shall be responsible for work schedules, systems and procedures which most efficiently utilize pharmacy personnel and resources.
- All personnel must possess the education and training needed for their responsibilities. Competence of all staff must be maintained through relevant continuing education programs and activities.
- Personnel must be selected and assigned solely on the basis of job-related qualifications and performance. The employment and discharge of pharmacy personnel shall be the responsibility of the director of pharmaceutical services. There should be an established procedure for orienting new personnel to the pharmacy and their respective positions. Procedures for the routine evaluation of pharmacy personnel performance should be established.
- Lines of authority and areas of responsibility within the pharmacy shall be clearly defined. Written job descriptions for all categories of pharmacy personnel should be prepared and revised as necessary.
- An operations manual governing all pharmacy functions should be prepared. It should be continually revised to reflect changes in procedures, organization, etc. All pharmacy personnel should be familiar with the contents of the manual.
- The director of pharmaceutical services should prepare periodic reports to the institution's administration containing qualitative and quantitative data on the pharmacy's activities for the period plus the current position of the pharmacy with respect to its long- and short-range plans. These reports require that an adequate data collection system be maintained.
- There should be an ongoing, formal program for assuring the quality of pharmaceutical services. This program should be based on process and outcome criteria.
- Hospitals provide services to patients 24 hours a day. Pharmaceutical services are an integral part of the total care provided by the hospital, and the services of a pharmacist should, therefore, be available at all times. Where around-the-clock operation of the pharmacy is not feasible, a pharmacist should be available on an "on-call" basis. The use of "night cabinets" and drug dispensing by nonpharmacists should be minimized and eliminated wherever possible.
- An efficient system of charging for drugs and services (including those not directly attached to the dispensing of a drug product) shall be implemented. A professional fee or per diem fee system should be used. Certain pharmaceutical services (such as pharmacist-conducted patient education programs) may be suitable for a discrete charge levied in addition to the customary fee for drugs and services.
- Some small facilities may not require, or be able to obtain, the services of a full-time pharmacist. However, it should be noted that the concepts, principles and recommendations contained in this standard apply to *all* hospitals, regardless of size or type. Thus, the part-time director of pharmaceutical services has the same basic obligations and responsibilities as his/her full-time counterpart in the larger institution.
- The relevant standards and guidelines of the American Society of Hospital Pharmacists and the Joint Commission on

---

[d] Any system of control which assures the quality of the outcome of the work performed by supportive personnel is deemed to be "appropriate."

Accreditation of Hospitals should be adhered to regardless of the particular financial and organizational arrangements by which pharmaceutical services are provided to the facility and its patients.

Standard II: Facilities

There shall be adequate space, equipment and supplies for the professional and administrative functions of the pharmacy.

- The pharmacy should be located in an area (or areas) convenient to the patients being served. The facility's communication and transportation systems should extend to the pharmacy.
- Space and equipment, in an amount and type to provide secure, environmentally-controlled storage of drugs, shall be available.
- There should be designated space and equipment suitable for the preparation of parenteral admixture and other sterile compounding and packaging operations.
- The pharmacy should have a private area for pharmacist-patient consultations. The director of pharmaceutical services should also have a private office or area.
- Current drug information resources must be available. These should include appropriate pharmacy and medical journals and texts, and drug literature abstracting and/or indexing resources.

Standard III: Drug Distribution and Control

The pharmacy shall be responsible for the procurement, distribution and control of *all* drugs used within the institution. Policies and procedures governing these functions shall be developed by the pharmacist with input from other involved hospital staff (e.g., nurses) and committees (pharmacy and therapeutics committee, patient care com-

mittee, etc.). In doing so, it is essential that the pharmacist routinely visit all patient care areas to establish rapport with their personnel and to become familiar with medical and nursing procedures relating to drugs.

- The pharmacist should maintain an up-to-date formulary of drug products approved for use in the institution. While the items to be included in the formulary are selected by the pharmacy and therapeutics committee (or its equivalent), it is the pharmacist's responsibility to establish specifications for these drug products and to select their source of supply. In doing so, it is advisable that written specifications for multisource items be prepared and utilized in the acquisition process.
- Policies and procedures controlling the use of investigational drugs (if used in the institution) shall be developed and followed. The pharmacy should be responsible for storing, packaging, labeling, distributing and maintaining inventory records of investigational drugs. It should also be responsible (in cooperation with the principal investigator) for providing information about these drugs.
- There shall be a procedure for providing drugs and pharmaceutical services in the event of a disaster.
- Written regulations governing the activities of medical sales representatives within the hospital shall be prepared. Sales representatives should receive a copy of these regulations, and their activities should be monitored. The use of drug samples within the institution should be eliminated to the extent possible. However, if the use of drug samples is permitted, they must be controlled and distributed only through the pharmacy.
- The pharmacist must review the physician's original order or a direct copy thereof, prior to dispensing any drug (except for emergency use). There should be no transcribing of medication orders by nursing or clerical staffs (except for their own records).
- A medication profile for all inpatients and all (or selected) outpatients shall be maintained and used.

- The pharmacist must institute and control procedures needed to insure that patients receive the correct drugs at the proper times. In accomplishing this, it is necessary that all drugs used in the institution (including i.v. fluids) be distributed by the pharmacy. All drugs must be packaged, labeled and distributed in a manner which meets applicable professional standards and legal requirements.
- An adequate system for controlling "controlled substances" must be maintained.
- In the interest of patient safety, all drugs dispensed by the pharmacy for administration to patients should be in single-unit packages and, to the extent possible, in ready-to-administer form. The need for nurses to manipulate drugs (i.e., withdraw doses from multidose containers, label containers, etc.) prior to their administration should be minimized; thus, the unit dose system of preparing and distributing drugs should be used.
- All preparation of sterile products (e.g., i.v. admixtures, piggybacks, irrigating solutions), except in emergencies, shall be done by pharmacy personnel.
- Floor-stocks of drugs should be kept as small as possible and limited to drugs for emergency use and routinely used, "safe" items such as mouthwash and antiseptic solutions. All drug storage areas within the hospital must be routinely inspected to insure that no unusable items are present, that all stock items are properly labeled and stored, etc.[c]
- There shall be a system for removing from use any drugs subjected to a product recall.
- When feasible, the pharmacist should prepare those drug formulations, strengths, dosage forms and packages which are not available commercially, but which are useful in the care of patients. Adequate quality assurance procedures shall be developed for these operations.
- A written stop order policy or other system of assuring that drug orders are not inappropriately continued shall be established.
- Policies and procedures for the use of medications brought into the institution by patients shall be established.

Standard IV: Drug Information

The pharmacy is responsible for providing the institution's staff and patients with accurate, comprehensive information about drugs and their use, and shall serve as its center for drug information.

- The pharmacist (in cooperation with the organization's librarian, if any) is responsible for maintaining up-to-date drug information resources (both in the pharmacy and at patient care areas) and using them effectively. The pharmacist, in addition to supplying specific drug information, must be able to furnish objective evaluations of the drug literature and to provide informed opinion on drug-related matters.
- The pharmacist must keep the institution's staff well informed about the drugs used in the institution and their various dosage forms and packagings. This is accomplished through newsletters, seminars, displays, etc., developed by the pharmacy. No drug shall be administered unless the medical and nursing personnel have received adequate information about, and are familiar with, its therapeutic use, adverse effects and dosage.
- The pharmacist must insure that all patients receive adequate information about the drugs they receive. This is particularly important for ambulant and discharge patients. These patient education activities shall be coordinated with the nursing and medical staffs and patient education department (if any).

Standard V: Assuring Rational Drug Therapy

The most important aspect of pharmaceutical services is that of maximizing ra-

---

[c] Examples of nursing unit inspection forms are available upon request from the American Society of Hospital Pharmacists.

tional drug use. In this regard, the pharmacist, in concert with the medical staff, must develop policies and procedures for assuring the quality of drug therapy.

- Sufficient patient information must be collected and maintained by the pharmacist to insure meaningful and effective participation in patient care. This requires that a medication profile be maintained for all inpatients and for those ambulatory patients routinely receiving care at the hospital. A pharmacist-conducted medication history from hospitalized patients will also be useful.
- All physicians' medication orders (except in emergency situations) must be reviewed for appropriateness by the pharmacist prior to dispensing the first dose. Any questions regarding the order should be resolved with the prescriber at this time and a written notation of these discussions made in the chart or copy of the physician's order. The nursing staff must be informed of any changes made in the order.
- The pharmacist, in cooperation with the pharmacy and therapeutics committee, should develop a mechanism for the reporting and review (by the committee or other appropriate medical staff group) of adverse drug reactions.
- Appropriate clinical information about patients must be available and accessible to the pharmacist for use in his/her daily practice activities.
- The pharmacist must review each patient's drug regimen on a concurrent basis and directly communicate any suggested changes to the prescriber.
- A formalized drug use review program, developed and conducted jointly with the medical staff, should be initiated and integrated with the overall hospital patient care evaluation program. This program should include, but not be limited

to, the use of antibiotics and other anti-infective agents.
- The pharmacist must actively participate in developing the hospital formulary. This is particularly important in small hospitals lacking the services of various medical specialists.
- The pharmacist shall be a member of the pharmacy and therapeutics, infection control, patient care, utilization review and other committees where input concerning the use of drugs is required.

Standard VI: Research

The pharmacist should conduct, participate in, and support medical and pharmaceutical research appropriate to the goals, objectives and resources of the pharmacy and the institution.

- The pharmacy should maintain a file of all investigational drug studies and similar research projects involving drugs in which the facility's patients are participants.
- The pharmacist should be represented on the institution's clinical investigation committee, or its equivalent, if there is one. Alternatively, the pharmacy should receive a copy of the research protocol for any study involving drugs and the facility's patients.

Supplemental References

The American Society of Hospital Pharmacists (4630 Montgomery Avenue, Bethesda, Maryland 20014) has numerous publications which elaborate on many of the concepts embodies in this Standard. They are described in the Society's publications catalog, available upon request.

46—Comprehensive Pharmacy Services in an 85-Bed Hospital

David J. Tanner

The purpose of this article is to describe the implementation and operation of a pharmacy program that provides a unit dose drug distribution system, a totally centralized intravenous admixture program and clinical services in an 85-bed hospital.

Caldwell County War Memorial Hospital of Princeton, Kentucky opened in 1951. After two expansions in the 1960s, the hospital currently serves 34 medical, 10 surgical, three pediatric, nine obstetrical, two intensive care, and 27 long-term care patients. There are eight physicians on the medical staff with 15 registered nurses and 21 licensed practical nurses serving the institution.

Previous Pharmacy Services

Prior to January 21, 1975, the hospital had a drug room operated by one full-time clerk who handled the buying and maintenance of the pharmacy stock. A consultant pharmacist provided services for approximately one and one-half hours daily, primarily to dispense extended care prescriptions and check floor stock medications.

The drug distribution system was bulk floor stock with no control of the amount of medication sent to each unit. The use of hypodermic tablets was practiced in the administration of several controlled drugs. There was no pharmacy and therapeutics committee, formal pharmacy-nursing interrelations, formulary management, phar-

macy monitoring of i.v. fluid therapy or emergency pharmacy services. Essentially, the pharmacy department was what it professed to be: a drug room, with no formal pharmacy services, serving only as a storage depot for medications.

Need for Change

A progressive administrator and medical staff saw the need for developing a more comprehensive pharmacy program in the institution. It would be idealistic to believe, however, that the advance in pharmacy technology through innovative approaches in drug distribution, i.v. therapy control and clinical pharmacy involvement was the primary stimulant to greater interest in pharmacy service. It would be less than honest not to admit that regulatory agencies, such as the Department of Health, Education, and Welfare (DHEW), the Standards for Pharmacy Services established by the Joint Commission on Accreditation of Hospitals (JCAH), and the development of PSROs, were the primary reasons for seeking a full-time pharmacist to develop a program that would satisfy federal and state laws and the minimum standards of DHEW and JCAH. This is not to say that increasing the quality of total patient care was not a consideration; this was thought to be a major benefit of adequate compliance with these regulatory agencies. Administration's first step was the recruitment of a pharmacist with adequate institutional experience.

Management Goals and Priorities

Management first had to consider the implementation of comprehensive pharmacy services and the development of professional rapport with other hospital staff. Standards set forth by the regulatory agencies indicated the initial steps. The director of pharmacy services would be responsible for participating in the development of a hospital formulary, and implementing the decisions of the pharmacy and therapeutics committee.[1] The pharmacist decided to pursue the economics of formulary management via a functional pharmacy and therapeutics committee[2] to provide an economic base upon which to build and justify the pharmacy programs needed. The establishment of this committee was the initial priority in developing interdepartmental rapport. The P and T committee established consisted of the director of pharmacy services (chairman), the hospital administrator, the director of nursing and a representative of the medical staff.

Realizing the importance of the P & T committee functions of the pharmacy director, both administratively and clinically, and realizing the small size of the institution, the concepts of what Smith refers to as the "microsystem," were useful in dealing with small group dynamics. The concept of visualizing a "microsystem" refers to the fact that committee members interact not only within the committee, but do so throughout the day, socially as well as professionally.[3] It was useful in such a limited environment to realize that direct interactions among committee members occurred daily and could indirectly affect a member's function within the entire group. By developing the necessary professional relations within the P & T committee, the director of pharmacy services was able to communicate directly to the medical staff

the objectives of rational, economic formulary management.

Departmental Organization

The pharmacy department was designed to provide discrete work areas to minimize cross traffic. The location of the pharmacy was chosen carefully and provides 450 square feet of space. The results of planning and design are represented by Figure 46.1. The areas are as follow: a unit dose dispensing area with ready access to stock not kept in the immediate area; an i.v. admixture preparation area, equipped with supplies, fluids and medications; an area to be used for the bulk packaging of unit dose solid and liquid oral drug products; eight-foot shelving, each unit with eight 12-inch shelves provides adequate storage of all bulk packaged unit dose products and supplies.

Economic Considerations

Crucial to the implementation of total pharmacy services in a small institution are the economics involved with the feasibility of such programs. The evaluator and implementor of such an undertaking must realize that it is impossible to compare the economics of the previous pharmacy services to the development of new pharmacy programs. In our current state of health care delivery a price tag has not been applied to the cost or value of quality health care achieved by total pharmacy services. It is, therefore, this author's opinion that evaluators and implementors of programs, especially those of pharmacy services, must be aware that the days of the pharmacy, radiology and laboratory departments assuming the major revenue contribution to the institution are declining because of a narrowing profit margin, resulting primarily from third party reimbursement trends and inflation.

Figure 46.1

Layout plan of pharmacy department.

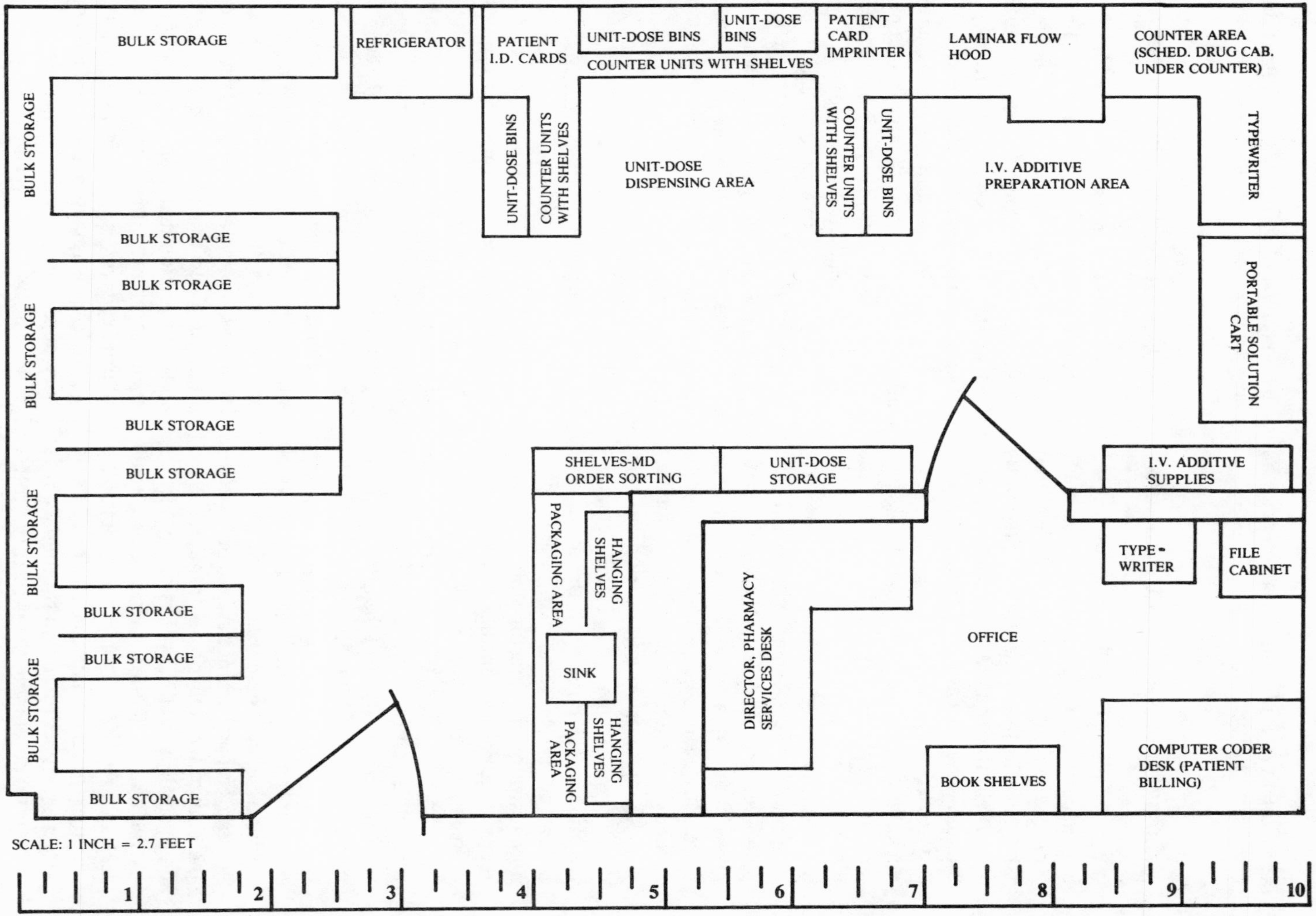

SCALE: 1 INCH = 2.7 FEET

Many third party agencies view the total economics of nonprofit institutions, and not separate departments, for their reimbursement schedules. One cannot overlook the reimbursement policies of third party agencies, since 87% of the revenue received for pharmacy services is essentially through these agencies.[4] This 87% stronghold is seen as a potential plus for pharmacy service development, for if narrowing profit margins are expected and the initial cost of program development can be contained in the implementation stages, then the economic feasibility of the programs can be justified through revenues generated by the pharmacy.

The initial revenue saved through inventory control, product deletion, product returns and the development of a closed formulary represented a saving to our institution of over $12,000 and a decrease in inventory from over 2500 to less than 1000 items. The new programs were then designed to fit a budget related to these savings. An in-depth plan and budget (including personnel, equipment, etc.) was submitted to the administrator for the renovation and building of a new pharmacy department. This author believes that any size institution can use this tactic to evaluate the amount of revenue available to use on new program development, without increasing expenses. Costs, including total renovation of the new pharmacy area, materials, fixtures, unit dose carts, and all equipment, were less than the inventory savings established through formulary management. This allowed only the pharmacy staff's salaries to decrease the profit of the pharmacy department in the implementation stages of program development.

Department of Pharmacy Services

The department of pharmacy services operates from 7 a.m. to 5 p.m. daily. The pharmacy director may be paged for an emergency 24 hours a day. Pharmacy personnel consists of one full-time director, two part-time pharmacists who alternate providing services two days per week, two full-time technicians providing unit dose and admixture services, one full-time administrative technician and two part-time hospital messengers. There is no outpatient dispensing, either in the emergency room or through the pharmacy. The director of pharmacy is also the director of central stores. Central stores personnel, a purchasing agent and a storeroom clerk, are not budgeted to the pharmacy department but are directly responsible to the director of pharmacy services. Renovation and reorganization to formalize pharmacy-central stores as a single department was begun recently.

The pharmacy director assumes many responsibilities in the institution which are felt to compensate for the pharmacy salary expenses not previously incurred by the institution. He functions as the hospital administrator in his absence. Committee involvement of the director of pharmacy includes the pharmacy and therapeutics committee (chairman), the pharmacy-nursing committee (chairman), and the infection control and patient care committees. This relationship to various groups enables the director to be aware of all facets of the hospital's operation and be involved with total patient care as it relates to other departments.

The pharmacy publishes a physician-oriented pharmacy newsletter. A structured format is followed in its monthly presentation. Use of the University of Kentucky Drug Information Center maintains the credibility of the referenced data presented.

The director of pharmacy is involved directly with the inservice programs presented in the institution. Routine programs are presented to the nursing and medical staffs relative to current therapeutics. Over 20 such presentations were presented during a recent nine-month period. Drug information services are supported by a well-equipped library with current text books and periodicals.

The establishment of a poison control center in the hospital emergency room was one of the first accomplishments of the new pharmacy involvement. This center is equipped with readily accessible antidotes and information on their use. Additionally, the director of pharmacy is on call for consultation in a poison emergency.

Unit Dose Drug Distribution System

The following represents our unit dose system in both philosophy and function.

Pharmacist-Nurse Oriented System. Beste described a unique pharmacist-nurse approach to unit dose drug distribution where the medication nurse is employed by the pharmacy department.[5] However, in our small institution, with limited professionals from which to draw, it was not feasible for the pharmacy department to hire the medication nurse because of other duties she performed on the nursing unit. The following concepts were employed to benefit from an active pharmacist-nurse-oriented unit dose program:

1. The medication nurse on all shifts is directly responsible to the director of pharmacy concerning all matters of medication distribution, procurement, storage or administration. This direct line of communication enables the medication nurse to become more involved with pharmacy procedures and concepts. It also saves steps in problem solving and allows the nursing staff to use the time saved for additional activities in patient care.
2. The day shift medication nurse is responsible to the pharmacy at the time of cart filling for comparing and reviewing the nursing patient profiles or medication administration record (MAR) with the pharmacy patient profiles for accuracy. The nurse

brings the MAR to the pharmacy when the cart is ready to be sent to the unit, and together with the pharmacist checks the contents of each patient's drawer for accuracy and ascertains that the MAR and pharmacy profile are identical. This procedure serves as our 24-hour check of orders written by physicians. The major benefit of this checking procedure is that it decreases the communication problems that might exist between pharmacy and nursing in the areas of generic drug use, formulary equivalents, new dosage forms, administration times, etc. Potential problems are clarified in the pharmacy, eliminating timely personal, written or telephoned communications. This procedure consumes a maximum of 15–25 minutes of the daytime medication nurse's time. This nurse is then responsible for communicating to the evening medication nurse pertinent facts concerning the pharmacy-nursing communications for that day. The evening medication nurse than briefs the night medication nurse.

3. Clinically-oriented dialogue is also a very important part of our pharmacist-nurse daily consultation. The medication nurse exchanges information with the pharmacist concerning the patient's clinical status. The nurse's observation of conditions that could be drug-related are communicated to the pharmacist at this time. The pharmacist, in turn, relates information concerning clinical signs of drug effects, toxicity or side effects for the medication nurse to use in her daily patient observations.

Nursing Units Served. There are three nursing units served—two acute care and one extended care. The nursing units are approximately equal in bed size. The two short-term units are provided with medications on a 24-hour basis. One cart is filled after the 8 a.m. medications have been administered and the other after the 12 noon medications have been administered. The long-term care unit of the institution is served every 72 hours; the cart is filled after the 8 a.m. medications have been administered. This frequency complies with the ASHP Statement on Unit Dose Drug Distribution.[6]

Type of Cart Used and Method of Transfer. The type of unit dose cart used is a light-weight, very mobile, non-cassette, self-contained unit with a double-locked controlled drug compartment. The entire cart is removed from the nursing unit for filling. The average time away from the unit is 60–70 minutes. Since prn doses of both controlled and noncontrolled medications are contained in the cart, requests for such medications while the cart is being filled are handled as stat orders (see below). This procedure causes little difficulty, averaging less than one such request daily.

Physician's Orders. The pharmacy department receives a direct carbon copy of the physician's order. The carbon copy contains all orders the physician writes for a particular patient. It was felt that to effectively use the pharmacy patient profile, the recording and monitoring of each patient's i.v. therapy, diet, laboratory tests, and treatments were essential.

Messenger Service. Since the institution is not equipped with a pneumatic tube system, an alternative method of receiving physician orders—a messenger service—was provided. The physical communication link between the nursing units and the pharmacy is provided by two three-quarter time hospital messengers. The messengers are directly responsible to the director of pharmacy; but they are budgeted to the hospital personnel budget and not the pharmacy, for the messengers provide routine pick-up and delivery service for all hospital departments. They also serve as responsible parties for the maintenance of the hospital's mail room. The messengers make routine rounds every hour. Approximately 20–30 minutes/hour are spent in activities external to the pharmacy. In the remaining time, they perform packaging activities, stat order deliveries, supply duties and clerical tasks in and out of the pharmacy.

Disposition of a New Order. The following sequence of events occurs when a new order is written on the nursing unit.

1. Immediately after the order is flagged, the ward clerk detaches the carbon copy, places it in the outgoing box for the hospital messenger to deliver to the pharmacy department on her hourly tour. The ward clerk is responsible for maintaining a chronological listing of new and discontinued medication orders. This document is not a permanent part of the chart, but a convenient form for the physician's reference. The chart will remain flagged until the medication nurse has transcribed the physician's order to the MAR.
2. The pharmacy technician, upon receipt of a new physician's order, will transcribe the order to the pharmacy patient profile, pull the medication indicated in the amount equal to the number of doses to supply the patient until the next cart filling and flag the profile which contains the order for the pharmacist to check for accuracy. After the order has been verified by the pharmacist, the medications are placed in an envelope, imprinted with the patient's name and room number for proper identification, for delivery to the nursing unit.
3. Upon receipt of the medication on the nursing unit, the medication nurse checks the medication received against the transcribed physician order on the MAR. The medication is then placed in the patient's drawer in the unit dose cart.
4. Maximum delivery time allowed for routine orders is 60 minutes.

Stat Orders. The following procedure is followed when stat orders are requested.

1. Immediately after a stat order is written by a physician, the ward clerk will detach the carbon copy of the order and place it in the outgoing box for the hospital messenger to relay to the pharmacy.

2. The ward clerk then telephones the pharmacy to request that the messenger pick up the copy of the stat order. If the messenger is not in the pharmacy department, she is paged to the appropriate unit. The order will be filled immediately and the medication sent to the unit via messenger.

3. Maximum stat delivery time allowed is 20 minutes from the time of the initial doctor's order to the administration of the drug. Actual stat delivery time has been 10–15 minutes. The number of stat orders averages eight/day.

Handling of New Medication Orders When the Pharmacy Is Not Open. The following procedure is followed.

1. A night drug cabinet is used to fill all medication orders that are written during nonpharmacy hours; there is no access to the pharmacy department by anyone but the director. The night drug cabinet has a representative stock of medications reflecting our physicians' prescribing habits. The maximum supply of medication for any one medication is 24 hours.

2. The charge nurse is responsible for obtaining such medication. The medication nurse observes the same functions of charting and monitoring of the patient profiles and medication as if the pharmacy had filled the order.

3. On the carbon copy of the physician's order (which will be sent to the pharmacy the following day) the medication that is retrieved from the night drug cabinet and placed in the patient's drawer is underlined and initialled by the medication nurse. This enables the pharmacy, when it receives the orders on the following morning, to see which patients have night drug cabinet stock and determine what medications are required for 8 a.m. administration. The cabinet medication is withdrawn from the patient's drawer when the cart is filled

the next day. The MAR is checked for the number of doses administered during the night for that particular patient at the time of cart filling and serves as a double check for charge information and dosage schedules.

Controlled Drugs and Preoperative Medications. These are maintained on a sign-out basis in the unit dose cart in the double-locked drawer. A conventional 25-flag document is used for charge purposes. This flag is sent to the pharmacy to document that a prn or a preoperative medication was given and is recorded appropriately for patient billing.

Floor Stock Medications. Since the hours of pharmacy operation are limited, it was necessary that several floor stock medications be maintained for convenience. These include iopanoic acid tablets, senna extract, bisacodyl suppositories, insulin, tuberculosis skin test, and histoplasmin skin test.

Packaging Program. The ASHP guidelines for single packaging of drugs are the criteria used to maintain adequate quality control in our packaging operation.[7] It is the policy of the pharmacy department that all doses be prepackaged and ready for administration upon delivery to the nursing unit. No multidose packages of drugs are issued to the unit if at all possible. We have become completely self-sufficient in our packaging needs. For solid orals we use the Medi-Dose system of packaging[a]; for liquid orals, the breech filling of Ped-Pod oral syringes is used[b]; and for injectables, we use the breech filling of Tubex syringes.[c] Labels for all three systems are prepared by a manual Monarch Ticko-press machine[d] with type set manually or by the use of customized rubber mats.

Patient Medication Charges. The charging of medications is the responsibility of the pharmacy administrative technician. Patient

---

[a] Medi-Dose, Inc., Sellersville, PA 18960.
[b] MPL Solopak Division, 1820 West Roscoe St., Chicago, IL 60657.
[c] Wyeth Laboratories, Inc., Philadelphia, PA 19101.
[d] Monarch Marking Systems Co., Dayton, OH 45412.

charges are totaled upon patient discharge, at 30 days for Medicare billing, and at the end of the month. The end-of-month procedure is for business office bookkeeping convenience.

Patient Identification. The pharmacy department receives a plastic embossed identification card for each patient upon admission. An imprinter now eliminates the timely use of a typewriter for patient identification. The card contains the patient's name, pay code, hospital number, computer number, age, sex and attending physician.

Pharmacy Patient Profile Maintenance. The pharmacy patient profile used incorporates a comprehensive ten-day medication profile and charge document. The unit dose technician records laboratory tests, daily diet, allergies, treatments, diagnosis and i.v. therapy on the profile. It was felt that only by thorough documentation of the patient's entire hospital stay could the pharmacy patient profile be a functional document useful to the pharmacist in daily profile reviews.

Patient Interviews. Although not directly involved with patient interviews, the pharmacy receives a copy of the nursing interview with the patient upon admission. This document provides the pharmacy with appropriate information on the patient's allergies, vital signs, weight, habits and similar data for appropriate documentation on the pharmacy profile. It is planned that the pharmacist will be involved directly in the future with patient interviews upon admission and discharge.

Patient Intrahospital Transfer. The medication nurse is responsible for communicating to the pharmacy department all patient transfers within the hospital. The medication nurse responsible for a particular patient's medication is responsible for the delivery of the patient's name-tag, MAR and medication to the new unit. A simple transfer form is used to communicate this change to the pharmacy.

Automatic Stop Orders. The night shift medication nurse is responsible for notifying physicians concerning medications that are due for renewal. This communication is handled by completing a form and placing it on the face of the patient's chart for physician review 24 hours before the medication order is due to expire.

Types of Forms Used. It was a cumbersome task to select the various forms for use in our unit dose system. The Parke-Davis Uni/Use form proved most satisfactory.[f] The short-term section of the institution uses a 14-day MAR and the long-term area uses a 31-day form. The pharmacy patient profile is thorough in its data base and is a 10-day form. Auxiliary forms include "medication not given," "medication renewal," and "patient transfer" memoranda.

Centralized Intravenous Admixture Program

Our first step was implementation of a centralized piggy-back i.v. admixture program for antibiotics. The success and acceptance by the medical and nursing staffs of this initial program was attributed to (1) standardization of all i.v. antibiotic therapy through predetermined protocols, (2) simplicity of ordering by physicians and (3) savings of nursing time in both the preparation and monitoring of i.v. therapy. Once the merits of a centralized admixture program were realized, transition to our program went smoothly. To complement the admixture service, the pharmacy department in May 1976 also will issue i.v. fluids without additives for a 24-hour supply upon physician's order. Floor stock i.v. fluids will be eliminated.

The following concepts and considerations represent this pharmacy department's approach to a centralized intravenous admixture program in a small institution.

[f] Parke, Davis & Co., 208 Welsh Pool Rd., Lionville, PA 19353.

Equipment. An Abbott three-foot Clean Air Center[8] is used in the pharmacy for the preparation of all i.v. admixtures. Labels for admixtures are printed by the machine used in the unit dose packaging program. The machine preprints common i.v. admixture strip labels, containing the dose, concentration, type of fluid and rate of infusion.

The Pharmacy Patient I.V. Admixture Profile. The unit dose technician is responsible for preparing this profile. After the transcription from the physician's order to the profile, the pharmacist checks the transcription and then gives the order to the admixture technician, who files the profile in a Kardex and color flags the pencil clock for one-hour prior to the time the admixture is due on the nursing unit. The profile form used is designed to give the pharmacist the maximum amount of useful information for monitoring the patient's i.v. therapy. . . . Upon discharge of the patient, or discontinuance of the therapy, the patient's i.v. admixture profile is pulled from the i.v. Kardex and placed in the patient's unit dose profile. At this time, the unit dose technician annotates the total number of admixtures prepared on the patient's unit dose profile for charge purposes.

I.V. Fluid Preparation. All i.v. fluids with additives are prepared for a 24-hour period in the laminar air flow hood in the pharmacy department during normal operating hours. The i.v. admixture technician prepares all admixtures using a protocol outlined in an i.v. admixture procedure manual prepared by the director of pharmacy. Latiolais,[8] Rapp[9] and the ASHP *Parenteral Drug Information Guide*[10] provided the initial data base from which the protocols were written. If any idiosyncratic problems occur with new or unfamiliar admixtures, the i.v. technician consults the director of pharmacy before their preparation. The technician prepares routine admixtures according to the stated protocol and leaves the empty

medication containers with the units of fluid for the pharmacist to check. After the pharmacist has checked that the preparation is correct, he places them in an outgoing box for the hospital messenger to take to the nursing unit for proper storage, and initials the i.v. profile.

I.V. Admixture Orders after Normal Pharmacy Operating Hours. A totally centralized i.v. admixture program without 24-hour pharmacist coverage has been a major problem. In our institution, we have overcome this obstacle by the use of an Abbott Saturn 17 15-inch laminar air flow hood located on one nursing unit. The hood is located near the night drug cabinet so that admixtures for any part of the hospital can be prepared before going to any nursing unit when the pharmacy is not in operation. The same procedure manual that is used in the pharmacy is on each nursing unit for reference. The nursing staff must consult the director of pharmacy before preparing any admixture that is not included in the routine protocol of the i.v. program. Medications for i.v. use are retrieved from the night drug cabinet only if a new order is written after the pharmacy is closed. If the order was written during the day and the admixture cannot be located, the pharmacy director must be contacted before another is prepared. The following protocol is used by nursing staff when handling the carbon copy of the physician's order for i.v. admixture ordered after normal pharmacy operating hours: (1) the medication is underlined and to the side is written "NDC", (2) the type and volume of fluid vehicle is specified, (3) the time the admixture was administered is noted on the carbon copy and (4) if more than one dose is taken from the cabinet, the number of doses and time each was administered is noted on the carbon copy of the physician's order. Less than 2% of the i.v. admixtures in our institution are ordered at times other than when the pharmacy is in operation.

---

[8]   Abbott Laboratories, Inc., 1400 Sheridan Rd., North Chicago, IL 60064.

Pharmacy-Nursing Relations in I.V. Admixture Therapy. Nursing and pharmacy work closely for the adequate attainment of quality i.v. therapy. The pharmacy and nursing directors formulated an i.v. admixture profile which we call the "IVAR" (intravenous administration record) to complement the MAR used in our unit dose program. This form . . . is useful in the appropriate monitoring of the patient's i.v. therapy. The form not only reflects the patient's routine fluid and all i.v. admixture therapy but also the patient's catheter care, fluid intake record and single order i.v. therapy. The IVAR allows nurses on each shift to know the exact status of the patient's i.v. therapy without having to sort through charts for the original order.

Patient Charges. The department of pharmacy services is responsible for all patient charges of fluids with additives in the institution. Patients are charged for only those fluids actually administered; therefore, both the i.v. additive and unit dose systems eliminate the need for credits.

I.V. Infusion Pumps. Three infusion pumps are used routinely for fluids which contain various additives that require rigorous control of administration. The pharmacy department is responsible for maintaining the pumps and regulating their distribution and use throughout the hospital.

Clinical Pharmacy Involvement

The following is an overview of the clinical involvement our hospital pharmacist assumes.

Pharmacy-oriented Centralized Hyperalimentation Program. The department of pharmacy services is totally responsible for preparing all total parenteral nutrition (TPN) solutions and the monitoring of patients on TPN therapy. The director of pharmacy monitors the patients' hospital stay in relation to their total alimentation needs. The physician, when requesting that a patient be placed on TPN therapy, contacts the pharmacy department and requests the director to review the patient's chart. The director then recommends to the attending physician the requirements of the individual patient's TPN needs. The pharmacist then writes the orders relative to the patient's TPN therapy indicating the proper laboratory tests to monitor, nursing care procedures, and the volume and rate of infusion. The physician reviews and signs the orders after consultation with the pharmacist. Once the patient has been placed on TPN therapy, the pharmacist is responsible for changing all TPN bottles and tubing, adjusting flow rates, and dressing the patient's catheter-tubing site on a 24-hour basis. The pharmacist receives all laboratory results pertinent to the patient's TPN therapy and records them on a flow sheet in the pharmacy, allowing for accurate adjustment of electrolytes, glucose and the volume of fluid infused on a daily basis. The pharmacist consults with the attending physician daily regarding the patient's TPN status and acquires a total clinical assessment of the patient.

Pharmacy Participation in Medical Emergencies. The director of pharmacy responds to all emergency codes when in the hospital and is paged frequently when out of the hospital. A thoroughly equipped emergency cart organized therapeutically by medical emergency is available at each nursing unit. The pharmacist must be knowledgeable about all medical emergency procedures, including cardiopulmonary resuscitation, and be aware of the priorities involved in different medical emergencies to adequately assist the physician and auxiliary personnel in a given medical emergency.

Twenty-four Hour Pharmacy Consultation. The director of pharmacy is on call around the clock for medical emergencies and consultation. He receives an average of 40 consultation requests per month. A pharmacist consultation request form (Figure 46.2) has been implemented recently to better document and formalize these physician-

Figure 46.2

Pharmacist consultation request form.

DATE: _____PHYSICIAN: _____

INFORMATION REQUIRED BY: DATE: _____TIME: _____

NATURE OF REQUEST

I. DRUG INFORMATION:
- DRUG NAME:_____
- TYPE OF INFORMATION REQUESTED:
  - Dosage forms .... □
  - Indications .... □
  - Side effects .... □
  - Efficacy of product vs. current therapy .... □
  - Pharmacokinetics (absorption, distribution, excretion, metabolism) .... □
  - Drug interactions .... □
  - Laboratory parameters to follow in therapy .... □
  - Dosing: adult or pediatric .... □
  - Cautions in therapy .... □
  - Pharmacology (mechanism of action, target organ, etc.) .... □
  - Other _____ .... □

II. CHART REVIEW: DRUG THERAPY CONSULT
- PATIENT: _____
- DIAGNOSIS: _____
- INFORMATION REQUESTED:
  - Alternative drug therapy for disease state .... □
  - Possibility of drug interference with laboratory data .... □
  - Possibility of drug-drug interaction .... □
  - Possibility of pharmacokinetic parameter interfering with drug therapy .... □
  - Side effects most frequent with current drug therapy .... □
  - Other _____ .... □
  - Comments or explanations: _____

III. DRUG THERAPY PROFILE PREPARATION REQUEST
- DISEASE STATE:
- DRUG THERAPY DESIRED (SPECIFY THERAPY TO BE INSTIGATED, IF KNOWN):

- PROFILE WILL CONTAIN: LABORATORY PARAMETERS TO FOLLOW, CONCOMITANT DRUG THERAPY IF REQUIRED, NURSING PRINCIPLES IN THERAPY MANAGEMENT AND PATIENT MONITORING, DOSING, AND OTHER PERTINENT INFORMATION.

IV. OTHER: _____

Return to Department of Pharmacy Services

pharmacist interactions. Physicians are encouraged to submit requests for both inpatients and outpatients. Requests are answered by telephone if the information is required in less than 24 hours. If more than 24 hours is allowed for information retrieval, formal consultations are typed and referenced similar to a radiology or pathology consult.

Formulary Latitude of the Hospital Pharmacist. To augment the hospital pharmacist's ability to monitor drug therapy through his chairmanship of the P & T committee and the ensuing formulary management, the medical staff bylaws state that the pharmacist can substitute similar therapeutic as well as nonproprietary products either as single entity or in combination for those products prescribed that are not formulary items. The pharmacist's professional judgment is used to determine whether the physician should be notified of the change before the substitution.

Patient Chart Review. The director of pharmacy, in accordance with DHEW regulations,[11] inspects and reviews patient charts monthly for the long-term section of the institution. Chart reviews in the short-term section are requested frequently by physicians when the assistance of the pharmacist is needed. This service is of particular value in a small institution because a physician is not on the premises 24-hours a day. In addition to requested chart reviews, the pharmacist, as delineated in the medical staff bylaws, is responsible for the routine monitoring of appropriate laboratory parameters when following anticoagulant and aminoglycoside therapy. The pharmacy receives a daily copy of each patient's laboratory results to assist in this responsibility. If appropriate laboratory tests inadvertently are not ordered the pharmacist has the authority to initiate the order. He also is given latitude to perform dosage and dosage frequency adjustments when monitoring aminoglycoside therapy based on appropriate laboratory parameters.

The use of a physician memorandum has been an effective method for informing the physician of aspects of a patient's therapy noted through chart and profile review. The physician memorandum (Figure 46.3) is a two-part no-carbon-required form which provides both the pharmacy and the physician a copy of the correspondence. When the memorandum is written, the original copy is detached and placed face down on the patient's chart for the physician to review. The carbon copy is retained in the patient's profile in the pharmacy. All profiles with such memoranda attached are filed separately to be used in a retrospective study to determine the significance of this information service.

Figure 46.3

Physician memorandum form.

PHYSICIAN MEMO
Pharmacy Patient Profile Review

Through review of _____. Pharmacy Patient Profile, the following observation may be of use to you in your clinical evaluation or plan.

_____
_____
_____
_____
_____
_____

Significance of Observation: VERY IMPORTANT □

POTENTIALLY IMPORTANT □

LITTLE IMPORTANCE BUT POSSIBLE □

Reference if Necessary: _____

Date: _____ Pharmacist: _____

The initial intent of the memorandum was to save both the pharmacist and the physician time in communicating information about medication, its use, misuse, and other factors directly affecting the patient. The medical staff appears to appreciate this mechanism for maintaining surveillance of all therapy in the institution. An order change rate or personal response to approximately 90% of all pharmacist recommendations corroborates their acceptance and appreciation of the system.

The medicolegal aspects of maintaining and using pharmacy patient profiles is complemented by this memorandum which documents physician consultation on pertinent matters concerning the patient's therapeutic regimen. The legal liability and responsibility of maintaining pharmacy patient profiles must be assumed automatically when implementing a unit dose drug distribution system.

Pharmacy Technician Course. Since formal pharmacy services could not be provided on a 24-hour basis, the need to educate the nursing staff in drug therapy was essential. It was assumed that in order to have progressive pharmacy programs, an adequate professional pool of technicians would have to be established in the event a vacancy should occur. Therefore, the pharmacy will initiate in June 1976 a 30-week pharmacy technician course conducted by the director with the assistance of the staff pharmacists. This 140-hour course has been approved by the National Association of Licensed Practical Nurses for continuing education credit. Over 50 persons have applied to take the course, 75% of whom are nurses.

Future Pharmacy Programs and Goals

A major goal of our department is to become even more of a key factor in the future delivery of primary health care in our institution. Increased clinical pharmacy involvement is the primary area of program development that will be pursued now that adequate service programs have been implemented. Programs currently in the planning and development stage include attendance at physicians' rounds, development of a retrospective and prospective drug usage review program, direct involvement with patient counseling (including admission and discharge interviews) and implementation of ambulatory pharmacy services.

The relatively new concept of quality

assurance programs for hospital pharmacies as outlined by Stolar[12] will be evaluated and implemented in stages to assess our programs. An active quality assurance program will be implemented as soon as possible for self-assessment of pharmacists and for data collection for drug usage studies. The goal of such a program in our pharmacy department is seen as a mechanism for assuring the patient, our peers and regulatory bodies that quality is continually being maintained.

Profiles in Perspective

Four variables are key factors influencing the success of pharmacy programs in small hospitals.

1. The one variable that will influence program outcome more than any other is the extent of the director of pharmacy's management and clinical expertise. One skill is not effective without the other. If there is a lack of managerial expertise, clinical programs are not economically justified; if there is a lack of clinical expertise, the absence of professional rapport and cooperation with medical and nursing staffs will decrease the efficiency of accomplishing management goals and objectives.
2. The degree of professional acceptance and functional latitude afforded the hospital pharmacist by the medical staff is the second variable. The confidence which the medical staff has in the hospital pharmacist is directly proportional to the extent of his individual management and clinical expertise as demonstrated in the first variable.
3. The adequacy of pharmacy-nursing relations is the third variable. Two factors contribute to the success of pharmacy-nursing relations: (1) professional acceptance of the pharmacist for his individual expertise in patient care and (2) the time spent in program implementation.
4. The fourth variable which directly affects pharmacy program implemen-

tation is the progressiveness of the hospital administrator's attitudes toward pharmacy services. The administrator must be convinced that the director of pharmacy has the managerial and clinical expertise to implement appropriate services economically and provide a higher quality of health care delivery in compliance with regulatory agencies. The degree of the administrator's confidence in the pharmacy director will be based on the following: what services the hospital pharmacist can provide with the least amount of revenue, the efficiency of formulary management and inventory control, the extent of professional acceptance by medical and nursing staffs, and the number of visible contributions of the pharmacy services to the total quality of health care.

It should be emphasized that these four variables are interdependent. There is no clear cut answer as to whether or not implementation of total pharmacy services in any given small institution is economically feasible, justifiable and functional.

Conclusion

The goal of comprehensive pharmacy services in any institution is to increase the quality of patient care. The contributions toward quality patient care by clinical pharmacy services,[13] unit dose drug distribution,[14-19] centralized intravenous admixture services[20-22] and formulary management[23-25] have been discussed in the literature. A study by Mikeal et al.[26] showed that larger hospitals tended to have higher quality pharmaceutical services than smaller hospitals. We would hope that the services developed in our department are counter to this trend. It is clear that quality assurance programs in hospital pharmacy are necessary to assure that all hospitals, regardless of size, provide adequate pharmaceutical services to patients.

Beyond the scope of this introductory article describing the pharmacy services provided in our small institution, is a thorough, long-term economic and functional evaluation of these services. This evaluation is currently being performed through a research grant, and the results will be reported at a later time.

References

1. Joint Commission on Accreditation of Hospitals: Standards for hospital accreditation (Dec) 1970.
2. Code of Federal Regulations Title 20, Ch III, part 405.1027 and 405.1127, U.S. Department of Health, Education, and Welfare, Social Security Administration.
3. Smith, M. C.: Survey shows hospital pharmacy in advisory role, *Mod Hosp 113*:114–118 (Dec) 1969.
4. Zellmer, W. A.: Hospital trends (editorial), *Am J Hosp Pharm 32*:1107 (Nov) 1975.
5. Beste, D. F.: An integrated pharmacist-nurse approach to the unit dose concept, *Am J Hosp Pharm 25*:397–407 (Aug) 1968.
6. Anon: ASHP statement on unit dose drug distribution, *Am J Hosp Pharm 32*:835 (Aug) 1975.
7. Anon: ASHP guidelines for single unit packages of drugs, *Am J Hosp Pharm 28*:110–112 (Feb) 1971.
8. Latiolais, C. J. et al.: Stability of drugs after reconstitution, *Am J Hosp Pharm 24*:666–691 (Dec) 1967.
9. Rapp, R. P.: Guidelines for the administration of commonly used intravenous drugs, *Drug Intell Clin Pharm 7*:38–42 (Jan) 1973.
10. Trissel, L. A., Grimes, C. R. and Grallelli, J. F.: Parenteral drug information guide, American Society of Hospital Pharmacists, Washington, D.C., 1974.
11. Conditions of participation relative to pharmaceutical services in skilled nursing facilities, *Fed Regist 39* (Jan 17) 1974.
12. Stolar, M. H.: Quality assurance for hospital pharmacy, part 1: basic concepts, *Am J Hosp Pharm 32*:276–80 (Mar) 1975.
13. Keys, P. W. et al.: Quality of care evaluation applied to assessment of clinical pharmacy services, *Am J Hosp Pharm 32*:897–902 (Sep) 1975.
14. Slater, W. E. and Hripko, J. R.: The unit dose system in a private hospital, part one: implementation, *Am J Hosp Pharm 25*:408–417 (Aug) 1968.
15. Slater, W. E., and Hripko, J. R.: The unit dose system in a private hospital, part two: evaluation, *Am J Hosp Pharm 25*:641–648 (Nov) 1968.
16. Lazarus, H. L., et al.: Unit dose—a survey of pharmacy drug control—two, distribution system, *Hosp Formul Manage 9*:23–36 (Nov) 1974.
17. Parker, P. F.: Unit dose system reduces error increases efficiency, *Hospitals 42*:24 (Dec) 1968.
18. Hynniman, C. E. et al.: A comparison of medication errors under the University of Kentucky unit dose system, and traditional drug distribution system in four hospitals, *Am J Hosp Pharm 27*:802–814 (Oct) 1970.
19. Rosenberg, J. M. and Salvatore, P. O.: Implications of a unit dose dispensing system in a community hospital, *Hosp Pharm 8*:35–39 (Feb) 1973.
20. Latiolais, C. J.: Teamwork: the key to success in i.v. therapy, *Am J I V Ther 2*:13–16 (Jun–Jul) 1975.
21. Cantrell, M. et al.: Improved techniques in i.v. therapy reduced contamination hazards, *Am J I V Ther 2* (Sep) 1975.
22. Schwarton, N.W. et al.: A comprehensive intravenous admixture system, *Am J Hosp Pharm 30*:607–610 (Jul) 1973.
23. Katcher, A. L.: Appraising purposes and functions of the P & T committee, *Hosp Top 47*:61–66 (Feb) 1969.
24. Francke, D. E.: Pharmacy service: what are the goals of the pharmacy and therapeutic committee?, *Hospitals 41*:99–100 (Oct) 1967.
25. Francke, D. E.: A strengthened pharmacy and therapeutics committee offers new opportunities for pharmacists, *Hospitals 41*:91–94 (Nov) 1967.
26. Mikeal, R. L. et al.: Quality of pharmaceutical care in hospitals, *Am J Hosp Pharm 32*:567–574 (Jun) 1975.

47—Reviewing the 1970s:
Hospital Pharmacy Practice

William A. Zellmer

As the 1970s draw to a close, it seems fitting to reflect on hospital pharmacy's progress during the past 10 years. What achievements will be attributed to this decade by future historians of hospital pharmacy?

From our current perspective, the 1970s have been remarkable for the consensus that has developed among practitioners regarding the essential features of hospital drug control systems. Also noteworthy has been the further innovation and refinement of clinical roles for hospital pharmacists.

Unit dose drug distribution and intravenous admixture services were pioneered in the 1960s. For the most part, the rationale and justification for these innovations also were well established more than 10 years ago. The debate over the desirability and feasibility of unit dose and admixture services in all hospitals carried over into the 1970s. However, sometime during the decade now ending, most hospital pharmacists internalized these concepts and became committed to implementing them. By the end of 1979, more than 60% of short-term hospitals are expected to have a partial or complete unit dose system, and over two thirds will have implemented at least a partial admixture service.[1]

Clinical pharmacy practice remained confined largely to teaching hospitals during the 1970s. In those institutions, the maturity and sophistication of clinical pharmaceutical services advanced markedly, as did the acceptance of such services by other health professionals. Pharmacists at a number of hospitals were successful in developing routine clinical services based on principles of pharmaceutical science (e.g., pharmacokinetic monitoring), giving greater credence to their efforts as specialized pharmacy functions. For the first time, pharmacy departments in the 1970s were confident enough to obtain hospital budget allocations specifically for clinical services and to charge for those services in patients' bills. Also noteworthy was the increasing involvement of pharmacists in clinical drug research.

Although few hospitals had a comprehensive clinical pharmacy program,[1] a distinct clinical thread ran through many of hospital pharmacy's priorities in the 1970s. Practitioners seemed to have a heightened sense of responsibility for the quality of drug therapy in their institutions. Evidence for this included increased pharmacist involvement in patient care audits, drug use review, and patient drug education. Some hospital pharmacists became more aggressive in pursuing restrictive drug-use policies through the pharmacy and therapeutics committee. (Overall, however, there was still much room for improvement in the selectivity of formularies.[2])

Increased attention was devoted to intravenous therapy, including the safety of admixture compounding procedures, the accuracy of i.v. fluid administration, and the merits of in-line filters. Studies of i.v. drug stability and compatibility continued unabated, although the quality of such studies improved noticeably compared with those of the previous decade.

Hospital pharmacists in the 1970s also

began taking a hard look at the value of their own services. Ongoing, systematic, objective assessment of a pharmacy department's programs was a development long overdue.

The dynamism of hospital pharmacy in the 1970s was striking. Most practitioners were genuinely committed to upgrading their services to patients. As a whole, the discipline could hardly have been characterized as complacent with its performance. The challenging practice standards of ASHP and JCAH, and the general innovativeness of the hospital field contributed to hospital pharmacy's progress. The most important factor, however, was the youth and enthusiasm of hospital pharmacists themselves. Hospital practice attracted a large number of new pharmacy graduates. According to the Bureau of Health Manpower, the number of hospital pharmacists doubled between 1966 and 1974. This steep growth curve extended through the whole decade. Many pharmacists well trained in ASHP-accredited residency programs were appointed pharmacy directors in key hospitals around the country. These enterprising practitioners joined a sizable corps already within hospital pharmacy who were committed to changing things for the better.

May the shakers and movers of the 1970s continue their ambition and commitment, and may we have more like them to carry us forward into the 1980s.

References

1. Stolar, M. H.: National survey of hospital pharmaceutical services—1978, *Am J Hosp Pharm 36*:316–325 (Mar) 1979.
2. Rucker, T. D. and Visconti, J. A.: How effective are drug formularies? A descriptive and normative study, ASHP Research and Education Foundation, Washington, D.C., 1979.

Related Readings in This Volume

11. Drug Usage Review in a Community Hospital
25. Prescription Errors
28. Clinical Pharmacy in Emergence Medicine
31. Intravenous Drug Therapy
32. Pharmacist and Hyperalimentation Programs
33. Clinical Pharmacy on Oncologic Service

Readings for a Broader Perspective

1. Schwerin, G. D., and Nelson, A. A. "Development of Pharmacy PSRO Criteria and Standards for South Carolina Hospitals," *Hospital Pharmacy* 13 (October 1978): 535, 541–542, 547, 550, 553–554.
2. Ashby, D. M., and Hoffman, R. P. "Current Status of Pharmacy Services in Large Hospitals," *Hospital Pharmacy* 11 (January 1976): 4, 8–10.
3. Pelissier, N. A. "What We Learned While Trying to Implement a Unit-Dose System," *Pharmacy Times* 44 (May 1978):50–54.
4. Ballentine, R., Primeau, J., McKinley, J. D., and Evans, S. "How We Provide Outpatient I.V. Additives to Cancer Patients," *Pharmacy Times* 42 (September 1976):42–45.

LONG-TERM CARE INSTITUTION

48—Geriatric Practice Provides
Professionalism and Prestige

John F. Aforismo

John F. Aforismo, R.Ph., 29 years old and just six years out of school, has acquired an extraordinary respect in the semirural suburbs that stretch north of Hartford, Conn. Doctors, usually a bit stiff about acknowledging a pharmacist as a collaborator, welcome his advice. Nurses have come to rely on him. One put it this way: "He doesn't just sell a product; he solves problems."

What endears John Aforismo to his colleagues on the health care team is that he is a cool and quiet professional. Seated at his desk in a little office behind his store on Elm Street in Windsor Locks, he smiles at such talk. "Professionalism is a state of mind," he says, quoting Dr. Henry Palmer, his mentor at the University of Connecticut School of Pharmacy.

Perhaps out of that state of mind he might have adapted a high professional pattern of practice to any situation that presented itself. But in fact Aforismo has developed a specialty that has enabled him to put to professional use all the skills he had acquired in five years of training. He is a specialist in providing pharmacy service to nursing homes. He serves five of them with a zeal and a skill that have earned him a growing reputation and have brought him to the attention of the governor of the state.

"You have to really like the job to give our kind of service," he says, "otherwise it won't work."

Aforismo owns his store in partnership with a classmate, George Troie, who prefers to tackle the business side of the enterprise and the off-the-street trade. Their venture, the Windsor Locks Medical Pharmacy, is housed in a modest brick medical arts building, where a dozen doctors maintain a part-time practice. The two partners employ a third pharmacist, Lori Overholt, who began as John's pupil in a clinical program for fifth-year students at the University of Connecticut. She loved the kind of pharmacy practice she saw at Windsor Locks, and the partners liked the way she took to it.

They also employ two high school girls in the afternoon and a part-time driver.

Behind the high counter, topped with an elaborately ornamental apothecary jar and a metal vase of straw flowers, are the card files that hold the key to their practice. Here are the profiles of every patient in every one of the nursing homes that retain what is somewhat grandiloquently called, "The Convalescent Home Service Division of the Windsor Locks Medical Pharmacy." The "Division" consists of John Aforismo with an assist from Lori Overholt.

Each patient's card bears the diagnosis, allergies, specialized diet, a list of medications past and present, and a summary of idiosyncracies, such as whether tablets must be crushed or taken in fruit juice.

That file is reviewed every 30 days to verify the latest orders signed by the doctor, to check the nurses' notes for reactions, and to evaluate the total medication regimen of each patient to see where drug combinations may spell dangers. "A doctor may not always bear in mind the total picture," Aforismo points out. "And the patient may change doctors."

If anything in the medication picture troubles the pharmacist team at Windsor Locks, a report goes off to the doctor in charge.

How does that service sit with the doctors and nurses? "They like it and so do we," Aforismo notes.

What launched the Windsor Locks Medical Pharmacy into its specialty was the unit-dose system, which enabled the nurses to do away with a cumbersome time-consuming routine that had been necessary to avoid medication error or contamination. Now each weekday afternoon a car leaves on its rounds carrying cards of heat-sealed plastic bubbles (blister packs), each of which contains the precise, double-checked dosage for the patient. The card is labeled with all the directions stipulated by the doctor, and the relevant indications and contraindications noted by the manufacturer, plus whatever other pharmaceutical data—such as possible side effects—might seem pertinent. The doses are dated. The nurse need only pop the bubble open at the patient's bedside.

The convenience of unit-dose helped to establish John Aforismo in his specialty. What keeps him there is a variety of services far beyond the delivery of medication. For that story, it is best to go to the homes themselves. Terry Burnham, R.N., director of nursing at Parkway Pavillion, recalls the time, two years ago, when John fought a scabies outbreak. Patients began reporting an unaccustomed itching toward the end of the day and they called Windsor Locks for advice.

"We had gotten used to calling on John for almost any problem," notes Parkway Pavillion's assistant director, Janet Green, R.N.

John and George showed up at seven the following morning with a full protocol. John had spent a good part of the evening in research and much of the night in drafting the policy. By the time the home's administrator arrived for work at nine, the crisis had passed. The suspected scabies victims had been segregated, and John was giving an in-service lecture to the staff on the recommended medication collected overnight from the pharmacy's sources.

"We still get calls for that policy of John's," says Nurse Burnham. "The state asked for it, and regularly other homes keep telephoning us for it."

At the moment Aforismo is at work on a study of the effects of indwelling catheters on the patient's urine. Another ongoing interest of John's is the waste involved in the mandatory destruction of medication in any health facility. The law in Connecticut, as in many other states, requires the destruction of medication left unused by a patient who dies or is discharged or is taken off a regimen.

Aforismo filed a report with Governor Grasso on his findings in several homes. The governor has now initiated her own investigation, listing the Aforismo study among others as source material.

At Prospect Hill, another of the convalescent and geriatric homes that dot the countryside near Hartford, the story is much the same. John Aforismo has wrought changes. He gives in-service talks not only to nurses but to nurses' aides on everything from sunburn and poison ivy to allergy. He serves on committees on infection control, antiseptic discipline, and drug distribution. He is there to answer questions.

Janet Edwards, director of nursing at Prospect Hill, recalls a behavioral problem that afflicted one of her geriatric patients. John studied the list of drugs ordered for the patient. He thought the problem might be caused by certain drug interactions and reported that idea to the doctor. The doctor agreed; the medication was changed and the problem solved.

Then there are the extras, for example, the fact sheets Aforismo mails out, each on a different disorder. Out of the file, the nurses pick one on epilepsy. It defines the disorder in terse outline, listing symptoms with medications commonly used.

There are also bulletins on new medications as they arrive in the store so that the medical staff can keep a file on what is available. Frequently, nursing directors ask John to be on hand when the state inspectors come. "They're always much impressed with him," says one nurse.

They may well be, and John Aforismo and the Windsor Locks Medical Pharmacy may be a model professional pharmacy, but does it pay?

John Aforismo's answer is enthusiastically affirmative. He and George Troie have been operating the Windsor Locks store for just three years. They gross $300,000 a year. Their nursing homes pay $10 an hour for consultations. They hope to add two or three more homes to their practice, with the help of Miss Overholt. They pay her $15,000 a year, $3,000 more than either of the partners can draw at present. But by the year's end they will be out of debt and making money, they say.

Of course, they have problems, Aforismo admits. Many of their nursing home patients are on welfare in one form or another. And they must wait 90 to 120 days for payment on prescriptions.

Committee meetings at the nursing homes consume five days out of every month, and John frequently makes rounds with the doctors. Technically the service is on call 24 hours a day. "We've made deliveries as late as one in the morning," John says.

The Windsor Locks Medical Pharmacy serves a minimum of 15,000 patients in the nursing homes and the general community. The five nursing homes have a total of 700 beds, and each is normally at 95% to 97% of capacity. That busy practice yields the business 60% to 70% of its gross.

John had come out of school in 1972 and into a chain apothecary store that confined its business to filling prescriptions. He opened his own shop at Newington, Conn., on an investment of $6,000. It was minimal, he grants, less than half of what one ought to put in, but he thought he might make do with a very low inventory since he had an obliging wholesaler an hour away. If a customer was in a hurry, John could always whip down and pick up what was needed. With little capital or sustaining power, the prospects were unpromising.

It was then that John spoke to Dr. Palmer, who suggested that he look into the situation of nursing homes in Hartford suburbia. He looked, liked what he saw, and proposed a joint service with George Troie who was skating on the thin edge of insolvency in Windsor Locks.

The scheme worked, although for about a year the two of them tried to run their separate stores keeping only the nursing home service in common. "That was a mistake," John grants. They gave up the Newington place and now are clearly making a go of it.

For John and his wife Shireen this is a moment of quiet triumph. They married when John was in his third year of pharmacy school. "Actually," says John, "Shireen put me through school and gave us our start." Shireen was a beautician and still keeps her hand in although she doesn't have much time, what with two children and a third on the way.

"She worked hard; now it's time for me to work," John says smiling.

John Aforismo is on the point of making it precisely as he wants to, with the professionalism he so admires. Wondering about the sources of that profound regard for the profession, we asked whether pharmacy ran in the family. John grinned. "I'll tell you how it was," he said. "I was registering at Connecticut U. I had no direction whatever, but I thought it would be better to pick a specific course of study rather than one in the liberal arts, what with a war on. That morning I had received a letter from a pharmaceutical company—I can't remember which—about careers. It popped into my mind, and I wrote down 'Pharmacy' as my choice. I have no regrets."

49—How We Serve the Elderly in Nursing Homes and Hi-Rise Apartments

L. Steve Lubin

Our pharmacy's nursing home program is a modification of the standard system. We call ours the "monitored dose" system; and with it, we have the capability of switching to a "controlled" or "unit-dose" system at any time, without major changes. The services we provide, in any case, are basically the same, but the flexibility comes from within the system itself. This program fully complies with all current Medicare-Medicaid standards.

Our current services include the following.

1. Holding monthly meetings with the nursing home administrator,
2. Conducting monthly meetings with the entire nursing staff,
3. Signing all charts, forms, and reports, and keeping current on all necessary paperwork,
4. Monitoring charts and medications as well as the condition of patients and their responses to medication,
5. Consulting with nurses and physicians regarding patient therapy and response,
6. Disposing of unused and/or discontinued medications promptly,
7. Consulting and advising on all medication delivery, and
8. Providing a pharmacy manual.

At the monthly meetings, we discuss certain disease states and the use of appropriate medications for them. We talk about patients and their response to the medications they are receiving. Our drug delivery system is also reevaluated, and the nursing staff makes a full evaluation of our services.

Medication Paperwork

Our nursing home program services two 100-bed facilities—the Hardin Guest Home for the Elderly and the Greater Community Senior Citizen Center—as well as two 20-bed senior citizen guest homes.

Our commitment to these institutions requires that we be responsible for all necessary paperwork pertaining to medication, and that we contact the doctor if there are questions concerning prescriptions. All forms are signed and updated, at least monthly.

Patient charts are monitored to ensure (1) that the doctor's orders were correctly interpreted, (2) that the proper medication was ordered, and (3) that ensuing reorders were copied correctly. Medications are also checked to assure that the correct drug—with proper directions—was dispensed. Unused medication is disposed of immediately, according to the pharmacy manual.

As mentioned, we call this medication delivery system "monitored dose" as opposed to a "controlled dose" or "unit-dose" system. The numerous checkpoints—monitoring the charts, checking the medication bins, charting the patient profile, etc.—assure that errors can be quickly spotted. Here is how the system works:

- Orders are phoned in by nurses—directly and *only*—to a pharmacist;
- Orders are filled and dispensed, by the pharmacist, in regular vials;
- The label includes patient information, drug name, directions, amount sent, and the date;
- A duplicate of the label is put on the patient profile chart. (We are presently experimenting with a reorder system, utilizing this duplicate label.);
- A 3-part ticket is made which shows the date ordered, the names of the patient and ordering nurse, and any charges.

All patient profile charts are carefully examined before any prescription is filled. We are monitoring proper usage, possible drug interactions & incompatibilities, and duplication of ordering. Generally, a 30-day supply will be sent to the patient, unless we are otherwise advised, or the usage is questioned. This enables convenient, once-a-month ordering, and ensures that the patient is receiving his medicine properly on a day-to-day basis. And it allows us to spot a problem if a patient's medication is reordered too soon, within this 30-day supply period. Narcotics and DEA (Drug Enforcement Administration) prescriptions are handled separately. For such medications, an individual

sheet for each prescription is prepared, and they are packaged separately and signed for by the receiving nurse.

The flexibility of the system enables any part of it to be modified to the nurse's, administrator's, or bookkeeper's wishes. For example: (1) Physicians' orders could be picked up and checked, instead of being phoned in, (2) the bulk of the ordering—for all the routine medications—could be done automatically by our checking the reorder sheets, and (3) a partitioned cart could be used to eliminate a drug storage room and to permit bedside dispensing.

As mentioned, this system can be converted either to a controlled dosage or to a true unit-dose system. We have examined all of the presently-available systems, and we have the capability to utilize them if it is deemed advisable.

Our preference for this "monitored dose" system is based on our studies of cost factors and patient billing. Aware of the limited funds of the individual patient, the high cost of nursing home care, and the amount of medication usually required, we believe every effort should be made to keep the medication costs per patient as low as possible.

Our pharmacy is in a position to use the "monitored dose" system more efficiently than others, because:

(1) No extra costs are involved, owing to the fact that this is our usual routine for filling prescriptions,

(2) We have the capacity to purchase a wider range of volume drugs in bulk packages, according to our normal methods,

(3) We have the ability to "special" price because we are a sound, independent business—not bound to making a certain percentage profit on each individual or prescription. This allows us some leeway in cases involving costly injectables, extended usage of expensive drugs, patients temporarily discontinued from Medicaid, the exceptionally poor or indigent patient, etc.,

(4) We credit patients for unused or discontinued medicines. These medications are

destroyed and written off as a business expense. However, only 2% of the dispensed prescriptions are returned for these reasons.

3 Methods of Billing

We offer 3 methods of billing, our preference being to bill the home—totally. In this case, each patient has a separate charge sheet showing date and ticket number, and accompanied by two copies of the charge ticket. The nursing home receives this itemized, alphabetical listing a few days before its billing period cuts off. Our statement is totaled, and ready to be included with each patient's bill.

Another choice is to invoice each patient individually, just as with a separate store charge account. Or, we can arrange to bill in any combination of these methods—to suit the needs of the patients and the institution.

Although it has rarely occurred, we do look to the nursing home administration for help in collecting delinquent accounts, when this becomes necessary.

In addition to serving nursing home and senior citizen guest home patients, we have developed another plan which we call our "Hi-Rise" program. Its purpose is to serve the elderly who live in 3 government hi-rise dormitories and two smaller apartment buildings sponsored by religious groups.

Professional Services & Purchasing Help

This free hi-rise program is divided into "professional services" and "consumer purchasing assistance." It is available to *all* residents of these buildings, whether or not they are our customers.

As in the nursing homes, our professional services for the hi-rise elderly consist of educating and counseling them, monitoring their medications, and screening them for various diseases—such as diabetes and hyperten-

sion. We give lectures at the residents' association meetings, set up personal—as well as general—consultation appointments within the building, and maintain patient profiles for each individual.

In addition, we check on—and carefully stress to each individual patron—the following points about the medicines taken:

- Correct usage,
- Results achieved—good or bad—and answering their questions about how to eliminate side effects,
- Possible medication interactions,
- Need for continuing to take medication, and duration of time it should be taken,
- General guidelines of what to do or avoid doing.

Our "consumer purchasing assistance" program is very popular with the elderly who reside in the hi-rise buildings—and many of them utilize only that part of our service. It is designed to assist those low- and fixed-income people who have limited access to transportation and shopping areas.

By offering special discounts, we keep our prices competitive with the senior citizen discount market. Other services we offer the elderly are: Cashing of monthly checks, accepting phone and utility bills, and writing money orders. But perhaps the most popular feature of our consumer program is the once or twice daily delivery service to hi-rise residents—made feasible by the high volume of deliveries we have to any one location at one time.

A Rewarding Experience

The programs which we have developed to serve large numbers of elderly patients have been a rewarding experience for us, both personally and professionally.

Our greatest reward, of course, comes from the knowledge that we are able to use our professional expertise to bring better health and peace of mind to patients who are often psychologically neglected.

Related Readings in This Volume

30. Senescent Drug Abuse
59. Drug Therapy in the Elderly
61. Cost-Benefit of Drug Monitoring in Skilled Nursing Facility

Readings for a Broader Perspective

1. Rawlings, J. L., and Frisk, P. A. "Pharmaceutical Services for Skilled Nursing Facilities in Compliance with Federal Regulations," *American Journal of Hospital Pharmacy* 32 (September 1975):905–08.

2. Devenport, J. K., and Kane, R. L. "The Role of the Clinical Pharmacist on a Nursing Home Care Team," *Drug Intelligence & Clinical Pharmacy* 10 (May 1976):268–71.

3. Kidder, S. W. "The Pharmacist's Responsibilities in Skilled Nursing Facilities," *Hospital Pharmacy* 12 (November 1977):547–50.

4. McKenzie, M. W., Pevonka, M. P., Stewart, R. B., Hood, J. C., and Kalman, S. H. "The Pharmacist's Involvement in the Long Term Care Facility," *J. Am. Pharm. Assoc.* NS 15 (January 1975):16–20.

5. Madaio, A., and Clarke, T. R. "Benefits of a Self-Medication Program in a Long Term Care Facility," *Hospital Pharmacy* 12 (February 1977):72–75.

RURAL AREA

50—Pharmacy Services in a Rural Community

W. Ray Burns

The Palmetto Family Health Care Center (PFHCC) is a rural health center located in an upper South Carolina community. As a non-profit organization, it was created in February 1976 to plan and develop health services for the Pacolet communities and surrounding areas. The 7,000 square feet in the facility are a result of local cooperation and participation. PFHCC resembles a private medical practice, but it is more comprehensive in that it affords patients the convenience of total primary care under one roof. Foremost in this concept is the development of an efficient, knowledgeable, and accessible family health team composed of individuals from the areas of medicine, nursing, dentistry, allied health, social work and pharmacy. The Center addresses itself to a broad scope of health care for patients that encompasses their physical, mental, and emotional well-being and growth.

The staff includes three family practice physicians, a family practice dentist, dental hygienist, health educator, nurse practitioner, administrative staff, other health-related supportive personnel, and a clinical pharmacist. This team provides a cooperative approach to the delivery of family health care. The pharmacist operates as a team member with special expertise in clinical pharmacy and serves with other team members in delivering comprehensive patient care. The pharmacist works on patient education, acute and chronic therapy compliance, monitoring chronic patients, calculating dosage, and screening for adverse reactions and drug interactions.

The family practice pharmacy, located in this innovative rural health center, employs five elements which Eckel suggested were necessary in an ambulatory setting:[1] (1) a restricted formulary; (2) an efficient drug purchasing system; (3) prepackaging of drugs in specific quantities; (4) utilization of the patient record as the dispensing order; and (5) an adequate record to assure patient compliance.

The Pharmacist's Professional Duties

The clinical pharmacist has a responsibility to both the patient and the physician. He tries to improve the delivery of health care to the patient and aids the physician in his continuing education and in planning therapy programs.

A drug history is taken when the patient arrives at the pharmacy consultation room. This history begins with the patient's profile card, a family medication record, which remains in the pharmacy and includes current medications, allergies, idiosyncracies and chronic diseases.

After the history is taken, the prescription

is reviewed by the pharmacist, who calculates the correct dose, the quantity required for treatment and the brand of the product to be used. The prescription is compared to the patient's profile card and screened for allergies, idiosyncracies and drug interactions. Next the prescription is reviewed with the patient. The patient is informed of the name and strength of the medication, the proper time of administration, the use and care of any special devices for its administration, products to avoid while on the medication, significant side effects, the length of time before results can be expected and the total length of treatment required.

After this step, the patient is given any printed information that is available to aid in understanding the diagnosis and the use of the medication. These aids are designed to improve patient compliance. Finally, questions are answered on the above information or any other factors important to the treatment experience. It is clearly defined that the pharmacist is involved with the education of the patient through the consultation process.

The pharmacist also has responsibilities to the physician. These include drug and poison information, drug calculations, product evaluations, product identification, the monitoring of hypertensive patients through monthly blood pressure checks and checks on compliance, follow-up on acutely ill patients, and follow-up on physician interpretation of cultures to ensure that the patient was maintained on the proper medication as indicated by culture and sensitivity tests.

To enable the pharmacist to provide these services, a library of pharmacy and medical textbooks is located in the health center. If information cannot be found from these sources, a cooperative program with a local hospital and the Medical University of South Carolina in Charleston can be utilized to obtain information through literature searches.

The pharmacist manages two follow-up programs in order to enhance patient compliance. The patient has the choice of having his medications filled in the Center or of taking them to another pharmacy. If the patient chooses to have the prescriptions filled at the Center, the pharmacy technician prepares the medication and the clinical pharmacist dispenses it.

The Pharmacy

The Pharmacy has three basic components: the consultation room, the dispensing area and the waiting room. A consultation room is used to counsel the patients in a pleasant, comfortable surrounding. The dispensing area resembles a professional pharmacy in which the medications are stored and prepared for dispensing. The waiting area is part of the Health Center's community waiting room. The entire pharmacy area consists of less than 300 square feet.

Dispensing of Medications

Dispensing a patient's medication at the Center has the following advantages:

1. *Convenience to the patient.* This feature allows patients to tend to the majority of their health needs, including prescriptions, without having to drive to several different locations for services.

2. *Savings to the patient.* The physicians follow a formulary which allows the pharmacy to purchase on volume contracts, thus obtaining discounts which are passed along to the patient. Also, all medications are dispensed at the cost of the medication plus a professional fee.

3. *Improvement in compliance.* The patient has a very good understanding of why he or she is taking the medication and what is expected of him or her from the physician and the pharmacist; the patient is more apt to follow any directions fully, thereby improving compliance.

4. *Assurance of a quality product.* Each product selected for our formulary is re-

viewed by the pharmacist for problems in bioavailability and for acceptance by the patient. The cost, dosage form and schedule are considered in the assessment of patient acceptance.

5. *Communication between pharmacist and physician.* Any question regarding a patient's medication can be resolved quickly and efficiently by both physician and pharmacist working in the same office.

Discussion

This role model for pharmacy services has been well received by the community, both in the professional and private sectors. The practice setting allows the clinical pharmacist and the other team members to interact in the treatment program of a patient and his family. It allows the pharmacist and physician to become integral parts of the health care team. The physician, amidst the complexities of therapeutics, has a close working ally in the pharmacist. The uniqueness of the system allows the pharmacist to concentrate on drug education and consultation, and rewards him for the time spent which is not directly related to the dispensing activity. The income for this consultation is derived directly from patient receipts whether the patient gets the prescription filled at the Health Center or not. For each visit to the Center, the patient is charged the Center fee. For this charge, the patient receives physician services and pharmacist consultation along with the health education services of a nurse practitioner. The consultation fee for the pharmacist services enables the pharmacist's salary to be based upon his availability to the patient and the physician, and not on how many prescriptions are filled.

This family practice pharmacy program is unique because it is located in a rural community. However, two other South Carolina pharmacists, Dr. Rick G. Schnantz, Florence Family Practice Center, Florence, and Dr. Robert E. Davis, Lexington Family Practice Center, Lexington, operate similar programs in their respective communities.

Reference

1. Eckel, F. "Community Oriented Pharmacy Services," *American Journal of Hospital Pharmacy* 30 (May 1973):425–27.

Readings for a Broader Perspective

1. Dolan, M. "Clinical Pharmacy in the Coal Fields," *American Pharmacy* NS 18 (January 1978):22–25, 38.
2. Dolan, M. "Primary Health Care in the Rural South," *American Pharmacy* NS 18 (October 1978):26–29.
3. Kurtzman, M., Heltzer, N., and Counts, R. "Model for the Development of Rural Pharmaceutical Services," *American Journal of Hospital Pharmacy* 34 (February 1977):163–67.
4. "Appalachian Practice—Rugged, Remote, and Rewarding," *Tomorrow's Pharmacist* 1 (December 1978/January 1979):4–6.

COMPUTERS IN PHARMACY

51—Computer Applications to Pharmacy Practice

Alan B. McKay and Thomas R. Sharpe

Picture, if you will, the community pharmacist of the not-too-distant future. The preponderance of his time is spent counseling with patients about various aspects of their health care. His daily activities are centered around a tastefully decorated patient counseling center which is readily accessible from the comfortable waiting area. Situated within easy reach are health information pamphlets, schedules for upcoming drug-related education programs, patient medication records and, at the pharmacist's side, a cathode ray terminal (CRT). The availability of the computer with its fantastic speed and vast storage capabilities has freed the pharmacist from many of the slow, repetitive chores that in the past effectively prevented him from assuming a true clinical role. The computer handles all of the information associated with prescriptions with computer speed, accuracy and versatility. When information for a new prescription is entered, the computer checks the patient's profile for possible drug interactions and allergic reactions; adds the new prescription to the profile; corrects the current store inventory for the dispensed prescription and automatically prices the prescription. Information such as drug-drug interactions, drug aller-

gies and contraindications and patient instructions appear on the computer terminal at the pharmacist's side, thus enabling him to evaluate and interpret possible problems and to counsel the patient on the appropriate way to take his medications.

Innovations as dramatic as computerization of community pharmacy operations are not without problems. One major barrier is the fear and distrust with which many individuals view computerization. Pharmacists are often ill-at-ease discussing the possible computerization of their pharmacy operations for a number of reasons, not the least of which is concern for the high cost that may be involved. Many pharmacists are also concerned about loss of control over pharmacy operations and fear of being displaced by this highly efficient machine.

This last fear is basically unfounded, however. No doubt, the computer can store tremendous amounts of information. It can also retrieve this information at incredible speeds. Nevertheless, a computer **cannot** "think," nor can it make decisions by itself. What it **does** do, however, is to provide comprehensive information to the decision-maker very quickly. Thus it represents a very sophisticated tool, but **only** a tool. It provides **support** for the pharmacist's professional judgments, rather than subsuming them.

Health Applications of Computers

Indeed, computers and other information processing technologies are playing an increasingly important role in systematic delivery of health care. Much of the progress in computer applications has occurred in institutional and ambulatory hospital settings where computers have been used to perform a number of operations. These include:

1. Record-keeping, payroll, billing, and the ordering of drugs and supplies (these functions presently constitute 50 percent of present computer applications).
2. Recording and analyzing the results of health screening examinations to detect diseases that might otherwise go unnoticed.
3. Monitoring critically ill patients in surgery and intensive care units.
4. Recording and interpreting the results of electrocardiograms (ECG's).
5. Giving doctors almost instant access to laboratory test results.
6. History taking and appointment scheduling.

One area of major interest has been in the automation of various ancillary services such as laboratory, radiology and pharmacy. Computer services in clinical laboratories are now commonplace. Systems have been developed for pharmacy inventory control, label printing and other administrative tasks, usually as part of a larger, computer-based system. A number of systems presently under development would assist in the communication of orders from patient care areas to the pharmacy and then would perform drug interaction screening.

While hospital computer applications are becoming more commonplace, computer applications in community pharmacy settings are in a period of relative infancy. In the past couple of years several innovative approaches have been developed that will be touched on later in this paper. First it might be appropriate to give the reader a clear, if somewhat concise, idea of exactly what is involved in the computerization of pharmacy operations.

General Concepts

Two terms with which the reader should be familiar are "HARDWARE" and "SOFTWARE." We will discuss each briefly and relate them to judgments concerning automation of pharmacy operations.

HARDWARE—Basically hardware refers to the physical equipment used in a computer system. It is generally made up of Input Devices for introducing data for processing, Output Devices for printing processed information, Storage Units (or memory) and the "heart" of the system: the Central Processing Unit (CPU). It has been the decreasing costs of hardware and the increasing sophistication in the computer field that has allowed the introduction of computer applications at the community pharmacy level.

Hardware configurations may take two forms. One form is time sharing. With a time sharing system, a large number of users (community pharmacists or departments within a hospital, for example) are connected to a very large computer. Each user shares in both the use and cost of the computer. The time sharing system is the most efficient method where large numbers of individual terminals can be hooked into the computer. This is the method found most commonly in hospital settings. The major consideration in utilizing a time sharing system is the low cost of operation for the number of users served. Another consideration is the ease with which the program can be updated and the almost limitless storage capabilities. They are also very reliable, and good central maintenance can insure minimal "down time." The most obvious shortcoming is the high cost of establishing the system.

A second configuration is that of the mini-computer. A minicomputer is a very small (both in terms of physical size and the number of functions it can perform) computer which is solely dedicated to the limited needs of a single user. While this type of computer is extremely efficient, it lacks the versatility of the larger computers and the capability of linking a large number of users into an integrated information system.

SOFTWARE—Computer software is the collection of instructions and programs that "tells" the computer what operations to perform, where to store information or processed data and what information to produce upon demand. Generally the software program is unique for a particular computer system and reflects the needs of the individual user. They may be leased along with the hardware or created to meet the specific needs of the user.

Applications to Pharmacy

With this brief introduction into computerization in general, we can now turn to specific applications of the computer to the field of pharmacy.

In general, pharmacy computer operations have been limited to the hospital setting. Experience has been growing in this area and programs are now commercially available from several computer companies. Less development has occurred in community pharmacy applications; but several companies, as well as some educational institutions, have been involved in organizing computer systems with community pharmacy applications. Listed below are some of the applications that have been made of computer networks in existing pharmacy programs:

1. Patient Profiles
2. Preparation of prescription labels

3. Generation of lists of automatic stop orders (Hospital)
4. DEA and narcotic inventory control
5. Generation of nursing drug administration lists (Hospital)
6. Investigational drug control (Hospital)
7. Poison control information—toxicology
8. General drug information
9. Parenteral compatibility control (Hospital)
10. Drug maintenance control programs
11. Formulary control—Inventory control
12. Automatic dispensing of drugs
13. Drug-drug interactions
14. Drug-laboratory interactions
15. Drug-allergy control
16. Comprehensive drug utilization program
17. Billing (including Medicaid and third party)
18. Drug recalls
19. Patient instructions
20. Continuing education
21. Computer check of credit cards

One application of particular concern is drug interaction screening. It is a difficult and cumbersome task for a pharmacist to accurately review all medication profiles for drug interactions on a routine basis. Pharmacists in the past have attempted to meet this challenge by developing charts and card files specifically designed for the rapid retrieval of drug interaction information. However, this is an extremely time-consuming procedure. Often these systems are retrospective in review, rather than prospective in analysis. This problem has created a growing interest as well as a real need for more efficient methods designed to retrieve and utilize knowledge of documented drug-drug interactions. A computerized system is ideal for this purpose. Once a master list of interactions is developed for the computer and placed in its storage, the computer can automatically screen for potential interactions each time a new drug is entered into a patient's profile. When such an interaction is encountered it can warn the pharmacist, who will then take the appropriate action based on his professional judgment.

Another factor creating an interest in the area of drug interactions is the professional liability of the pharmacist and the physician. The failure to detect and/or avoid a serious harmful effect to the patient resulting from a drug-drug interaction may make the physician and pharmacist potentially liable for legal involvement. If reviewing a patient's medication profile is the duty of pharmacists in a particular locale, then this will undoubtedly become part of the legal standard in the care for patients throughout the country. When this is the standard of practice for pharmacists the consumer will expect the prudent pharmacist to perform this function regularly and accurately.

A Community Pharmacy Concept

With these general considerations of pharmacy computerization in mind, let's look at one specific example. In October of 1974 the University of South Carolina initiated a community pharmacy computer project that was headquartered at the Family Practice Center of the Medical Center. It was introduced as a test program to determine the feasibility of a computer network operating out of community pharmacies in the Charleston, South Carolina area. At about the same time interest developed in the Atlanta area among several community pharmacists and at Mercer University School of Pharmacy as to the feasibility of establishing an Atlanta Metro Community Pharmacy Computer Network. With the assistance and cooperation of the University of South Carolina a consulting firm was contracted to conduct a feasibility study and, upon its completion, twenty-nine community pharmacies agreed to participate in the System for five years. Working through the University of South Carolina, Mercer obtained consultant services and an option to use the software program that is presently being used in the Charleston project. Some of the features offered by the proposed Atlanta program include:

1. Profile system on each patient.
2. Automatic screening of each new pre-

scription for interactions and flagging the interaction for the pharmacist to interpret, as well as providing a short paragraph of explanation and citing references for the interaction.

3. Label generation for new prescriptions and refills.

4. Lists patients due for refills on a day-to-day basis to allow for patients on maintenance drugs who are overdue for refills to be contacted.

5. Provides patient instructions for each prescription filled.

6. Maintains up-to-date inventory on a per unit basis.

7. Inventory system will interface with wholesaler computer in some cases for simplified drug orders, or in all cases it will provide a daily printout of all drugs that fall below a present minimum for that store.

8. Provides Medicaid requests on a print-tape to be forwarded to the state Medicaid office. (In South Carolina the computer directly interfaces with the state Medicaid computer and can communicate Medicaid claims at night when the store is closed and demands on both computers are minimal.) Billing is then done on a weekly basis rather than the two to three month lag that exists in some states (and with **no paperwork involved**).

9. Toxicology information as well as immediate notification of drug recalls from the main computer, enabling an immediate and thorough screening of all patient profiles for patients on these drugs.

10. Continuing education on a Programmed Learning format available on request.

These are just a few of the features provided. Intangibles that have been mentioned by the pharmacists committed to the system include fear of the malpractice situation without the computer, competitive edge and the cost saving factor.

The Atlanta program will be purchasing the hardware for the pharmacies at cost of

$250,000 and it will be housed near the School of Pharmacy. Costs to the individual pharmacies will vary but the figure for an average pharmacy in the Atlanta Program has been quoted at approximately $450.00 per month. This figure is for a five year contract and includes services of the main computer and any updates on the program during the five year period. The cathode ray tube (CRT) and line printer may either be purchased or leased separately. Incidentally, the line printer will print out ready-to-mail bills on demand right in the pharmacy at a cost of 4 cents per patient plus postage. This includes two copies for the patient as well as one for the pharmacy.

Conclusions

Rapidly declining costs of the computer hardware and growing expertise in the community pharmacy setting are making the advent of the computer a matter of a few years at most. With this in mind, perhaps it is time for us to consider some of the possible effects on our profession.

The computer can free the pharmacist from many hours of repetitive, unproductive labors, and enable him to perform many professional services for his patients that now are provided in the very limited fashion dictated by the limitations of time. Computerization will give the pharmacist a comprehensive knowledge of the drugs in his inventory as well as pertinent information pertaining to drug utilization. This knowledge can give him an invaluable capability as a consultant to physicians on drug prescribing and toxic overdoses.

Perhaps more importantly, the computer can serve as a strong impetus to continued competence. For the first time continuing education can become a reality for the vast number of practicing pharmacists who rarely have time to participate in continuing education programs. Programmed learning sessions covering a large number of current pharmacy topics to be utilized by the pharmacist at his leisure, can be brought into the community pharmacy via the computer. Through the computer the pharmacist will be able to keep abreast of his rapidly changing profession. Just as the information concerning the drugs in his pharmacy are updated on the computer, so too will his expertise in dispensing those drugs.

Readings for a Broader Perspective

1. Lauer, J. "The Computer Can Be the Strongest Tool Ever Used by Practicing RPh's," *American Druggist* 177 (March 1978):50, 52.
2. O'Brien, T. E., Swihura, S. J., and Standish, E. L. "How We Computerized Our Unit-Dose Dispensing," *Pharmacy Times* 44 (November 1978):85–86.
3. "Computerized Systems Help RPh's Cope With Paperwork," *American Druggist* 179 (January 1979):40, 42.
4. Knight, J. R., and Conrad, W. F. "Review of Computer Applications in Hospital Pharmacy Practice," *American Journal of Hospital Pharmacy* 32 (February 1975):165–73.
5. Braunstein, M. L., and James, J. D. "A Computer Based System for Screening Outpatient Drug Utilization," *J. Am. Pharm. Assoc.* NS 16 (February 1976):82–85.
6. Pennebaker, G. "Calculated to Make a Molehill Out of a Mountain," *California Pharmacist* 24 (September 1977):20–25.
7. *American Pharmacy* NS 20 (March 1980): 44–47.

MINORITIES IN PHARMACY

52—Black Pharmacists in the U.S.
. . . How Their Status is Changing

Ira C. Robinson and Rosalyn C. King

America needs some 12,000 black pharmacists today in order to provide the manpower required to deliver a level of pharmaceutical services availability equal to the present capability for non-black communities. Yet, only some 2,000 black pharmacists were found to be available in the U.S., according to the most recent report of the Pharmacy Manpower Information Project.

On the surface, it appears that some significant degree of progress has been made in the direction of narrowing this gap between need and reality. Yet, a detailed analysis reveals that relative progress in providing additional black pharmacists and/or better integrating them into the mainstream of American pharmacy has fallen far below expectations.

Negligible numerical increases in black pharmacist manpower in the U.S. over the past decade have been inadequate to reflect a concomitant increase in the proportion of this minority group among the general pharmacist population. While there is evidence of a new kind of dedication to the task of increasing enrollment and graduation of black pharmacists by many of our pharmacy college deans, only the future will tell whether their dedication is matched with adequate understanding of the problem and directional intensity.

There are, however, several important ways in which the status of black pharmacists in America is changing. This report will briefly discuss these, and related problems, issues and needs which significantly impact on temporary and long-term progress in this vital area.

Background

During 1973, some seven states and the District of Columbia had 100 or more practicing black pharmacists within their boundaries. The states were California, Florida, Illinois, Michigan, New York, Ohio and Texas. While California claimed some 211 black pharmacists and Illinois claimed some 182, black pharmacists represented only 1.9 per cent and 3.3 per cent of the states' pharmacists, respectively. Approximately one-third or 150 of D.C.'s practicing pharmacists were black. It is interesting to note that three of the four predominantly black colleges of pharmacy are located within the seven jurisdictions in which the largest numbers of black pharmacists are located. Ten states shared the distinction of having five or fewer practicing black pharmacists within their boundaries, although the black populations in these states ranged as high as 350,000.

In general, black pharmacists have become assimilated into all facets, though not at all levels, of pharmacy practice in America. As is the case with the general pharmacist population, black practitioners are distributed by a vast majority in community practice with the next larger percentage concentrating in institutional practice. Beyond these two principal practice loci, black pharmacists are distributed in such small numbers as to be virtually non-existent either as employees or as employer/managers.

Community Practice

Within community pharmacy, chain store units have made remarkable inroads into our more rural communities as well as into our major urban centers. Within major urban centers, black pharmacists have been heavily recruited by the major pharmacy chains over the past five to 10 years. Simultaneously, there has been a steady decline in the number of black-owned independent community pharmacies.

The number of black-owned chains (three units or more) has increased minimally during this same time period. Actually, the relative size and percentage of chain operations owned by black pharmacists have actually diminished due largely to the lack of fiscal and management resources on the part of would-be black pharmacist entrepreneurs, as well as those already in operation, *and* to the proliferation of the more affluent multistore chains such as Walgreens, Eckerd, Peoples Drug, Drug Fair, Thrift Drugs. . . . Some of these are becoming well established in the more rural areas of states such as Florida.

To date, we have been able to identify some 10 black-owned pharmacy chains in the U.S.: Ar-Ex Pharmacies (four units),

Los Angeles, Calif.; Hilton Court Pharmacies, Inc. (four units), Baltimore, Md.; Jack's Apothecaries (four units), Houston, Tex.; Medic Drug Marts (three units), Atlanta, Ga.; Nelson's Prescription Laboratory (three units), Detroit, Mich.; Physicians' Drug Center, Inc. (three units), Detroit, Mich.; Prescription Arts Pharmacy (three units), Detroit, Mich.; Professional Pharmacy (three units), Washington, D.C.; Swain's Drugs, Inc. (four units), Chicago, Ill.; and Washington Park Pharmacies, Inc. (three units), Ft. Lauderdale, Fla.

Institutional Practice

For the purpose of this paper, *institutional practice* refers to the hospital or nursing home (extended care center, convalescent home) as the locus of practice. Then, among the 16,000 institutional practitioners in the U.S., approximately three per cent of 491 were found to be black. This indicates that the representation of this minority group in hospitals and nursing homes is greater than in the overall practice of pharmacy in this country.

Virtually half of our black institutional practitioners were found to be employed in private hospitals, approximately one-fifth in each of federal and non-federal governmental hospitals, and less than two per cent in nursing homes. While more than one-fourth of black pharmacists choose institutional pharmacy as a career, slightly more than one-seventh of the majority pharmacist population did so. There exist no current data to indicate positive change in this area over the past few years or so.

Industrial Pharmacy

In the industrial and wholesale pharmaceutical markets, black pharmacists have successfully scaled the economic barrier on few occasions. Earlier established industrial firms owned by blacks have collapsed within the past five to seven years in Washington, D.C., Atlanta, Philadelphia, and Los Angeles.

Coastal Pharmaceutical Co. of Norfolk, Va., appears to be the sole black-owned industrial pharmacy facility in operation in the U.S. today. While Coastal does no manufacturing itself, it distributes some 30 generic and specialty pharmaceutical products to retail and government markets.

Of those firms which folded within the past five to seven years, all were principally repackagers and distributors of products of contract manufacturers.

Two Washington, D.C.-area firms are presently in their initial stages of establishment. One of these intends to engage in extensive repackaging operations while the other plans the total manufacture of a limited line of generic and specialty therapeutic products, some repackaging and contract pharmaceutical research and development services. One suburban Maryland firm has engaged in its own research and development, production, marketing and distribution activities with cosmetics since 1977 under the principal ownership and management of a black pharmacist.

Drusupco of New Orleans represents the first broadline black-owned drug wholesaler in the U.S. Having become established over the past three years, Drusupco now distributes pharmaceutical products for some 40 of the major pharmaceutical manufacturers. Detroit has spawned the second black-owned and operated wholesale pharmacy firm, Midwest Wholesale Drug Co., which began its operations in 1976 with a single manufacturer's product line. It now represents some 25 of the nation's major manufacturers.

Government Scene

Of the 13 federal agencies relating to health, the Veterans Administration employs the largest number of pharmacists—1,300. Blacks comprise approximately seven per cent of this number. According to 1975 data, the U.S. Public Health Commissioned Corps employed some 345 pharmacists. It is estimated that about three per cent or 10 of these may be classified as minorities: four blacks, two Spanish-surnamed, three Orientals and one native American. The federal government employs some six percent of all practicing pharmacists.

While black pharmacists remain underrepresented in the federal government, several of these have attained middle to senior management positions in the Veterans Administration and in the Surgeon General's Office. For instance, Edgar Duncan, a pharmacist, served for several years as Assistant Surgeon General of the U.S. Another black pharmacist, Albert Bryant, serves in the Veterans Administration central office in Washington, D.C.

D.C. Leads

At the state level, the District of Columbia has without question led the nation in its appointment of black pharmacists to leadership positions on the board of pharmacy. The current D.C. Board of Pharmacy president and secretary are black, as have been the secretary and a majority of board members for many years.

States such as Florida, Illinois, Louisiana, Maryland, New York, North Carolina, Indiana, and Texas are among those to lead in accepting black pharmacists into what may be considered to be one of the last and strongest bastions of racial prejudice in modern pharmacy—the regulatory boards. In fact, several of these have elected or appointed blacks as presidents of their boards in the South: Florida (Monroe Mack, Tampa); Louisiana (James Wilson, New Orleans); and Texas (Albert Hopkins, Sr., Houston). Countering this degree of progress is the fact that the vast majority of states have no record of ever having had a black pharmacist sit on their regulatory boards. A black non-pharmacist has been appointed to the California board.

Associations

Mary M. Runge, the first black candidate for the presidency of the American Pharmaceutical Assn., has previously served as president of the California Pharmaceutical Association (CPhA). A community pharmacist in Oakland, Calif., Ms. Runge has also served as the first and only black member of the national accrediting body for pharmacy colleges, the American Council on Pharmaceutical Education.

Another black pharmacist, Byron Rumford, has previously served as vice speaker and parliamentarian of the APhA House of Delegates. The American Society of Hospital Pharmacists proved to be a leader in recognizing and accepting blacks when it selected Wendell T. Hill, Jr., Pharm.D., then of Michigan, as its president during 1972. Since 1972, the American Association of Colleges of Pharmacy (AACP) has elected Ira C. Robinson, one of the authors and then dean of the Howard University pharmacy college, to five consecutive terms as secretary-treasurer of its Council of Deans; and Patrick R. Wells, Ph.D., dean of the Texas Southern University pharmacy school, to its board of directors.

Own Groups

Black pharmacists, having been removed from the mainstream of political activity and professional recognition in the predominantly white professional associations, established their own national and local organizations. Among these is the National Pharmaceutical Association, formed out of desperation by a group of black pharmacists in 1947. This association indisputably serves definite social and educational needs of this minority pharmacist group. It publishes a quarterly journal and has an affiliated student group.

A more recent addition to the field is the National Pharmaceutical Foundation, organized in 1972. The Foundation was established to complement the activities of all existing local and national professional organizations in improving the access of blacks to opportunities in education, employment and entrepreneurship. With executive offices in Washington, D.C., NPF has sponsored two national conferences on the progress and problems of black pharmacists in America; and has more recently established a national clearinghouse on opportunities for minorities in pharmacy (Project C.H.O.M.P.).

By far the largest of the local or metropolitan black pharmacist organizations is the Chicago Pharmacists' Association, which boasts a membership of some 230. Other successful examples of such local organizations are the Central Los Angeles Pharmacists' Association, the Houston Pharmaceutical Association, the Detroit Pharmaceutical Association, the North New Jersey Pharmaceutical Association and the Progressive Pharmacists' Association of New Orleans.

Education

During the fall of 1977, a total of 3,002 minority pharmacy students were enrolled in the nation's colleges. Of these, 984 or 32.8 per cent were black. Of the 984 black pharmacy students enrolled, 533 or 54.2 per cent were located in the four predominantly black colleges—Florida A and M, Howard, Texas Southern and Xavier Universities. The majority of black pharmacy graduates continue to be produced by these four colleges.

During 1976–77, with 62 of the 72 accredited colleges of pharmacy reporting, 202 black Americans and 98 foreign blacks were graduated nationally at the baccalaureate level. Three black Americans and two foreign blacks completed programs of study for the Pharm.D. degree; no black Americans and two foreign blacks earned their master's degree; and two black Americans and three foreign blacks earned the Ph.D. degree during the 1976–77 fiscal year.

Master's

Florida A and M University initiated the offering of a master's degree program in pharmacology and Doctor of Pharmacy degree program during 1977. It stands alone among the predominantly black colleges of pharmacy in offering post-baccalaureate and graduate degree programs in pharmacy.

Unfortunately, neither of our black colleges offers graduate programs leading to the Ph.D. degree. These colleges have a special responsibility to provide such programs at the earliest possible moment, especially since one of the most serious deficiencies of current programs for the recruitment and retention of minorities in the health professions is the glaring absence of appropriate role models with whom aspiring young black health professionals can identify.

Problems

The stresses and strains of urban living are no better evident than in the practice of pharmacy in ghetto urban settings. Since a disproportionate number of black pharmacists practice in such settings, they are constantly beset with such problems. For example, they and fellow pharmacists in areas as widely separated as Watts in Los Angeles, Miami/Ft. Lauderdale, and New York City have had their business insurance cancelled or rendered possible only through payment of exorbitant fees, where available at all.

Intensifying the anguish and economic losses of these pharmacists are the periodic robberies to which they are frequently subjected. Many of their locations being in or near pockets of poverty-stricken Americans, these pharmacies are particularly vulnerable to wholesale shoplifting activity.

Black pharmacists seeking to begin or expand a community pharmacy, or wholesale or manufacturing operation face an almost insurmountable problem of lack of financial resources. Unfortunately, the U.S. Small Business Administration programs seem not to be there for the "small" businessman in that the agency normally requires a business history and/or a reasonable percentage of the total financial resources from the applicant. The vast majority of black pharmacists have neither.

Issues and Needs

It is evident that a significant "few of the few" have recently gotten into the mainstream and contributed to the leadership of our profession. This is a salute to the courage and stamina of these black pharmacists and to certain groups and individuals within the profession at large. It is also evident that the issues and problems facing black pharmacists may or may not face the majority pharmacy group, and when these are common to both groups, they may not assume the same priority interest among the former group. For instance, the absence of an organized national effort to assist black pharmacists in obtaining finances to enable them to establish or expand their own independent or chain pharmacy, wholesale or industrial operations must assume one of the highest levels of priority in the black pharmacist community. The matter of expanded national and local programs of financial assistance to enable aspiring young black pharmacists to enroll and complete pharmacy studies is among the most critical issues facing the future of the black pharmacist in America.

This is to say that all of the critical issues currently facing the profession of pharmacy must necessarily concern black pharmacists as well. However, for example, federal legislation which will assure adequate levels of financial aid to incoming minority pharmacy students must assume a higher level of priority among black pharmacists than the sexual make-up of the incoming student body.

Degrees

Whether a single degree or two different degrees is/are offered by the nation's colleges of pharmacy is considerably less salient than the relative static enrollment levels for black pharmacy students. The question as to whether there will be pharmacist reimbursement for services over and above the cost plus profit for the medication dispensed must be subordinated to the wider concern for the availability of the black pharmacist in today's and future medically underserved communities in America, in entrepreneurial/management positions in the wholesaling and pharmaceutical manufacturing industries, in senior management/executive levels in our federal governmental agencies, in leadership positions in our nation's professional associations, and in faculty and administrative positions.

All pharmacists are affected by the changing status of the black pharmacist in America. We must, therefore, all jointly seek effective solutions to the most critical issues facing this minority group.

Readings for a Broader Perspective

1. *National Pharmaceutical Association Journal*, various issues.

PROBLEMS AND ISSUES IN PHARMACY

53—Competency in Pharmacy: Where Are We?

Samuel H. Kalman

From all the clamor about the competency of pharmacists and the rush of the profession to do something about it, the public and government are apt to conclude that it is the pharmacist's competence which is solely responsible for the inadequacies in the medication system and the way in which drugs are used.

It goes without saying that the second party in the transaction, the patient, also must be held partly accountable for the widespread misuse of drugs. And in some instances, the third party, to the extent that insurance programs promote the misuse of drugs, should shoulder responsibility.

Further, it should be clear that the pharmacist's performance is not influenced solely by his competence. His actions cannot be judged independent of the many variables which make up the medication system.* The pharmacist may be supremely competent, but could perform poorly for a variety of reasons—fatigue, tension, pressure, just being too busy. Or, the observed lack of performance may be due to administrative/managerial/legislative decisions that impede appropriate service.

Concurrently, we cannot allow the consuming public to equate the poor state of its health to the delivery process. In a recent talk, Aaron Wildavsky[1] made the following statement: "Speaking of the delivery of health services is a fundamental misnomer, as if defining a (medical) process by its (health) purposes could, by some verbal sleight of hand, guarantee achievement. Health can be delivered only in small part; it must largely be lived. What can be delivered? Medical services and medicines, although, of course, that is no guarantee they will be used." Pharmacists are trained to provide services associated with the proper utilization of medications which are intended to *assist* the patient in getting well. This is far from delivering *health*.

If the competency of the pharmacist is to be put on the firing line, let's judge him on the functions which he should perform and for which he can be held uniquely accountable, not on outcomes which are, for the most part, beyond his control.

The pharmacist's competency is at issue when one is able to say that an action he takes to provide a service is inadequate and

* The term "medication system" here means the process which begins at the receipt of the prescription order and ends with dispensing of a drug and monitoring follow-up.

that the inadequacy is directly related to an absence of specific knowledge or skills. The knowledge and skills which the pharmacist should possess are those needed to perform, optimally, the functions which constitute the contemporary practice of pharmacy.

Defining Contemporary Practice

The American Pharmaceutical Association, jointly with the American Association of Colleges of Pharmacy (AACP), is conducting research to determine what constitutes the contemporary practice of pharmacy. Under contract, Educational Testing Service of Princeton, New Jersey has developed (with representative input from the profession) a comprehensive inventory of responsibilities of the pharmacist. At this writing, the inventory is being readied for sampling 5,000 pharmacists nationwide. This work will provide some insights into the basic service (functions) of pharmacy practice. At that point, acceptable ranges of performance, i.e., standards of practice, will need to be established. Based on these standards of practice, determinations will be made about the necessary knowledge, skills and abilities—competencies—which are requisite to providing acceptable, basic service.

It is important to understand that these criteria (functions or services) and their associated standards (allowed variance from criteria) will only cover basic or core functions. Individual practice settings (e.g., mental health institutions, IV additive programs in hospitals) often have unique characteristics. The pharmacist practicing in such settings will be looked to for pertinent services which, although specific to the setting, are still within the purview of pharmacists. These services, however, are not covered by the APhA/AACP research.

A recent issue of *The Internist* carries a short article entitled "Clarinetists, Carpenters, and Physicians." The opening paragraph reads: "The word 'incompetent' whether applied to a physician, a clarinetist, or a carpenter, implies that there are standards of competence to measure against. While this is clearly true for woodwinds and woodworking, it is not so in the case of medicine."[2] Nor is it the case for pharmacy until the earlier mentioned research is concluded and universally acceptable practice standards are adopted. Such practice standards are in the future.

What Can We Do Now?

What can the profession do now? Two things. The first is related to providing a means by which pharmacists may determine, on a personal level, where gaps exist in their knowledge and skills. The recent Boston study[3] reveals startling omissions of pharmacy service which comprise basic pharmacy tasks and are directly related to the pharmacist's knowledge: failing to check for penicillin allergy; failing to tell patients taking sulfisoxazole to ingest the medication with a full glass of water; failure to package and label medications in full compliance with state and federal law [among others]. These types of omissions cannot be tolerated. These tasks and services constitute the basic functions of the profession.

The second is to find out how patients form their opinion of pharmacy practice and either correct wrong perceptions or encourage pharmacists to begin to provide those services which patients feel are an integral part of the pharmacist's service: providing chairs for patients, being available for patient consultation [to name only a couple].*

In determining their individual educa-

* The School of Pharmacy, University of North Carolina, recently conducted a study[6] which found that patients place a high value on such amenities and view them as part of total pharmacy service. Patients consider both competency-related and noncompetency-related services in the same category. In effect, the pharmacist often may be judged as incompetent by failing to provide a service which is not at all related to his knowledge.

tional needs, pharmacists may seek out the resources of the colleges of pharmacy and the professional associations. Alan Knox has suggested[4] that continuing education personnel, who are located in the colleges of pharmacy and elsewhere, serve as "linkage-agents" between the learning resources and pharmacy practitioners, thereby facilitating the pharmacists' access to appropriate resources. In this regard, it is noted that many continuing education personnel are currently fulfilling this role.

Those responsible for educational activities should keep in mind the primary role of the pharmacist as it has been historically approached. In this regard, Margaret M. McCarron, in writing *An Approach to Clinical Pharmacy*,[5] provides some guidance: "The clinical pharmacist can help to define (his) role by understanding the problems that he is equipped to solve. He should not try to perform functions that are unrelated to his own professional skills and competencies. The logical role for him is in the area of his expertise—drugs, drug use, and drug information." Dr. McCarron ends her article by saying, "There are many problems related to drugs and drug therapy, and effective solutions are needed. Is it not reasonable to expect the pharmacist to truly *expand* his role, remain concerned with drugs and their use, and add a new dimension to patient care by developing programs to prevent problems related to drug therapy, prevent drug-induced illness, and help to improve the quality of drug therapy by application of modern drug knowledge to the daily care of patients?" Although Dr. McCarron may have had in mind those pharmacists who are being trained in more clinically oriented programs, the same "advice" holds for all pharmacists when the term "clinical" is used to mean *"patient-centered."*

Further, in searching out areas to keep pharmacists updated in their knowledge and skills, we should guard against the tendency to fall for the "new roles" syndrome. Today, with more frequency than ever, we hear about new roles for pharmacists. The push for new roles, many which are inappropriate for pharmacists, can have sorry effects for the profession. It causes an uneasiness in pharmacists who feel that they must begin to provide superfluous services to remain competitive; it creates confusing impressions about the pharmacist and obscures his key role; it wrongly ascribes titles to what are merely new opportunities and uses of technology to effect better practice. This is not to say, however, that innovative programs which are concerned with the unique role of pharmacists should not be supported.

A few words about our point number two—determining patient perceptions of pharmacy.

One of the best ways to find out how patients perceive the role of the pharmacist is to ask them. The North Carolina consumer study[6] used a questionnaire as a device to gain insight into pharmacy operations from the consumer's perspective. The self-administered, anonymous questionnaire asked questions about consumer receptivity and satisfaction with pharmaceutical service and its cost, pharmacy patronage motives, travel time and distance from the pharmacy, and certain demographic characteristics. The study was viewed overall "as a favorable device for offering comments on how to better the delivery of pharmaceutical service."

There is no doubt that the public's view of the pharmacist shapes its opinion of him and his services. This point is dramatized by the recent order to French pharmacies (by the Health Ministry) to stop selling such items as film, hair rollers, toys [and other items], "to prevent French pharmacies from deteriorating into novelty and notions supermarkets, as many in America have."[7]

In view of the foregoing, it seems appropriate to mention the current, highly successful program of the APhA Academy of Pharmacy Practice—"The Pharmacist, the Pharmacy, and Professional Body Language." This multi-media program (which was developed with the generous support of

Lederle Laboratories) is scheduled, at this writing, for presentation at ten state association meetings during 1977. It provides an opportunity for pharmacists to understand how their actions, those of their personnel and the nonverbal language of the pharmacy itself can have positive effects and create favorable public perceptions of pharmacy.

Where Are We?

In the fall of 1975, recognizing that practice standards were still in the future, the profession requested the American Council on Pharmaceutical Education (ACPE), as the nationally recognized accrediting agency in pharmacy, to accept responsibility for developing a program to assure quality in pharmaceutical continuing education. In accepting this responsibility, the Council recognized "that pharmacy is moving resolutely to more clearly defined practice standards, which, when adopted by the profession, will be used as the basis for determining criteria to measure the competence of pharmacists. When these practice standards are available, they may be used to develop additional criteria by which providers are recognized."[8]

However, it should not be inferred from the above that earned continuing education credit is equal to competence. The ACPE-CE provider approval program is in line with one of the recommendations contained in the *Final Report of the AACP/APhA Task Force on Continuing Competence in Pharmacy:*[9]

For the present and until additional methods of assuring continuing competence of pharmacists are developed, reliance should be placed on continuing education. In view of the need for this reliance for the indefinite future, imaginative and innovative programs of continuing education should be developed; and an effective organization for *and adequate financing of continuing education should be accorded a high priority.*

This recommendation is based on the assumption that, "Although participation in continuing education does not by itself automatically assure that the practitioner is thereby maintaining his competence, at this stage in the development of means to assure continuing competence it is the most effective method available by which the practitioner may update and enrich his qualifications."

This is where we are!

References

1. Wildavsky, A.: Can Health Be Planned? Or, Why Doctors Should Do Less And Patients Should Do More: Forecasting the Future of Health System Agencies, 1976 Michael M. Davis Lecture, University of Chicago (Apr. 23) 1976.
2. The examining room: clarinetists, carpenters, and physicians, *The Internist 17*: 16 (Sept.) 1976.
3. Massachusetts Consumers' Council: Cutting Corners at the Corner Drug Store: An Investigation of Pharmacy Practices in Greater Boston, Massachusetts Consumers' Council, 100 Cambridge Street, Boston, Massachusetts, 1976.
4. Knox, A. B.: Continuing education of pharmacists, *J. Am. Pharm. Assoc. NS 15*: 442–447 (Aug.) 1975.
5. McCarron, M. M., editor: Principles of Clinical Pharmacy Illustrated by Clinical Case Studies, Drug Intelligence Publications, Inc., Hamilton, Illinois 1976, p. 4.
6. Gagnon, J. P.: North Carolina Prescription Consumer Study, University of North Carolina School of Pharmacy, Chapel Hill, North Carolina 1976.
7. Shearer, L.: French druggists restricted, *The Washington Post Parade Magazine* Feb. 13, 1977.
8. American Council on Pharmaceutical Education, News Release, Oct. 28, 1975.
9. AACP/APhA Task Force on Continuing Competence in Pharmacy: Final report, the continuing competence of pharmacists, *J. Am. Pharm. Assoc. NS 15*: 432–437 (Aug.) 1975.

54—We Have The Capability To Do So Much More Than We Do!

Ricke D. Waldman

When offered the opportunity to write an article for the 40th birthday anniversary edition of the Nebraska MORTAR & PESTLE, my first reaction was that no one is going to want to hear my opinions of what I feel is the most important problem facing our profession. Our biggest problem, you see, is our own fault. I don't think the general public thinks we are any more professional than the grocer or the manager of the discount shopping center. This is because many pharmacists are not "professional" pharmacists.

Unfortunately, I think I am speaking of the majority when I say that our profession has talked about concern for health care and applying expertise in health care when the main concern has been financial gain. Of course I am not suggesting that pharmacists are overpaid but the tactics used by many so-called "professionals" to insure their salaries is far from professional practice.

I believe the almighty dollar (i.e. the Love of Money) has degraded the professionalism of Pharmacy to a critical low. I don't think we can be called a profession any more than the grocery business when a pharmacist will ignore or overlook regulations on refilling a penicillin prescription for a cold(??) because a patient "knows that it works" lest the patient go to another pharmacy the next time. That is not professionalism!!

Unfortunately, the medical profession is dictated by much the same philosophy and consequently the doctor passes the disease right on to the pharmacist. After all, it is tiring to hear the doctor or even a receptionist say time and time again, without much thought, "ya, go ahead and refill it!" without even considering the potential for misuse.

I am ashamed that we have allowed our profession to get to the point where we don't get paid for what we know and can do, or worse yet, for what we learned but have forgotten, all because we aren't expected to use the knowledge, don't have the time to use it or aren't allowed to use it. We are overpaid for what we do and the public knows it, but we are underpaid for what we **could** do!!

Our profession is now desperately trying to revive a dying horse that is infected with people who have allowed the $$ dollar sign $$ dictate their moral character. We see campaigns to improve the public image of our profession, when the public knows we aren't using the knowledge we have . . . properly!

I realize many pharmacists have been able to establish professional pharmacy service and have been successful, but the majority are more concerned about merchandising a product or just putting in their time and getting paid. I am very disillusioned by the meetings I attend because the speakers and the majority attending entertain with vulgar word usage and smoking cigarettes . . . a picture of the moral character and concern for health of our profession!

I am a pharmacist because I feel I have something to offer my patients by explaining to them how a medication can help them or how the medication can hurt them. I provide as much service as I can in the time I have available with the **patient's** welfare as first consideration. Everything else falls into place.

55—Understanding Pharmacy Manpower in Terms of Society's Needs

Donald A. Dee

Some pharmacy observers around the country may wonder—how can a state pharmaceutical association publicly criticize apparent excessive manpower production and simultaneously support a request for funding a new college of pharmacy building with an integral requirement for increased enrollment? The answer is that associations, like people, can be schizophrenic. Or, as one pharmacist has observed, "They just don't understand Minnesota politics!"

Or, maybe pharmacists don't really understand pharmacy manpower as it relates to society's needs. Does anyone?

The rumors run rampant. As a group of new applicants for pharmacy licensure conclude their board of pharmacy exams, some "jokingly" comment that they are looking for employment. A possible conclusion would be that of oversupply. Reality? In a short time, all are employed.

Some pharmacists are upset over the rapid increases in undergraduate enrollment since 1970. However, a closer analysis of the makeup of the enrollment produces some data that create uncertainties. For example, some college entering classes consist of 50 percent or more female students. Will the female pharmacy graduate of 1978 practice pharmacy on a full-time basis for 35 or 40 years as might be expected of the male graduate of 1955? With the societal changes that have taken place in recent years and appear to be still taking place, more and more women are opting for a lifelong career in their chosen field and an increasing number fall into the categories of breadwinner, head of the household or self-supporting single person.

Let's consider some figures other than data on female practice potential. Pharmacy is not the only profession to have experienced a significant enrollment increase in the past decade. Recent Department of HEW statistics on health manpower indicate that pharmacy has had an 80 percent increase between 1965 and 1975. In the same time frame, enrollment in medical schools has increased approximately 70 percent and in schools of osteopathy nearly 120 percent. Dentistry, nursing and other health professions have experienced a similar growth. However, that growth throws additional elements into the equation. In 1975, the ratio of physicians to population was approximately 160 per 100,000 population. Projections indicate that that number will increase to 200 by 1980 and to 240 by 1990. If the prescribing trends, which have been fairly constant since the end of World War II, remain constant through 1990, more and more prescribers are going to be writing more and more prescription orders. That will require more and more pharmacist dispensing, input, control, supervision, monitoring and informational services.

The current president of the Minnesota State Pharmaceutical Association has articulated MSPhA philosophy on the manpower situation. As a former member and president of the Minnesota State Board of Health, he also has commented on a number of occasions that the broad public health knowledge of the pharmacist should be brought to bear in a number of public health and administrative positions which previously have been filled by nonpharmacists. And that is precisely what is happening, perhaps because pharmacists' horizons are broader than before and perhaps because there are more pharmacy graduates looking for positions. In Minnesota alone, I would estimate that there are 75-100 positions which were not even in existence five years ago which are currently filled by pharmacists. Government positions such as the head of the health maintenance organization unit of the state health department and the head of the utilization review division within the state welfare department are examples. In the private sector, corporations providing consultant pharmacist services have been organized. Recently, pharmacists have also become involved in formal drug information services, poison control centers, and have increasing authority as therapeutic advisors and decision-makers. New roles for pharmacists are opening up and, therefore, traditional ratios of pharmacist/population do not apply when nontraditional functions are performed. Does under-employment represent the issue or should we be more concerned with underutilization of the pharmacist's talents and expertise?

Lest you be misled into thinking that pharmaceutical association executives are blessed with rose-colored glasses, let me express some other thoughts on the matter of pharmacy manpower.

No state pharmaceutical association represents graduates of only one college of pharmacy. In fact, I would guess that few, if any, state associations have even a majority of members who are graduates of a single college of pharmacy. Under those circumstances, it is politically hazardous for any state association or its leadership to criticize a single college of pharmacy. On the other hand, if a pharmacy association—including national and local as well as state associations—detects a problem or a problem trend within the colleges of pharmacy, it is the responsibility of the association leadership to draw attention to the problem so that it can be solved. That can be done through any of several means. I prefer the most direct one—a face-to-face discussion between the association leadership and the dean and other faculty leadership of the college of pharmacy. We are fortunate in having that kind of a relationship in Minnesota even though both parties certainly reserve the right to disagree.

The rub comes when a college of pharmacy in an adjacent state is apparently producing pharmacists far in excess of the needs of that state. How proper is it for a pharmaceutical association in State A to be critical of manpower production in a college of pharmacy in State B? Especially when a sizable number of graduates of State B's college are members of State A's pharmaceutical association? Obviously, the pharmaceutical association in State B should be discussing that matter. So, the leadership of State A's association might well draw the problem to the attention of the leadership of the association in State B. When apparently nothing happens in the way of discussion, let alone resolution of the issue, State A could legitimately make use of the pharmacy press to let rank and file pharmacists on both sides of the state borders know of the situation.

How proper is it for a state to be training

more than ten times the number of pharmacists needed for its own attrition replacement? Has the quantity and quality of faculty improved proportionately to the quantity of students? Because of tuition reciprocity, I am aware that students in at least one state can attend a college of pharmacy in another state at approximately 40 percent of the tuition they would have to pay in their home state. Should a state subsidize the education of out-of-state students with no payback in sight?

Among the more galling observations I've heard in this entire subject area is that it is "insolent" for a pharmaceutical association to question the colleges regarding enrollment numbers. I feel it "insolent" for a representative of the American Association of Colleges of Pharmacy to call an association of pharmacists "insolent" for merely suggesting that colleges reassess their recruiting and enrollment activities. If pharmacy associations won't raise questions in this area, who will? The answer is that no one else will, until individual pharmacists tell their state and federal legislators that governmental subsidy must cease until more opportunities are available. Those legislators, looking at governmental appropriations, would then force program cutbacks.

Then there is a moral ethic which comes close to reconciling the immovable object and the unstoppable force. Is it ethical for a college of pharmacy to recruit and provide a talented young person with a pharmacy education if the opportunities for practicing that profession in the near future may be limited? Countering that question is the rhetorical question—Isn't it the responsibility of a college of pharmacy to offer interested and qualified students the *opportunity* to pursue the career education of that person's choice? That is an issue on which educators and practitioner-oriented associations might take different sides.

But a seeming excess of pharmacy manpower production is not going to be curtailed voluntarily by colleges of pharmacy,

nor are pharmaceutical associations going to create instant solutions to these long-range issues. Among the people we all need to inspire to create opportunities are those who are in college now or have recently graduated. I have had conversations with pharmacists who have said that they contacted every pharmacy in a given area only to find that there were no employment openings. When asked if they had considered any alternatives, they replied that they had not. To cite an example of pharmacists not considering other options, I am aware of an association which advertised in the public press for a health field association executive. They received nearly 100 responses—from teachers, social workers, insurance salesmen and people with a host of other backgrounds. In a discussion with me regarding pharmacy manpower, that association's chief executive expressed his dismay that not one pharmacist had applied. It would seem that we have not instilled into the fledgling pharmacist the concept of looking at a sufficiently broad number of options in addition to more traditional pharmacy activities.

I commented earlier on the potential value to a state in subsidizing the training of nonresident pharmacy students. Let's consider also the role of the state pharmaceutical association regarding state funding of a college. As capitation fees from the federal government diminish and disappear, the colleges once again become more reliant on state legislatures. While I would advocate a position of cooperation between state association and college administration, I would also observe that associations have more political clout and lobbying expertise than any college of pharmacy. The establishment of tuition fees, state appropriations to finance operational expenses, and voluntary contributions by alumni and friends of the college are all decided by organizations or individuals outside of the college. Associations can be helpful to a college in this regard. They can also severely harm a college if the adversary role is chosen. And I would choose the latter role only as a last-ditch resort.

I believe that mere disagreement on one issue with a college of pharmacy should not create a barrier for discussion on other topics. Associations need the colleges because without them, advancement of the profession would be extremely limited and slowed to the point where we would fall further and further behind the rapid changes taking place in health care delivery. It is the responsibility of the colleges, in addition to providing a quality professional education for future pharmacists, to probe new areas of activity, authority and responsibility for those pharmacists. It is the role of the association, as I see it, to oversee college activities and to provide a leash when the cry of academic freedom leads the college too far astray.

If these brief observations have caused you to reflect that health manpower in pharmacy is a complex issue, then I have accomplished my goal. Try answering my phone when a pharmacist calls saying he is concerned about excess manpower. Ask him to give you a listing of the names of pharmacists he knows are qualified, looking for a position and unable to find one. Chances are he can't name one. But the perception continues nonetheless.

And to show you how cyclical issues in pharmacy can be, I recently came across an article in the *Minnesota Pharmacist* reporting on a speech presented by APhA past president Max Eggleston at the University of Minnesota. The headline caught my attention. It read "Eggleston Says Proper Distribution of Pharmacists Would Solve Shortage." That was published in June 1969, less than seven years ago. It is quite possible that in fewer than seven more years, we will once again be concerned with manpower shortages, instead of a potential excess. The standards of measurement will need to change, however, to include the newer professional functions also being assumed by pharmacists. An understanding of the profession's resources, including manpower, is essential to develop those new measurement instruments.

56—Report of the Study Commission on Pharmacy, II: Pharmacy and the Pharmaceutical Industry

William A. Zellmer

In part, the Report of the Study Commission on Pharmacy[1] seems to be based on the premise that the pharmaceutical industry is a component of the profession of pharmacy.[a]

[a] For example, in its conception of pharmacy as a knowledge system (p 13), the Report includes the activities of the industry ("translates knowledge into technology, uses some knowledge to create prod-

Considering the historical development of pharmacy practice and the American drug industry,[2] and the number of pharmacists employed by the industry,[3] it is understandable why one might hold this viewpoint. In reality, however, pharmacy and the pharmaceutical industry are separate social institutions. As independent health professionals, pharmacists should think of their role as distinct from that of the industry, and they should be active in practicing and promoting this distinction. Further, this distinction must be understood by colleges of pharmacy—the primary audience of the Report of the Study Commission—because it has an obvious bearing on the training of future pharmacists.

Many pharmacists undoubtedly believe that their profession encompasses the pharmaceutical industry. It is not uncommon to encounter appeals to the "fraternal instincts" of pharmacists in arguments calling for their support of some political or economic position of the industry. On the other hand, some valid criticisms of drug companies are sometimes misapplied to the profession of pharmacy.[4]

A substantial portion of the general public believes that the pharmacist and the industry are closely aligned. For example, the Dichter study of consumer opinion showed:

> Fifty-two percent of the responses indicated the pharmicist to be most closely allied with the drug manufacturer, compared to 13% indicating alliance with the patient. It is clear that the pharmacist is seen as being more concerned with his source of supply than with his patients. The pharmacist is also perceived to be more closely allied with the drug manufacturer than with the physician (22%).[5]

The purpose of contemporary pharmacy is the advancement of rational drug therapy.

This purpose is incompatible with certain goals of the industry which include the promotion of drug product sales to generate profits and returns on investment. The patient-oriented roles to which pharmacy aspires (e.g., drug product selection, patient education and counseling, drug information services, management of drug therapy for chronic illnesses) require the pharmacist to be an independent practitioner. In order to establish and maintain his credibility, the pharmacist must be free from any hint of alliance with the manufacturers and distributors of drug products.

Of course, it is in the public interest for pharmacy and the industry to cooperate and work together, whenever possible, for the benefit of health care. But they must approach these interactions as independent forces, not as separate elements of a health profession.

The Report of the Study Commission on Pharmacy is correct when it says that "pharmacy should be defined basically as a system which renders a health service by concerning itself with knowledge about drugs and their effects upon man and animals."[6] But care must be taken to discriminate between the activities of drug manufacturers and the purview of the profession of pharmacy. The compounding of drug products is now largely a function of the industry. The techniques of compounding must still be taught in colleges of pharmacy because this skill will be needed for some time to come by general practitioners. But the in-depth knowledge needed for product formulation in industry and research centers should be taught as one of the differentiated roles discussed by the Study Commission. The primary objective of colleges of pharmacy must be to train patient-oriented pharmacists—pharmacists who can actively and independently pro-

ucts, devices, and instruments"). When the Report states, "a substantial share of the knowledge of pharmacy is translated into a product that is a drug," it places the functions of drug manufacturers within the walls of pharmacy. When it tabulates "the largest and most active" "associations and groups of pharmacists," the Report includes the Pharmaceutical Manufacturers Association (p 83–84).

mote rational drug therapy. The achievement of this objective will be hastened if we are careful not to confuse the pharmaceutical industry with the profession of pharmacy.

References

1. Study Commission on Pharmacy: *Pharmacists for the Future*. Health Administration Press, Ann Arbor, Michigan, 1975.

2. *Ibid*. p 10–11.
3. *Ibid*. p 17.
4. Burlage, H. M. and Burlage, R. K.: Wall i: profit product—"the noble exploiters," in *The four walls of pharmacy—professional power with and for the people*, Vantage Press, New York, New York, 1974, p 43–52.
5. Dichter Institute for Motivational Research, Inc.: *Communicating the value of comprehensive pharmaceutical services to the consumer*, American Pharmaceutical Association, Washington, D.C., 1973, p 26.
6. Study Commission on Pharmacy, *op cit*, p 14.

57—Magnifying the Impact of Clinical Practice by Automated Drug Reviews

Martin Jinks and Joseph L. Hirschman

Introduction

Because of recent advancements in automated drug utilization review (DUR), and due to the general unfamiliarity of most clinical practitioners with computer technology and third-party administrators, this thesis will be approached from an elementary perspective. The discussion will begin with an overview of the present status of DUR in ambulatory patients and will then focus on the growth of Medicaid drug benefit programs and the related emergence of private companies which administer these programs utilizing automated DUR techniques. A brief review of the levels of automated DUR will be included. Finally, arguments expounding the future potential role of clinically trained pharmacists in this "business" setting will be presented, with emphasis on the significant impact such specialists can have on patient care. In short, the authors wish to share their experience and to proselytize to the pharmacy profession the advancing opportunity for clinical pharmacists in an evolving health care environment.

Drug Utilization Review in Ambulatory Populations

Achieving effective DUR in ambulatory patient populations presents a special problem. Due to a lack of institutionalization, pharmaceutical services are fragmented among a multitude of providers. There exists no organized, centralized medical data collection system linking pharmaceutical services from multiple providers, i.e., pharmacist(s) and physician(s), to the individual patient. The absence of comprehensive tracking capability severely limits the ability to focus clearly on drug use problems in ambulant patients. Even simple DUR tools, such as drug profiles, are relatively useless. They are maintained by less than 50 percent of community pharmacies. Even more disconcerting, Nelson et al.[1] showed that only one of 48 pharmacists who maintained profiles identified a well-known drug interaction when serially presented with the prescriptions for entry onto the drug profile. This may indicate that even when the manual data collection system functions, community pharmacists are too busy, unknowledgeable or unwilling to intervene when common problems arise, and that even under ideal conditions, problem detection and monitoring could be improved. When one also considers that patients obtain prescriptions or medications from several different providers, a practice that renders many conscientiously maintained profiles incomplete, it is safe to say that neither physician nor pharmacist could accurately specify a given ambulant patient's current drug use patterns with certainty.

The status of cross-sectional ambulatory patient DUR is presently a limited one due to the fragmentation of services and information. Current DUR in ambulatory settings consists mainly of the inspection of each individual prescription by a pharmacist, who ascertains that the prescription meets legal standards, is accurate, and contains minimum accounting information. In this manual review system, standards of service are determined by legal regulation, and the pattern of drug usage observed does not go beyond each prescription being filled.

Some commercially available electronic data processing (EDP) systems that function as patient profile systems have become available to pharmacists recently. These have the added advantages of speed, accuracy and automated drug use problem identification, such as potential drug interactions. However, these EDP systems share the limitations of manual systems in that they are incomplete when patients utilize services from multiple providers.

In recent years, a most important incentive has nudged providers of pharmaceutical services toward responding to the challenge of DUR. At present, 25 percent of recipients of health care are covered by Medicaid programs, and these recipients consume over one-third of all health services. Over 10 percent ($11 billion per year) of total health care expenditures are for drugs.[2] It soon became clear to those in government that because a growing share of costs of pharmaceutical services is being derived from tax dollars, they had a responsibility to hold down costs. The pressures of great numbers of eligible recipients and huge volumes of prescription claims requiring processing have led to the creation and growth of new specialists in the health care industry, mainly corporations and state agencies which combine EDP expertise with knowledge of the health care and drug delivery systems. State agencies either administer the disbursement of Medicaid drug benefits directly or they contract with private companies to serve as the fiscal liaison (i.e., claims processor) between state government and pharmacy providers. Private companies possessing these collective resources are known as fiscal intermediaries (FIs). The level of participation of FIs in DUR and other program monitoring ranges from little involvement other than claims processing, to sophisticated computerized reporting and consulting with state agencies, to total FI responsibility for DUR and peer review support. FIs are most commonly reimbursed on a "fee per claim processed" basis, but other arrangements, such as fixed price contracts, have been tried. The relative merits of these contracts and arrangements have significant implications for DUR and are worthy of extended discussion in a separate paper.

Drug Utilization Review by the Fiscal Intermediary

Almost all ongoing, broad-population DUR in ambulatory patients has evolved within the fiscal intermediary context. The basic function of the FI is to screen drug claims for government or commercial drug benefit programs. This involves editing the claim (prescription) for accuracy of information, auditing the claim for recipient eligibility, checking for duplications and appropriate billing, and reimbursing the provider. Obviously, EDP capability is a prerequisite to performing these functions. This basic DUR activity, performed routinely by FIs, is called "claims review."

The impact of smoothly operating "claims review" as a program control quickly reaches a plateau, since it only addresses the clerical aspects of filling out a claim. This limitation has stimulated FIs, either independently or at the behest of contracting state agencies, to exploit the unique data collection opportunities available for computer manipulation in a Medicaid program. Unlike the individual pharmacist's profile, the computer profile of a Medicaid recipient is a virtual mirror of all pharmaceutical services obtained and all providers involved. Exact products and dates of services are included. In addition, summation of group statistics by recipient, provider and drug therapeutic class are easily compiled through automated assimilation of claims (i.e., prescription) data.

Thus in addition to claims review, administrative screening review and professional review mechanisms were devised to control drug use and costs in Medicaid programs. Administrative screening review involves looking at specified quantitative criteria, such as limits on total dollars per month, total claims per month, claims within the same therapeutic class per month. number of providers per month. . . . Patient profiles which exceed a given limit are then forwarded for professional review. Professional review is performed by staff professionals hired by the FI to render opinions on Medicaid claims which fail administrative criteria. Professional review also incorporates the use of professionals to establish fixed criteria, such as upper dose limits on duration of therapy for a given drug. These fixed criteria become predetermined measures against which existing drug use rates and costs are compared. Professional review has a disadvantage in that no attempt is made to determine local standards of practice, and it does not include program providers in the decision making process.

The final mechanism for DUR found in a few FI drug programs is peer review. Laventurier defines peer review as "a hierarchical system of specialists (e.g., pharmacists) who study data, investigate professional patterns which vary from the usual, and communicate the results of their investigation and recommendations to their peers with the view of sharing valuable information about the health status of the community, and of individual patients."[3] This definition applies, of course, to all utilization review and not only DUR. Very importantly, peer review is conducted by committees of *local* professionals who *provide services* to the drug program whose practitioners are being reviewed. Criteria setting and control by local providers of pharmaceutical services, rather than by FI staff, differentiates peer review from professional review.

The peer review mechanism is most appropriate for monitoring quality issues, i.e., rational prescribing and dispensing. So called "quality" DUR problems exist because they are usually in the "gray areas" of prescribing and subject to local standards. For example, one committee may choose to review long-term antiparkinson agents which are routinely prescribed with antipsychotics prophylactically to treat extrapyramidal side effects, while another committee may feel more comfortable reviewing only long-term, prophylactic antiparkinson agents in patients receiving a combination of phenothiazines and tricyclic antidepressants. While both cases are legitimate review areas, the latter is easier to defend, to document, and perhaps to change prescriber behavior. It is extremely important to recognize that, because of limited legal power to act, the main recourse of the FI to improve Medicaid drug use with regard to quality issues, other than arbitrary limits, is to communicate with, and educate, the provider(s) through peer review decisions.

The Drug Utilization Review Specialist—Ambulatory Clinical Pharmacy on a Grand Scale

In ambulatory populations, the impact of clinically trained pharmacists has produced hardly a ripple in changing patient expectations, irrational prescribing habits, drug interaction and adverse drug reaction prevention, and improving patient compliance. The problem remains that the pharmacists in the community who dispense, and physicians who prescribe, are forced to make drug-related decisions in the absence of a total patient drug history. Even when clinical pharmacists do work closely with patients and/or prescribers in the clinic or in community practice, their impact is limited to the relatively small number of patients within their sphere of influence.

The advancement of EDP techniques and the unique position of the FI has opened up new opportunities for clinical pharmacy

specialists in ambulatory patient care. Patients who receive care in third-party financed drug programs are in a closed system, that is, the automated claims processing system allows health practitioners access to the total drug history of any program recipient. Because of EDP technology, the last major hurdle to effective ambulatory DUR, namely the incomplete drug history, has been minimized. Problems remain, of course, with unsupervised OTC drug use or in the rare instance when Medicaid patients purchase drugs from private resources. Nevertheless, the potential for broad impact on drug utilization patterns of ambulatory patients is greatly enhanced. Considering the fact that large state Medicaid programs may have over one million recipients eligible for drug services, that several hundred thousand patients may utilize the program each month, and that every single patient profile history is reviewed electronically every month, the impact of computerized DUR is indeed on a grand scale!

Given an idealized system of automated data collection with sufficient administrative and professional support, what specifically would the role of the clinically trained pharmacist (let's call him a "DUR specialist") be in ambulatory patient DUR?

Professional Review

Without a peer review network, there are three major areas in which a DUR specialist, working on the FI staff, can contribute to a professional review level of DUR: (1) problem identification, (2) criteria setting, and (3) program evaluation and integrity.

Regarding problem identification, the DUR specialist utilizes the broad-based data collected to examine rates, trends and costs of drug use patterns. Overutilization patterns (e.g., patients obtaining excessive amounts of narcotic analgesics) and underutilization patterns (e.g., patients not complying with an established antihypertensive regimen) can be identified, and computer techniques devised to isolate problem patients and/or providers.

Criteria setting is a second major area of contribution. It provides a mechanism to detect, without prejudice, cases of suspected drug misuse. Criteria attach value judgments to the drug data and represent what their developers think are optimal use patterns. For example, the DUR specialist may determine that the utilization of a barbiturate hypnotic daily for more than two months, or the chronic use of liquid concentrate antipsychotics in patients concurrently taking oral solid dosage forms, is inappropriate and requires a computer patient profile to be generated for review. The DUR specialist may also establish the automatic generation of profiles for those physicians who routinely prescribe daily, long-term (e.g., more than six months) antianxiety drugs to an exceptionally high percent of patients compared to his or her peers. Once a profile is generated from this criteria, the profile is reviewed by the DUR specialist and the providers contacted when appropriate. The intervention process involves an explanation to the provider of the perceived problem and a credible defense of the DUR specialist's contentions, through literature documentation, cost comparisons [and other means].

Criteria effectiveness must be constantly monitored, and thus evaluation and maintenance of program integrity is a third major function of the DUR specialist. Follow-up on individual patients whose medication use has caused definitive DUR action will demonstrate whether desirable change in patient, pharmacist, or physician behavior has resulted. Computerized summation of total program utilization also assists the DUR specialist in tracking outcomes related to problem solving efforts within specified drug or therapeutic classes. Tracking these impacts is also important because EDP is expensive, and specific DUR activities must be carefully selected with cost/patient benefit in mind. Problem areas which are marginal or intractable should be given low priority, and acute quality of care or economic problems should receive concentrated effort. The pharmacist DUR specialist has perhaps the best perspective of any health professional to select these high impact, drug use problem areas. Finally, the DUR specialist has a responsibility to temper any overzealousness of nonpharmacist staff who attempt to apply cost-saving DUR techniques that are not in the best interests of the program recipients.

Peer Review

In the presence of a peer review network, the role of the DUR specialist is greatly expanded. First, he acts as a stimulus for establishing local criteria. This is done by alerting the peer review committee (PRC) members to computer identified and selected drug use problems, and requesting that the PRCs establish criteria to address these problems. The criteria setting process can be facilitated by the DUR specialist supplying guidelines, based on experience and literature documentation, for the PRCs to base DUR decisions upon. The DUR specialist may even conduct seminars or utilize other educational tactics to bring PRC members up to date in state-of-the-art therapeutics. The PRCs may accept, modify, or reject the guidelines according to local standards of practice and perceived ability to effect change in the "gray areas" of therapeutics. To many, adapting therapeutic guidelines to accommodate local standards is an inversion of the ideal process, but the approach is a pragmatic deference to the forces to resist change within the current ambulatory drug use environment.

Once criteria are established by the PRC, the DUR specialist continues to act as a drug information resource, providing support material to the PRCs. The support material documents recommendations of the PRCs in their communications with program providers after criteria are deviated from and a patient profile generated.

Well informed committees are essential to effective peer review, because their power to act is limited to informing and educating providers. A key effort of the DUR specialist is the provision of ongoing contining education to the PRCs, and to all program providers, through newsletters, presentations and other media. Community practitioners serving as PRC members often lack confidence in their knowledge of therapeutics and feel insecure in making DUR decisions without continual reinforcement for, and documentation of, their problem solving activities.

Drug Utilization Review Deficiencies and Future Needs

Before concluding, some deficiencies and future needs relating to clinical pharmacy activity in ambulatory patient DUR by FIs deserve mention. Perhaps the greatest deficiency of ambulatory population DUR conducted by FIs is that most FIs are either drug program specialists or administer drug programs in isolation from other services. Therefore, they do not have access to total patient information, such as diagnoses, procedure outcomes, etc. There are a number of barriers to obtaining complete information, not the least of which is the issue of patient and provider confidentiality. Comprehensive automated programs exist, notably the federally specified Medicaid Management Information System (MMIS), which capture total patient information. Portions of MMIS collect drug data suitable for DUR purposes, but DUR reporting at the individual ambulatory patient level is uncommon in MMIS due to the technical expense and the lack of clear evidence of improved cost-benefit. However, it is illogical to separate review of pharmaceutical services from other services, and a trend towards requiring comprehensive DUR in third-party programs that includes drug use data is gaining momentum. The implications and challenges for the

DUR specialist in a reporting system which includes not only drug history but also total diagnostic and laboratory information, are enormous. Indeed, this capability is a prerequisite for meaningful, broad based outcome measurements of ambulatory DUR impact.

A related future need is to look critically at automated DUR by FIs to determine cost-effectiveness. Some literature exists pertaining specifically to DUR by FIs in Medicaid drug benefit programs, and the information indicates significant dollar savings.[4] However, the methodology and statistical treatment of these data is questionable, and further study is needed to corroborate the evidence.

A major deficiency with this form of pharmacy practice is that it is entirely retrospective in nature. Intervention is after the fact, whereas clinical or community pharmacy is often prospective and preventive. However, given that retrospective DUR identifies and reduces problems of drug misuse, it can be considered to have preventive features also.

Thirdly, DUR specialists with clinical practice experience will find a void in patient contact in the FI environment. Despite knowing there is great potential for impacting significantly on improving patient care, the lack of feedback from the recipients of one's efforts is a real problem.

Finally, because pharmacy revenues are related to volume of prescriptions dispensed, a conflict of interest exists within the pharmacy profession in the performance of peer review functions. Effective DUR results in an overall reduction, or at least change, in drug use. Since community practitioners are reimbursed a "dispensing" fee, the question arises whether pharmacists will ever become fully committed to peer review (i.e., reduced income often) as long as this reimbursement model exists. Not until pharmacists are paid *not* to dispense inappropriate medications will the pharmacist-entrepreneur wholeheartedly become involved in the many marginal areas of drug therapeutics. To date, pharmacists have enthusiastically participated in peer review, but one must wonder if, in the future, they will (or should) continue to contribute to peer review activities altruistically.

Summary

The high costs and rates of drug utilization in our society have been amply documented. The entry of government financing and the emergence of the fiscal intermediary to administer third-party drug programs attest to both a perceived need for cost controls and effective DUR.

DUR in ambulatory populations has been a particularly vexing problem because of the lack of a complete patient drug history and other data collection capabilities. The FI, using EDP technology, has been able to minimize this barrier to DUR data collection requirements in third-party environments.

In doing so, the FI has opened up significant opportunities for clinically trained pharmacists as therapeutic consultants. These DUR specialists function as FI staff persons to perform DUR tasks, such as drug use problem identification, criteria setting, program evaluation, and as a drug information resource to the peer review network.

References

1. Nelson, A. A. et al.: Evaluation of the Utilization of Medication Profiles, *Drug Intell. Clin. Pharm. 10*:274–281 (May) 1976.
2. Knoben, J. E.: Drug Utilization Review: Current Status and Relationship to Assuring Quality Medical Care, *Drug Intell. Clin. Pharm. 10*: 222–228 (Apr.) 1976.
3. Laventurier, M. F.: A Prototype Pharmacy Foundation Peer Review Program, *Calif. Pharm. 19*:36–38 (May) 1972.
4. Yarborough, F. F. and Laventurier, M. F.: Peer Review Works Via a Committee of Seven: Six Pharmacists Plus One Physician, *Pharm. Times 40*:58–63 (Mar.) 1974.

58—Why Today's MD's Have High Regard for Pharmacists

Karl Neumann

Physicians seem to be developing a new respect for pharmacists, an attitude that has been missing for a long time.

For many decades now, physicians have had the center stage in the health care field all to themselves. The limelight has shone on no one else. Much of the reason for this attention, almost adulation, that physicians have received from the public is as much the result of default by pharmacists, nurses and others, as anything the practicing physician did. For while medicine has made tremendous strides forward, the average physician in practice—the one the public comes in contact with—is hardly responsible for the progress. Yet, medicine somehow is full of smug, complacent physicians in practice, while pharmacy is crowded with individuals with professional inferiority complexes.

Treadmill. The great strides forward in pharmacology did not help the practicing pharmacist. In fact, it helped put him behind the eight ball. The new potent medications were produced in the laboratory. Unlike the physician, the average pharmacist became dissociated with the progress. For a time, pharmacists were on a treadmill, going nowhere, and, more recently, in a rut bemoaning their lack of progress. Somewhere along the line, as pharmacists are the first to admit, they, in their own eyes, lost much of their image of professionalism.

But all of this may be changing now.

Example. Recently, on rounds at a major New York teaching hospital, a group of physicians—several residents and four older physicians in their forties—were interrupted by a young man whose name plate said "pharmacist intern." He proceeded to point out that a medication that had just been added to a patient's IV bottle was incompatible with other substances in the bottle. The pharmacist intern backed his statement with hard facts and the bottle quickly came down.

The older physicians had never seen a pharmacist intern before and weren't sure where he had come from. But, they all agreed that they would be happy to see him around again.

Not isolated. A check of other physicians revealed that this was not at all an isolated incident. At more and more hospitals, pharmacists routinely check patients' charts for drug incompatibility, attend medical conferences and rounds, and carefully go over medications kept in wards. In one hospital, pharmacists make their own ward rounds and whenever physicians can, they

join the pharmacists. Much of the stiff formality of former years is gone.

In many hospitals, physicians, nurses and pharmacists are on a first name basis. Virtually all medical residents have kind words for pharmacists.

Outside hospitals, too, pharmacists seem to be assuming new roles. Young pharmacists, say several physicians, seem to be well versed in drug interactions and side effects. They seem more eager to ask patrons questions about medications they are taking, rather than wait for patrons to ask them. In some areas, pharmacy students have worked with physicians on community health programs—immunization, blood pressure testing, and others.

Better informed. Several physicians remarked that young pharmacists seem better informed and more eager to help. One doctor said that he is more prone to let pharmacists decide on drug therapy than he was in the past. Another physician felt that pharmacists are doing a better job in instructing patients than previously.

Physicians may have to move off center stage and make some room under the spotlight for the pharmacist.

Doctors queried at a pediatric convention not too long ago said that pharmacists seem to be challenging their prescriptions with increased frequency. With what appeared to be admiration for pharmacists, they noted that the latter are usually quite correct.

The doctors were especially impressed by pharmacists' knowledge about interactions and side effects, and by the patient profiles they maintain.

As pediatricians, they commented favorably about pharmacists alerting women to the dangers which ingested drugs may present to the developing fetus, or to the breast fed infant.

59—Drug Therapy in the Elderly: Is It All It Could Be?

James W. Cooper Jr.

Now that there is a legal mandate for pharmacists to provide consultant services to skilled nursing facility (SNF) patients, 78 percent of whom are over 65, it is time to review some of the research dealing with the elderly and to propose further areas of needed documentation. This paper focuses on the "real world" drug-related problems of the elderly in acute, long-term and ambulatory settings and documents solutions to these problems.

The need to move from crisis-oriented to prevention-oriented health care delivery leads to some searching questions: Is rational, economic and safe medication usage a reality for the elderly? Can we ascertain and affect the incidence of drug-related problems in the primary care population segment that uses more drugs per person than any other age group?

In our terminology, a drug-related problem may be defined as improper or inappropriate patient drug usage or an undesirable drug effect. Using this working definition, a review of some of the pertinent reports focusing on both the institutionalized and the ambulatory elderly patient may lend insight to the magnitude of the problem, to attempted and working solutions and to areas of needed research.

Rationality of 'Geripharmacotherapy'

While 84–87 percent of elderly ambulatory and 95 percent of institutionalized elderly patients are reported to be taking prescription drugs, in 100 consecutive nursing home admissions 64 percent of the patients' primary diagnoses were inaccurate; 84 percent of the secondary diagnoses were either lacking or inadequate.

The inadequate performance in identifying clinical and therapeutic problems of the chronically ill aged was remarkably consistent, regardless of whether patient referral was from a general or psychiatric hospital, the patient's home or another nursing home. If the pre-admission diagnosis is incorrect in so many patients admitted to long-term care facilities, how can the pre-admission drug therapy be rational?

Within nursing homes a recent report found that 25 percent of prescribed drugs were not considered effective or needed or given for their FDA-approved use. Another group found that the *least* mentally impaired and *most* physically active nursing patients were the most heavily "drugged" with neuroactive substances. A recent physician survey demonstrated generalized medical lack of interest in the care of ill aged patients in institutions.

Drug-prescribing patterns in a 250,000 patient SNF population were reported recently. At the same time a call went out for vigorous promotion of expanded pharmacist involvement in providing drug information and regimen review, as well as reasonable reimbursement for these services.

Response to Elderly Inpatient Needs

A manual system for drug utilization review of 10 most commonly used drugs in the SNF (amitriptyline hydrochloride, aspirin, chloral hydrate, chlordiazepoxide, digoxin, hydrochlorothiazide, methyldopa, milk of magnesia, nitroglycerin and thioridazine) has been published. For each drug a purpose for the review, assumptions, required data, data sources, criteria for use, possible problem areas, abstract form and supporting references are provided.

Professional associations have published monographs on long-term care facility pharmaceutical services and monitoring drug therapy, a manual for pharmacists providing drug information and inservice training and a workbook for development of a pharmacy policy and procedures manual for SNFs.

Numerous investigators have documented the effectiveness (cost and otherwise) of the consultant or clinical pharmacist in reducing the number of drugs per patient, adverse reactions, medication errors and cost and in improving pharmacist-physician communication as well as elderly patient status.

Patient Errors, Compliance and Education

Patient errors of commission and/or omission in the self-administration of drugs in ambulatory elderly patients are common. One report found that 59 percent of an elderly outpatient population with chronic illnesses made errors in the self-administration of prescribed medications and more than 25 percent committed potentially serious errors. In another study of ambulatory patients who self-administered drugs in an SNF and in a hospital a 60 percent error rate was seen in those who received drugs without instructions, whereas only a 2.3 percent error rate was seen in instructed patients.

The need for supervision of the elderly patient receiving long-term drug therapy was recently reemphasized in a study in which 20 percent of randomly selected elderly patients taking medications had no recorded contact with their physician for six months or longer. Another survey of elderly patients (conducted in their homes) found that many stored their drugs improperly, tended to hoard drugs and did not have enough explicit instructions regarding indications for taking the drugs. Although many drugs were obtained directly from pharmacists, their advice was rarely sought.

Adverse Reactions and Interactions

In patients more than 60–70 years old, the risk of drug reaction is 1.5 times that in adults 30–40 years old. The elderly have also been shown to have a higher frequency of hospital admissions due to adverse reactions than younger patients.

The most comprehensive study of inpatient drug use and adverse reactions is yielding published data concerning the relationship of age to hospitalized patient adverse reaction rate. A study of seven nursing homes found that almost 25 percent of the patients risked a potential drug interaction. With the pharmacist consultation, however, the incidence of adverse reactions and potential interactions in the elderly may be reduced. Probable digoxin toxicity was found to be decreased from 19 percent to 10 percent in elderly inpatients by pharmacist prediction of digoxin toxicity using pharmacokinetic principles.

Drug-Related Problems and Hospitalization

Looking at only adverse reactions and interactions appears to be merely the tip of the iceberg. Almost one third of the patients (65 or older) admitted to two small community hospitals were found to have drug-related problems that influenced their need for admission. Fully two thirds of the problems of these elderly patients were classified as *misuse* of drugs (poor compliance, covert multiprescriber usage, dietary indiscretion/ inadequacy with drug therapy and therapeutic ineffectiveness or inappropriateness of prescribed therapy). The remaining problems were caused by adverse response to preadmission drug therapy.

Why Patient Needs Are Not Met

We are just beginning to realize the scope of elderly patient problems with drug therapy. However, the problem of patient errors in self-administration of drugs was documented more than 15 years ago (1962). The lack of specific training in clinical pharmacology and geriatrics in many medical schools has brought specific recommendations from the American Geriatrics Society, and current health care legislation is addressing the lack of sufficient general clinical training in pharmacy schools.

That there is no specific accreditation requirement for geriatric experience in baccalaureate or PharmD programs is a paradox—the skilled nursing facility is the first area in which the clinical involvement of the pharmacist is mandated. Long-term care clinical education programs are expanding, however, in the nation's pharmacy schools.

The time lag in advancing medical science findings to the "standard of care" level for elderly patients is a further concern, e.g., predicting creatinine clearance and digitalis and aminoglycoside dose requirements based on the elderly patient's decreasing renal function.

We know very little about bioavailability in drugs in aged ill patients. Pharmacokinetic changes in distribution, metabolism and excretion are beginning to receive attention.

Today 90 percent of our elderly are out in the community. Planners should use the virtually untapped resources of the nation's pharmacists in planning elderly patient home health or day care pilot programs.

Future Service and Research

Specific questions need resolution. Can we affect planning and funding agency attitudes as well as practitioner attitudes toward the elderly patient's perceived or unrealized needs? Can the accuracy of diagnoses and subsequent rationality of "geripharmacotherapy" be improved? If therapeutic acumen is increased, can effective drug distribution, utilization and review be developed? Can the adverse reaction rate be affected in ambulatory and institutionalized elderly populations? Can elderly patient hospital admissions due to drug-related problems be reduced?

These questions are represented as a challenge to the health care professions to find meaningful solutions to the specific problems of our nation's elderly patients.

60—Third Party Prescription Programs—
A Pharmacist's Comparison

C. Morgan Jones

In its infancy, I viewed the dispensing of prescriptions paid in part or entirely by a third party as an occasional service extended to a few established customers. Times have changed however, and the past ten years have seen an increase in the number of patients desiring third party payment of prescriptions, resulting in an increase in the number of carriers handling these programs.

The dispensing fee has not increased much, if at all, in spite of the inflationary costs of filling a prescription. A $2.00 fee added to a 1977 ingredient cost certainly does not return the same percentage that a $2.00 fee did on a 1976 ingredient cost. The fact that there is less and less margin to work with is reflected by those that discount the co-pay. Ten years ago, a $2.00 co-pay was commonly reduced by as much as 25% to $1.50. Today, however, most large chains in the Columbus market are discounting the $2.00 or $3.00 co-pay by a mere 11¢. That is either a 5.5% or 3.7% discount. This token discount is no doubt extended to maintain a discount image.

My pharmacy is a 5,000 square foot, large-volume, general mix store located in a medium-sized suburban shopping center of nine businesses. The community is upper-middle class, white collar. It is primarily residential, consisting of single family homes with moderate concentration of apartments and condominiums interspersed. The following material is based on a careful review of my records for the nine month period, April 1976 through December 1976, and is summarized on Table 60.1.

Carriers

I am currently signed as a provider to five private carriers—Medi-Met, PCS (Pharmaceutical Card System, Inc.), Aetna, Blue Cross and PAID [Paid Prescription, Inc.]; and one government carrier—Veterans' Administration. Included in Table 60.1 is a second government carrier, Workers' Compensation. Effective September 1976 (halfway through this survey), I no longer accepted prescriptions billed to the Industrial Commission. My reason for discontinuing Workers' Compensation is the recent arbitrary nature of their decisions about which drugs would be covered. Also, they took longer than any other carrier for reimbursement. As an alternative, I bill the patient directly (my usual and customary charges) for the prescription and offer to supply and complete the required C-17 forms for the patient to submit himself.

My policy has been to provide every carrier dictated by the patients' needs. I have not been selective or critical as to which carriers I would provide. I have only been interested in becoming a provider to satisfy my goal of full service to all. The fact that two carriers, PCS and PAID, charge an annual fee did not deter me from applying as a provider, although I believe it is improper that the providers must underwrite a portion of the carrier's administrative expenses.

Total Number of Claims Submitted

Table 60.1 lists my seven carriers in decreasing order by the total number of pre-

Table 60.1

	Total number of claims submitted	Average number of days for payment	Number of claims increased/Total dollar increase	Average number of claims decreased/Total dollar decrease	Number of claims delayed	Average number of days delayed	Number of claims rejected	Average reimbursement per claim	Average co-pay per claim	Total reimbursement per claim
Medi-Met	451	20	1/1.00	56/$ 9.85	13	48	6	$ 4.79	$1.90	$ 6.69
PCS	384	22	12/$2.49	49/$12.06	23	52	6	$ 4.41	$1.50	$ 5.91
Aetna	297	35	4/$ .50	37/$10.49	7	86	0	$ 4.53	$2.00	$ 6.53
Blue-Cross	172	22	1/$ .05	1/$ .10	8	69	0	$ 4.55	$1.80	$ 6.35
PAID	141	40	0/0	101/$18.34	10	105	0	$ 5.92	$1.20	$ 7.12
Veterans' Administration	97	54	0/0	0/0	0	0	0	$ 9.06	0	$ 9.06
*Workers' Compensation	65	78	0/0	0/0	2*	?*	1	$12.68	0	$12.68

* Workers' Compensation includes only five months of activity, before I stopped accepting them. Within this time-span, there were two claims submitted which have not been paid as of 4/15/77. Overall, I have 14 claims amounting to $204.40 that have been outstanding for as long as three years.

scriptions submitted for payment in this nine month period. I filled a total of 1,607 third party prescriptions, which accounted for 5.7% of my total prescription volume.

Average Number of Days for Payment

I consider the length of time for payment to be from the day a batch of claims is mailed until the day a check is received. In reality, this time may be an additional thirty days because I bill once a month, and a claim may be generated just after a batch is processed. The table shows Medi-Met to be the fastest payer, while the Veterans' Administration takes almost three times as long.

Number of Claims Increased Per Total Dollar Increase

The number of claims in which payment increased from the time it was submitted, is small in number. I do my best to keep current with as many price changes as possible, keeping my mathematical errors to a minimum. The claims increased by Medi-Met, Aetna, Blue Cross and four by PCS, were due to my own mathematical errors—to the carrier's benefit. The carriers had been on the job, caught my errors and increased my payment. Payment by PCS was increased on eight claims due to price increases of the ingredients used, of which I was not aware. This leads me to believe that PCS maintains its own current price list and pays accordingly, regardless of the amount submitted.

Number of Claims Decreased Per Total Dollar Decrease

Medi-Met, PCS and Aetna all decreased about the same percentage of claims, anywhere from 12.4% to 12.8% of those submit-

ted. Of the 142 claims decreased by these three carriers, four were due to my mathematical errors and fourteen were instances where the carriers just were not keeping abreast with current prices. The other 124 were due to the fact that these carriers will not recognize (or are not capable of handling) the situation in the central Ohio market area, where the drug wholesalers are adding an additional 10–12% to the wholesale list price of federally controlled drugs. This is to account for their increased security and bookkeeping requirements.

The PAID situation is most perplexing. PAID has apparently negotiated a variety of contracts with program sponsors, possibly due to the competition from other carriers. PAID has six plans, three of which allow the provider to bill at average wholesale costs, and three which request billing at actual acquisition costs. Their manual also states that the pharmacist's dispensing fee varies with the state and the patient's employer. All of this results in much confusion on the pharmacist's part. PAID does not update or give ample information in their manual. Fortunately, the other carriers are more consistent and maintain readable manuals. The net result is that I am not sure what my acquisition cost or dispensing fee is on each claim. For this report I based the number of reductions upon an average wholesale cost with a $2.00 dispensing fee. Based upon this $2.00 dispensing fee, (which happens to be the lowest I know of by private carriers) they decreased payment on 72% of the claims submitted.

PAID has Group I and Group II providers. The Group I provider offers a minimum of services and has a dispensing fee of about $1.95 to $2.00. The Group II provider offers a variety of services such as patient records, patient consultation, longer hours, emergency service and delivery, and is therefore entitled to a higher fee of about $2.20. The provider must apply to be considered as a Group II provider, filling out a form giving details of services and samples of patient prescription records. When I originally applied to PAID as a provider, I requested Group II status. PAID accepted me as a Group I provider. I permitted this pass initially since my business with PAID was insignificant; but in January 1976, I applied for reclassification to Group II status. In May 1976 I was informed that I was accepted as a Group II provider, and would be receiving payment as such. This never developed. In December 1976, I wrote again noting that I had been accepted as a Group II provider but was not being paid as such. In response, they acknowledged receipt of all my former correspondence and said they would take steps to correct the error.

Only Aetna provides a form for the provider to contest the decreased reimbursement. This form, called NORAC (Notice of Reduced Acquisition Cost) can be filled out to substantiate the acquisition cost as originally submitted. Upon returning the NORAC with the next batch of claims, one should be reimbursed by the amount which was decreased. I have done this several times, but have never received the additional payment or acknowledgement that it was under consideration.

The reduced acquisition costs are more of a nuisance than an economic burden. It is not worth the time of researching my costs, xeroxing my invoices and mailing them to the carrier involved, in hopes of getting a few additional cents. I think the carriers realize this too.

Number of Claims Delayed

I had a total of 61 claims delayed. Of these 61 delays, thirteen were due to my error in completing the claim form and four were apparently caused by excessive charges for medication, since my reimbursement was reduced in each. The other 44 were paid as submitted. The majority of delayed claims were for reasons unknown to me. I assume it was either because the drug involved was relatively new, or there was a recent price change. In any case, the fact that so many claims were delayed is another nuisance. Compounded prescriptions, which do not have an NDC code and are not included in any list of legend drugs, totally baffle the carriers. This results in either a delay or rejection.

PCS and PAID delayed the highest percentage (6–7%). I attribute this to two areas. First, they have the most confusing forms to fill out (indeed, they were the only ones to be delayed because of improper completion of forms). Secondly, nothing can be omitted from the form. Patient's age, sex, drug name, NDC number, days supply, quantity and directions cannot be overlooked.

The new claim form of PAID allows for the entry of two claims on one form. However, when one claim is delayed on that form, the accompanying claim, even if acceptable, is also delayed. Hopefully, with the acceptance of the universal claim form on April 1, 1977, some of these problems will be eliminated.

Average Number of Days for Delayed Payment

I consider the length of time for delayed payment to be from the day the claim was originally mailed until the day it was finally paid. It is frustrating when it takes a minimum of seven weeks to receive payment, especially when that delay is not the pharmacist's fault.

Number of Claims Rejected

A total of twelve claims were rejected, all for valid reasons, according to the terms of the various contracts signed with the carriers. One must be on his toes at all times to prevent these rejections. Of the twelve, five were for prescriptions of non-legend drugs, three were for dispensing a quantity exceeding that which is permitted, three were for dispensing drugs not covered and one was because the dispensing date was in error (used the original date on a refill).

Dealing with five carriers and the myriad of plans of each, one is tempted to just dispense the 34-day supply to all and play it safe.

Norlutate is considered an oral contraceptive and cannot be covered regardless of use.

Average Reimbursement Per Claim

A total of $8,508.03 was received for 1,607 claims, for an average of $5.29 per claim.

Average Co-Pay Per Claim

Four of the carriers have various option plans, where the employees of different companies have co-pays ranging from $0.00 to $2.00. As an example, my PCS patients were 50% at $2.00 co-pay, 1% at $1.50 co-pay and 49% at $1.00 co-pay.

Total Reimbursement Per Claim

Considering both the carrier's reimbursement and the co-pay portion paid at the time of dispensing, the average price per third party prescription was $6.86. My average for *all* prescriptions dispensed (third party and self-pay) was $5.53. The preliminary 1976 Lilly Digest stated the average prescription price as $5.60. Three explanations for this apparent anomaly of $1.33 between third party and self-pay are: first, 9% of my prescriptions were for oral contraceptives at an average price of $2.60, considerably below the average for all other prescriptions. Since oral contraceptives are not paid by third parties, they are not calculated into the average third party prescription price, resulting in a higher average price for third party prescriptions. Secondly, patients know their privileges under the various programs and utilize

the maximum quantities available for a single co-pay. This results in a larger average prescription for those filled under third party programs. Thirdly, pharmacists are well aware that a justified and equitable dispensing fee would be in the $2.60 to $2.80 range. In a survey for the year of 1976, compiled early in 1977, my prescription costs yielded a $2.65 dispensing fee *not* including profit. No third party carrier presently begins to approach these needs.

Each and every third party prescription may not be billed to the carrier by an amount equivalent to my usual and customary charge to a self-pay patient. However, the charge realized from a third party prescription did not vary significantly from my usual and customary charge to a self-pay patient. To substantiate this, I sampled all of my Aetna prescriptions and found that 297 were dispensed for $1,938 or an average of $6.53 per prescription. If these same prescriptions had been dispensed to self-paying patients at usual and customary charges, they would have yielded $1,918, for an average of $6.46 per prescription.

Generalities

In one instance, Veterans' Administration took 142 days to pay a batch. After a telephone call, it was explained that the office was moving and my batch had been misplaced. On at least one occasion, Medi-Met paid for one batch before payment for an earlier batch was made. Blue Cross on one or two occasions, made payment for claims which I did not submit and did not belong to me. PCS mailed another pharmacy's check to me. Instances like these make one wonder what type of controls and work schedules these carriers maintain.

PAID, PCS and Blue Cross on occasion failed to acknowledge all claims submitted within a batch. Payment for the one or two strays always followed.

Medi-Met's payment voucher is quite easy

to read. I wish the others were equally decipherable.

PCS, on several occasions, sent back several forms that were supposedly in error, when actually there was nothing wrong. I noticed with several of the carriers that a claim may be delayed for a long period of time, when the exact claim for the refill will be paid routinely. Frequently the price on an original filling will be decreased, but on a claim for the refill it will be honored; when in both instances the acquisition cost was the same. This can only be an indication of the slowness by the carriers in concurring with the current costs.

Summary

It is frustrating that I am on the end of a one way street and cannot negotiate with a carrier. Instead I am offered a "take it or leave it" approach. The national average of third party prescriptions is 25%, with many providers filling 80% to 90%. Obviously, they are not in a position to "leave it." This view has been aired repeatedly by many pharmacists through the country, but at the risk of being redundant, my review of third parties would not be complete without mentioning this "thorn" in pharmacies' side.

In conclusion, I would hope that pharmacists throughout the state will be encouraged to evaluate their own data systematically. Have it in a ready, retrievable form so that when called upon—whether it be for an audit by the carrier, the signing of a new contract with a carrier, or at the request of the newly-formed OSPA committee on third party prescription programs, this information will be available.

61—The Potential Cost-Benefit of Drug Monitoring Services in Skilled Nursing Facilities

Pharmacist Review of Drug Regimens Can Reduce Costs, Improve Patient Care

Samuel W. Kidder

The performance of monthly drug regimen reviews by pharmacists in skilled nursing facilities can reduce costs through the reduction in average monthly prescription use, and through the reduction in hospitalizations resulting from adverse drug reactions. The reduction in prescription use alone could save Medicare and Medicaid from $3.2 million to $37.2 million per year. National hospital cost reductions resulting from adverse drug reactions in skilled nursing facilities are hard to estimate, but they do exist, and whatever their magnitude they are *in addition* to those resulting from reduction in prescription use. Both these cost reductions can be brought about while *improving* the quality of drug therapy in these facilities. Data to support each of these quality and cost assertions are presented below.

Prescription Reduction Effect

[Table 61.1] shows the reduction in unnecessary prescriptions that was brought about through the performance of drug regimen reviews by pharmacists in six different skilled nursing facility studies and one study of patients in an institution for the mentally retarded. It is important to note that these reductions were brought about as a result of recommendations by the pharmacist to attending physicians.

The prescription reduction effects cited in [Table 61.1] provide considerable evidence that drug regimen reviews performed by pharmacists can provide recommendations to physicians that appropriately *reduce drug utilization in the range of 0.9 to 2.44 prescriptions per patient per month*. The most frequent reduction would probably be about 1.5 prescriptions per patient per month.

If these average prescription reductions are applied nationwide to each Medicare and Medicaid skilled nursing facility patient

month, one can obtain an estimate of the range of savings that could accrue to these programs as a result of drug regimen reviews.

The annual gross savings for the 0.9 prescription reduction amounts to $19.8 million. For the 2.44 prescription reduction the annual gross savings is $53.8 million. The cost of performing these reviews is reported to be 13 cents and 14.37 cents per patient day. If this cost were averaged to 15 cents per patient day, the monthly per patient cost would be approximately $4.50, and the annual cost for all Medicare and Medicaid patients would be approximately $16.6 million.

The annual net savings to the Medicare and Medicaid programs would therefore amount to $3.2 million for the 0.9 prescription per month reduction and $37.2 million for the 2.44 reduction. By reasonable inference it may be stated that savings of this magnitude could be realized if the drug regimen of every skilled nursing facility patient were adequately reviewed by pharmacists.

If the same drug monitoring process were applied to intermediate care facility patients, an additional net savings ranging from $3.5 million to $40.9 million could be realized.

Table 61.1

Pharmacists	Number of Patients or Beds	Average Prescription Reduction Per Patient	Average Net Prescription Reduction Per Patient
Cheung & Kayne (Southern Calif.)	517 patients	From 6.8 to 5.6	1.2
Rawlings & Frisk (Idaho)	260 patients	From 7.7 to 6.1	1.6
Hood (Florida)	40 patients	From 7.6 to 6.7	0.9
Marttila (Minnesota)	20 patients	From 7.2 to 5.6	1.6
Lofholm Northern Calif.)	55 beds	From 6.8 to 4.6	2.2
Cooper & Bagwell (Georgia)	142 patients	From 7.22 to 4.78	2.44
Ellenore & Frisk (Idaho)	475 patients	From 2.4 to 1.5	0.9

Reduction in Hospitalization

Cost savings that can result from a reduced rate of hospitalization caused by inappropriate drug therapy are not easily documented. Three studies do, however, provide some insight into the magnitude of such savings.

In the work that Cheung and Kayne performed in 1972, 68 hospitalizations were avoided when potential adverse drug reactions were detected through drug regimen reviews. An expert panel of physicians judged that these adverse drug reactions would have resulted in hospitalizations, and the authors estimated that these hospitalizations would have resulted in expenditures of $49,000.

In a 1977 study of 9,117 hospital admissions, Morse and LeRoy identified 489 admissions that had a high probability of being drug induced. Of the 489 admissions, 113 were formerly skilled nursing facility patients. The authors estimate that 45 of these admissions could have been avoided through the performance of drug regimen reviews, and that the avoidable hospitalizations resulted in expenditures of $53,000.

In a more recent study of 147 patients by Thompson and Floyd eighteen adverse drug reactions were avoided. These adverse drug reactions would have resulted, as judged by the attending physicians, in hospitalizations. The authors estimate that the *annual* savings resulting from prevention of hospital readmissions amounted to $8,989.20.

The Thompson and Floyd study was conducted over a 31-month period and the average monthly number of patients monitored was 92. This means that 2,852 (92 x 31) patient months were monitored by the pharmacists. The 18 adverse drug reactions that were avoided during those 2,852 patient months yields a rate of 6.31 avoidable adverse drug reactions that would have resulted in hospitalization per 1,000 patient months. The Cheung and Kayne study yields a rate of approximately 33.53 per 1,000 patient months.

It would be tenuous to apply these rates nationwide and project total Medicare and Medicaid hospital savings because validating studies that would allow for such projections have not been performed.

Our lack of complete knowledge of the magnitude of these savings does not however mean they don't exist. Suffice it to say that if the ratio of avoidable adverse drug reactions that would require hospitalization were only one per 1,000 patient months (certainly a conservative estimate), then *Medicare and Medicaid annual savings would amount to approximately $5.1 million*. These savings would be *in addition* to the *net* savings (after paying the pharmacist for his monitoring services) that result from reduction in prescription use.

Quality Improvements

The dollar savings that could result from drug regimen reviews are an objective measure of improvement in the financing of long term care. Quality of care is not as easily measured. But patient care is bound to be improved if patients are not exposed to unnecessary drug therapy, since such therapy exposes the patient to unnecessary risks. This is particularly true if these risks are likely to expose the patient to adverse drug reactions that necessitate other therapies, extended length of stay, or even hospitalization.

Conclusion

The information presented in this paper provides strong evidence that the reviews performed by pharmacists of the drug regimens of skilled nursing facility patients can bring about substantial cost savings to the taxpayer. These reviews, which are an extension of the drug consultant services pharmacists have traditionally provided, can bring about these savings while *improving* the quality of patient care.

But public recognition of the value of this service is lagging. Presently only six states—California, Idaho, Nevada, Maine, New Jersey, and Massachusetts—formally provide any recognition of the value of this service in Medicaid reimbursement. This is true even though Federal regulations require that the service be performed, and Federal statute (Section 1902(A)(13)(E) of the Social Security Act) requires reimbursement to skilled and intermediate care facilities to be based on a "reasonable cost related basis."

Unless there is greater public recognition

of the value of this service it is likely that pharmacists will only be able to perform cursory drug regimen reviews. In this event, the patient as well as the taxpayer will be the ultimate losers.

Notes

In 1974 Federal regulations (Federal Register Vol. 29, No. 12, Thursday, Jan. 17, 1974, pages 2238–2257) required the pharmacy consultant to conduct a drug regimen review for each skilled nursing facility patient at least monthly.

62—Independent Buys Antibiotics for More Than 200 Drug Stores

Robert Brody

Between filling prescriptions, Phil Giannino bargains with antibiotics manufacturers over the phone. The pharmacist fires off bids for pharmaceuticals and improvises, in the give-and-take, like a boxer with quick feet.

"I practically live on the phone," jokes the 32-year-old drug retailer, who owns two drug stores called Harry's Prescription Pharmacy, in Palos Heights, Ill.

But Mr. Giannino isn't buying antibiotics only for his own stores. He's doing it for 237 other drug stores as well—167 independents and the rest chains, including Newman Drugs, Oak Drug and Arlen Pharmacy, all in Illinois. He is the unpaid president of the Pharmacy Buying Council of Illinois, a wholesaling type of operation he founded in Oct., 1977.

Last summer, Mr. Giannino met with Ernie Lequatte, president of the Illinois Pharmaceutical Association and Don Vaught, its former president, to talk about forming a buying organization. They endorsed the concept and launched a promotional drive.

For openers, they mailed brochures displaying a special logo to every drug store in the state. The brochure promised retailers a chance to purchase various antibiotics at uncommonly low prices. As expected, Mr. Giannino was soon getting dozens of inquiries from drug store owners.

Requirements

To receive service from the Pharmacy Buying Council of Illinois, a drug retailer is required to order at least $100 worth of antibiotics from a selection of 47 products. A check must accompany all orders. Only orders from Illinois pharmacists are accepted.

Some co-ops and wholesalers prefer to bill purchasers after delivery, taking the risk of receiving late payment, if any at all. Buying groups, Mr. Giannino charges, tend to form a fraternal atmosphere that can spell ruin. He says members of those groups are tempted to exploit friendships with colleagues in charge of purchases as a means of gaining leverage.

The inconvenience of advance payment is balanced, however, by the absence of a fee for the buying service. Mr. Giannino arranges all purchases without charge.

Purchasers are obliged to furnish their Drug Enforcement Administration numbers—just to ensure that they are licensed to handle pharmaceuticals. The buying group ships orders on receipt of a check and guarantees delivery of goods in three to five days.

With those primary guidelines, the organization is attracting an average of two new customers a week. Brochures subsidized by the Illinois Pharmaceutical Association are being sent around to attract still more.

Merchandise

Mr. Giannino says he buys only antibiotics manufactured by Beecham, Bristol and Lederle. Since last October, he reports, Beecham alone has received more than $80,000 in orders from the Pharmacy Buying Council of Illinois. Those who use his service get 500 250-mg capsules of Totacillin for $18.27, considerably below what they would pay by buying direct, or through a wholesaler.

Mr. Giannino, who notes that antibiotics are "the fastest-moving pharmaceuticals in a drug store," attributes the lower prices, in part, to reliance on the United Parcel Service for distribution. The cost of UPS service is borne by retailers. Eventually, he says, the wholesaling group may dive into the OTC market as well—preferably by bidding on well-recognized brand-name products. The retailer favors dealing with easily identified items. He intends to stay away from narcotics, however.

Why has he established the buying council? Chains buy at advantageous prices and create hardship for independents, he says, citing one manufacturer who allegedly gives a Chicago drug chain a 20% discount on all orders, while charging higher prices to retailers whose stores have a smaller sales volume.

Rival Wholesalers

The retailer is critical of some drug wholesalers, too, for charging service fees that bite into a store's profit margin.

"These wholesalers promise you the moon and give you nothing," Mr. Giannino gripes. But if a wholesaler came along with lower prices—on a par with those given to chain—he states he would voluntarily abandon the Pharmacy Buying Council of Illinois. As of now, however, he has no such plans.

"I'm still in the pharmacy business," he insists. "I'm not interested in becoming a big wholesaler. But I also don't care to get ripped off."

"I'm tired of being pushed around," says the combative retailer, who worked for the Osco and Walgreen chains shortly after graduating from the University of Wyoming pharmacy school.

"Why should the big stores get all the business? Independent drug stores are going broke like crazy! If I'm going to stay in this profession, I want to make a decent living. But until some manufacturers and wholesalers stop playing games with prices, nobody among us will."

Still, rather than lapsing into resignation, he keeps moving straight ahead.

Storage

Mr. Giannino stores a backlog of merchandise ordered for retailers in a cramped 48-sq.-ft. room in his professionally oriented pharmacy. But he has begun to negotiate for a shopping center storefront with a 300-sq.-ft. cellar that would double as a small-scale warehouse. Stores participating in the council would help cover rental costs of the space.

"I feel the council is going to grow," he predicts. "In fact, it'll probably double this year."

Further expansion, he observes, will come largely as a result of three policies: sticking to brand-names, demanding payment for goods in advance of delivery, and increasing product selection. Some medium-sized Illinois chains, he adds, are already nipping at the bait.

The Outlook

"Buying groups are the thing of the future," he says. "It's almost the only way for independents to survive high costs. Our organization charges nothing to buy or to belong, but eventually we will—a reasonable charge. I don't have profit in mind, but I can see profits will come from this."

Every weekday, Mr. Giannino calls manufacturers to inquire about prices and put in preliminary bids. He negotiates with sales-men and regional managers, making notes and changing bids. Polishing off a deal usually takes three or four phone calls.

"Sure, it takes time and a lot of work," he points out. "But it's worth it. All you have to do is stay on the phone."

Readings for a Broader Perspective

1. Appel, W. F. "Economic Security for Pharmacists—Free Lunch?" *J. Am. Pharm. Assoc.* NS 17 (May 1977):278–81.
2. "The Question of Ancillaries," *California Pharmacist* 24 (March 1977):4–5.
3. Johnson, R. C. "Overview and Objectives of Drug Program Management," *California Pharmacist* 25 (January 1978):19–24.
4. Allaben, J. W. "What Is the Role of Pharmacy Technologists?" *Pharmacy Times* 43 (November 1977):52–54.
5. Weiss, J. A. "How Unit-of-Use Dispensing Results in Timesaving R_x Efficiency," *Pharmacy Times* 42 (January 1976):43–46.
6. Gourley, D. R. "The Pharmaceutical Orphan: The Small Hospital," *Hospital Pharmacy* 10 (December 1975):502.
7. Zellmer, W. A. "The Will and the Power to Change the Public's Perception of Pharmacy," *American Journal of Hospital Pharmacy* 33 (August 1976):765.
8. Apple, W. S. "The Washington Phenomena," *J. Am. Pharm. Assoc.* NS 16 (August 1976): 446–52.
9. Siler, W. A. *Death by Prescription.* Nashville, Tennessee: Sherbourne/Charter House Publishers, Inc., 1978. 263 pp.
10. Silverman, M., and Lee, P. R. *Pills, Profits and Politics.* Berkeley, California: University of California Press, 1974. 403 pp.

WOMEN IN PHARMACY

63—Special Strengths of the Woman Practitioner

Angèle D'Angelo

Many changes are now taking place which will affect pharmacy significantly. Females are entering the profession in dramatically increasing numbers. The once less than 10 percent figure has changed to close to 40 percent enrollment of females in pharmacy colleges across the country. Hopefully, this increase will be the solid force needed to strengthen the role of women pharmacists and bring about public acceptance.

To understand the special strengths of women in pharmacy we must first look at the women who entered the profession when there were no visible female role models. Since intellectual capacity and the ability to learn are not dependent upon hormone production, there is no need to dwell upon the established fact of the female ability to master the scientific knowledge required to become a pharmacist. However, the women who made it through the pharmacy curriculum to graduation had to have some special qualities over and above the intellectual capacity to learn the course material.

The first women in pharmacy faced several hurdles which were not encountered by their male colleagues. The camaraderie usually enjoyed in college had to be limited to the few females in class or perhaps to a special male in the class. On the whole it was usually lacking. The rigors of the curriculum plus the lack of the emotional support of camaraderie usually produced a pharmacist deeply knowledgeable about the course content. Thus, this early barrier produced a positive outcome.

Secondly, arriving into the professional world, the female pharmacist was not readily accepted. She constantly had to prove that she was as competent as a man.

Another problem these women faced was that of combining a career and marriage. Some of the women in pharmacy at that time had no intention of marriage. Those that did put their careers into mothballs. Those that tried to combine a pharmaceutical career plus marriage in the days before women's lib had to have special qualities plus strong determination. To exist in this dual role, her professional performance had to be superior or she would soon find herself replaced. In addition, her household responsibilities were usually never lessened. Thus she had to develop an enlarged capacity to handle the work load as well as the emotional problems. She did not have the luxury of being able to hide behind the customary psychological defenses women usually used at that time. Her ability to perform well in spite of these handicaps opened the doors for females in pharmacy today.

The contemporary female pharmacy student has visible role models as well as female faculty members to help counsel her. She must now realize her special female attributes and cultivate them to achieve new dimensions.

Today every pharmacist, male and female, should be clinically involved. Clinical pharmacy is that personal health science that brings patient and practitioner into a close relationship. A pharmacist is no longer concerned only about the drug entity per se. Rather, his concerns are broadened to include the drug as it affects a particular patient. This would encompass, but not be limited to, the physical, mental and emotional well being of the patient. Thus, an important part of clinical pharmacy is communication with the patient. Sometimes this is deeper than the spoken word. Understanding the patient, his fears, and also anticipating his needs require a special sensitivity.

While it would be unfair (and probably untrue) to state that such abilities are limited to females, it is true that they are often much more visible in women. The sexual stereotypes of the "emotional female" and the "rational male" have hindered women in many areas of professional development, but have helped them in some areas. Women in our society have been encouraged to cultivate the important human attributes of communication, empathy, and sensitivity to another's emotions. Proper utilization of these attributes is vital to the patient-pharmacist relationship. In this area of communication, women pharmacists have something very important to offer to their male colleagues—they can serve as effective role models. As women have in the past destroyed the stereotype that they are less intelligent and competent, men can now destroy the stereotype that they are inherently less sensitive and emotional.

Pharmacy educators are becoming increasingly aware of the need to develop the communication skills of all clinical pharmacists. Evidence of this can be seen if one looks at the pharmacy college curriculum. In it there are psychology courses which deal with how to conduct a patient interview and courses within other behavioral sciences which try to create an awareness in all pharmacists for the special needs of clinical pharmacy.

Another special strength which women pharmacists have to offer the profession, also in the area of communication, is that of communicating with female patients. Women patients are much more willing to discuss with a female pharmacist such things as vaginal suppositories and oral contraceptives. They are also much more willing to discuss their children's medical problems and medications.

Women in pharmacy today are no longer severely hindered by the problems which faced their predecessors. They share the camaraderie of other female colleagues and are becoming accepted by society both in the professional world and as working wives and mothers. Hence women are now in a much better position to contribute their special strengths to clinical pharmacy, particularly in the area of the patient-pharmacist relationship emphasizing communication and understanding.

Readings for a Broader Perspective

1. Kronus, C. L. "Women in Pharmacy: Trends, Implications and Research Needs," *J. Am. Pharm. Assoc.* NS 17 (November 1977): 674–79.
2. Mercer, F. L. "34% of Women RPh's Experienced Employment Discrimination," *Pharmacy Times* 44 (October 1978):88–90.
3. Donelson, J. H. "Women in Pharmacy—We've Only Just Begun," *American Journal of Pharmacy* 150 (September/October 1978): 165–68.
4. Kimble, M. A. "The Sleeping Woman," *Drug Intelligence & Clinical Pharmacy* 9 (March 1975):153.
5. Kirk, K. W., and Henderson, M. L. "Expectations of Female Pharmacy Students," *J. Am. Pharm. Assoc.* NS 15 (November 1975): 622–23, 651.

Chapter Four

Past, Present, but Mostly Future

The five articles selected for this chapter are designed to introduce a broader perspective for interpreting the professional duties and problems that were treated earlier. Several of these provide an important historical review of how patients have been served by pharmacists in the past. Most, however, focus on expanded roles for the pharmacist in coping with the requirements of an increasingly interdependent and dynamic delivery system.

Readers can draw their own conclusions about how professional pharmacy services should be structured to ensure the efficient provision and appropriate use of drug therapy. The impact of the readings as a whole, though, suggests that the status quo (practice stressing distributive functions where paper and telephone are the major vehicles of professional communication) is unlikely to dominate the way pharmacy is practiced in the future. Given this probability, a career in pharmacy could be exciting for those who are challenged by technical complexity, service to mankind, and the opportunity to influence how the profession meets these responsibilities.

64—The Pharmacist

"To be a pharmacist is to be in the forefront of the constant endeavors against human misery to fellow man."—Quote by George F. Archambault

Just as the roots of the history of pharmacology are veiled in myth and legend, so also are the beginnings of those who first dabbled in creating medications. Although some of the drugs are the same, the 20th-century pharmacists resemble the "magicians" of the past in occupation only. *RPh* here explores the evolution of the pharmacist and his transformation from the priestly sorcerer who relied chiefly on magic and the assistance of gods to today's highly skilled professional who places his faith in science.

Ancient

Medicine, magic, religion, and pharmacy were closely connected in ancient civilizations. In Egypt, where the Pharaoh drew authority directly from the gods, life was pervaded by the supernatural. The priesthood and medicine intertwined, the physician being assigned responsibility for the preparation of drugs.

Later the compounder emerged as a specialist; he was designated as *urma* and performed his duties in a special room of the temple, the *asi-t*. By about 1000 B.C. the Pharaoh had created an official with the title of Superintendent of the Office for Measuring Drugs. Indicated is that his duties were more concerned with religious ceremonies, festivals, or funerary rights than with therapy.

In Mesopotamia, medicine and pharmacology were priestly functions: the *asu*, one of three classes of healing priests, was originally a diviner but came to be knowledgeable about drugs. The three priesthoods guarded their spheres of knowledge as caste secrets, but folk remedies proliferated among the common people; herb dealers hawked their wares from public stalls and the marketplace became a traditional site for the exchange of old wives' remedies.

The Greek period in medicine saw the gradual emergence of a class of preparers of medicines. The master pharmacologist of ancient Greece was Pedanius Dioscorides (ca 40–90). He compiled a vast lore on herbal remedies and drugs into five books under the general title of *De materia medica*; this most important book on drugs was a treasurehouse of pharmacy that remained a standard work for centuries.

Dioscorides classified more than 600 remedies from plants, about 50 mineral preparations and some 80 treatments with animal substances. He discussed each drug's source, mode of preparation, its effects and therapeutic uses. He also drew on the accumulated knowledge of diverse cultures.

Arabia

During the flourishing period of Arabian medicine, pharmacy began gradually to be separated from medicine. However, many physicians continued to dispense drugs and many pharmacists continued to diagnose and treat patients. The greatest clinician and scholar was Abu Bakr Muhammad ibn-Zakaria (Rhazes 865–925). He served as director of the Baghdad hospital, [and] performed original chemical and alchemical experiments. He was also a prolific writer who produced more than 200 works, including a monumental encyclopedia of medicine and pharmacy called *al-Hawi*, known in Western literature as *Liber continens*.

The latter part of the tenth century produced two great Persian figures born five years apart: Abu'l l-Rhaihan al-Beruni in 975 and Abu Ali al-Hussein ibn Abdallah ibn Sina (Avicenna) in 980. Both contributed greatly to pharmacological literature.

Al-Beruni was a man of obscure origins. Apparently orphaned at an early age, he was befriended by nomadic tribesmen, then adopted by a noble family. He was variously a poet, linguist, astronomer, mathematician, physicist, and geographer. Toward the end of his long life he turned to pharmacology and produced a massive compendium entitled *Knowledge of Drugs*, which lay buried in Asian archives for nearly a thousand years; about 40 years ago a partial text was rediscovered by Western scholars. Along with a rich *materia medica* it describes the drug trade that flowed between Arabia and the East and it unravels historic nomenclature by listing the names given to the same drug in different languages. Noted are some 900 Persian, 700 Greek, 400 Syrian, and 350 Indian terms.

Avicenna was another eclectic genius who lived adventurously as physician, chemist, poet, philosopher, diplomat, roisterer. He produced at least a hundred books and treatises, including the classic *Canon of Medicine*, a five-volume tome that summed up the accumulated medical knowledge of the time. Translated into numerous Latin editions, it served as an important medium for transmitting many of the original Greek precepts to medieval Europe.

Perhaps the greatest of the Arabian pharmacological scholars was Abdullah ibn al-Baitar (1197–1248) of Málaga. He was trained as a botanist, traveled throughout most of the Arabian empire to study medicinal plants, and combined personal observation with diligent research. His observations were recorded in the monumental *Corpus of Simples*, which described some 1800 vegetable, 145 mineral, and 130 animal drugs. Al-Baitar quoted the findings of 150 previous writers and he added to the literature 300 newly identified medicinal substances.

Middle Ages

Medieval pharmacy was intimately linked with religion, and monks followed the recommendation of Cassiodorus: "Learn to know the properties of herbs and blending of drugs, but set all your hopes upon the Lord." In some monasteries the task of preparing medicine was assigned to a monk versed in the art; alternatively it might be a general duty shared by the monks.

A towering figure in conventual medicine was Hildegard of Bingen (Ste. Hildegard, 1098–1179). The daughter of Germanic petty nobility, she became a nun at the age of 14, rose to be prioress, and eventually founded her own convent at Rupertsberg near the Rhine. Hildegard was a practical medical practitioner who organized a school for nurses and took a keen interest in botanical remedies. She grew more than 40 kinds of medicinal plants, used more than 60 other types that her nuns gathered from field and forest, and imported some two dozen more from distant lands.

Hildegard wrote two important medico-pharmacological works entitled *Liber simplicis medicinae* and *Liber compositae medicinae*; in the 16th-century an edited version

was republished as the *Physica*. The remedies she cited were largely a compilation of earlier writers, such as Pliny, but her writing reflected her own wide-ranging curiosity and vigorous mind. It displayed also that special compound of sense and superstition that characterized the age; she urged proper diet and exercise, endorsed many practical therapies, but also believed that epilepsy could be cured by placing an emerald in the patient's mouth.

The Dominican Albertus Magnus (1193–1280) was a noted teacher at the University of Paris; he was called Doctor Universalis for his extensive knowledge of philosophy, astronomy, geography, zoology, botany. He was the first to use the word alkali in its present sense, and one of the first to describe chemical reactions in terms of affinity.

A favorite pupil of Albertus was Thomas Aquinas, a great theologian and philosopher who added his own small footnote to pharmacology. Aquinas was the first to use the word amalgam in describing the combination of mercury with another metal. Another pupil was Petrus Hispanus who became Pope John XXI, the only physician-pope. *Thesaurus pauperum (Treasury of the Poor)*, attributed to him, dealt with dietetics and therapy. The work mixed shrewd empirical observations with a belief in some of the curious nostrums of the age; one of the remedies he recommended was an *Aquae mirabilis* in which filings of gold, silver, and copper were suspended in the urine of a boy. Later as pope he reportedly installed an alchemical laboratory in the Vatican.

While priestly druggists heeded the words of Cassiodorus, others experimented with remedies that were unique or exotic, if not effective. The juice of the rose, which provided herbalists with a decoction for purging "hot humors," was used also as a remedy for "shaking and trembling of the heart." The root of the lily was pounded and mixed with honey as an antidote to ulcers of the head and scalp; alternately it could be boiled in vinegar and applied to warts and corns.

John of Gaddesden practiced in the early 14th century and was physician to England's Edward II. He wrote *Rosa anglica*, so called because it was divided into five parts like the five sepals of the rose. For hemorrhage he recommended swine excrement and for epilepsy the bladder of a goat extracted while full of urine and baked in an oven.

In the Kingdom of the Two Sicilies sometime between 1231 and 1240 the Holy Roman Emperor issued an edict that officially recognized the pharmacist. The main import of the regulation was to separate the pharmacist from the physician, supervise pharmaceutical practice, and to require that pharmacists be bound by oath.

In the early 15th century the Italian physician Saladin di Ascoli published a book, probably the first in Europe for pharmacists, in which he outlined the duties and obligations of the pharmacists. He warned his readers to fortify themselves against unethical acts, such as dispensing abortifacients, selling poisons knowingly for harm, substituting ingredients that would be detrimental to the patient, or making other changes in a prescribed medication without the physician's consent.

Renaissance

Pharmacy evolved into a well-established profession during the Renaissance, a movement abetted by the growth of guilds, the spread of licensing and regulation, and the development of standards in education and training. Moreover, the role of the pharmacist improved with advancements in therapeutics and chemical art, especially the complexities of distillation.

An important event occurred in 1558 when the apothecaries of Montpellier petitioned that university for a course in pharmaceuticals. The apothecary guild provided a grant for the project and the course was taught by Bernhardin de Ranc, a master apothecary, the first of his profession to teach at a European university. Half a century later a chair of surgery and pharmacy was established at Montpellier and in 1675 Louis XIV created there a chair of pharmaceutical chemistry.

In Paris the apothecary Nicolas Houel founded the *Jardin des apothicaires* in 1576 under a royal ordinance. During the centuries that followed the institution was supported and enlarged by the Paris apothecary guild and was used as part of the guild's apprentice training system.

Throughout the Renaissance most pharmacists were trained by the apprentice system. In London the applicant had to serve a seven-year apprenticeship, then pass an examination that dealt with "election of simples and preparing, dispensing, handling, commixing and compounding of medicine." In Venice a student spent five years as an apprentice and three years as a pharmaceutical clerk before taking a similar examination.

Sharp rivalries grew up between physicians and pharmacists over their prerogatives and status; in France, Germany, and England there were acrimonious disputes that dragged on through much of the period. The physicians complained that pharmacists dispensed medical advice and pharmacists charged that physicians sold medicine. In England additional friction rose when apothecary shops were placed under the regulation of the Royal College of Physicians; pharmacists often flaunted the college's authority and in 1696 the physicians responded by opening a London dispensary for the poor under their own management. The controversy that followed was satirized by Dr. Samuel Garth in *The Dispensary*, a poem that poked fun at both sides, but the apothecaries eventually won the struggle.

Recognition

The progress of pharmacy differed according to countries but throughout much of

Europe in the 18th century there was more efficient regulation and increased status. Former medieval guilds evolved into professional societies, the first pharmaceutical journals were founded, and educational standards were improved.

Prussia led the way with an edict in 1725 separating pharmacists into two classes and establishing licensing requirements for each. Those of the second class were allowed to operate only in small towns and were required to pass an examination after serving five years as apprentices and six years as clerks. To obtain an unlimited first-class license, the pharmacist had to serve a similar round as apprentice and clerk, then attend courses in chemistry, botany, pharmacology. Instructions were given at the Collegium Medicum in Berlin; the chair of pharmaceutical chemistry was held there by a series of distinguished professors, including Caspar Neumann and Martin Klaproth.

Spain granted pharmacists a standing comparable to that of physicians and established a governing board to regulate the profession. Training was mostly through apprenticeships, variously four to eight years in different regions, but formal instruction was offered by the Madrid College of Pharmacists; by mid-century the college had acquired both a laboratory and a botanical garden. Similar schools later grew up at Barcelona, Zaragoza, Cádiz, Cartagena. Spanish law at one time prohibited the practice of pharmacy by women.

In Paris the apothecary guild twice launched abortive attempts to create a pharmaceutical college; both efforts failed because of strong opposition from the medical profession. Louis XVI finally granted the pharmacists recognition as an independent profession in 1777 and established the Collége de Pharmacie to serve as both an educational center and governing board. The college set standards for examination and licensing and a clear line was drawn between pharmacists and herbalists; the latter were limited to trading in roots and herbs that required no compounding or chemical preparation.

English pharmacy evolved in a somewhat haphazard fashion, beset by the bitter feud between pharmacists and physicians that had begun in the previous century. The quarrel came to a head in 1703 when the London College of Physicians brought suit against a pharmacist named William Rose, charging him with selling medicine without a prescription. Rose was convicted but the House of Lords reversed the verdict and handed down the far-reaching opinion that it was in the public interest for pharmacists to be allowed to give advice on medical matters. Thereafter apothecaries became increasingly general practitioners of medicine. The apothecaries for their part complained of unfair competition from a motley group of grocers, chemists, and apothecaries who did not belong to accredited guilds.

In Scotland and Ireland the pharmacists became associated with surgeons and drifted into general medical practice among the poor. A 1721 law allowed all Scottish pharmacists to join the corporation of surgeons without special examination, the only requirement being an extra license fee of £50. In Ireland apothecaries and surgeons were usually members of the same guild, but Dublin apothecaries became an exception by forming an independent guild in 1745. Surgery was also taken up by some English apothecaries and they made it a practice to hang saws, knives, and forceps on the shop walls as a sign of their additional function.

America

At the beginning of the 19th century, pharmacists in the United States still learned their art as apprentices and were subject to little or no regulation. The first attempt to organize the profession occurred in Philadelphia in 1821 when physicians denounced the unpredictable quality of medicines. Aroused pharmacists met at Carpenter's

Hall for a series of tumultuous meetings. In the process they formed America's first association of pharmacists, drew up a professional declaration of independence and code of ethics, moved to establish an educational system.

In 1822 this association inaugurated night school courses on chemistry and materia medica, and pharmacy, which grew into the present Philadelphia College of Pharmacy and Science. During the next half century local societies offered similar instruction courses in Boston, New York, Baltimore, Cincinnati, Chicago, and St. Louis.

In 1868 the University of Michigan established the first pharmacy department sponsored by a state institution, which evolved into the School of Pharmacy eight years later.

The University of Wisconsin established the second state university school of pharmacy (1883), at the special request of the state's pharmacists. In 1892, the school became the first in the United States to offer a four-year course in pharmacy and soon thereafter became the first to offer graduate degrees in pharmaceutical fields.

Outstanding among 19th-century pharmacists was William Procter, Jr., often called the Father of American Pharmacy. Apprenticed to a local Philadelphia pharmacist at the age of 14, he was graduated from the Philadelphia College of Pharmacy six years later. Before his unanimous election to the first chair of pharmacy at his alma mater in 1846, he had owned and operated his own pharmacy, written for the *American Journal of Pharmacy*, which he edited for 22 years, contributed significantly to the founding of the American Pharmaceutical Association, and served on the revision committee of the *United States Pharmacopoeia*, an organization with which he was associated for 30 years.

Procter epitomized a proud minority who were creating an independent profession. By the turn of the century the local druggist, or community pharmacist, had become a familiar figure, a pillar of the middle-class community. Besides giving helpful advice and filling prescriptions, he was expected to administer first aid to the occasional minor injuries of neighborhood children. During prohibition druggists were the only legitimate wholesale dealers in medicinal alcohol and in some areas there was heavy traffic in prescription whiskey. The mortar and pestle were the traditional symbols of the druggist's trade, but he came to be associated just as much with the soda fountain where he daily dispensed malteds and ice cream sodas. He knew his regular customers by their first names and was genuinely concerned about their health problems, and his store often was as much a center of community activity as a center for dispensing drugs.

The New Breed

Emerging in the latter half of this century is a "new breed" of pharmacist. Better informed on drug incompatibility and side-effects than the average physician, the new generation of pharmacists has the potential to receive a high professional status on a new basis.

New directions are being taken in education. An emphasis has been placed on producing a clinical pharmacist for a clinical mode of practice: patient-oriented, trained in drug evaluation, drug interaction, and drug abuse, better able to deal with a public that many feel is over-reliant on drugs and poorly informed of their adverse effects. Introduced into curriculums at pharmacy colleges are courses that focus on the patient-pharmacist relationship and on the psychological and sociological aspects of pharmacy practice. Last-year pharmacy students often spend as much as 50 percent of the academic year in hospital settings becoming familiar with the practical aspects of the pharmacy and working with patients. The future pharmacists may be expected not only to dispense medications, but to monitor and evaluate drug-therapy programs, counsel patients on the proper use of medications, and to provide a source of continuing health care once the patient has left the physician's office.

Controversial since 1974 is the minimum educational requirement for entry into professional practice. The American Association of Colleges of Pharmacy defeated a proposal last year that would have made the more extensive, clinically oriented Pharm.D. degree the prerequisite for the practice of pharmacy. A number of students are continuing on for this professional doctorate, and an even larger number of practicing pharmacists are returning to school for further education.

The "drug revolution" has generated a new flood of legislation not only from Congress but from state legislatures, 40 of which have passed generic drug laws that allow physicians and pharmacists to substitute generic drugs for equivalent brand-name agents. This runs counter to 20th-century prescribing custom, and an AMA survey indicates that the majority of physicians resist substitution without their permission. Complicating the issue are questions concerning liability in the event a patient experiences adverse reactions to a substituted drug.

Women and Pharmacy

A few women in the early 18th century became pharmacists through apprenticeships. Elizabeth Greenleaf founded a pharmacy in Boston as early as 1727 and Elizabeth Marshall, who learned pharmacy from her father, took over from him after 1804. In Kentucky the Louisville College of Pharmacy for Women opened in 1883, but came to an untimely end in 1896.

The role of women in pharmacy tended to follow a general social trend, with only a few in practice at the turn of the century. They did not begin to enter the pharmacy profession in greater numbers until the early 1940s when the manpower demands of war resulted in a shortage of pharmacists and colleges of pharmacy welcomed them into the fold. By 1965, women made up a mere eight percent of the country's pharmacists. In a recent national study on the practice of pharmacy, 19 percent of responses to a questionnaire came from women and more than half of these had entered the profession within the last five years. But even more significant are attitude changes within the field of pharmacy toward women: The American Pharmaceutical Association elected its first woman president in 126 years in 1978.

Future

A 1975 Study Commission on Pharmacy defined pharmacy as "a system that renders a health service by concerning itself with knowledge about drugs and the effects upon people and animals." Thus pharmacists are following other health professionals in the trend toward specialization and they are needed in such medical areas as oncology, pediatrics, and geriatrics, in the industrial and cosmetic sciences, and in research. Nuclear pharmacy has recently been recognized by the American Pharmaceutical Association as a board specialty, and it has set an example for other specialties to follow.

Summing Up

By French pharmacist George Lepine: "Saturn endowed Janus with two faces. I do not know what god—or what demon—has judged us worthy to possess three: we are scientists, we are artisans, and we are also merchants."

65—Approaching the Future of Community Pharmacy

Michael A. Schwartz

Community pharmacy, it seems to me, is the one area of pharmacy practice where we are floundering with regard to the role of the practitioner, his economic status, his professional image, the education required and the future. In most other traditional areas of pharmacy, the hospital, the industry, etc., we can clearly see roles which pharmacists will play, we have well-defined educational programs, and we can make reasonable predictions about the future. Not so with community practice.

I would like to explore with you some of the reasons why I think we are in this state of limbo and then offer some suggestions as to how we must proceed if we are to not only survive professionally but also make a meaningful contribution to society. And, of course, these two goals are inextricably bound together.

At the outset, I want to make it clear that the views I will express are strictly my own. I offer them here primarily as food for thought and as a basis for continuing discussion. I hope that out of this dialogue will emerge concrete proposals for implementation to improve community pharmacy practice and education.

We are all aware of the changes which have taken place in community pharmacy over the past several decades. Prior to World War II we saw the community pharmacist as primarily an independent owner of a small retail operation, spending a good deal of his time compounding prescriptions, selling mostly health related merchandise, and prob-

ably spending a good deal of his time in personal interaction with patients. The latter often earned him the title of "Doc." He was, for the most part, generally satisfied with his role in society and felt himself to be a necessary and worthwhile contributor to the welfare of his community.

In the thirties, the schools of pharmacy shifted from a Ph.G. to a B.S. program that was to remain the standard for education for over twenty years until the 5-year program began in 1960.

Today, of course, the situation is quite different in a number of significant ways:

1. There is virtually no compounding of prescriptions;
2. More than half of the nation's pharmacists are employees; and
3. The small independent practice is virtually gone with many more larger independents and chains replacing them.

In addition, there are two other factors which affect the community pharmacist:

1. He practices in virtual isolation within the four walls of his pharmacy and has little day-to-day contact with other pharmacists. His contact with physicians is mostly by telephone. He has little opportunity for the kind of interaction possible when numbers of professionals work together, as in a hospital, and has as a result become very provincial.
2. There is a considerable body of evidence to show that the community pharma-

cist is not viewed as a professional involved in health care by the public, by government agencies, by other health professionals or even by pharmacists themselves.

Economics of Professional Practice

It is my contention that the *primary* reason for the present status and image of pharmacists is economic. An examination of some statistics may make this clear. The state of Pennsylvania is used as an example. In Pennsylvania, there are 10,857 pharmacists residing in the state of which 10,047 are in practice; 8,422 are in community practice. With a population of 9.85 million, there are 84.3 pharmacists per 100,000 people. The national average is 63.4[1] Pennsylvania is certainly not moving toward the national average as judged by present enrollment in its four colleges of pharmacy.

In 1972, graduates numbered about 270; in 1973 and 1974 there will be about 370.[2]

At present, there are 980 pharmacists age 65 or over and another 1000 age 60–64. There are apparently more than enough students enrolled to replace those lost by death and retirement. Can we conclude from all these figures that there are too many pharmacists in Pennsylvania *at present*?

Another way of looking at the situation is to try to assess the volume of professional practice: If Pennsylvania is a representative state then according to national averages with about six prescriptions per person per year and about 10 million people, there should be about 60 million prescriptions filled per year. This means on the average, there are about 7200 Rx/pharmacist/year or 24 per day, and that each of the 2800 pharmacies fills about 21,000/year or about 70 per day.

Assuming the average professional fee to be about $2.00, then the average pharmacist earns $48 per day from prescriptions and the average pharmacy, with three pharmacists, earns about $140 per day. Since the professional fee includes overhead, I think we can fairly conclude that there is not sufficient prescription volume to allow each pharmacist to earn a reasonable living solely from professional activity.

I cite these figures merely to show why, I think, pharmacists have been forced to become merchants, to add to their establishments a growing variety of non-health-related merchandise. It has been done simply in order to make a living. I feel that if there were only half the number of pharmacists at the present time in Pennsylvania, there would not have been the same trend toward mercantilism over the years and there would have been less likelihood of our becoming viewed as merchants.

Need to Develop New Professional Roles

While I feel that economics has had the *most* influence on the present status of community pharmacy there are other factors which have undoubtedly contributed. Most important among these is the fact that pharmacy organizations and individuals have largely failed to recognize the need to seek new professional roles as their primary compounding role faded. The schools, until very recently, must be considered equally guilty on this score as must the boards of pharmacy. The latter have generally stubbornly maintained the traditional view of the pharmacist's role and this is reflected in their examinations which seem to stress many areas that educators now would like to eliminate from their curricula but feel that to do so would be a disservice to their students who must pass the board examination.

At the same time, drugs have become a greater source of problems than ever before and there has arisen a need for someone with expertise in drug therapy to apply it in the routine use of drugs. The most logical person to fill this need because of his education, experience and location in the community, is the pharmacist.

So much for a brief review of the past and glimpse of the present with which we are all too familiar. What concerns us now is new direction for community pharmacy in the future. Since we are discussing the future, which is synonymous with the unknown, much of what I will say might be considered speculative. I will offer some concrete suggestions on the one hand and on the other hand merely point out problems which need discussion and resolution. I do hope to show you, however, that the same economic factors which have been operating *against* us in the past will operate in our favor in the future and that community pharmacy is facing a potential professional golden age in the present decade if we are astute enough to grasp the opportunity to take advantage of it now.

Clinical Role and Professional Future

My entire argument hinges on the premise that a clinical role is the only acceptable professional future for pharmacy. This was stated eloquently by T. Donald Rucker[3] at a recent seminar in Iowa when he said that the practice of clinical pharmacy must become recognized as the "cornerstone of professional service." Without providing a complete definition of "clinical pharmacy" it can be said that its objective is to apply the pharmacist's specialized knowledge of drugs so as to optimize patient health in matters relating to drug therapy. It certainly implies that pharmacy practitioners exercise judgment concerning a new regimen of drug therapy for a given patient in the light of that patient's state of health and current drug therapy.

The most important determinant of how a role is evaluated by society, and hence how it

is rewarded, is the degree to which it calls for the exercise of high level knowledge, judgment and discretion. In addition to the normally higher monetary remuneration, society also grants to a profession high prestige and the privilege of self-regulation. These privileges are not granted to merchants or non-professional service people. If pharmacists are indeed professionals their first allegiance must be to measures that support patient well-being. This must be made clearly visible to society and the measures referred to must be of value to society. The present role of the community pharmacist does not meet these requirements; the clinical role will.

Goals

In order to convert community pharmacy from its present state to one which meets these standards of a well recognized profession, I believe there are certain essential goals which must be achieved. Let me first list these and then suggest some means by which they may be achieved by organized pharmacy in Pennsylvania.

1. Separation of the pharmacy from the drug store.
2. Assurance to the public of high level professional services important to their health.
3. A public relations program to interpret these services to the consumer.
4. Political action—a positive approach to participation in changing the health care system.

I have not listed these in any order of priority since I feel all are essential and all can be worked at simultaneously. In fact, as you will see, they overlap in many ways.

Separation of Pharmacy from the Drug Store

First, consider separation of the pharmacy from the drug store. By my usage of these two terms I am obviously defining them as different entities. I suggest that the term drug store be applied to any establishment selling a variety of merchandise traditionally associated with the large drug store as we know it today. The term pharmacy on the other hand should be reserved for a site of professional practice by a pharmacist. My "drug store" would not be allowed to dispense prescription drugs or any non-prescription items requiring the supervision of a pharmacist in their sale. The latter would be solely reserved for the pharmacy.

This concept is not new. Several years ago Donald E. Francke suggested the same thing.[4] He described the drug store "as a commercialized jungle which dulls and tarnishes and blunts the professional drive of pharmacists as they seek to practice their profession within its walls." I think this is an accurate description especially as applied to our more recent graduates. Clearly the large commercial drug store cannot be associated by the public with the practitioner serving the health needs of society. The fact that a health professional is practicing in such an environment is largely obscured by the commercial atmosphere and the public is confused over the actual role of the pharmacist. It is essential that this confusion be changed to a clear picture in the mind of the consumer of the pharmacist's important health team role.

In a paper published in the February 1972 issue of the *Journal of the American Pharmaceutical Association*[5] I advocated, rather than complete physical separation of the pharmacy from the drug store, a separate *identification* of these two entities even if they were able to coexist within the same walls. My reason for this compromise approach was the difficulty of attempting to change the laws in 50 states. However, today we are considering only one state and I recommend to you that everything possible be done, including changing the law if necessary, to achieve a complete physical separation of the pharmacy from the drug store.

Services to be Provided to Society

Of course, a mere change in environment, while essential, cannot alone bring about the desired changes in pharmacy practice. There must be a concomitant general upgrading of the level of value of services provided by the community pharmacist to society. This was well expressed by George Griffenhagen in a recent editorial[6] when he said, "Two decades ago, a pharmacist might have identified pharmaceutical services as maintaining a full inventory of pharmaceuticals and providing emergency service, delivery service and charge accounts. But most of these activities under today's standards can be looked upon more as good pharmaceutical administration rather than as unique professional services."

Griffenhagen goes on to list professional services as:

1. Patient medication record system;
2. pharmaceutical services to nursing homes;
3. professional guidance to the self-medicating public;
4. adverse drug-reaction reporting;
5. monitoring drug interactions; and
6. product selection.

In the paper by Rucker referred to earlier,[3] are listed six areas in which the author thought community pharmacists could make a case for compensation under national health insurance.

1. Dispensing;
2. clinical pharmacy;
3. institutional services;
4. first level clinical medicine;
5. peer review; and
6. public health.

Time does not permit me to review these and I refer you to Rucker's paper and other recent literature for detailed descriptions. The important point is that these services are considered to be needed, are of value in that compensation may be gained for them and they can be performed by an adequately trained pharmacist. I believe the burden falls upon the organized profession to take whatever steps are necessary to insure the public that they will receive these services and that they will be performed with a high level of expertise.

Interpreting Services to Public

My third essential is a public relations program to interpret these services to the public. We are generally aware that our public image is not that of a practicing professional. With this image it is very difficult if not impossible to achieve a level of confidence in the pharmacist as a provider of sophisticated health related services. Thus, our economic status and professional image suffers. We do not attract the best young people into the profession and we gain an inferiority complex ourselves.

On the other hand, I have observed that consumers, especially leaders in the current consumer movement or revolution, are not dogmatic about price alone, and once shown the potential value of clinical pharmacy services, actually become better advocates of clinical pharmacy than certain pharmacists. Consumerism is not merely a reaction to high prices but also to poor quality of product and poor service. These cannot be considered separately. I have had occasion in the last few months to talk to at least three consumer groups at length about what they should expect from their pharmacist and why these services are necessary. In every case I felt I had convinced them that the pharmacist can play an important role in maintaining their health, in assuring them quality drug products, and in protecting them from adverse effects of drugs.

Pharmacy's Role in Health Care

The fourth essential I list is a positive action program of gaining and utilizing political influence to insure that pharmacy will have a role in new health care organizations and systems. In the past it has been characteristic of organized pharmacy (and, in fact, some other professions) to virtually ignore voices from outside the profession until they pose a direct threat through proposed legislation. Then our organizations have attempted to staunchly defend our position, and often were the loser. It would be wasteful to attempt here to point out some of these many instances and I will assume that all of you here are quite familiar with a number of them. It is clear that we cannot ignore the thrust of society's demands for adequate health care, of the consumer's desires for quality service at reasonable cost or of the government's determination to respond to these needs.

We know there will be some form of national health insurance soon. We know there will be attempts at least to reorganize the health care delivery system. The federal administration is funding experiments with Health Maintenance Organizations, for example, and several bills on HMO's are under consideration in congress. Are you aware of their provisions for pharmacy services?

If we are to insure that the public receive high quality pharmaceutical services, organized pharmacy—not the government nor anyone else—must establish the criteria and standards of performance. If we do not, standards will be set by others and we will be forced to comply with a set of circumstances not of our own making. Thus, our involvement is essential.

If I were to stop I could be accused of merely adding to the rhetoric which seems to surround many, if not most, meetings of pharmacists. Let me, therefore, list for you some of the steps which I believe each of the groups represented here might take in order to achieve these essential goals.

State Pharmaceutical Societies

First, the state pharmaceutical society. If the Pennsylvania society is typical, it has only about 20–30 percent of the state's pharmacists as members, is understaffed and under-funded, and is dominated by older pharmacists most of whom are owners of independent pharmacies. These factors in general have caused societies to be more business-oriented, to be unable to take the time to explore new roles and, because of lack of funds, to be usually committed only to "putting out fires." Yet, the state society must become the prime driving force for change if the goals we seek are to be reached. As I see it, the society must do the following:

1. Seek legislation to separate the pharmacy from the drug store.

2. In order to assure the public of high level professional services the society must attempt to induce pharmacists voluntarily to perform these services which include:
   a. Maintenance and proper utilization of patient prescription records;
   b. consultation with patients regarding prescription and OTC medication; and
   c. participation in continuing education.

If, however, pharmacists are reluctant to perform them, I believe they must be forced to do so through regulation or legislation.

The state society can help its members in any number of ways, including:
   a. Establish local journal clubs and study groups using recent graduates as discussion leaders;
   b. convert its journal into a clinically oriented publication;
   c. establish regional meetings at which clinically oriented programs are presented; and
   d. consider the establishment of a state-wide computer based patient record system to which all members would have access.

The state society should also establish a peer review system in order to achieve self-regulation through which the public can gain confidence in the pharmacist's professional competence.

3. In the area of public relations it is essential that the consumer become fully aware of the nature of clinical pharmaceutical services, of the ability of the pharmacist to perform these services and of the importance of these to health. Somehow the society must finance and carry out a public relations program which will do this.

4. In order to assure that clinical pharmacy practice is a component of whatever new health organizations evolve it is essential that organized pharmacy become involved now while these are in the planning stages. This requires political action, for example, in securing appointment of pharmacists to government and quasi-government agencies which are doing this planning, such as regional medical program, comprehensive health planning, etc. It requires that you maintain close liaison with legislators, that you seek to appear before those legislative committees which are considering health related legislation.

I think, too, that state societies should be involved in research projects and demonstration projects of new models for provision of pharmaceutical services such as HMO's, foundations, etc.

Schools of Pharmacy

Next, the schools of pharmacy. What is called for today is a total commitment by the schools to training a skilled clinical pharmacy practitioner. I think that the schools in Pennsylvania have generally accepted the clinical pharmacy concept and are moving toward it at varying rates in their educational programs. If they are like my own school, they feel constrained by two factors: the five-year program and the outdated state board exams. Ideally, of course, there should be no time requirement for education of a pharmacist and we should instead have a performance requirement. That is, as soon as a student can demonstrate both the knowledge and clinical skill necessary to practice he should graduate and commence practicing. Realizing that, at least for the present, such a method is not feasible, I suggest the schools must do the following:

1. Define the product they wish to produce. That is, establish minimum knowledge and performance standards for the practice of pharmacy using, of course, clinical practice as the base line.

2. Establish curricula needed to produce that product. In doing this, we should not start with any preconceived notions of 4-year, 5-year or 6-year programs nor should we simply repackage our traditional courses.

3. Be prepared to implement these new curricula and to change them as new needs are recognized.

The schools should also seek to suitably retrain those practitioners who have not had clinical training and to provide in the future a suitable pattern of continuing education so that practitioners will be able to maintain at least minimal competence.

Finally, the schools should be conducting research in professional practice probably in conjunction with the state society and other groups where collaboration is either necessary or desirable. By this, I mean the evaluation of new roles, new techniques and new organizational patterns.

State Boards of Pharmacy

In considering the role of the state board of pharmacy, it must be kept prominently in mind that the board does not exist to serve the pharmacy profession but, in fact, to protect the public by insuring at least minimum standards of practice. I believe the board can best serve the public today by defining pharmacy practice as a clinically based practice and then using its powers to insist on *quality* clinical practice. The powers of the board generally lie in three areas:

1. Examination for licensure;
2. periodic relicensure; and
3. inspection.

The board should, therefore, (1) convert its examination to one which tests the clinical skills and knowledge of the candidate, (2) require clinically oriented continuing education, (3) establish requirements that will insure clinical practice of pharmacy, such as patient records, and (4) use its inspection power to monitor practice. The board should also consider requiring the separation of the pharmacy from the drug store as being in the public interest.

The suggestions I have offered are basic and pertain directly to the essential goals I enumerated earlier. I am sure each of you could add to the list.

In considering possible implementation of these suggestions you must be prepared for a great deal of resistance from pharmacists. Perhaps some of it can be overcome when we consider the future. I remarked earlier that the very economic forces which are defeating professionalism in pharmacy today can do just the opposite in the future.

Future Possibilities

I will show you that within this decade of the seventies there will be more than sufficient volume of professional practice so that every pharmacist will be able to earn a comfortable livelihood by practicing his profession full time. Without this change in economic pattern, I believe it would be impossible to accomplish the four goals I keep alluding to as essential.

Let us examine the potential in prescription volume alone. It is projected by any number of knowledgeable and capable authorities that by 1980 prescription volume will be more than double what it is today, that is there will be on the order of 2.6 billion prescriptions per year. If we assume that community pharmacy manpower remains about the same as it is today, then the average pharmacist will fill about 50 prescriptions per day in Pennsylvania. Nationwide, the figure is closer to 70 per day and some authorities calculate an even higher figure.

Add to this the responsibility for OTC drugs and we have a clear manpower shortage. There seems to be no doubt that we will be forced to reorganize the drug distribution system by introduction of automation and/or subprofessional personnel just to serve the minimal needs of society for safe distribution of drugs.

The important point is, however, that the need to be a merchant will no longer exist. We can, therefore, sell the concept of total devotion to professional practice to pharmacists on economic grounds as well as on public need.

With increasing use of drugs, the need for clinical pharmacy practice will become even more apparent as problems traceable to drug therapy grow in dimension. In addition to the growing volume of prescription drug usage we are also witnessing a growth in development of prepaid comprehensive health care. This concept has the obvious potential of freeing the pharmacist from the burden of "making a sale" in order to earn income and can therefore, be an important factor in promoting clinical pharmacy practice because it clearly separates the transfer of a commodity (the drug product) from the services necessary for that transfer.

Society is already showing a great reluc-tance to pay for pharmacy services through third parties unless these services can be shown to supply an important contribution to health care. A total commitment to clinical pharmacy practice is called for in order to make community pharmacy the important contributor to health care which it can be and which is needed. This can be done without sacrifice of economic gain and I hope community pharmacists will urge their local, state and national organizations to get started.

References

1. Licensure Statistics, Census, National Association of Boards of Pharmacy, Chicago, 1971.
2. Report on Enrollment in Schools and Colleges of Pharmacy, First Semester, Term, or Quarter 1971–72, *Amer. J. Pharm. Educ. 36*, 120 (1972).
3. Rucker, T. D.: The Pharmacist and National Health Insurance—Potentials and Problems, paper presented to University of Iowa Pharmacy Management Seminar, Iowa City, Feb. 17, 1972.
4. Francke, D. E.: Let's Separate Pharmacies and Drugstores, *Amer. J. Pharm. 141*, 161 (1969).
5. Schwartz, M. A.: The Drugstore and Pharmacy, *J. Amer. Pharm. Assoc. NS 12*:66 (1972).
6. Griffenhagen, G. B.: editorial, *J. Amer. Pharm. Assn. NS 12*:55 (1972).

66—Clinical Pharmacy: The Past, Present, and Future

Don C. McLeod

Origin of Clinical Pharmacy Practice

When surveying the literature of pharmacy, it is evident that the clinical pharmacy movement has budded and blossomed within the past decade. The germs of clinical pharmacy have existed for several decades in the better hospital pharmacy departments in the country. The motivation and philosophy which led hospital pharmacists to activate pharmacy and therapeutics committees, to push and struggle for formularies of the best pharmaceuticals and to identify and eliminate causes of medication errors is closely akin to the philosophy sustaining the clinical pharmacy movement. The hospital is an organized health care setting in which, under common administrative guidelines, medical care professionals have come together to provide medical care. It is not surprising that those pharmacists trained in this environment are the ones today providing leadership in clinical pharmacy practice, both in hospitals and organized health care settings outside of the hospital.

Francke has shed some light on this germination of clinical pharmacy as follows:

> Using the term clinical in a very broad sense, formal training for clinical practice in hospital pharmacy developed quite apart from the colleges of pharmacy. Whitney at Michigan in the 1930's and Clarke at The New York Hospital in the 1940's were pioneers in this field. I recall the great frustration and disappointment expressed by Mr. Whitney because he could not interest

either the dean or the faculty of the college in the prospect of using the tremendous interdisciplinary teaching facilities of a great university hospital for the education and training of undergraduate pharmacy students. This situation began to change in the late 1940's when Flack at Jefferson Hospital in Philadelphia, Purdum at Johns Hopkins and myself at Michigan developed programs which combined residencies and advanced degrees. However, these programs affected only a few graduate students and had almost no effect on the instruction of undergraduate students.[1]

An abortive attempt at "clinical" pharmacy education was begun at the University of Washington during World War II. In an editorial in 1969 announcing a change in title of the journal *Drug Intelligence* to *Drug Intelligence and Clinical Pharmacy*, Francke has described this effort as follows:

> One of the most dramatic events of recent years is the emergence of the concept of clinical pharmacy and its belated adoption by colleges of pharmacy as an educational tool. It is sad to have to say, however, that it was the narrow provincialism of pharmaceutical educators themselves which held back the development of the concept of clinical pharmacy for more than a quarter of a century. Clinical pharmacy as an educational tool was begun by Professor L. Wait Rising of the University of Washington in 1944, but was disapproved by resolution by both the American Association of Colleges of Pharmacy and the American Council on Pharmaceutical Education in 1946. This action abruptly terminated an imaginative research program in teaching methods without even giving the professor

who originated it, the students taking the course, or the pharmacists participating in it an opportunity to be heard. The value of the clinical pharmacy experiment at the University of Washington was again brought to the attention of pharmaceutical educators in 1953 by Professor H. W. Youngken, Jr., then at the University of Washington, but the idea lay dormant for many years until recently resurrected.[2]

The doomed efforts of Professor Rising were aimed at community pharmacy practice, and it is not known if his concept of clinical pharmacy would coincide with the more advanced concepts of today.

In an article entitled "Evolvement of Clinical Pharmacy," Gloria Francke[3] has carefully chronicled the use of the term "clinical pharmacy." It is beyond the scope of this article to highlight all events, but it seems clear that certain early uses (in the 1960's) did not connote clinical pharmacy as it is intensely practiced by some today. It appears to me that the flowering of clinical pharmacy closely paralleled two events in hospital pharmacy practice. One was the development of unit dose drug distribution systems in many hospitals in the late 1960's. Another activity associated with the clinical pharmacy movement was the development of the drug information center concept in the early 1960's. Drug information, along with radiopharmacy, were the first easily identified specialty areas in pharmacy practice.

I vividly remember attending the sessions of the ASHP at the APhA Annual Convention in Las Vegas in 1967. I had just obtained the B.S. degree in pharmacy and had entered a hospital pharmacy residency under H. A. K. Whitney, Jr. Prior to the residency, even though I had worked two summers in a university teaching hospital, I had never heard of clinical pharmacy, of Pharm.D. programs, or any "exciting new roles" for the hospital pharmacist. At the Las Vegas meeting, young pharmacists charged with implementing unit dose drug distribution systems were talking about the sort of problems and

experiences they were undergoing, and many talked about making rounds with physicians as a part of their daily routine. I also became aware of Pharm.D. programs such as the ones at the University of Kentucky and the University of California at San Francisco. While the elder statesmen of hospital pharmacy inspired awe in me at that time, it was this evolving "clinical pharmacy" as practiced by some younger pharmacists that captured my imagination in the coming months and years. I believe that there are hundreds of hospital pharmacists who can relate similar stories.

Since the early clinical pharmacists were predominantly found in or associated with advanced residency and graduate (Pharm.D. and M.S.) programs in university teaching hospitals, it was natural that the schools of pharmacy soon became a ground of contention. It took about one morning of medical rounds or the presentation of the patient data at grand rounds to convince even the most astute hospital pharmacy resident that most of his curriculum had been for naught. The depression that resulted is not described in psychiatric texts. In the more hearty, the German concept of "angst" probably best described the feeling pervading those first few formative years. It was evident that pharmacy school curricula had to be drastically changed, hospital pharmacy practice had to undergo a revolution and residency training in most hospitals had to be upgraded.

Given the tremendous clinical handicaps resulting from inadequate pharmacy education, it is surprising how rapidly the clinical pharmacy movement has advanced. Responsive chords in many students and young practitioners were clearly struck, and the federal government, through capitation grants to schools of pharmacy, gave considerable support to clinical pharmacy education and practice at a critical time. Many of the things that were merely dreams to young clinically aspiring pharmacists less than a decade ago are now a reality in many locations. There are still the skeptics in academia and in practice, and the uninitiated in the other health professions, but solid accomplishments are rather commonplace in many hospitals and clinics.

Current Scope of Clinical Pharmacy Practice

When one surveys major advances in medical practice, it is obvious that most of them occur in university teaching hospitals. The origin and early development of clinical pharmacy practice has likewise taken place in the academic medical care institution. Today a large portion of the clinically trained pharmacists still practice, and often teach, in the major teaching hospitals. On the contrary, there are still many university teaching hospitals where pharmacy is relatively undeveloped.

Thus far, the exodus of the clinically trained pharmacist into nonuniversity settings has been rather small when the vast number of hospitals, health care institutions and organized health care programs are considered. It seems that schools of pharmacy will soon be somewhat saturated with clinical faculty, and that more clinically trained graduates will be going into community hospitals and other nonacademic settings. This is a necessary development if clinical pharmacy is to truly be an important development in medical care. At this time, only a relatively few community hospitals are actively recruiting clinical pharmacists to function as specialists within the pharmacy department. When "clinical pharmacists" are sought, the director of pharmacy frequently does not envision high-level clinical pharmacy practice.

The most common clinical pharmacy practice model encountered in the teaching hospital is that of a clinical pharmacist (often on the school of pharmacy faculty) providing intensive services to a small group (12–30) of patients on a medical or pediatric teaching service. This pharmacist makes rounds with the medical staff, follows closely the diagnostic proceedings and therapy of patients on the service and teaches students and residents about cases encountered. This is the only model of clinical practice many students encounter, and there is considerable difficulty relating to this role model since there are only a few ongoing practice responsibilities and the day is spent largely with academic matters. This role model has some personal rewards for the practitioner-educator, but it alone cannot suffice in the majority of hospitals. This is the practice model currently in vogue in many university teaching hospitals.

A variation of this model is the docent program at the University of Missouri in Kansas City. Here the clinical pharmacist is separated from the traditional pharmacy department. The clinical pharmacy practitioner-educator serves as faculty for medical and nursing students as well as pharmacy students. In the Kansas City program, the docent team provides continuing services, both inpatient and ambulatory, to a defined group of patients. A shortcoming in this model is the continued existence of a traditional pharmacy department largely separated from the clinical activities.

Another clinical pharmacy practice model is that associated with unit dose drug distribution services provided from a decentralized pharmacy in the patient care area. Unit dose systems have been the impetus to clinical pharmacy evolvement in many teaching hospitals as well as community hospitals. Unit dose was an entree into the patient care area which spared the pharmacist the trauma of announcing he was there for clinical reasons. It allowed him to sharpen slowly his clinical abilities and to begin making inroads gradually with the medical staff. Unit dose systems forced the pharmacist to become intimately involved with the nurse, the physician, the medical chart and, to some degree, the patient. It was this arena that spurred many of the younger and more ambitious pharmacists to pursue clinical pharmacy practice.

While unit dose systems forced the pharmacist into the patient care area, it has proven difficult for a pharmacist to work in the satellite pharmacy and maintain a close clinical involvement with patient drug therapy. The magnitude of technical and supervisory activities tends to consume the time and energy of the pharmacy staff, unless there are a great many pharmacists or ample technical staff. Even with adequate supportive personnel, a clinical program of quality is not easy in the presence of a unit dose drug distribution system as operated in most hospitals having the system. Only through wise management, proper recruitment of clinical staff and much hard work will the clinical program have a large impact on rational drug therapy. Safer handling and administration of drugs will ensue, but often with little meaningful clinical involvement with the physician and the therapeutic decision-making process.

The hospital outpatient clinics have been the grounds for a logical extension of the clinical pharmacy concept. Proper choice of drug therapy, and patient education and compliance, were properly a concern of the pharmacist, and many articles have described activities directed toward these matters. As pharmacists began taking medical school courses in many of the Pharm.D. programs and gaining acceptance for their expertise in drug therapy, it is not surprising that a few began managing the chronic drug therapy of selected patients. This is being done in some U.S. Public Health Service Indian Hospitals and in other organized health care settings providing comprehensive services. Common diseases managed by the pharmacist have been hypertension, diabetes and tuberculosis. If clinical pharmacy is going to make its maximal input into improving rational drug therapy, a signifi-

cant involvement in ambulatory and community medicine must be developed. If this occurs it will be an outgrowth of the hospital clinical pharmacy programs, not a development within the drugstore establishment.

There are now several easily identified clinical pharmacy specialties developing. The drug information specialist was an important precursor to the clinical pharmacist, and he is probably the most entrenched specialist in most comprehensive clinical pharmacy programs. The drug information center is a sanctuary removed from direct clinical activities, and many drug information specialists have no ongoing clinical responsibilities. In a few hospitals, a competent drug information specialist may exist without a direct clinical pharmacy program. In other hospitals, the drug information specialist is an integral part of the clinical pharmacy team and provides an important support service to enhance the overall quality of pharmacy programs. Some drug information centers provide services on a regional basis, both to the medical and pharmaceutical community.

Pediatrics is a natural area for pharmacy specialization, and the pediatric pharmacist was probably the first identifiable clinical pharmacy specialist. There are now at least a few dozen pediatric clinical pharmacists who have gained acceptance by their colleagues in pediatrics. One factor contributing to the rather rapid entrance of the clinical pharmacist into pediatrics has been the generally cordial welcome extended by pediatricians. Of the various medical specialists, the pediatrician has been very supportive of a team approach to medical care, and generally has not acted in a threatened or condescending way toward the clinical pharmacist. This is the only "break" the well-prepared and ambitious clinical pharmacist needs.

Psychiatric clinical pharmacy has become a viable practice in several locations around the country. Again this is an easily identified specialty area in medicine, and community mental health centers have developed all over the country in response to the mental health needs of the community. The best examples of clinical psychiatric pharmacy are in the mental health centers. One of the hallmarks of the community health center is well-organized, interdisciplinary teamwork. There is also a shortage of psychiatrists in many places to deal traditionally with all the patients. Medication is the main therapy afforded most mental patients, and this therapy is often poorly controlled. The forte of the clinical psychiatric pharmacist is drug therapy control and patient assessment. In some community mental health centers, the clinical pharmacist conducts clinics (e.g., lithium and fluphenazine maintenance) and schedules patients back to the pharmacy clinic for reassessment and medication maintenance. The pharmacist, working under policies of the community health center and backup of psychiatrists, may discontinue or alter doses of drugs, initiate new therapy or refer the patient to the psychiatrist. This is wise use of a long-established health professional in an area where the number of new job descriptions of various counselors, aides, therapists, etc., is almost astounding.

Another specialty area being developed in clinical pharmacy is clinical pharmacokinetics. Clinical pharmacokinetics is a tool, like pharmacology, in which every clinical pharmacist should have a basic understanding and familiarity so that well-established knowledge can be applied to every patient. Clinical pharmacokinetics is also a very complex science that is in every way as difficult to master as cardiology, for example. Every physician should know basic cardiology, but not every physician is a cardiologist (or clinical pharmacokineticist). The Department of Pharmaceutics of the School of Pharmacy at the State University of New York at Buffalo has established the first post-Pharm.D. specialty training program in clinical pharmacokinetics. Levy[4] and Gi-

baldi[5] have described the philosophy of this concept. To function competently in clinical pharmacokinetics, specialized training in the pharmacokinetic laboratory is definitely indicated. Also, considerable clinical medicine experience is needed if the specialist in clinical pharmacokinetics is to advise and work with the physician in clinical matters. The Pharm.D. graduates at Buffalo (and some other programs) have the clinical medicine experience, and with intensive training in the laboratory, it is felt that selected Pharm.D. graduates should be competent in clinical pharmacokinetics. Quite a few clinical pharmacists are now applying pharmacokinetic concepts, often with computer aid, but this alone is not enough to make them specialists in clinical pharmacokinetics. The scientific arm of the pharmacokinetics laboratory is needed as well.

In the long run, clinical pharmacy must prove to be a viable practice outside of the hospital and its clinics. For a meaningful clinical pharmacy practice to develop in the community, pharmacists trained clinically in the organized health care setting (largely hospitals) must spread their practice concepts outside the health care institution. The ferment will not come from community pharmacies, nor will the thrust of clinical pharmacy programs be aimed at the solo medical practitioner and his patients. Particularly favorable settings should be the group family practices now forming throughout the country. At least one article has described a clinical pharmacy practice as a part of a group family practice in Iowa.[6] This is an exciting possibility and could be the largest specialty practice of clinical pharmacy in the future. If this development takes place, the family practitioner of clinical pharmacy will provide needed nourishment to the health care system and to the clinical pharmacy movement. This clinical pharmacist should be a versatile person capable of providing good drug information, managing the drug therapy of many patients and serving as a drug therapy educator to the patient and health care team. Many clinical pharmacists should prefer this role to that of the clinical pharmacist in the hospital.

There are many aspects of clinical pharmacy practice that have been described in the literature. Many of these activities are common to all clinical pharmacy practices, or serve as subspecialty activities for a few clinical pharmacists. The advent of total parenteral nutrition (TPN) a few years ago proved to be a clinical entree for many hospital pharmacists. With the technique being new and involving considerable sterile compounding, many pharmacists were quickly part of the decision-making process for the prescribing and monitoring of TPN therapy. Many of the traditional elements of pharmaceutical compounding were at once combined with the clinical assessment of the patient.

Antibiotic usage studies have been an avenue for the pharmacist to develop ongoing clinical activities in the hospital. Several pharmacy-initiated programs have been described, and the results of these programs have advanced the cause for clinical pharmacy and have improved drug therapy.

Adverse drug reaction detection and reporting has been another route for the involvement of the pharmacist in clinical matters. Early articles in the pharmacy literature brought attention, as did medication error studies, to the need for persons knowledgeable and primarily concerned about drugs to become more involved with the drug use process. This sort of need was manifested a few years later by the tremendous attention brought to drug interactions. Although the sudden interest in drug interactions now seems shallow, since many of the interactions were beneficial and almost all are predictable if the pharmaceutical sciences are known, the publicity was beneficial toward increasing sensitivity to drug therapy problems.

Many pharmacists now serve as an integral part of the cardio-pulmonary resuscitation (CPR) team in hospitals. This involvement can be merely technical (supplying drugs ready-to-administer and recording drug usage) or can involve the pharmacist as an initiator of therapy and a therapeutic advisor throughout the procedure. This is the sort of "blood and guts" activity that vividly dramatizes the clinical involvement of the pharmacist, but alone is not a sufficient practice base.

There are several activities that pharmacists frequently undertake in order to insure appropriate drug therapy. One of these is the taking of medication histories from selected patients upon admission to the hospital or prior to clinic treatment. Nonlegend as well as prescription drugs may be the source of drug-induced diseases or abnormal physical and laboratory findings. Another activity is drug therapy counseling at discharge from the hospital or after initiation of therapy in the clinic. Patient medication compliance, prevention of adverse reactions and toxicity, and general patient enlightenment are reasons for medication counseling.

In some hospitals, clinical pharmacists are deeply involved with rather narrow clinical programs, e.g., monitoring of anticoagulant therapy. Probably the most publicity yet garnered for clinical pharmacy in the lay press dealt with the case of Richard Nixon. The following account from the *New York Times* on November 5, 1974 documents well one activity of the clinical pharmacy program at Long Beach Memorial Hospital and the application of clinical pharmacokinetics:

Latest Bulletin on Nixon

LONG BEACH, Calif., Nov. 4—Following is the text of a bulletin issued at 9:15 a.m. today by Dr. John C. Lungren, personal physician to former President Richard M. Nixon, at Memorial Hospital Medical Center, on his patient's condition:

Former President Nixon still continues

to show gradual improvement. His vital signs are stable.

We will attempt careful ambulation today in his room with help. During this activity he will be closely monitored.

We're still concerned that the minor effusion still persists in the left lung (effusion means presence of a minor amount of fluid in the lung which is probably secondary to irritation of the diaphragm from the hematoma).

We're still working with hematologists in the department of pathology to rule out any abnormality in his blood analysis to account for the platelet deficiency.

He remains under sub-intensive care.

Upon Mr. Nixon's rehospitalization, I asked Dr. William Smith, director of pharmacy services at Memorial Hospital Medical Center and an assistant clinical professor, U.S.C. School of Pharmacy, to use the best scientific method to determine how Mr. Nixon handles the anticoagulant drug Coumadin. This request was made on Thursday morning, Oct. 24.

Dr. Smith on that day assigned two pharmacists of his staff who have specialized in anticoagulant drugs the task of analyzing the previous anticoagulation program of Mr. Nixon.

In addition, he telephoned a colleague, Dr. William Barr, professor and chairman, department of pharmacy and pharmaceutics, Medical College of Virginia, to see if the special computer systems they have been developing could be used to determine the parameters of how Mr. Nixon handles the drug.

Since that time, our Dr. Smith, Dr. Barr and a staff of their pharmacokinetics laboratory have completed and tested several computer programs using both digital and analog computers.

Last week, I received an initial computer generated plot of Mr. Nixon's anticoagulation program through Oct. 27, which has proven very useful.

The computer programs will assist us in deciding the importance of such parameters as: absorption rate, blood level drug concentrations and relationships to laboratory tests, and elimination rate of the drugs, all specific to Mr. Nixon. These parameters now have been tentatively determined but require verification by actual drug blood level studies. Blood samples have been drawn and will be sent to Vir-

ginia early this week for assay. With this data, the computer will provide us with several drug dosing curves from which we can select the best anticoagulation program specific for Mr. Nixon.

I would like to add, Dr. Smith informs me that the analog computer programs for anticoagulant drugs and several other drugs will soon be available on site at Memorial Hospital Medical Center for future patients. Every patient from here on out who gets admitted on anticoagulation therapy will have this new service available to them.

The pharmacy staff and drug information service at Memorial Hospital continues to assist with reviewing all drugs for Mr. Nixon for possible reactions and interactions and serving as resources for drug-related questions.

Issues in Clinical Pharmacy Practice

Existence and Definition of Clinical Pharmacy

In an editorial in July 1972, Whitney asked if the masses of American pharmacy were suffering from the "Ostrich syndrome" (otherwise known as "head-in-sanditis") or if the masses were simply being responsive to inept leadership.[7] This satire was prompted by the report of the Task Force on the Definition of Clinical Pharmacy, Institutional Pharmacy and Group Practice which was adopted by the American Pharmaceutical Association House of Delegates in 1972. This report contained in part the following now infamous statement: " . . . pharmacy should not be identified as 'clinical pharmacy,' and pharmacists should not be identified as 'clinical pharmacists.' "[8] In reaction to the same report, Provost has written:

Although I agree philosophically with the Task Force statement and the APhA's official position, I recognize that it is a good example of organized pharmacy spitting in the wind. And the wind being created by clinical pharmacy is the briskest that has ever swept the profession. Since we have textbooks and journals with "clinical pharmacy" in their titles, departments and professors of clinical pharmacy in schools of pharmacy, and clinical pharmacist job titles in actual practice, it doesn't make much sense to try to reverse or deter the use of an established term. The situation is reminiscent of resolutions of past years against outpatient dispensing.[9]

From cloistered vantage points, some have questioned the seriousness and intent of the clinical pharmacy movement. At the same time others have engaged in polemics. During this while, several hundred pharmacists, largely based in health care institutions, have brought about an entire new direction to pharmacy practice and a whole new dimension to pharmacy education. The existence of clinical pharmacy is not an issue to the hundreds now practicing it intensively.

There likewise has been considerable speculation and debate over a definition of clinical pharmacy. Those now practicing an advanced kind of clinical pharmacy and continually experimenting with new practice concepts can be eternally grateful that organized pharmacy largely twiddled its pestles and did not straight-jacket the concept with a definition in its infancy. A definition worthy of the movement will probably come in time, but at the present it is sufficient to merely be "in love" without trying to reduce all the emotions, feelings and acts to a definition of 25 words or less.

Brodie has conceptualized the role of the clinical pharmacist as follows:

> The pharmacist is available in the patient care area on a 24-hour basis. He takes the patient's drug history on admission and instructs him in the home use of medication on dismissal; he maintains a complete pharmaceutical service record, monitors drug therapy and relates it to clinical laboratory tests and adverse drug reactions; he is available to the physician when he plans the drug regimen and assists the nurse in managing the drug portion of patient care plans for which she is responsible. In addition, he becomes a continually available source of drug information, usually reinforced by an organized drug information service. The pharmacist is responsible for analysis and confirmation of drug orders for patients and for the filling of orders by qualified technicians, and is available to the nurse prior to the time of administration of medications. The pharmacist does not assume an independent role in the planning of drug therapy, but coordinates his efforts with those of the nurse and . . . physician.[10]

There are parts of this conceptualized role which some would wish to expand, clarify or modify, but it largely covers the roles most clinical pharmacists now perform.

Clinical Pharmacy—Specialty or General Direction?

In a 1972 article still relevant today, Provost has questioned whether clinical pharmacy is a specialty practice or a general direction in pharmacy.[9] At the present, some pharmacists are full-time clinical pharmacists while others are only marginally involved or not involved at all. Some have tried to equate clinical pharmacy with hospital pharmacy, but all leaders in hospital pharmacy have gone out of their way to emphasize that clinical pharmacy practice should transcend any environmental barrier. Those leading clinical pharmacy practitioners have no thoughts of trying to limit the clinical pharmacy movement to the hospital or its clinics. Those hospital pharmacists performing only dispensing functions must know that they are not clinical pharmacists if they have read recent issues of the *American Journal of Hospital Pharmacy* or *Drug Intelligence and Clinical Pharmacy*.

If proper leadership existed in most hospital pharmacies, clinical pharmacy could be a general direction for all of hospital pharmacy (this would not exclude other segments of organized pharmacy from becoming more clinical). In very few hospitals has every pharmacist been expected and required to be a clinical practitioner. Most hospitals with clinical pharmacy services still have some pharmacists who merely dispense or perform relatively low level administrative services. The existence of the traditional pharmacist in the face of trained clinical pharmacists with an advanced degree (usually Pharm.D. or M.S.) tends to create a caste system in pharmacy. While both are pharmacists, there often exists much misunderstanding between the two. The basic problem in this dilemma is inadequate leadership on the part of directors of pharmacy. It seems that the profession and the clinical pharmacy movement would be better off if all pharmacists were either practicing clinically or performing high-level management functions. There should be no friction between these two pharmacists; since each complements the other. If this does not come about, a sizeable number of clinical pharmacists in the hospital may be employed outside of the pharmacy department in the future. This will tend to dilute the pharmacy image of the clinical pharmacist and insure the continued stagnation of many pharmacy departments.

Clinical Pharmacy Versus Clinical Pharmacology

Provost has pointed out the close similarity of clinical pharmacy and clinical pharmacology by noting quotations taken from a WHO publication entitled "Clinical Pharmacology: Scope, Organization and Training." This article states:

> The clinical pharmacologist may be concerned with research on the monitoring of adverse effects . . . The clinical pharmacologist is also concerned with monitoring the therapeutic use of drugs and the pattern of drug prescribing, including indications, contraindications and suitability. His interests may also involve research in . . . errors by patients in following directions for taking drugs and dispensing errors. . . .

> Clinical pharmacologists should play an active part in planning the provision and dissemination of information about drugs.

> The analysis of drug levels in body fluids has been shown to be important for the care of individual patients. The clinical pharmacologist has an essential role to play in the practical application of pharmacokinetic data.

> Clinical pharmacologists can fulfill an important service by surveying prescribing patterns and the incidence of adverse reactions. His general pharmacological interests and experience make him the most suitable person to coordinate the detection and quantification of adverse reactions to drugs in hospitals.[9]

Provost goes on to say that one could substitute the word "pharmacist" for "pharmacologist" in all of the preceding quotations and the publication from which they were taken could easily become a treatise on clinical pharmacy.

A clinical pharmacologist is usually a physician with an additional training of about two years duration in clinical pharmacology which prepares him for the scientific study of drugs in man. In an editorial, Francke[11] has stated that there are only about 40 clinical pharmacologists in the U.S. who have both the M.D. and Ph.D. degrees. Francke says that a clinical pharmacist could adequately do 90% of the functions of the clinical pharmacologist, and that if the two work together they would be able to perform even better than they now can.

Charles Walton, one of the most respected pharmacy educators giving sustenance to the clinical pharmacy movement, has written an article entitled "Clinical Pharmacology and Clinical Pharmacy: A Necessary Alliance for Practical Advances in Rational Drug Therapy."[12] Walton suggests that the two groups should work together for mutual benefits, with the clinical pharmacologists serving as strategists and the clinical pharmacists as tacticians in the advancement of rational drug therapy. In this article, Walton stated the case for the need of the American College of Clinical Pharmacology to open its membership to selected clinical pharmacists. This undoubtedly caused anxiety among many physician-pharmacologists and some pharmacy leaders, but it seems to be a wise strategy to promote closer teamwork between the two groups.

The Pharmacist As a Primary Practitioner: Will a Search for Relevance Lead to Subservience?

Some clinical pharmacists have begun providing primary health care in a variety of clinic and ambulatory settings. This is quite common in the USPHS Indian hospitals. Pharmacists are now providing continuing care to patients with hypertension, diabetes, mental illness, tuberculosis and other chronic conditions primarily managed pharmacologically. While this activity by pharmacists is new and exciting, it is not necessarily strengthening to the pharmacy profession. Nurse practitioners and physicians' assistants also perform these activities under the auspices of the physician.

Most pharmacists, even those with the Pharm.D. degree, are not well-trained in physical diagnosis and patient assessment techniques. If the pharmacist is to be a provider of primary health care, he should be educated and trained for this activity, and the patient population should be well-chosen so that the provision of primary health care blends well with the foremost goal of insuring safe and rational drug therapy for a broad base of patients. If this foremost goal is abandoned, clinical pharmacy will lose its identity in an amorphous conglomeration of assistant and allied health practitioners.

Justification of Clinical Pharmacy Services

If clinical pharmacy is to be a continuing movement and sustaining force in pharmacy practice, the patient and his fiscal representatives must be convinced that the benefit is worth the cost. The clinical pharmacist or his employer should be able to gain reimburse-

ment directly for his services (outside the dispensing process and drug cost). While some data have been generated which document the cost benefit of the clinical pharmacist, more data are needed.

It has been encouraging to learn that in a few areas of the country third party payers are reimbursing specifically for clinical pharmacy services unrelated to the dispensing of drug products. Hopefully, detailed reports will soon be published, thereby promoting widespread acceptance of this practice.

Along with adequate reimbursement mechanisms, a legal basis for clinical pharmacy practice needs to be developed in each state. If clinical pharmacy is to be truly important, it must have a responsibility to the patient and health care system which, if unfulfilled, results in legal action against the practitioner and the health care institution.

If the legal basis of practice is developed and reimbursement mechanisms accepted, the next step is for licensing and accrediting bodies to require certain standards of clinical pharmacy practice, particularly the presence of qualified practitioners as a minimum. Qualifications are probably best determined through a self-imposed certification process for the clinical pharmacy specialists and generalists.

Issues in Clinical Pharmacy Education

There are currently several smoldering issues confronting clinical pharmacy education. One is the faculty status of practitioner-educators. If practitioners are going to serve as faculty members they should have academic credentials and be deserving of equal voice with the basic scientists in pharmacy education. Some clinical pharmacists should eventually rise to be full professors, without qualifying titles, and some should become deans of schools of pharmacy, just as physician-educators become professors of medicine and deans of the schools of medicine.

Another issue in pharmacy education is whether or not every pharmacist should be trained clinically. If clinical training is to be of a good quality, several prerequisites must be met. The academic capabilities of the student must be quite high, students must be indoctrinated with a clinical practice philosophy early in their education and a large number of clinical faculty members must exist who can precept the student, often one faculty member for one or two students. These prerequisites are not generally being met, and many B.S. graduates have not had adequate clinical training for the present health care system, let alone systems of the future. Schools of pharmacy do not have adequate faculties to train all students well clinically. Many are hardly giving proper attention to a few Pharm.D. students in a post-B.S. program.

The curricula of schools of pharmacy is a matter in need of considerable innovation. Clinically oriented courses are generally being added in the last year or two of the curriculum, but by this time many students are stone-deaf toward clinical pharmacy and professionalism in general. The course titles in the school catalog look rather appropriate, but the parts have not been assembled in a synchronous fashion and quality is often lacking. Pharmacology, medicinal chemistry and pharmaceutics have been taught in isolation from each other and from the clinical situation.

Another issue in pharmacy education is the adequacy of the role models portrayed by clinical pharmacy faculty. Schools of pharmacy have placed clinical faculty in hospitals so that model clinical practices could be developed, around which the faculty would teach students and residents. Many of these "clinical services" have been eight-hour, five-day-a-week programs which halt completely during vacations and holidays. The faculty activities have usually not been well-integrated with the pharmacy de-

partment. There has often been no real responsibility to the pharmacy department, the medical staff, the hospital or the patient. Pierpaoli has expressed concern about this situation in a recent editorial entitled "The Rise and Fall of Clinical Pharmacy Education."[13] It is of utmost importance that realistic role models be implemented in all teaching programs. It seems rather naive to believe that someone right out of a struggling Pharm.D. program can immediately set himself up as a therapeutic consultant to medical specialists who have been in training for almost a decade. A thorough search for the most qualified and experienced clinical pharmacists must be undertaken. A goal should be for the clinical pharmacy faculty to be considered as peers and colleagues of the clinical medicine faculty.

The Quest for Quality in Clinical Pharmacy Practice

There are many critical factors along the pathway to quality in clinical pharmacy practice. For the continued growth and maturation of clinical pharmacy, schools of pharmacy and their affiliated hospitals hold the key to excellence. Practice, in general, will be no better than the educational process of the schools of pharmacy and the training programs of the teaching hospitals. In an invited lecture at the 1975 annual meeting of the American Association for the Advancement of Science, Dean Michael Schwartz outlined the following characteristics necessary for quality in pharmacy education:

1. All schools of pharmacy should be components of academic health science centers, which should include at least schools of medicine and nursing.
2. Each school of pharmacy should have strong basic science teaching and research programs in at least its major disciplines, i.e., pharmacology, medicinal chemistry and pharmaceutics.

3. Within each academic health science center there need be only one department of pharmacology with its primary base in the school of pharmacy, but serving the teaching needs of all professions.
4. Schools of pharmacy should undertake responsibility for supervising the entire continuum of education and training of all pharmacists and supportive personnel.
5. The full-time clinical faculty should be subject to the same standards of scholarship and expertise by which their counterparts in academic clinical medicine are judged.
6. Each school of pharmacy should have one or more faculty member taking part in the research efforts of the academic health science center in socioeconomic aspects of health care delivery.[14]

Schwartz further suggested that the single most powerful tool available to build an educational structure based on excellence is accreditation. He stated the need for a high level of minimum standards so that weak schools could not continue. Other suggestions were that scholarly effort by clinical faculty must be supported and rewarded, and that a system of certification of specialties should incorporate the highest standards and judgments by peers, and that the certification be carried out in a rigorous manner.

The American Association of Colleges of Pharmacy and the American Council on Pharmaceutical Education should give immediate attention to establishing rigorous standards for the Pharm.D. programs in existence. These programs are supplying much of the clinical pharmacy manpower, but the quality of graduates varies tremendously. Some programs have strong clinical pharmacokinetics and medical school components, while others are void in these courses. Some have extensive residency or clerkship requirements, while others do not.

Residency training in clinical pharmacy needs to undergo considerable evolution over the next few years. It seems that clinical pharmacy residencies should be confined largely to progressive teaching hospitals and the ambulatory programs of these hospitals. Furthermore, many believe that clinical pharmacy residencies should take place in those pharmacy departments offering high quality comprehensive pharmacy services in which the total services are well-integrated into a continuum of service. Very few departments currently meet this criterion. As a result, many residents fail to appreciate the enormous teamwork and talents needed for total services. A critical matter in those hospitals with pharmacy residencies is to elevate the level of practice of *all* pharmacists so that residents are being trained to practice as the entire staff is practicing. The dichotomy between what residents are being taught and what they see practiced must cease if true quality is to be obtained.

A matter of considerable importance is the development and eventual certification of clinical pharmacy specialties. Currently, drug information, pediatric clinical pharmacy, psychiatric clinical pharmacy, family clinical pharmacy, clinical pharmacokinetics and radiopharmacy are logical specialty areas in which practitioners are now identified. The impetus and planning of the certification process should come from those pharmacists functioning as specialists. The specialty examining board should be composed of roughly the following persons: several clinical pharmacists nationally recognized in the specialty, at least two prominent physicians closely allied to the specialty, a pharmacy educator of national prominence and a health care administrator or planner. Except in unusual circumstances, a candidate for certification should have completed a Pharm.D. or clinically oriented M.S. program and should have completed a clinical residency or fellowship in the specialty. This initial certification should not be controlled by any pharmacy organization.

Clinical pharmacy must develop into a challenging and rewarding practice if it is to succeed. My own view is that the scope and depth of knowledge and skills in the domain of clinical pharmacy is of such a magnitude that many years of intensive learning are required to master the field. There are no overnight successes. Intellectually, there is no dead end to clinical pharmacy unless imagination and ambition are lacking. It is imperative that many excellent practitioners remain in the clinical arena for a lifetime. Only then will the practice truly advance and become established. I have heard many young clinical pharmacists remark that they can not visualize themselves in their practice when they turn 35 or 40 years of age. The reason for this uncertainty is the lack of a colleague and peer relationship with the physician and the absence of a substantial scientific practice base. It is important that the substance of clinical pharmacy practice sustain the qualified pharmacist through a career of clinical pharmacy practice, often in a specialty area.

In order for clinical pharmacy practice to grow and become established, a new breed of hospital pharmacy department head is required. If clinical pharmacy is to become the practice standard and its practitioners rewarded and encouraged, directors of pharmacy in large part need to have been trained clinically. They must realize the planning, sacrifices and hard work necessary to develop a comprehensive pharmacy program that is clinically based. They must support well, both professionally and financially, those who achieve clinically as well as administratively.

In the long run, the success of clinical pharmacy will be proportional to its contribution to patient care and public welfare. It must have the consent of other health care practitioners, health care administrators, third-party insurance firms, the government and the public. There are many determinants of quality, and a concerted effort by practitioners, educators and department heads is needed to advance clinical pharmacy practice.

References

1. Francke, D. E.: The importance of an historical perspective, *Drug Intell Clin Pharm* 8:55 (Feb) 1974.
2. Francke, D. E.: Drug intelligence and clinical pharmacy, *Drug Intell Clin Pharm* 3:157 (Jun) 1969.
3. Francke, G. N.: Evolvement of clinical pharmacy, *Drug Intell Clin Pharm* 3:348 (Dec) 1969.
4. Levy, G: An orientation to clinical pharmacokinetics, *In* Levy G. (ed): Clinical pharmacokinetics, American Pharmaceutical Association Academy of Pharmaceutical Sciences, Washington, DC, (Oct) 1974, p 1.
5. Gibaldi, M.: The clinical pharmacokinetics laboratory of the School of Pharmacy of the State University of New York, *In* Levy G. (ed): Clinical pharmacokinetics, American Pharmaceutical Association Academy of Pharmaceutical Sciences, Washington, DC, (Oct) 1974, p 11.
6. Juhl, R. P. et al: The family practitioner-clinical pharmacist group practice, *Drug Intell Clin Pharm* 8:572–575 (Oct) 1974.
7. Whitney, H. A. K., Jr.: The ostrich syndrome in American pharmacy, *Drug Intell Clin Pharm* 6:245 (Jul) 1972.
8. Report of the Task Force on the Definition of Clinical Pharmacy, Institutional Pharmacy and Group Practice, *J Am Pharm Assoc NS* 12:306–312 (Jun) 1972.
9. Provost, G.: Clinical pharmacy: specialty or general direction? *Drug Intell Clin Pharm* 6:285–289 (Aug) 1972.
10. Brodie, D. C.: Drug utilization and drug utilization review and control, National Center for Health Services Research and Development, p 41 (Apr) 1970.
11. Francke, D. E.: The clinical pharmacist and the clinical pharmacologist, *Drug Intell Clin Pharm* 6:207 (Jun) 1972.
12. Walton, C. A.: Clinical pharmacology and clinical pharmacy—a necessary alliance for practical advances in rational drug therapy, *J Clin Pharmacol* 1:1–7 (Jan) 1974.
13. Pierpaoli, P.: The rise and fall of clinical pharmacy education, *Drug Intell Clin Pharm* 9:97 (Feb) 1975.
14. Schwartz, M.: Educational needs for pharmacy practice in the year 2000, *Drug Intell Clin Pharm* 9:447–451 (Aug) 1975.

67—Clinical Pharmacy—Past, Present, and Future

Harry C. Shirkey

Introduction

It is said that those who do not pay attention to or learn from history may be forced to relive it. Early in our history, the professions of medicine and pharmacy were identified but not separated. They were intertwined to the benefit of patients. As time went by, the separate functions of the two professions became rather clearly delineated, although each performed to a small extent the functions considered to belong to the other. That is, some physicians dispensed while some pharmacists prescribed. In each case, the patient generally did less well, since neither professional was adept in the other's field. Now we see medicine and pharmacy moving closer together. Pharmacists today are living in an exciting and dynamic era; that of the development of clinical pharmacy. Pharmacists are reshaping their profession and making history! Clinical pharmacy has breathed new life into pharmacy.

As a pharmacist and physician I am very proud that, in a small way, I have been able to participate in the clinical pharmacy movement. I am personally indebted to two pharmacy deans who allowed me to take my pharmacy classes to the clinics, the wards and the patient amphitheaters. One of them was Dean Joseph Kowalewski (University of Cincinnati) who, in the late 1940's, was fortunately an iconoclast. Pharmacy at that time was in its "glamorous isolation" where pharmacy and medical education and their students' exposures were separated! By breaking this tradition, pharmacy students in 1948 were able to see a patient anesthetized before their very eyes in a surgical amphitheatre. The planes and stages of anesthesia were dramatically taught and easily remembered. Clinical exposure as part of life is better and longer remembered than learning from textbooks. In that situation pharmacology had strong clinical support.

Later, in 1961, the pharmacy students of Samford University [in Birmingham AL] had regular "laboratory" classes and participated in the therapy of children at the hospital.[1] This clinical union, encouraged by Dean Woodrow Byrum, continues today. Young pharmacists, physicians, nurses and others were being educated together at under- and post graduate levels. The goals of the hospital were being reached—excellence in patient care, education and research as they complemented and supplemented each other for quality, and continuously improving, child care.

Patients are the best teachers. One critically ill little black girl of five was carried to the hospital in severe heart failure. She had been in the hospital less than a month before and was sent home on medicine. Fluid was filling her lungs, her heart rate was extremely rapid, she gasped for air; her senses were dulled. She had congestive heart failure. Without delay of treatment, pharmacy students saw (inspected), listened and heard (auscultated), percussed and felt and touched (palpated). Two weeks later, this lovely "teacher" bounced a ball down the aisle of the same room. Not one student recognized her. Treatment was dramatic! The pharmacy students then recognized the power of their drugs which had not been given previously at home (lack of compliance).

Is There Justification for New Roles?

Let it clearly be recognized that pharmacy leaders, practitioners and educators, over the years have developed pharmacy from an apprenticeship system through progressive yearly increments of academic education of one, two, three, four, five and six years. Then, in recent years, came the tremendous blow! "Technicians can do your work." "Count and pour; lick and stick" no longer was professional. Has it not been well known for a long time that most of the training the "corner druggist" needs could be obtained on the job? The "ninety day wonders" of the Armed Services have always supported the need for and the value of technicians. Years of military experience have proven that pharmacy has the ability to train technicians in short courses to work efficiently under the supervision of a pharmacist.

Now, were the schools of pharmacy to train fewer pharmacists to direct the work of many technicians? *No!* The highly, although not clinically, trained students and graduates were to become part of the policy-determining and therapy-directing team. Scientists should act after collecting data. After escalating the pharmacy curriculum (without data for need), pharmacists were previously led down a cul-de-sac. Pharmacists have become "technicians!" Has clinical pharmacy obtained its new "strength" from a similar philosophy? Or is there data? What is the proof of the clinical pharmacist's value in the health care system? The cost of health care is such that the value of clinical pharmacy must be worthy of the cost—i.e., to the patient. Do we have data? Ideally, clinical pharmacy should reduce costs. How much more cost can be loaded on the back of the sick?

Should Pharmacists Prescribe?

Can the role of the clinical pharmacist be cost justified better if prescribing is one of the functions? For that matter, should the clinical pharmacist even be the drug expert, or should it be left to the clinical pharmacologist? What is a clinical pharmacologist? He is usually a physician with special training and experience in the animal laboratory, the bench laboratory but principally with patients (bedside care and research), and especially as related to drugs, as part of a total treatment regime. He, by training, examination and license, can both *diagnose* and *prescribe* and supervise or consult in the treatment of disease (all aspects).

The M.D. clinical pharmacologist has probably already been trained in a subspecialty of medicine or surgery with a minimum of about twelve to fourteen years of education after high school. The clinical pharmacist may have a minimum of about half this time. Obviously the quantity of the latter should be greater to fill unmet needs. The lesser education and different orientation of the clinical pharmacist makes his contribution greatest as part of a *team* necessitating competent medical diagnosticians.

Even though less trained than pharmacy graduates today, pharmacists have long prescribed for people who came directly to them for care. Funny that the suggestion of pharmacists prescribing sounds new; historically "counter prescribing" was then frowned on. Why should it be considered more ethical today? The clinical pharmacist should not "go it alone" in prescribing drugs. How can he, when he has not been trained to diagnose?

Should Pharmacists be Taught Diagnostic Skills?

Almost completely missing from the vast number of articles on clinical pharmacy is a discussion of how any meaningful treatment depends on *precise* diagnosis. This is a *critical* point because many are suggesting that pharmacists prescribe medications.[2-6] Many who suggest this would have the pharmacist "play physician," not as part of the team. Too, most pharmacists have not had training in clinical pharmacy.[7] I am worried! Are we rediscovering "counter prescribing" by the pharmacist without diagnosis? There are those who push the concept of pharmacists' prescribing—the politicians and others who promise comprehensive health care. Care in volume but not necessarily the best! Quality health care depends on diagnosis to ensure a possibility (no guarantee) of adequate therapy. Will we as pharmacists allow "less than the best" to substitute something for the promises? Or, worse yet, is the patient's self-diagnosis to be the basis of treatment?[8] Will television direct therapy? Will the clinical pharmacist stem the tide? Team work should be recognized as important for the *survival* of clinical pharmacy as an entity. It can contribute its richness to patient care.

Precise diagnosis permits (does not ensure) proper therapy (drug therapy included). A physician makes a diagnosis using all or part of the following:

I. **History.** A skillfully trained historian gains clues from symptoms, the progress of disease, genetics, and many other points to suggest the area of diagnosis to be considered. A check list of questions with answers is a poor substitute, especially if taken by one not particularly adroit in this important diagnostic technique.

II. **Physical Examination.** During the physical examination, the history may be strengthened by more pertinent and directed questions, and at any point strengthening of all points may be made.

A. **Inspection.** This is a most important part of the physical examination. The accomplished diagnostician can properly evaluate a grimace, an inappropriate smile, and weave it into a final answer as it fits into the diagnostic picture. Various scopes allow vision into ear, eye, mouth, rectum, vagina, peritoneum, joints, and other areas.

B. **Palpation.** The touching of the patient. Touch is a fantastic device of communication as well as necessary in feeling for masses, normal or abnormal. The soft or firm edge of the liver, the tip and notch of the spleen. The tone of the rectal sphincter, the palpation of abdominal masses with one finger in the rectum or vagina and a hand on the abdomen—these are part of the clinical assessment.

C. **Auscultation.** Listening with the unaided ear or with the stethoscope permits the hearing of normal or abnormal lung, heart, or bowel sounds, as it does the abnormal bruit, listening anywhere over the body, revealing an abnormal communication between artery and vein.

D. **Percussion.** Like tapping a barrel for sounds, this technique is another dimension of physical examination.

III. **Laboratory.** The expansion of diagnosis by the many available laboratory aids permits correlation with the history and physical examination and may redirect attention to any of the above for new discovery. Normal and abnormal tissues and fluids can be submitted to multiple laboratory examinations. Yes, the skillful clinician chooses **few** among the many tests, especially since cost is a factor in health care, and they are requested to strengthen or refute his working diagnosis. Test results themselves rarely "make" the diagnosis. Recent development of new techniques for expanded x-ray diagnosis, electrocardiography, non-invasive echoencephalography, and other procedures, continue to demand re-education to improve diagnostic acumen.

IV. **Course and Treatment.** The progress of the patient after institution of therapy may be of cardinal importance in making a precise diagnosis and in monitoring therapy as a diagnostic and treatment tool.

V. **Autopsy.** While of no life value to the patient, the autopsy has great value, either to similar patients with the same symptoms (early in an epidemic) or as one of a series of similar cases to be studied together subsequently. The autopsy may be the ultimate method of diagnosis.

In a situation where a diagnosis is made without the benefit of all the available information there is always a risk of catastrophe. A child with but mild respiratory symptoms may have only one or two petechiae, seen only after the clothing is removed for examination, or by careful inspection and search of the skin or well illuminated mouth or throat. Delay in correctly diagnosing the child's condition may bring death within two or three hours. In a different situation, a rectal finger examination may reveal a curable cancer in the person with otherwise "simple" constipation. Astute interpretation of the history alone directs the need for an easily performed rectal examination. These examinations are denied to the pharmacist acting alone, but are part of the team's resources.

Taking congestive heart failure, for example, the elements of history, physical examination, laboratory examination, and of course response to treatment, which are all necessary for diagnosis, are the same elements which are required for proper monitoring of the patient's therapy. Modalities of treatment include bed rest, the proper position in bed, manipulation of diet, oxygen and other drugs, psychotherapy and possibly parenteral fluids. Drugs *alone* are weak friends to the therapist.

Who is in Charge of the Patient?

In some clinical situations, the physician responsible for the patient may choose the clinical pharmacist to direct and monitor the drug therapy, or for that matter, all therapy. This should be because of the already proven expertise of the clinical pharmacist, the lesser capacity of the physician, or both. There will be variable situations. Overwork

and lack of physicians should not be the reason for such responsibility. If a greater number of physicians need to be trained, or they need to be trained more adequately, then such training is the answer.

There are many kinds of therapists in hospitals. In fact, there is great danger of the patient being partitioned[9] by a number of interested advocates of their profession, through pride and an understandable aggressiveness for a place in the sun. For each ship there must be one and only one person totally responsible—the Captain. All patients deserve the same total *quality* of care and direction. The ship's captain wisely shares his decision-making and the execution of required duties with his crew, especially certain ones who have by *excellence proven* their capacity. But there must be one captain. Who would you choose to be the captain?[10,11] No group needs to be on the "back of the bus"[11] in a well functioning team.

All licensed professionals must realize that their license, with its privileges and limitations, comes from the people (only indirectly from a professional society or board). The captain of the patient's care could, for example, be a social worker, who chooses certain "providers" of care as seen by that individual's limited experience and training. I have seen social workers act poorly as referring physicians but excellently as team members. The physician, by reason, license, and responsibility, must be the team captain. Only he can work alone, should that be necessary.

Should the resurgence of the pharmacist's interest in patients make him the captain of the team and should he choose the "providers"?[10-12] The profession could gain greater medical and surgical skills, gain political clout and become pharmacist-physicians. We already have divisions in medicine—allopaths, homeopaths, and osteopaths. One leader in organized pharmacy related to me personally that pharmacy-physicians were a distinctly possible product of the clinical pharmacy movement. If that were to be the consummated goal, then the vacuum of what *was* pharmacy would need to be filled by some other named health profession. Is this a goal? If it is, a number of students and present pharmacy practitioners would balk. Others who feel it is will be greatly disappointed. There is still not a solid front for clinical pharmacy, as dynamic as the field is and as much genuine energy is being expended. New responsibilities bring new risks, legal problems and more malpractice suits.[13-15] Who will sign the death certificates?

Are we training individuals in clinical pharmacy to act as team members or to go out alone to practice? Again, if quality of care is of less importance than the quantity or prestige of our practitioners, the answer could be that those trained in a hospital setting would practice as individuals or in small groups, *without* the continuing presence of a physician. Would we push our graduates to treat without diagnosis, then arm them with inferior OTC drugs? What would be the chance of success? The physician could be called "when needed." This system has failed where incompletely trained medical students so acting call "when needed." They knew not that they didn't know. *Will pharmacists?* Some advocate treatment by pharmacists of now neglected groups (American Indians,[12] psychiatric[16] and nursing home patients[17]). Is pharmacy going to allow the government or other groups to force it into second class status, or should the needs be met adequately to give this country the best care in the world, where pharmacists *contribute* to first class patient care and where pharmacists are *first* class?

When the Drug Research Board of the National Research Council heard representatives of clinical pharmacy, it was quite clear that there was a great divergence of opinions as to what clinical pharmacists should do. The spectrum of variability of human responses was evident. Some clearly placed the welfare of the patients first—even above

survival of pharmacy as we knew or know it. Others described a non-captained team with all crew. All of them correctly pinpointed defects in the present health care delivery system. With the passing of time, the answer to what clinical pharmacists should do becomes clearer.

The Future is Today

For clinical pharmacy, opportunities are rapidly unfolding, especially in hospitals. Hospital pharmacists when involved with patients are active as clinical pharmacists. Hospital pharmacists and their technicians should be part of the entire clinical pharmacy program. There needs to be one pharmacy head in each institution. Certainly *not* a committee. Areas of strength should be continuously monitored. If a Drug and Poison Information Center is receiving few calls or even many insignificant ones, it cannot be performing a vital function. It may even be poorly filling a vacuum which would otherwise gain sufficient attention to gain support for a fine center. Continuance of excellent activity in this and other areas where clinical pharmacists have offered significant contributions permit even greater recognition of pharmacy as a profession. It is of great importance for the pharmacist to be in all patient environments to see what he can contribute. I still see many instances where excellence in drug therapy can fail. For example, one may still see the clinical nurse with her mortar and pestle pounding on tablets to disintegrate them. There are many more situations which require constant attention in hospitals, since naive new populations of students will arrive to be educated and will imitate what they see and do.

There seems to be a clear need for the clinical pharmacist to go *outside* the university hospitals. How far he should go is not clear. How far he should *not* go is clearer. Large clinics require and deserve the talents of clinical pharmacists. The same is true for large and even small hospitals. While some small hospitals cannot afford a full-time pharmacist, they cannot afford to be without pharmacy service and direction. Part-time clinical pharmacy direction should be available to all.

What of the community pharmacy? Pharmacists in a community can be closely related to physicians, but still cannot know what has transpired during the diagnostic steps described previously, and the directions for treatment. How can they know what to supplement, what to duplicate, in supplying information to patients? Functioning alone, advice given to patients may cause problems of great import. It is certainly unsafe to assume that either the physician omitted the important facts, or if he did cover them, to assume that the pharmacist will do better. Are these data? Will there be less of adverse reactions, greater compliance? Wishing will not make it so.

Should clinical pharmacy exposure (patient exposure) be part of every pharmacy student's background? I unequivocally say, "Yes"! Otherwise, pharmacists can go to their shops (perhaps part of a department store or drug store environment) and lose themselves. Yes, even for the "technician," because he must relate his experience to the nature of his work—it relates to life and death. Ultimately all effort leads to the patient!

References

1. Susina, S. V., Adams, W. H., Shirkey, H. C. and Byrum, W. R.: The Hospital: A Pharmacology Laboratory for Pharmacy Students, *Am. J. Pharm. Educ.* 28:216–218, 1964.
2. Penna, R. P.: The Medicine-Pharmacy Interface—Harmony or Dissonance, presented to the Pharmaceutical Manufacturers Association, Ponte Verda, Florida, May 1, 1972.
3. Anon.: Lee Predicts Coming Era of Pharmacist Prescribing, *A PhA Weekly*, Vol. 15 April 1976.
4. Dahl, C. F.: Insight into the Issue "Clinical" Pharmacy, Special Meeting APhA House of Delegates, Cincinnati, Ohio, Nov. 10, 1972.
5. Werble, W. (Ed.): Pharmacist Will Prescribe Drugs, *Drug Research Reports (The Blue Sheet)* 14:RN3, 1971.
6. Whitney, H. A. K. and Covington, T. R.: The Future Impact of Clinical Pharmacy on Parenteral Drugs and the Industry, *Bull. Parenter, Drug Assoc.* 25:87–97 (Mar.-Apr.) 1971.
7. Dolezal, J. F. (Letter): Pharmacists Don't Know All the Answers, *N. Engl. J. Med.* 295:110 (July 8) 1976.
8. Bicket, W. J.: Autotherapy, the Future Is Now, *J. Am. Pharm. Assoc.* NS 12:560–564 (Nov.) 1972.
9. Moser, R. H.: The Partitioning of the Patient, *House Physician Reporter* (Dec.) 1971.
10. Anon.: Challenge to Pharmacy in the 70's, *Public Health Service Publication No. 2146*, U.S. Department of HEW, Rockville, Md., 1970.
11. Apple, W. S.: "Pharmacy's Lib," *J. Am. Pharm. Assoc.* NS 11:528–533 (Oct.) 1971.
12. Anon.: The Pharmacist as a Provider of Primary Health Care (unpublished). U.S. Dept. of H.E.W., Indian Health Service, March 14, 1974.
13. Fink, J. L. III: Some Legal Issues Presented in Clinical Pharmacy Practice, *Drug Intell. Clin. Pharm.* 10:444–447 (Aug.) 1976.
14. Barker, K. N. and Valentino, J. G.: On a Political and Legal Foundation for Clinical Pharmacy Practice, *J. Am. Pharm. Assoc.* NS 12:202–206 (May) 1972.
15. Kent, R. F.: Pharmacists Face More Malpractice Suits, *Medical Tribune*, Nov. 19, 1975.
16. Evans, R. L., Kirk, R. F., Walker, P. W. et al.: Medication Maintenance of Mentally Ill Patients by a Pharmacist in a Community Setting, *Am. J. Hosp. Pharm.* 33:635–638 (July) 1976.
17. Devenport, J. K. and Kane, R. L.: The Role of the Clinical Pharmacist on a Nursing Home Care Team, *Drug Intell. Clin. Pharm.* 10:268–271 (May) 1976.

68—Pharmacists for the Future: The Report of the Study Commission on Pharmacy

What are the roles of pharmacists likely to be in the future and how should they be trained to meet the needs of society? One response to this question is available from the report of the Study Commission on Pharmacy that was issued in December of 1975. Because this comprehensive investigation treated a number of related issues, the summary of the findings of this expert panel is included here.

1. The Study Commission recognizes that among deficiencies in the health care system, one is the unavailability of adequate information for those who consume, prescribe, dispense and administer drugs. This deficiency has resulted in inappropriate drug use and an unacceptable frequency of drug-induced disease. Pharmacists are seen as health professionals who could make an important contribution to the health care system of the future by providing information about drugs to consumers and health professionals. Education and training of pharmacists now and in the future must be developed to meet these important responsibilities.

2. The Study Commission advances the concept that pharmacy should be conceived basically as a *knowledge system* which renders a *health service* by concerning itself with understanding drugs and their effects upon people and animals. Pharmacy generates knowledge about drugs [and] acquires relevant knowledge from the biological, chemical, physical, and behavioral sciences; it tests, organizes and applies that knowledge. Pharmacy translates a substantial portion of that knowledge into drug products and distributes them widely to those who require them. Pharmacy knowledge is disseminated to physicians, pharmacists, and other health professionals and to the general public to the end that drug knowledge and products may contribute to the health of individuals and the welfare of society. . . .

3. The Study Commission believes that a pharmacist must be defined as an individual who is engaged in *one of the steps of a system called pharmacy*. We cannot define a pharmacist simply as one who practices pharmacy. Rather, he must be defined as one who practices a *part* of pharmacy which is determined by the activities carried on in one of the subsystems of pharmacy. A pharmacist is characterized by the common denominator of drug knowledge *and the differentiated additional knowledge and skill* required by his particular role. . . .

4. The Study Commission believes that the system of pharmacy must be described as being both effective and efficient in developing, manufacturing, and distributing drug *products*. However, the system of pharmacy cannot be described at present as either effective or efficient in developing, organizing, and distributing *knowledge and information* about drugs. When pharmacy is viewed as a knowledge system, it must be judged as only partially successful in delivering its full potential as a health service to the members of society. . . .

5. The Study Commission recommends that major attention be given to the problems of drug information to find who needs to know, what he needs to know, and how these needs can best be met with speed and economy. . . .

6. It is the opinion of the Study Commission that in spite of the real and multifaceted differentiation in the practice roles of pharmacists, there is a *common* body of knowl-

edge, skill, attitudes, and behavior which all pharmacists must possess. In a practical and detailed sense the objectives of pharmacy education must be stated in terms of *both the common knowledge and skill and of the differentiated and/or additional knowledge and skill required for specific practice roles.* This can be done only by stating a series of limited educational objectives which if met in sequential order will accomplish both common and differentiated objectives. . . .

7. The Study Commission recommends the following three component educational objectives for pharmacy education:
  a. The mastery of the knowledge and the acquisition of the skills which are *common* to all of the roles of pharmacy practice.
  b. The mastery of the additional knowledge and the acquisition of the additional skill needed for those differentiated roles which require additional *pharmacy* knowledge and experience.
  c. The mastery of the additional knowledge and the acquisition of the additional skills needed for those differentiated roles which require additional knowledge and skill *other than pharmacy.* . . .

8. The Study Commission recommends that every school of pharmacy promptly find the ways and means to provide appropriate practice opportunities for its faculty members having clinical teaching responsibilities so that they may serve as effective role models for their students. . . .

9. It is the opinion of the Study Commission that the curricula of the schools of pharmacy should be based upon the *competencies* desired for their graduates rather than upon the basis of knowledge available in the several relevant sciences. . . .

10. It is the opinion of the Study Commission that the greatest weakness of the schools of pharmacy is a lack of an adequate number of *clinical scientists* who can relate their specialized scientific knowledge to the development of the practice skills required to provide effective, efficient, and needed patient services. The Study Commission recommends that support be sought for a program to train a modest number of clinical scientists for pharmacy education. . . .

11. The Study Commission emphasizes that pharmacy is a knowledge system in which *chemical substances and people called patients* interact. Needed and optimally effective drug therapy results only when drugs and those who consume them are fully understood. We suggest that one of the first steps in reviewing the educational program of a college of pharmacy should be weighing the relative emphasis given to the physical and biological sciences against the behavioral and social sciences in the curriculum for the first professional degree. . . .

12. The Study Commission believes that those schools of pharmacy with adequate resources should develop, in addition to the first professional degree, programs of instruction at the graduate and advanced professional level for more differentiated roles of pharmacy practice. . . .

13. It is the opinion of the Study Commission that the optimal environment for pharmacy education is the university health science center for the full range of knowledge, skill, and practice can be found there. However, the Commission does not believe that it is practical or in the public interest to recommend that all colleges of pharmacy must be so located. Alternative arrangements, if effectively utilized, can provide an acceptable environment for the education of students at the baccalaureate level. . . .

14. It is the opinion of the Study Commission that all aspects of credentialling of pharmacists and pharmacy education and the quality of pharmacy education would be enhanced by the services of a National Board of Pharmacy Examiners. The Commission recommends that the National Association of Boards of Pharmacy, the American Council on Pharmaceutical Education, the

American Association of Colleges of Pharmacy and those professional organizations contemplating specialty certification, join in the formation of a committee to study the necessity and the feasibility of creating a National Board of Pharmacy Examiners and to recommend appropriate functions, activities, and organization.

Readings for a Broader Perspective

1. White, E. V. "A Family Pharmacist Takes a Critical Look at the Report of the Study Commission on Pharmacy," *Drug Intelligence & Clinical Pharmacy* 11 (February 1977): 94–101.
2. Gosselin, R. A. "The Future of Pharmacy," *American Journal of Pharmaceutical Education* 40 (August 1976):223–27.
3. Goyan, J. "Pharmacy Education in the 21st Century," *California Pharmacist* 24 (August 1977):26.
4. Boutwell, H., Garner, D. D., and Smith, M. C., "A Futurible Model for Community Pharmacy Practice," *J. Am. Pharm. Assoc.* NS 14 (January 1974):31–33; 40.
5. Smith, M. C. "Drugs of the Future and the Future of Drug Distribution," *American Journal of Hospital Pharmacy* 31 (July 1974): 677–83.

Chapter Five

Opportunities for Non-Practitioners

As it is noted in Table I-1, more than 9,000 pharmacy-trained graduates in 1973 held full-time positions in a variety of settings where direct patient care was not a primary objective of their employment. If this estimate could be adjusted for (a) under-reporting, (b) non-practitioners holding administrative posts but enumerated in practitioner-oriented categories such as "large chains" or "hospitals," and (c), the net increase in pharmacy graduates since the previous survey, it seems probable that the current figure exceeds 12,000.

With an employment base of this magnitude, normal replacement demand alone suggests job possibilities for pharmacists seeking a different means of professional expression. Moreover, in the judgment of the editor of these readings, the rate of growth in many of these areas is likely to exceed that for practitioners generally. This favorable outlook for those interested in positions as non-practitioners must be tempered to reflect the fact that some may require additional study beyond the first degree in pharmacy. Nevertheless, both practitioners seeking advancement opportunities, as well as pharmacy graduates interested in specialized areas of contribution, will want to examine the material below.

Your quest for guidance, though, is hampered by our lack of basic knowledge about the role of pharmacists as non-practitioners. Consequently, treatment of this topic is uneven and, of necessity, confined to information readily available.

Job Titles of Non-Practitioners

Table V-1 enumerates job titles held by pharmacy-trained graduates that have been compiled from personal knowledge and announcements appearing in professional or trade publications. While the 14 major categories are thought to be reasonably complete, a comprehensive survey probably would yield sufficient new entries to more than double the reported number of over 260.

In reviewing this list, it is essential for you to remember that some positions may call for prior experience as a licensed practitioner. These include the store supervisor or district manager employed by a chain drug firm, the director of a pharmacy department in a large hospital, and the executive director of a state board of pharmacy. Most of the remaining positions listed are probably filled by pharmacy graduates who have entered these posts directly or who acquired additional training.

Several titles may reflect similar responsibilities. Under the heading *Government— State & Local*, "Coordinator, Pharmacy Services," "Pharmaceutical Coordinator," and "Pharmacy Consultant," probably signify assignments involving the administration of prescription drug benefits within a health insurance program. On the other hand, a single entry, "Professional Representative" under *Pharmaceutical Manufacturing*, accounts for more than 2,000 pharmacists who are employed in this capacity. In addition, the reading on Pharmacist-

Table V-1

Selected Job Titles Held by Pharmacists as Non-Practitioners, Classified by Area of Employment

BUSINESS FIRM; CONSULTANT
Director of Research, Private Health Care Consulting Firm
Division Manager, Programs & Analysis, (Professional Health Systems)
Executive Director, Citizens Alliance for VD Awareness
Executive Vice President, Private Health Care Consulting Firm
Manager, Health Care Software
President, Computer Products & Services
President, Private Health Care Consulting Firm
President, Professional Health Research
Sales Representative, Computer Products & Services
Vice President, Private Health Care Consulting Firm

CHAIN DRUG STORE
Executive
Assistant Vice President & Director of Professional Relations
Assistant Vice President, Special Services
Assistant Vice President, Store Operations
President
Vice President and General Manager
Vice President, Professional Operations (or, Professional Relations)
Vice President, Purchasing and Distribution
Vice President, Store Operations

Store Operations
District Manager
Division Vice President—Pharmacy Operations
Divisional Vice President
Store Supervisor (responsible for 12 to 20 individual stores)

Other Positions
Assistant Director of Drug Purchasing
Director of Drug Purchasing
Director of Professional Operations (or, Professional Personnel)
Director of Special Projects
Director of Third Party Administration
Drug Buyer
Pharmaceutical Buyer
Regional Director of Professional Operations

EDUCATION
College
Assistant to the Dean
Assistant Dean
Associate Dean
Dean
Director of Externship
Director, Pharmacy Extension Services (or Continuing Ed.)
Instructor
Librarian
Professor (Clinical staff, however, function as both practitioners and non-practitioners.)

High School
Drug Ombudsman
Teacher—Science Department

GOVERNMENT—FEDERAL
Administration (HHS)
Acting Chief—Program Review Branch
Acting Chief, PSRO Branch

Acting Director, Division of Survey & Certification
Director, Office of Pharmaceutical Reimbursement
Hospital Administration/Pharmacy Consultant
Pharmacist Consultant
Pharmacy Consultant, Office of the Surgeon General
Pharmacist Director
Program Analyst, Division of Health Protection, OHC
Project Officer
Regional Pharmacy Consultant
Rural Health Systems Branch Project Officer
Senior Advisor for Extramural Affairs
Senior Facilities Certification Program Specialist
Special Assistant to the Principal Regional Official

Drug Purchasing (DOD, VA, AID)
Drug Procurement Specialist

Regulatory Agencies (FDA, FTC, DEA)
Chief, OTC Studies, FDA
Chief, Product Quality Branch, Division of Drug Quality, FDA
Commissioner, FDA
Deputy Associate Director, Bureau of Drugs, FDA
Director, Division of Compliance, FDA
Director, Office of Voluntary Compliance, DEA
Prescription Drug Labeling Officer
Prescription Drug Labeling Specialist
Special Assistant to the Director of OTC Drug Evaluation, FDA

Research (Department of Agriculture, FDA, NIH)
Pharmacologist
Research Pharmacist

Supervision of Patient Care Services (DOD, PHS, VA)
Colonel, Medical Service Corps
Director, Pharmacy Division
Major, Medical Service Corps
Pharmacy Liaison Officer, PHS

U.S. Congress (Staff, GAO, OTA)
Member, House of Representatives
Member, Senate
Policy Analyst, OTA
Staff Analyst
Staff Investigator, Manpower & Welfare Division, GAO

Other (HHS Regional Office, other)
Administrative Assistant, Medical Service Corps
Assistant Chief Counsel for Environment & Health, SBA
Chief, Pharmacy Section, CHAMPUS, DOD
Pharmacist Consultant (10 Regions)
Policy Planning Consultant, Long Range Health Planning, Ottawa
Research Analyst
Science Information Specialist, National Library of Medicine
Supply Officer, Medical Service Corps
VA Scholar
Vice President, U.S.A.

GOVERNMENT—STATE & LOCAL
Health Department
Director, Bureau of Pharmaceutical Services, Los Angeles County Health Dept.
Director, Drugs & Therapeutics Branch, Ontario Ministry of Health
Health Planning Consultant to State Health Coordinating Council
Manager, Support & Special Services, County Health Department
Secretary, State Department of Health & Welfare
State Registrar & Director of Public Health Statistics

Insurance Programs (Medicaid, Workmen's Compensation)
Administrator, Prescription Drug Section
Assistant Chief of Medical Facilities
Assistant Chief, Operations
Assistant Director, Medicaid Program
Assistant Pharmacist Consultant
Chairman, Pharmacy Committee
Chief, Bureau of Health Care
Chief, Division of Pharmaceutical Services
Chief Medical Care Specialist
Chief, Pharmacy Section
Chief of Provider Assistance
Chief, Volume Purchase Plan Section, Medicaid Division
Coordinator, Pharmacy Services
Deputy Director
Director, Medicaid Pharmacy Program
Director of Pharmacy
Director, Pharmaceutical Services
Drug Program Coordinator
Medical Care Program Pharmacist
Pharmaceutical Consultant III
Pharmaceutical Coordinator
Pharmaceutical Director
Pharmacist Consultant
Pharmacy Practice Consultant
Program Management Officer
Program Manager
Senior Consulting Pharmacist
Senior Pharmacist
Senior Social Services Medical Assistance Specialist
Special Policy Consultant to Director, Medicaid Bureau
Staff Specialist
Supervisor, Supplies Program
Utilization Review Unit Specialist

Licensure Agencies
Assistant Executive Director
Director
Executive Director
Executive Secretary
Investigator
Secretary

Mental Health Department
Assistant Commissioner of Interagency Affairs, New York City
Manager, Pharmacy Service Center, Office of Support Services

Other
General Treasurer, State of Rhode Island
Judge, Probate & Juvenile Court, Cheboygan County
Lt. Governor
Member, State House of Representatives
Member, State Senate

HEALTH CARE PROVIDER (Hospital, Health Maintenance Organization, Medical Care Facility, etc.)
Advisor, Drug Abuse Counselling Center
Computer Programmer
Director, Ambulatory Care Center
Director, Drug Information Service
Director, Hospital
Director, Nursing Home
Director, Pharmacy Department
Executive Coordinator for Pharmacy Services (HMO)

Executive Director, Family Health Care Center
Research Associate
Systems Coordinator, Department of Pharmacy, University of Texas System Cancer Center

LAW
Partner
Staff Attorney
Senior Patent Attorney

NON-PHARMACIST PRACTITIONER
Dentist
Physician*
Podiatrist
Veterinarian

PHARMACEUTICAL MANUFACTURING
Executive
Corporate Patent Counsel
Executive Vice President
Medical Department Administrator
President
President, Scientific Division
Vice President—Corporate Planning
Vice President—Sales

Librarian

Marketing and Sales
Associate Marketing Analyst
Director, Chain Store Sales and Planning
Director, Corporate Marketing Research
Director, Technical Affairs
District Manager
Government Administrator
Manager of Marketing Planning
Product Manager
Product Manager, In-Line Products
Professional Representative
Senior Marketing Analyst
Technical Writer

Production
Associate Product Manager
Chief Pharmacist
Director, Drug Information & Clinical Pharmacy Section, Medical Bioavailability Unit
Head, Materials Control
Industrial Pharmacist
Manager, Tablet Technical Services
Packaging Manager
Pharmaceutical Formulations & Process Engineer
Pharmaceutical Quality Inspector
Pharmacist; Process Development
Production Manager
  Injectables
  Liquids & Syrups
  Packaging Specialist
  Sterile Products
  Tablets & Capsules
Production Supervisor
Production Support Pharmacist

Regulatory Affairs
Director Regulatory Affairs
Labeling Specialist

*The President of the American Medical Association in 1972 received his first degree in pharmacy.

Manager Regulatory Affairs
Regulatory Coordinator

Research and Development
Analytical Chemist
Assistant Director
Clinical Associate
Clinical Research Associate
Department Head, Analytical Development
Director, Dept. of Pharmacokinetics & Biopharmaceutics
Director, Pharmaceutical Development
Director, Pharmaceutical Research
Director of Product Development
Group Leader, Physical Pharmacy
Group Leader, Pilot Plant Section
Manager, Technical Information Services
Medical Research Associate
Pharmaceutical Chemist
Principal Scientist, Package Development
Product Development Pharmacist
Research Fellow
Research Pharmacist
Stability Testing Specialist

Trade Relations/Health & Welfare Programs
Assistant Director, Medical Assistance Programs
Coordinator of Health & Welfare Programs
Director, Pharmacy Affairs & Health Programs
Director, Pharmacy Relations
Director, Professional Relations
Director of Trade Relations
Manager Customer Affairs
Manager of Health & Welfare Programs
Manager of Pharmacy Affairs
Manager of Pharmacy Communications
Manager of Pharmacy Relations
Manager Professional Affairs/Relations
Washington Representative, Pharmacy & Health Affairs

PROFESSIONAL/TRADE ASSOCIATIONS
National (APhA, ASCP, ASHP, NARD, PA, PMA, and others)
Associate Director, Minnesota Medical Association
Assistant Director, Pharmacy Management Institute
Associate Executive Director for Professional Affairs
Associate Executive Director for Scientific Affairs
Director, Bureau of Communication and Publication Services
Director, Bureau of Professional and Education Services
Director of Clinical Practice
Director, Drug Reimbursement Programs
Director, Federal Legislative & Regulatory Affairs
Director, Meeting and Convention Services
Director, Pharmacy Management Institute
Director, Professional Services
Director, Public Affairs
Director of Special Projects
Editor; Assistant Editor
Executive Director
Executive Vice President
President
President, American College of Hospital Administrators
Scientific Consultant
Senior Assistant Editor
Senior Clinical Science Writer
Senior Vice President
Vice President
Writer/Analyst, FDA Class Labeling Project

State & Local
Director, Continuing Education
Director, Drug Utilization Review, State Pharmacy Foundation
Executive Director
Executive Secretary
Executive Vice President
President
Secretary

PUBLISHING
Professional/Scientific Press
Editor
Associate Editor
Assistant Editor
Vice President

Public Press
Medical/Science Writer

Trade Press
Editor
Assistant Editor
Associate Editor
Pharmacy Editor
Reporter
Research Director
Staff Writer

THIRD-PARTY INSURANCE PROGRAMS (Private)
Director of Claims Processing
Director of Client Services
Director of Marketing and Client Services
Director of Operations
Director of Pharmacy Services
Manager, Professional Relations (Blue Shield Plan)
Pharmacy Consultant, Administrative
Pharmacy Consultant, Field Audit
President
Senior Pharmaceutical Consultant
Vice President, Government & International Affairs
Vice President, Health Care Information Services
Vice President, Professional Services

WHOLESALING—PHARMACEUTICAL
Corporate Buyer—Pharmaceuticals
Planning Projects Manager
Promotions Buyer
President
Vice President & General Manager, Distribution Center

OTHER
Bank Director
Director, SPCA
Executive Director, Art Institute of Chicago
Executive Director, United States Pharmacopeia
Manager, University Bookstore
President, Mueller Chemical Company
Proprietor, Wholesale Wine Company
Research Scientist, Non-Profit Research Institute

Lawyers (73) indicates that these specialists fill positions in association work, industry, government, teaching, and other areas in addition to the practice of law. Table V-1, therefore, should be viewed as more illustrative than definitive of various jobs available for non-practitioners. With this caution in mind, students can use this list as a beginning reference for more intensive exploration. For further details, contact a college placement counselor or the employers signified by the major categories and subheadings listed below.

Area of Specialization

We now revert to a standard format based upon readings which describe areas of importance for pharmacy graduates who wish to use their technical skills as non-practitioners. Table V-2 outlines six activities where readings are available for this purpose. In considering these possibilities, it should be noted that employment opportunities are likely to be strong for pharmacists who wish to coordinate and monitor the testing of drugs in patients. (Reading 71). Moreover, if Federal legislation should require that Phase IV testing be conducted for significant drugs upon their introduction to the market, the demand for qualified coordinators will increase further.

Students seeking expanding markets for their talents also should give special atten-

Table V-2

Pharmacists as Non-Practitioners. Classification System and Reading Codes

	Reading Code
Drug Ombudsman	69
Pharmaceutical Manufacturing	70–72
Pharmacist-Lawyers	73
Pharmacy Librarianship	74
Professional Association Executive	75–76
Quality Assurance	77

tion to Quality Assurance (77) and the collateral readings that are indicated. If national health insurance legislation is passed, and comprehensive drug benefits are included, pharmacists, with appropriate training, could be expected to hold full-time positions in evaluating prescribing, dispensing and compliance patterns.

Individuals interested in a description of selected positions held by several of the more than 150 pharmacists employed by the U.S. Food & Drug Administration are urged to consult: "Pharmacists in the FDA," *American Pharmacy* NS 20 (January 1980):28–32. Regardless of the non-practitioner area pursued, it is well to ask how the academic program in pharmacy will enhance your ability to advance. Many of the positions noted in this chapter represent executive posts where preference will be given to pharmacists with unique qualifications.

DRUG OMBUDSMAN

69—Alternative Employment for Pharmacists

Dale L. McGowan

After graduating from pharmacy school, most of us have begun a career in dispensing, administration, or clinical work in either a retail or hospital environment. Other graduates have turned to manufacturing, research, detailing and teaching. More recently, consulting pharmacists have found employment with drug information centers, state and federal government, and private corporations such as insurance companies. Finally, a few of us have gone to work in drug treatment centers designed to deal with the increasingly difficult problem of drug abuse. My employment as a drug ombudsman is a new alternative associated with drug abuse and is the subject of this article.

A drug ombudsman is a liaison person who facilitates communication, often between drug users and non-users. As a high school ombudsman, I increase communication between students and faculty at Davis High School in Modesto, California. I'm paid on the teachers' salary scale and work the same times of the year—but no teaching or counseling credential is required.

After graduating from U.C. School of Pharmacy in 1970, I went to work as a retail pharmacist but soon grew tired of the paper-shuffling "clerical work". My search for a job more personally satisfying brought me to Modesto where the school district was concerned about the growing number of young drug users. We created the ombudsman position, and I went to work with a commitment to establish personal relationships with students and faculty and to deal with potentially destructive drug use being caused by the frustrations of students' personal problems.

Is it presumptuous for lay therapists such as pharmacists to expect therapeutic results? I don't think so. The high school students often see the psychiatrist as a threatening institutional figure with whom they cannot "level". I have found it best to offer "counsel" as opposed to psychiatric help. Also, there is a large number of kids who need someone to talk to and very few qualified people to listen to them. Many of these students badly need an authentic, interpersonal relationship but don't have one at home, school, or elsewhere.

The drop-in center, a comfortable room near the center of the school grounds, is a place for individual and group discussion or simply "rapping". If requested by students, I offer drug information and education such as class lectures and articles in the school paper. Chemical analysis on a confidential basis is done for students with capsules, tablets, and powder that may be adulterated. First aid and "talk-down" are available for drug overdose. Under the direct supervision of the principal, the ombudsman gives the faculty feedback on how the students feel about classes, teachers, rules, parents, and other issues. I attend faculty meetings and aid in preparing and evaluating drug-related programs at the high school.

The ombudsman works with community services to help integrate city programs. I enlist the help of workers from other drug treatment centers and agencies such as crisis lines, drop-in centers, law enforcement, churches, health service, social welfare, family and social services, legal agencies, and various lay services. Other facets of my service include referral service, consultant work for other drug treatment centers, and participation in city and county councils relating to drugs.

There are problems in the transition from pharmacist to ombudsman. The greatest difficulty for me is in learning how to talk to students, teachers, and parents without alienating them. Often the people I counsel are sensitive and defensive so the development of a trusting relationship with me is essential. I have corrected part of this problem by insisting that students come to me on their own (no referrals) and that they accept the fact that they are coming because of their problems. Students often want to give me the responsibility for solving a problem, and I emphasize that they must take responsibility for themselves. It works best for me to listen to students and accept their feelings. Students find it easier to talk with an authentic person; that is, a person who experiences the reality of himself by knowing himself, being himself, and becoming a credible, responsive person. He must not be isolated from the many problems around him; to the contrary, a good ombudsman needs to be concerned, compassionate, and committed to improving the students' quality of life.

If the ombudsman alternative sounds promising to you, I hope you will pursue it. If not, I hope you will be aware of drug abuse and the value a pharmacist can be to the community. You are needed.

PHARMACEUTICAL MANUFACTURING

70—Competency Characteristics of the Industrial Pharmacist[1]

Ravindra C. Vasavada

What is industrial pharmacy? A search of the literature reveals there to be no simple, descriptive and generally accepted operational definition. Who then are industrial pharmacists? Here history may be helpful. Although the origins of "manufacturing pharmacy" can be traced back to the community pharmacy in Europe and America(1), the actual start of large-scale manufacturing of drugs and drug products began in the USA in the period of 1820–1840. As the pharmaceutical industry became more established and entered the modern era of growth and complex organization with attendant differentiation of functions, the term "industrial pharmacy" with broader connotations appears to have gained a measure of acceptance. Nevertheless, the somewhat restrictive term of "manufacturing pharmacy" still continues to enjoy wide usage.

Societies of industrial pharmacists had their origins in Europe. In 1955, the International Pharmaceutical Federation created a section of industrial pharmacy in which membership was restricted to pharmacists employed by pharmaceutical industry. Cooper(2) provides an interesting account of this development. He states: "For the first time in the history of pharmacy there came into existence a group dedicated to the promotion of the professional and scientific interest of the thousands of pharmacists employed in industry." The concerns of this group were directed towards increasing productivity and the quality of pharmaceutical products and studying the impact of emerging technology on the practice of industrial pharmacy, pharmacy research and the supply of raw materials.

On this side of the Atlantic, pharmacists' contributions to pharmaceutical industry were finally recognized in 1960 when the American Pharmaceutical Association created the Section of Industrial Pharmacy(3). Under the revised structure created in 1966, this section is now a part of Academy of Pharmaceutical Sciences. These historical events recognize the emergence of a new professional role for pharmacists.

From such a historical perspective, one could simply regard all professional pharmacists employed in pharmaceutical or allied industries as "industrial pharmacists."

One finds varying definitions of the word "pharmacy." Webster(4) defines pharmacy as "the art of preparing, preserving, compounding, and dispensing drugs, of discovering new drugs through research and of synthesizing organic compounds of therapeutic value." On the other hand, a medical dictionary(5) recognizes pharmacy only as "the art of preparing, compounding and dispensing medicines." "The art and science of preparing and dispensing drugs"(6) is an even more succinct statement. These definitions relate to "industrial pharmacy" in that, both compounding and dispensing are included. The Study Commission on Pharmacy(7) has cited the following definition of "pharmacy": "The art and science of compounding and dispensing of drugs or medicines." This is certainly a valid definition if one recognizes that both "compounding" and "dispensing" comprise a series of steps. As well enunciated in the Millis Report(7), compounding can be separated into the following series of steps: (*i*) discovery or invention, (*ii*) formulation, (*iii*) safety, (*iv*) efficacy, and (*v*) manufacture. Today, some or all of these steps are performed in pharmaceutical manufacturing establishments by pharmacy-trained individuals. However, many other disciplines are also involved.

While we have defined the limits wherein an acceptable definition of "industrial pharmacy" may lie, a precise wording is still difficult. Perhaps such must await a legal identification of the functional roles of pharmacists working in pharmaceutical industry in this country. If the present trend towards increasing regulation continues, and the professional pharmacy organizations seize the opportunity, this may not be long in coming. In The Netherlands, production and control of pharmaceuticals must be supervised by a full-time pharmacist, although exceptions are permitted in special cases. The duties of an industrial pharmacist are clearly defined by law. He is responsible for development of final specifications for production and control and their implementation during production(8).

In an industry which developed as an outgrowth of pharmacy, pharmacists today are outnumbered by chemists, biochemists, pharmacologists, microbiologists, and other nonpharmacist specialists. Although relatively small in number,[2] today one finds pharmacists (with or without any specialized education) in a wide variety of roles in research and development, quality control, production, clinical and regulatory affairs, and marketing and sales of pharmaceuticals. An excellent discussion of many of these roles has been presented by Cooper(9). In the area of pharmaceutical research and development, the pharmacist is ideally suited for so-called "product development" because of his diverse training directed towards an understanding of the therapeutic agents and their mode of use. A development pharmacist may actually be involved in one or more of the following areas:

(*i*) "Establishment of those physiochemical properties of drug substances and dosage forms which will influence their uniformity, stability, and physiological availability.

(*ii*) "Development of final formula and full-scale manufacturing process for all forms of administration of new drugs.

(*iii*) "The improvement of existing formulas and processes in terms of quality or cost on the basis of scientific investigation.

(*iv*) "The evaluation of new raw materials with potential value in pharmaceutical formulation, *i.e.*, excipients, solvents, preservatives, *etc.* . . .

(*v*) "The preparation, packaging, and control of new drugs during the entire period of clinical investigation.

(*vi*) "The scientific investigation of the stability and recommended storage conditions for all new products.

(*vii*) "The scientific investigation of merits and faults of new equipment preliminary to routine use in pharmaceutical production.

(*viii*) "The investigation of suitability of proposed packaging materials and containers."

The production function generally involves a variety of activities, including production planning and inventory control, warehousing, manufacturing and packaging. "Except in relatively small companies, the pharmacist generally serves in a supervisory capacity with emphasis upon technical skills in actual manufacturing operations or administrative abilities as he assumes broader departmental responsibilities."(9) More specifically, "pharmacists in charge of production units, supervise employees, plan schedules, work with engineers to modernize process and equipment, help develop sales forecasts in production plans and estimate needs in manpower and materials."[3] Since pharmaceutical products affect human lives, rigorous compliance with manufacturing protocol, and concerned awareness of their safety, quality and efficacy is essential. A trained pharmacist appreciates this principle and is ideally suited for a supervisory role in production areas.

Quality control is an essential part of the manufacture of drugs. Pharmacists and others working in analysis and control are concerned with developing and implementing methods to establish and maintain quality in each dosage unit of every product manufactured or being developed. Many pharmacists are employed as quality-control inspectors involved in physical and chemical testing of raw materials, drug substances, dosage forms, and packaging components. Advancement leads to supervisory and management roles.[3] While chemists are preferred for laboratory functions, graduate pharmacists are preferred in administrative control activities such as liaison with regulatory agencies, reviewing control procedures, auditing of control records and complaint analyses primarily because of their broad scientific background and their comprehension of the pharmaceutical as a unique product (9,10).

Since the drug salesperson commonly known as detail person or professional service representative is responsible for communication regarding drug products with prescribers (physicians) and dispensers (pharmacists), a trained pharmacist should be favored for this position. However, only about 10–15 percent of detail persons are pharmacists, because starting salaries are lower than in competitive positions(10).

The Pharmaceutical Manufacturers Association has recently announced a new program to acquaint pharmacy faculty with pharmaceutical industry practices and policies.[4] The National Pharmaceutical Council and several pharmaceutical firms have also made commendable efforts to disseminate the roles for the pharmacist in pharmaceutical industry. In this regard, the NPC Summer Internship Program[5], plus several films and publications[6](11–13) may be cited. All of these developments are most encouraging and they should help in eventual identification of unique roles for the industrial pharmacist.

From the vantage point of one involved in developing an educational program in industrial pharmacy and of one also interested in the identification of terminal behavioral objectives, it appears that industrial pharmacy is today where clinical pharmacy was 10–20 years ago. Yet this analogy may not be entirely appropriate since even today, informed individuals argue as to what constitutes clinical pharmacy. In its current popular usage, clinical pharmacy *is* pharmacy while industrial pharmacy must be regarded as a specialty or subcategory of the profession.

Competency-based education is a rational approach to education consistent with the scientific method most pharmaceutical educators practice or attempt to emulate. To quote Rosinsky(14), "Competency-based education has taken the teaching/learning process and systematized it." In developing a new program in industrial pharmacy at the University of the Pacific, it soon became apparent that realistic competency-based criteria were necessary to guide the program. A series of visits to universities with existing programs[7] and discussions with practicing pharmacists and others [in] industry[8] were conducted systematically. The information thus acquired was developed into a working set of competencies in consultation with certain of the staff of the University of the Pacific.[9] Items (*iii*)–(*x*) of the competency statements detailed below presently serve as the goals for the graduate program in industrial pharmacy at the University of the Pacific. These interrelated competency statements assume that the industrial pharmacist is fundamentally a pharmacist. Therefore, this individual must possess those attributes described in the competency statements developed by the California State Board of Pharmacy(15). In addition, this individual must have certain extra competencies associated with his/her projected activities in the pharmaceutical industry or related environment. These competencies represent goals to be addressed by an educational program, graduate or undergraduate, seeking to produce an individual with the knowledge and skills of an *industrial pharmacist*. What are these competencies which qualify a pharmacist to add the adjective "industrial" to his or her professional title?

(*i*) This pharmacist appreciates that a pharmaceutical as a product is unique—it is a chemical or a combination of chemicals specially formulated for a specific therapeutic effect in living subjects possessing the etiologic, pathologic and other diagnostic parameters for a particular disease, ailment or condition. His exercise of responsibility and judgment during the handling and manipulation of drugs and drug products at any stage of development of manufacture reflects comprehension of this knowledge.

(*ii*) This pharmacist is able to characterize the physical, chemical and biopharmaceutical properties of chemical compounds intended for use as drugs or as components of a drug delivery system, using known procedures and with reference to appropriate standards.

(*iii*) This pharmacist is able to participate and contribute to the development of final formula, pilot-plant and scale-up techniques. His overall functions result in the development, manufacture and distribution of a drug product which is safe, effective and of uniformly high quality.

(*iv*) This pharmacist is able to evaluate the equipment and packaging materials to be used during the manufacture of a specific drug product.

(*v*) This pharmacist is able to perform stability studies on drugs and drug products and is able to determine proper storage conditions.

(*vi*) This pharmacist is able to participate and contribute in the preparation, packaging and control of new drugs and drug products for clinical investigation. He is able to design and coordinate clinical trials under the overall supervision of a qualified clinician. He is capable of analyzing and interpreting the data from clinical studies as to appropriateness of their experimental design and statistical validity.

(*vii*) This pharmacist is capable of technical control of manufacturing operations so that a product of uniform high quality consistent with the requirements of the master formula and the Food and Drug Administration is assured. He is able to process solid, liquid and semi-solid dosage forms in his daily practice.

(*viii*) This pharmacist knows his physical plant and equipment and is capable of problem solving in collaboration with other scientists, engineers and maintenance staff.

(*ix*) This pharmacist is able to supervise quality-control operations during manufacturing, packaging and storage of drugs and drug products consistent with regulatory requirements and master formula. He understands the organization, function and practice of quality control in the pharmaceutical industry including the role of regulatory agencies such as the Food and Drug Administration.

(*x*) This pharmacist participates in the development of specifications, assay methods, test procedures for raw materials, packaging components, finished drug products and packages. He is able to analyze quality-control information with respect to appropriateness of sampling design and overall statistical validity. He is able to carry out such activities as inspection and auditing of control records, complaint analysis, in-process control review, label control and liaison work with regulatory agencies, research, clinical and production departments.

(*xi*) This pharmacist will be able to perform appropriate studies and/or tests to improve the existing product and processes, when presented with a specific objective.

(*xii*) This pharmacist communicates effectively regarding appropriate drug and drug product matters with other pharmaceutical industrial personnel, pharmacists, clinicians and with regulatory agencies.

(*xiii*) This pharmacist maintains his expertise and keeps abreast of advances and changes in his area of specialization. He is able to review and evaluate literature in his field.

(*xiv*) This pharmacist participates in the generation and dissemination of new knowledge.

Upon reviewing these competencies, a number of questions arise, *e.g.*, where and how does one acquire such competencies? Can certain competencies best be gained during the undergraduate pharmacy curriculum or *via* internships in pharmaceutical companies? Should being a pharmacist be a prerequisite? These are fundamental questions requiring considerable study and discussion. These and related aspects must be examined in the light of recent changes in the basic pharmacy curriculum. Traditionally, at least a course in pharmaceutical technology has been a part of the pharmaceutics curriculum in many schools of pharmacy. This often has given way to make room for clinical content. While some schools have had a program or multiple set of courses primarily geared to prepare a research-oriented scientist, several other potentially rewarding roles for the pharmacist in industry are not reflected in these curricula. Today pharmacists no longer play the important role in the pharmaceutical industry which normally would be expected of them—an observation made some 17 years ago(16), yet valid today. Further examination and study of the largely untapped and neglected potential for pharmacists in pharmaceutical and related industry is sorely needed.

Notes

1. Presented in part to the AACP Section of Teachers of Pharmacy, Minneapolis MN, July 1976.

2. In 1972, the number of registered pharmacists employed in pharmaceutical industry was 5,076. This represented 3.9 percent of the national total of pharmacists. However, since a license is not required for employment of pharmacists in pharmaceutical industry, a significant number of individuals with a degree in pharmacy are not included in this survey. Source: *Licensure Statistics, Census*, National Association of Boards of Pharmacy, Chicago IL (1973).

3. Ruggiero, John S., in *Career Directions for Pharmacists—Symposium*, Rutgers College of Pharmacy, New Brunswick NJ (1975) pp. 15–22.

4. *PMA Coordinated Industry Program for Pharmacy Faculty*, Pharmaceutical Manufacturers Association, 1155 Fifteenth Street N.W., Washington DC 20005.
5. *The NPC Pharmaceutical Industry Summer Internship Program*, National Pharmaceutical Council Inc., 1030 Fifteenth Street, Washington DC 20005.
6. *Opportunities for Pharmacists in Industry*, Merck Sharp and Dohme, West Point PA (1975).
7. The author visited the industrial pharmacy facilities at the University of Iowa, Purdue University, University of Tennessee, University of Wisconsin, and University of Florida, and interviewed the faculty in charge of the industrial pharmacy programs or courses. The contributions made by G. S. Banker, G. E. Peck, S. L. Hem, V. F. Smolen, D. O. Kildsig, P. F. Belcastro, all of Purdue University; by B. B. Sheth, University of Tennessee; by L. D. Bighley, J. L. Lach, and E. L. Parrott, University of Iowa; by J. T. Carstensen, University of Wisconsin-Madison; and by C. H. Becker, University of Florida, are gratefully acknowledged.
8. Author acknowledges helpful comments from discussions with practicing pharmacists and others in the pharmaceutical industry, in particular, P. Freiman, B. Poulsen, H. Mitchner, R. Kuromoto, all of Syntex Laboratories; S. Ericksen, Allergan Pharmaceuticals; S. Horn, Riker Laboratories; R. L. Sundberg, A. Asano, J. Marvel, all of Johnson and Johnson; W. McKeehan, J. Boylan, both of Eli Lilly Laboratories; C. H. Newman, E. R. Squibb and Sons Inc.; E. A. Holstius, Burroughs-Wellcome; L. M. Wheeler, Parke-Davis, M. Gamerman, Schering Corporation; W. T. Hensler, Sandoz Pharmaceuticals; and I. Lerner, Hoffman-LaRoche Inc.
9. Professors D. Y. Barker, P. N. Catania, D. G. Floriddia, M. H. Malone, K. M. Mills, and M. Polinsky.

References

1. Sonnedecker, G., *Kremers and Urdang's History of Pharmacy*, J. B. Lippincott, Philadelphia PA (1976) p. 326.
2. Cooper, J., *J. Am. Pharm. Assoc., Pract. Ed.* 18, 368 (1957).
3. *Op. cit* (1), p. 204.
4. *Webster's Third New International Dictionary*, G. and C. Merriam Co. Springfield MA (1966) p. 1694.
5. *Dorland's Illustrated Medical Dictionary*, 25th ed., W. B. Saunders, Philadelphia PA (1974) p. 1175.
6. *The Random House Dictionary of English Language*, College ed., Random House, New York NY (1969) p. 995.
7. *Pharmacists for the Future, The Report of the Study Commission of Pharmacy*, Health Administration Press, Ann Arbor MI (1975) p. 15.
8. Polderman, J., *Pharm. Weekblad*, 99, 984 (1964).
9. Cooper, J. in *Remington's Pharmaceutical Sciences*, 15th ed. (edit. Anderson, J. T.) Mack Publishing Co., Easton PA (1975) pp. 37–46.
10. Smith, M. and Knapp, D., *Pharmacy Drugs and Medical Care*, Williams and Wilkins, Baltimore MD (1972) p. 25–27.
11. Jones, C. H., *Pharm. Times* (June 1975), 62.
12. Bloor, P., Hardinsky, B., Eaves, T., Trice, A. E., Tall, D., Wellock, P. and Jafee, G., *Pharm. J.*, 213, 559 (1974).
13. Saroyan, R. L., *Pharm. Times* (February 1973), 44.
14. Rosinsky, E. F., *Am. J. Pharm. Educ.*, 39, 557 (1975).
15. Day, R. L., *ibid.*, 39, 569 (1975) *N.B.* p. 572.
16. Cooper, J., *Am. J. Pharm.*, 132, 158 (1960).

71—Research and Development (R & D) of New Drugs

Prepared by the Office of Customer Affairs, Sandoz, Inc.

Introduction

Research and development (R & D) of new drugs is an essential part of the pharmaceutical industry's contribution to advances in medicine. A return on their investments is essential for continued viability, and patent protection allows time to regain investments made in this process.

Pharmaceutical research and development is a vast and complex array of disciplines, procedures and decisions. Our goal is to provide you with an overview of the various procedures followed in developing a drug for patient use and obtaining marketing approval through the New Drug Application.

Basic Considerations

After an active compound has been either isolated from natural substrates or synthesized from chemical entities, the process of assessing its safety and efficacy as a new therapeutic drug is lengthy and expensive. The financial commitments required to do research on a new drug and file a New Drug Application (NDA) with the Food and Drug Administration (FDA), are often staggering. Therefore, skillful planning and a selective decision process is mandatory. This also facilitates the development of the safest and most effective drug in the shortest possible time.

Basically, drug research and development stages, or phases as they are called in the pharmaceutical industry, are divided into two major categories; the pre-clinical research completed before testing in humans is begun, and the clinical research which comprises four phases of study in humans.

At two points in this total research program a company must submit its research data to the FDA for review and approval before further research is conducted. The first submission of data is known as an IND (Notice of Claimed Investigational Exemption for a New Drug); it includes all the pre-clinical data available on the drug, a description of the studies to be conducted in humans, and an agreement to submit progress reports on all the studies as the research program is conducted. The IND must be filed with and not be objected to by the FDA before a new drug may be distributed in interstate commerce for testing on human beings.

The second comprehensive submission of data to the FDA is known as the NDA (New Drug Application) and it includes all the data generated in the first three phases of clinical research (the three phases will be described later) which substantiate the safety and efficacy of the drug for its intended uses. Also included in the NDA is all the available information on chemical and pharmaceutical manufacturing; quality control; and basic research in pharmacology, toxicology, metabolism, teratology, bioavailability and drug interactions. To more fully appreciate the depth and intensity of the research that must be conducted before an NDA is filed, we will discuss more fully the two basic categories of the research program, i.e., pre-clinical and clinical, as shown in the diagram [Fig 71.1].

Our description is based generally on the

Figure 71.1

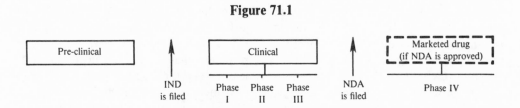

basic procedures followed by Sandoz, however, these procedures are common to research and development throughout the pharmaceutical industry.

Pre-Clinical

The initial pre-clinical work begins in the chemistry labs. The principal objective is to conceive of and synthesize new, patentable chemical compounds with biological activity of potential medical value. The first step, then, is the identification and synthesis of the new compound in the chemistry lab. The preliminary research is done by the analytical chemists to determine compound stability, salt forms and molecular structure. The chemical development department, which prepares larger quantities of the compound, at this time also synthesizes the compound and does stability tests. Secondary testing is conducted by the biology department to confirm initial observations of pharmacologic activity, evaluate the compound further in more specific tests, rule out the possibility that the desired effect is secondary to an undesired effect, and determine therapeutic ratio and dose-effect relationship as well as duration of activity and development of tolerance. If the results of this testing are favorable, expanded biological research is conducted. It includes additional pharmacologic studies in support of claimed primary activity and preliminary toxicity studies. At the same time, the chemical development department works to improve its processing of the compound to prepare a large batch of the compound. In the pharmacy and analytical research area, work is started on an initial stability screen.

The purpose of the screen is to set initial specifications for the new drug substance, purity for toxicity samples, identify impurities in the new drug substance and gather further analytical data.

Generally, at the completion of this work, a company will decide whether or not they want to proceed with testing in humans. This decision is based upon biological results, chemical development, the patent status, clinical considerations, pharmaceutical research and development plans, drug regulatory requirements, market needs, market research and financial considerations.

If the decision is to proceed with testing of the compound, expanded work in the pre-clinical phase continues in toxicology/pathology, drug metabolism, pharmacology, chemical development and pharmacy and analytical research. This research is conducted to verify the safety and efficacy of the drug in animals so that the drug can be tested in humans with a high degree of safety assured. At this stage, the data are compiled in the document known as an IND which must be filed with the FDA and approved by them before the clinical research phases can be started.

Clinical Research

Clinical research, as you probably know, is the formalized study of the efficacy and safety of drugs for the treatment or prevention of diseases or symptoms of diseases in humans. Although it is not a new practice, only within recent years has the science of planning and conducting well-controlled drug studies been developed to its high degree of reliability and verifiability. Certainly no one will dispute that history has shown us that the public must be protected from ineffective and potentially dangerous drugs and remedies developed and sold by charlatans. Over the years, the tremendous advances in chemistry and pharmacology, and the development of more rigid scientific methods of testing drugs in animals and humans have enabled the pharmaceutical industry to evaluate the already available drugs and test thoroughly all new drugs before allowing them to become generally available in the clinical practice.

As pointed out earlier, clinical research comprises three phases before the NDA is filed and the drug marketed. The three phases are continuous but in some instances do overlap. Each phase will be discussed separately.

Phase I

In Phase I, the initial tests of the new drug generally are conducted in normal human volunteers, but in some instances, effects of the drug are studied in patient conditions for which the drug is indicated. The object of these early tests is to determine in a limited number of normal human subjects the safety and tolerance of a single dose; a single day's dosage; and multiple, escalating doses over a specified interval. Also in Phase I, the ADME (absorption, distribution, metabolism and excretion) study of a single, safe dose is performed. The results of this study are the basis for the pharmacokinetic profile of the drug.

Phase II

Once the safe dose range of the drug is established in normal human subjects during Phase I, the Phase II research on the compound begins. Phase II studies are conducted in a limited number of patients with the disease for which the drug is to be used to determine the safety and efficacy of the drug in these patients. These studies are to be well

controlled and require that the safety and efficacy of the drug be compared to that of placebo, and with standard competitive products when desirable. During Phase II at least one multiple dose absorption, distribution, metabolism and excretion study is conducted. The optimum dosage of the drug is also evaluated. If the most desirable formulation of the drug, i.e., tablet, capsule, delayed release formulation, syrup, concentrate or injectable, has not been selected previously, it is done at this time. This may require further bioavailability studies to determine the relative rates of absorption, peak level in the blood and rate of disappearance from the blood of the various formulations.

At the conclusion of Phase II, all the available data relating to the drug including chemistry, pharmacy development, toxicology, pharmacology, clinical research, and market research are compiled and evaluated for the company's management which decides whether or not to proceed to Phase III, the final and most extensive phase of the development of the drug before the NDA is filed.

Phase III

Phase III comprises extensive clinical trials in which experienced physician-investigators treat select patients with the drug essentially as they would if it were approved for general medical use. However, these studies are conducted under "double blind" conditions, that is, neither the patient nor the physician know whether the patient is receiving, the test drug or a control agent— either placebo or a standard active medication widely used and accepted for the same indications, or both. Phase III may be conducted in 100–200 patients or in several thousand depending on the type of drug and the nature of the indication.

These clinical studies in Phase III are designed to provide definitive evidence of safety and efficacy of the drug for the disease under investigation. They are planned and conducted in such a way as to determine the maximum clinical data on the drug from predetermined patient population.

During the course of all clinical studies, thorough and efficient monitoring is required at regular intervals by clinical research personnel to ensure adherence to the protocol by the physician-investigator and completeness and accuracy of the case report forms. Documentary evidence of diligent monitoring is required by FDA.

The NDA (New Drug Application)

As we noted already when all the pre-clinical and clinical studies in the R & D Program for a particular compound have been completed and analyzed, and clinical and statistical reports written, all the data relating to the total development of the drug are compiled in one comprehensive document—the NDA, and submitted to the FDA. The NDA generally comprises numerous volumes and is assembled under the supervision of a company's drug regulatory affairs department which is a company's liaison group with the FDA.

They make sure the NDA is compiled according to the FDA guidelines and that it contains all the available information concerning the nature of the drug and its preparations and effects. These data are grouped into four main areas, namely, chemical manufacturing, pharmaceutical manufacturing and quality control, pharmacology/toxicology, and clinical research. The latter includes not only efficacy and safety data, but also full referencing of claims to be included in the proposed package insert.

At this point it is interesting to compare this description of the NDA and what goes into its development to the far less exacting requirements of information for an Abbreviated New Drug Application (ANDA) which only includes manufacturing, quality control, stability and, in some cases, bioavailability data. ANDA's obviously require

less time, effort and expense than NDA's since no clinical studies are required.

If the NDA meets all the FDA requirements and provides substantial evidence of the efficacy and safety of the drug, approval by FDA for marketing the drug is given. However, this may take years; the median time for FDA approval of an NDA is about 24 months. Once approval is given, the drug is marketed but research does not stop. Instead it moves into the so-called "Phase IV."

Phase IV

In Phase IV, clinical studies are conducted to provide further scientific information on the efficacy and safety of the drug and to compare the efficacy and safety of the drug with other marketed drugs used for the same indication(s). Even after the drug has been on the market for 10 or more years, Phase IV studies are conducted to update clinical data related to safety and efficacy of the drug to maintain an up-to-date profile on the drug for reference of the company and the FDA. Phase IV studies are also conducted to provide clinical data that can be used by the company to show the physician differential drug effects, long-term effects and the side effects profiles of the drug and the competitive products so that he can decide on the best drug for his particular patient.

Conclusion

As you can see from this brief overview of pharmaceutical research and development, considerable time and effort is expended to develop new drugs for improving patient care. The phases of research described here frequently take a decade or more. But despite the time and expense involved, the benefits of improving life or reducing suffering are of significant value to the patient and every member of the health-care team, to warrant continued pharmaceutical research and development.

72—Opportunities for Pharmacists
in Industry

Merck Sharp & Dohme

The pharmacist's future at Merck Sharp & Dohme [MSD] can bring fulfilling involvement in all phases and functions, including leadership at the top.

Today, over 300 men and women with pharmacy degrees are working at all levels of management, including executive directorships, and in all areas of our large and complex company—Research, Production, Sales, Marketing. We have pharmacists as our Executive Director of Pharmaceutical Research, Director of Field Operations and Director of Trade Relations. We have pharmacists serving as Region and District Sales Managers: over 300 pharmacists in our force of Professional Representatives and many more who are analysts in our Market Research area.

Merck & Co., Inc., our parent company, is a company planning for the future—doubling sales every six years—embracing more than 25,000 employees—investing over $500 million on new plants and facilities since 1964 (now at 60 plants throughout the world)—channeling more than $150 million a year for research and development.

At Merck Sharp & Dohme, we make almost 150 different prescription drugs and vaccines to prevent or treat disease. Among these are products of original advances in medicine, developed in the MSD Research Laboratories.

Merck Sharp & Dohme pharmacists are chosen for the positions they hold, not only on the basis of their pharmacy degrees, but for compelling qualities of mind, experience

and character that can best contribute to the ongoing development of the company. Personal qualities we consider essential include the ability to communicate, both orally and in writing, poise, and the capacity to work harmoniously with people. The ability to organize and administer is requisite for promotion to higher levels. A strong mathematical background, with thorough grounding in statistics, is invaluable.

Since many of the positions pharmacists hold at MSD can be filled equally well by non-pharmacists, a man or woman with a pharmacy degree, combined with these primary qualifications, has a decided advantage.

Research and Development

The pharmacist in Research and Development must be sensitive, innovative, adaptable, eager to learn new concepts and to develop original ideas.

Most pharmacists in the Research Laboratories are concerned with fundamental studies of the basic physical and chemical properties of new compounds and with applying their findings in the development of formulations and practical production methods for new dosage forms. They analyze the effect on drug action of physical characteristics such as particle size, binders and coatings; even the type of container.

Other pharmacists are involved in helping to prepare reports on clinical trials with

Adapted from a monograph with the same title and reprinted with permission of the publisher, Merck Sharp & Dohme.

experimental compounds for submission to government agencies.

The pharmacist in Research and Development is a member of a laboratory team. He has much opportunity for exposure to new techniques and principles, and he confronts one challenging problem after another. He learns from his co-workers by collaborating closely with specialists in other disciplines. Encouragement is given to publish his work and to participate in the activities of professional societies.

Five important assignments for pharmacists in the Research Laboratories are outlined below.

TITLE: Research Pharmacist
EDUCATIONAL REQUIREMENTS: Bachelor's Degree in Pharmacy.
NATURE AND SCOPE OF WORK: Solution of specific, generally short-range problems in his discipline. Careful observation of experiments and variances from expected experimental results. Compilation of pertinent literature data as assigned using reference volumes. Preparation of data for inclusion in project reports. Maintenance of specific records covering all aspects of his attack on a problem, insuring that all entries are properly witnessed. Assembly of apparatus for experiments. Work normally confined to one laboratory with little necessity for collaborating with others.

TITLE: Research Fellow
EDUCATIONAL REQUIREMENTS: Ph.D. Degree, plus several additional years of experience.
NATURE AND SCOPE OF WORK: Solution of complex research problems. Assistance in the design and implementation of research programs. Planning and scheduling of experiments and development of personnel assigned specific responsibilities within the program. A Research Fellow is required to be cooperative and responsible in dealings with others, both within and outside his own group.

TITLE: Director, Pharmaceutical Development
EDUCATIONAL REQUIREMENTS: Ph.D. Degree, plus eight to ten years of related work experience.
NATURE AND SCOPE OF WORK: Planning and implementation of laboratory and pilot scale research directed toward developing pharmaceutical dosage forms, especially tablet and capsule products, for clinical use and suitable processes for pharmaceutical production. Responsibility for activities of four work units involving fifteen or more pharmacists and supporting technicians, hourly workers and clerks. Coordination of process developments and their demonstration to operating areas both in the U.S. and abroad. Responsibility for pursuing the development of new materials, new equipment and new techniques for pharmaceutical processes.

TITLE: Director, Pharmaceutical Research
EDUCATIONAL REQUIREMENTS: Ph.D. Degree, plus eight to ten years of related work experience.
NATURE AND SCOPE OF WORK: Planning, directing and controlling the overall research aspects of the Pharmaceutical Research and Development Department. Involves the planning and guiding of research activities leading to the development of detailed data and information on the chemical, physical and formulation properties of new drug compounds; development of new materials and concepts for pharmaceutical formulations; development of dosage forms and processes for sterile, topical and fluid products; and development of specialized drug delivery systems. Responsible for planning, directing and controlling the activities of the biopharmaceutics unit. Chairs the company bioavailability team and closely guides its activities. Responsible for the activities of five work units involving fifteen or more pharmacists and chemists plus supporting technicians and clerical personnel.

TITLE: Medical Research Associate
EDUCATIONAL REQUIREMENTS: Bachelor's Degree; M.S. desirable, plus minimum of three years experience in pharmaceutical industry sales at the territory level, and one year of experience in handling hospital accounts (see section on pharmacist assignments in Sales & Marketing).
NATURE AND SCOPE OF WORK: Responsibility for developing and implementing projects to establish rapport with leading physicians in private practice in teaching institutions and major hospitals. Mainte-

nance of liaison between clinical investigators and responsible physicians in MSDRL Medical Affairs area. Support and assistance in planning, controlling and administering all clinical projects. Development of effective communications on new concepts and on MSD and competitive research projects and marketing plans.

Production Operations

The pharmacist in Production must be a leader . . . manager.

Production problems are always immediate and often urgent. Getting the production job done requires working with and through people. The successful production Supervisor, Manager or Director is not only task-oriented, but has a sound understanding of people and an ability to communicate clearly to them to enlist their enthusiastic support.

Pharmacists in Merck Sharp & Dohme operations head up production units, supervise employees, plan schedules and budgets, work with engineers to modernize processes and equipment, help develop sales forecasts into production plans, and estimate needs in manpower and materials. Among the challenges the pharmacists in production face, are the ultra high standards imposed on all normal process work to assure cleanliness and prevent product contamination.

Quality Control procedures are of the most exacting nature, designed to provide maximum protection to the patients whose lives are so intimately affected by the medicines we make. Many pharmacists enter production at Merck Sharp & Dohme through the position of Quality Control Inspector.

Once having learned the paramount importance of the quality standard to our operation, some pharmacists choose to move into more advanced Quality Control positions involving the testing of products from raw materials to finished packages, or the review and approval of labeling and advertising copy. Some pharmacists move into supervisory and management slots in our manufacturing and packaging areas. Other pharmacists become key members of our Process Engineering and Development team whose responsibility is assuring smooth production of manufacturing processes developed by Research.

The pharmacist's ability to administer is as important as his technical ability in a production job. There is supervision of people, involvement in union and personnel matters, and scheduling of manpower and flow of materials for maximum efficiency. The ability to communicate clearly with both the written and the spoken word is critical.

Academic background is only part of the preparation required for success in production. Success also depends on the versatility, social skills and managerial abilities of the individual.

Six significant assignments for pharmacist in production are described below.

TITLE: Pharmaceutical Quality Inspector
EDUCATIONAL REQUIREMENTS: Bachelor's Degree.
NATURE AND SCOPE OF WORK: Control checking and inspection to evaluate quality of material and methods. Quality troubleshooting of material and methods. Quality trouble-shooting in Pharmaceutical Production, Warehousing and Printing areas. Facilities inspection of other companies doing manufacturing or packaging for MSD.

TITLE: Production Supervisor
EDUCATIONAL REQUIREMENTS: Bachelor's Degree, plus two years of experience in Pharmaceutical Manufacturing or Quality Control.
NATURE AND SCOPE OF WORK: Direct supervision of manufacturing or packaging unit. Development and conduct of training programs for hourly employees. Review and updating of manufacturing, safety and quality documents. Investigation and analysis of cost variations and establishment of corrective systems.

TITLE: Superintendent-Pharmaceutical Manufacturing

EDUCATIONAL REQUIREMENTS: B.S. Degree, plus minimum of five years supervisory or allied staff experience, preferably including a minimum of two years of experience as a Production Supervisor.

NATURE AND SCOPE OF WORK: Responsibility for overall supervision and coordination of all Pharmaceutical Manufacturing Departments consisting of up to 75 hourly employees and four to six supervisors. Participation in solution of problems in areas of manpower and equipment utilization, quality control conformance, and technical service. Development of plans and recommended changes in organization, equipment, processes and manning to assure cost reduction, more adequate control of operations, and quality improvements.

TITLE: Production Manager, Pharmaceutical Manufacturing

EDUCATIONAL REQUIREMENTS: Bachelor's Degree, plus five to seven years of responsible supervisory or managerial experience.

NATURE AND SCOPE OF WORK: Responsibility for conformance by manufacturing areas to performance standards, budgets, schedule completion, quality, profit improvement, housekeeping, security, safety, labor regulations, and Good Manufacturing Practice regulations. Planning and recommendation of organization changes (structural and numerical) necessary to changing production requirements. Solution of technical, mechanical, scheduling and personnel problems of many degrees of complexity.

TITLE: Pharmacist-Process Development

EDUCATIONAL REQUIREMENTS: B.S. and M.S. in Pharmacy, plus three to five years of experience in pharmaceutical production, research and development.

NATURE AND SCOPE OF WORK: Assignment to specific phases of projects to improve manufacturing procedures in pharmaceutical manufacturing. Responsibility for the preparation and accuracy of new product formulas, pilot lot formulas, revised and rework formulas. Participation in transition of new products from laboratory to production scale operations. Responsibility for serving as pharmaceutical consultant during the development of new packaging techniques or packaging components. Conduction of experimental work on portions of long range pharmaceutical technology projects, such as direct compression, flow patterns in coating pans, increased tablet production rate, and so on.

TITLE: Manager, Pharmaceutical Process Engineering and Development

EDUCATIONAL REQUIREMENTS: Ph.D. in Pharmacy, plus eight to ten years experience in Pharmaceutical Production or Development.

NATURE AND SCOPE OF WORK: Responsibility for supervision and direction of a resident technical staff that plans and carries out programs involving process and equipment projects for Pharmaceutical Production, and a technical development machine shop that services the West Point plant site. Development of new equipment and processes for the improvement of manufacturing and packaging operations. Direction of pilot plant runs and the transfer of new products from MSDRL or other Customer Divisions to Pharmaceutical Production. Responsibility for writing all new production formulas based on scale-up of Research processes. Preparation of capital forecasts for department. Recruiting, training, and direction of Engineers, Pharmacists and other specialists.

Sales and Marketing

The pharmacist in Sales and Marketing: Analyst . . . Strategist . . . Information Specialist.

Merck Sharp & Dohme's internal Marketing staff develops and coordinates strategy for increasing sales, improving distribution methods and discovering and developing markets for both new and established products.

Marketing offers the pharmacy graduate two principal areas of growth . . . Marketing Research and Product Management. A graduate with one year of statistics may start in Market Research, where his job is essentially that of fact finder and analyst. Using the latest methodology, the new analyst may conduct market evaluation studies, determine customer attitudes, or develop criteria for the design of sales territories.

The analyst can advance to supervisor posts within Marketing Research, or he may move into product management, where he is responsible for planning the marketing strategy for important products or product lines and analyzing marketing reports from the field.

Pharmacists also hold key positions in the Sales staff at our West Point headquarters, directing the management of Sales regions, planning the introduction of products to the doctors, arranging educational briefing sessions for the Professional Representatives, and keeping them posted on product information. About 33% of the MSD Professional Representatives hold pharmacy degrees.

The principal responsibility of the Professional Representative is to give the medical profession complete and accurate information.

Clarity and ease in oral communication is an essential qualification of the Professional Representative. All MSD Professional Representatives receive intensive training from one of the industry's most sophisticated training teams.

Six important assignments for pharmacists in Sales and Marketing are summarized below.

TITLE: Professional Representative
EDUCATIONAL REQUIREMENTS: Bachelor's Degree.
NATURE AND SCOPE OF WORK: Calls regularly on assigned physicians and hospitals to communicate to them balanced, accurate and complete information on MSD products. Calls on hospital and retail pharmacists to provide information and assure the availability of MSD products in his territory. Completes all training courses required to continually update his product knowledge. Provides professional, public and trade relations services in accordance with established company policies.

TITLE: District Manager
EDUCATIONAL REQUIREMENTS: Bachelor's Degree, plus minimum of five years of field sales and sales administration experience.
NATURE AND SCOPE OF WORK: Monitors competitive, market and product situation in sales district, and gathers and communi-

cates market intelligence to company management. As first-line sales supervisor, maintains approved manning levels and effective deployment of sales staff, and ensures maintenance of high levels of expertise of assigned Professional Representatives. Establishes plans, programs and objectives working in conjunction with both Region Manager and Professional Representatives to assure implementation of marketing goals in district.

TITLE: Product Manager, In-Line Products
EDUCATIONAL REQUIREMENTS: Bachelor's Degree; M.B.A. desirable. Minimum of five years experience in various Sales or Marketing activities.
NATURE AND SCOPE OF WORK: Responsibility for developing marketing promotion programs, forecasting sales requirements, maintaining indepth knowledge of markets, creating marketing strategy plans for assigned products, participating in development of company's long-range plans, and maintaining liaison with all areas of company activities involving his products.

TITLE: Manager of Marketing Planning
EDUCATIONAL REQUIREMENTS: Bachelor's Degree; M.B.A. or equivalent desirable, plus minimum of seven or eight years of experience in various marketing or planning activities.
NATURE AND SCOPE OF WORK: Responsibility for planning and directing Marketing strategy, advertising programs, and sales promotion for assigned products with sales objectives exceeding $100,000,000. Provides direction to a staff of three to five Product Managers. Coordinates execution of all promotional programs for assigned products.

TITLE: Associate Marketing Analyst
EDUCATIONAL REQUIREMENTS: Bachelor's Degree.
NATURE AND SCOPE OF WORK: Responsibility for providing solutions to specific marketing problems through the application of appropriate marketing research methods and techniques. Conducts investigations to define specific marketing research problems. Develops research plans for securing data to solve problems, including sampling procedures, statistical methods, and form and questionnaire design. Coordinates data gathering, including personal interviews

with individuals, usually physicians and paramedical personnel. Summarizes, analyzes and interprets data for general management.

TITLE: Senior Marketing Analyst
EDUCATIONAL REQUIREMENTS: Bachelor's Degree, plus three to five years of experience in a marketing research position, or an M.B.A. with two to four years of experience in a marketing research position.
NATURE AND SCOPE OF WORK: Responsibility for design, conduct and reporting of studies requiring a broad understanding of the various facets of the ethical pharmaceutical marketing process. Defines marketing problems and delineates individual marketing research assignments. Develops and recommends methods for assembling data on sales, costs, inventories, and other matters, into forms most usable for interpretive purposes consistent with cost considerations.

Trade Relations

The pharmacist in Trade Relations: Planner . . . Communicator . . . Policy Formulator. The Trade Relations area of Merck Sharp & Dohme offers unique opportunities for pharmacists in working with other pharmacists in every segment of the profession.

TITLE: Director of Trade Relations
EDUCATIONAL REQUIREMENTS: B.S. in Pharmacy; plus minimum of ten to twelve years experience involving a broad background in Sales and Marketing activities in the drug field and a demonstrated knowledge of the factors involved in dealing with trade associations and organized groups in the field.
NATURE AND SCOPE OF WORK: Develops and recommends programs to maintain and improve the business atmosphere in which the MSD sales staff functions. Communicates the objectives of company policy and marketing programs to our larger customers, wholesale drug executives, retail and hospital pharmacy executives and hospital administrators. Administers the company's pharmaceutical advertising program and budget.

TITLE: Manager of Pharmacy Relations

EDUCATIONAL REQUIREMENTS: B.S. in Pharmacy.
NATURE AND SCOPE OF WORK: Responsible for implementing Trade Relations programs under supervision of the Director of Trade Relations.

Health and Welfare Programs

The pharmacist in Health & Welfare Programs: Monitor . . . Communicator. Pharmacists in Health & Welfare Programs are responsible for monitoring developments in the field of Third Party Prescription Payments and pharmacy legislation—to advise on company policy on state and private formularies.

TITLE: Manager of Health & Welfare Programs
EDUCATIONAL REQUIREMENTS: Bachelor's Degree.
NATURE AND SCOPE OF WORK: Develops and recommends programs to establish and maintain effective liaison with individuals involved in public assistance and private sector third party prescription drug programs. Confers with officials of federal and state government and executives of private insurance carriers to encourage a climate favorable to physician's freedom of choice in prescribing. Works closely with the MSD Field Sales Force. Recommends appropriate action by MSD based upon information acquired by personal contacts and those of Coordinators of Health & Welfare Programs.

TITLE: Coordinator of Health & Welfare Programs
EDUCATIONAL REQUIREMENTS: Bachelor's Degree.
NATURE AND SCOPE OF WORK: Develops effective liaison with all persons responsible for Third Party Payment for drugs in either the public or private sectors. Initiates meaningful contacts with high-level executives of federal and state governments—Blue Cross and Blue Shield—executives of major insurance companies. Regularly contacts state medical and pharmaceutical societies and all persons on Formulary Committees. Communicates meaningful information to the Manager of Health & Welfare Programs.

[Note: Although the job descriptions furnished above have been prepared by a single manufacturer, similar positions are likely to be found among most of the firms in the drug industry.

Readings for a Broader Perspective

1. a. "Clinical Studies—Reading and Evaluating." b. "Quality Control—Sampling Techniques and Practices."

These introductory essays may be obtained by writing: C. Earl DeRamus, R.Ph., Office of Customer Affairs, Sandoz Pharmaceuticals, East Hanover, NJ 07036.

2. Petrick, R. J. "The Industry—An Inside Story," *Tomorrow's Pharmacist* 2 (February /March 1980):15–18.

3. Clarke, F. H. (ed.) *How Modern Medicines Are Discovered.* Mt. Kisco, N.Y.: Futura Publishing Co., 1973. 177 pages.

4. Clarke, F. H. (ed.) *How Modern Medicines Are Developed.* Mt. Kisco, N.Y.: Futura Publishing Co., 1977. 144 pages.

PHARMACIST-LAWYERS

73—Pharmacist-Lawyers

Joseph L. Fink III

In the past, various estimates of the number of pharmacist-lawyers have been made but most have been based on personal estimates with no attempt made to identify these professional hybrids and inquire about them. Estimates have ranged from a low of 75–150[1] to as high as 400–500.[2] In the only study found in the literature, Professor William Curran of the Harvard School of Public Health reported 141 persons with degrees in pharmacy and law.[3] In that study conducted for the Commonwealth Fund, he also found 205 persons with law and medical degrees, 32 with degrees in law and public health, 25 dentist-lawyers, and 14 persons holding degrees in hospital administration and law.[3]

The study reported here was undertaken to locate as many pharmacist-lawyers as possible, to yield a profile of the group, to note their work activities and to investigate interest in both professions.

Methodology

To collect names and addresses of pharmacist-lawyers, letters were sent to 52 state pharmacy association executives, 48 state board secretaries and 73 faculty members, usually in pharmacy administration, one at each college of pharmacy. Returns were received from 73 percent of both association executives and board secretaries as well as 53 percent of the faculty members. For survey purposes, a pharmacist-lawyer was defined as one who has graduated from a school of law as well as a school of pharmacy. Licensure as a pharmacist or admission to the bar was not required to be considered a pharmacist-lawyer. The resulting address list served as the starting point for the survey.

A questionnaire was sent to each person believed to be a pharmacist-lawyer with a cover letter explaining the purpose of the survey with a postage-paid reply envelope. Those responding were asked to list other pharmacist-lawyers so that the address list was constantly expanding. As a further method, a letter to the editor was published in *Pharmacy Times*[4] requesting information on the location of members of the cross-professional group.

The questionnaire included questions on age, schools of pharmacy and law and years of graduation, degrees held other than pharmacy and law, location of pharmacy licensure and bar admission, primary work activity and professional memberships. Further, questions were included on factors influencing the respondents to enter law school as well as the most pressing problems facing pharmacy and the law.

Results

A total of 216 questionnaires were mailed to persons reported to be pharmacist-lawyers and 38 were mailed to students at accredited law schools reported to be pharmacy graduates. The return rate for pharmacist-lawyers was 134 (62 percent) while that for pharmacist-law students was 26 (68 percent) yielding an overall return rate of 63 percent. Although the 134 were confirmed by their responses to be graduates of both pharmacy and law schools, the total number of pharmacist-lawyers is estimated at 175 to 200 due to the number of persons reported and known to be dual graduates who did not complete the questionnaire. Moreover, there are probably a number who were not located by the method used here.

Pharmacist-lawyers were found in 37 states and the District of Columbia, with the greatest number located in New York. . . .

Sixty-four percent of those responding in the pharmacist-lawyer group were under age 40, indicating that the group is relatively young. As would be expected, 88 percent of those attending law school were under age 30. However, it is noteworthy that 12 percent of those currently attending law school are over 30. Of special interest is an 81-year-old judge in Montana who became a pharmacist by apprenticeship and a lawyer through self-instruction and clerkship.

Among the 134 law graduates responding, 51 colleges of pharmacy, or slightly over 2/3 of the colleges in the continental United States were represented with two other colleges no longer in existence also represented. One pharmacist-lawyer entered pharmacy by way of an apprenticeship. With comparable diversification, the 26 pharmacists currently attending law school represent 19 different colleges of pharmacy.

Consistent with the relative youth of the group, the data indicated that nearly 40 percent of the lawyers graduated from pharmacy school during 1961 or later and nearly 75 percent graduated in pharmacy during the 1950's or later. Law school requires three or four years depending on whether study is full-time or part-time. By tabulating the instances in which pharmacy graduation preceded law graduation by more than four years, we can approximate what proportion of the respondents did not go directly to law school. Sixty-five percent of the law graduates did not go directly to law school. One person completed his law degree 36 years after he finished pharmacy. For the students, 40 percent did not go directly to law school, indicating an increase in the tendency to enter law school directly from pharmacy school. One current student will see 21 years pass between his pharmacy and law graduations. Diversity is seen in the law schools attended; 75 law schools were represented by the responding graduates while 20 are attended by the 26 students. There are 149 law schools accredited by the American Bar Association.[5] There were a number of law schools which had graduated more than one pharmacist-lawyer, but the schools with the greatest numbers were—Georgetown University (7); University of Maryland (6); SUNY-Buffalo (6); University of Wisconsin (4). Data concerning year of graduation from law school indicate that increased interest in law began in the mid-fifties and increased greatly by the mid-sixties, 85 percent of the pharmacist-lawyers responding having received their law degrees after 1956. Of interest is one respondent who entered pharmacy after attending law school, graduating in pharmacy 16 years after finishing law. He remarked that he did so because he was "running my father's pharmacy after World War II and decided to practice pharmacy rather than law." His was the only instance where law study preceded that of pharmacy.

Nineteen (14 percent of the pharmacist-lawyers hold degrees other than their basic degree in pharmacy (BS or PharmD) or law (LLB or JD) but four of the 19 earned an advanced degree in law (LLM) as their other degree. Eight, or nearly 31 percent of the current students hold degrees other than their basic pharmacy degree. Four in the lawyer group hold PhD's while two law students do. Table 73.1 . . . lists these degrees.

Nearly all respondents hold pharmacy licenses, probably as security; only one lawyer and one law student do not hold pharmacy licenses. However, seven percent of the law school graduates have not been admitted to the practice of law.

Table 73.2 . . . presents a breakdown of the chosen work of those responding. Eight possible answers were presented based on the career opportunities outlined by Steeves[2] and Woods[1]—practice of pharmacy, practice of law, pharmacy association work, work in the pharmaceutical industry or

Table 73.1

**Degrees Held Other Than Basic Pharmacy
or Law Degree**

Degree	Pharmacy-Lawyers Number	Pharmacy-Law Students Number
BA (Bacteriology)	1	—
BA (Biological Sciences)	—	1
BA (Chemistry)	1	—
BA (Psychology)	—	1
BS (Chemistry)	2	1
BA (Zoology)	—	1
LLM	4	—
MBA	2	1
MS	5	1
PhD	4	2
Total	19	8

Table 73.2

**Primary Work Categories for Pharmacist-Lawyers
and Law Students**

Activity	Pharmacy-Lawyers Number	Percent	Pharmacy-Law Students Number	Percent
Practice of pharmacy	15	11	6	23
Practice of law	71	53	11	42
Pharmacy association work	8	6	—	—
Pharmaceutical industry	8	6	—	—
Government service	11	8	2	8
Teaching in pharmacy school	8	6	2	8
Teaching in law school	1	1	—	—
Other	10	7	—	—
No response	2	2	5	19
Total	134	100	26	100

Note—Students were asked to respond with their expectations upon graduation.

government service, teaching in a school of pharmacy or law, or other activities.

Nearly 53 percent of the graduates practice law while 11 percent engage in pharmacy practice and 8 percent are in government service, a distant second and third. Seven percent are in other fields while six percent are in pharmacy association work, six percent in the pharmaceutical industry and six percent are teaching in schools of pharmacy. A smaller portion (42 percent) of the students said they intended to practice law and 23 percent said they would practice pharmacy. This variation may be due to misinterpretation of the question by the students in that some appeared to state present activity rather than the prospective response sought. In addition to the categories listed above, the following occupations were present among the law graduates—two judges, three pharmacy chain executives, one bank president, one hospital administrator, one businessman, one state legislator and one attorney for a health insurance plan. Twenty-six of the 71 who practice law as their primary activity indicated that they practice some pharmacy as well.

Eight of those graduates responding indicated that they do part-time teaching in a pharmacy school although it is not their primary activity. This represents six percent of the law graduates which contrasts with slightly over 11 percent of the physician-lawyers who teach on a part-time basis.[6] As of December 1971, there were 38 persons with law degrees teaching in colleges of pharmacy,[7] most on a part-time basis, but it cannot be determined how many also hold degrees in pharmacy. Since letters were sent to one faculty member at each college of pharmacy it is expected that nearly all dual-degree holders in pharmacy academia have been included.

The number of memberships in professional organizations was tabulated to indicate professional ties. Membership in bar associations was higher than in pharmacy organizations for the law graduates but the opposite was true for the students. The interest in pharmacy organizations appears to be inversely related to the amount of time the respondent has been out of pharmacy school, since the law students are more recent pharmacy graduates. However, the 46 percent membership level for lawyers in the American Pharmaceutical Association and 39 percent for state pharmacy associations is in line with the fact that 45 percent of the law graduates do not practice law as a primary activity. Therefore, those not practicing law probably have that greater interest in pharmacy which leads to pharmacy memberships. Despite the response that 42 percent of the students intend to practice law upon graduation, only 31 percent hold student membership in the American Bar Association which requires a very nominal membership fee.

Of 134 pharmacist-lawyers responding, four percent were women. A higher percentage was seen with the students—12 percent women. Both of these figures are higher than the national figure of three percent of the attorneys in the nation being women,[8] but the proportion of women holding the MD-JD combination (four percent) is very close to that for women pharmacist-lawyers.[9]

Factors influencing these pharmacy graduates to enter law school are listed in Table 73.3. The law graduates listed interest in law first, with lack of stimulation in pharmacy second, and desire to work for pharmacy in an administrative or legislative capacity third. The students ranked lack of intellectual stimulation first above job flexibility with lack of professionalism in pharmacy coming in third. Although no student listed interest in law as a reason for entering law school, it can be assumed to be present. This lack of mention can best be explained by noting that the question was open-ended without a list of possible responses.

In Table 73.4 . . . are compiled the responses to the question, "What do you see as the most pressing problem facing pharmacy?" Both groups placed greatest importance

Table 73.3

Factors Influencing Pharmacy Graduates' Entry to Law School

Factor	Pharmacist-Lawyers Number	Percent	Pharmacist-Law Students Number	Percent
Interest in law	27	20	—	—
Lack of intellectual stimulation in pharmacy	21	16	7	27
Desire to work for pharmacy in an administrative or legislative capacity	16	12	2	8
Self-improvement	12	9	—	—
Job flexibility	10	7	5	19
Interest in business	8	6	—	—
Economics	6	4	1	4
Lack of professionalism in pharmacy	5	4	4	15
Member of family or friend	4	3	1	4
Faculty member in pharmacy school	3	2	1	4
Desire for something less scientifically oriented	1	1	3	12
Desire to teach law in pharmacy school	1	1	1	4
Desire to change basic institutions in our society	1	1	1	4
Long hours	1	1	—	—
Interest in politics	1	1	—	—
No response	17	12	—	—
Total	134	100	26	100

Table 73.4

Primary Problem Facing Pharmacy

Problem	Pharmacist-Lawyers Number	Percent	Pharmacist-Law Students Number	Percent
Merchandising versus professionalism	46	34	12	46
Government regulation	15	11	4	15
Organizational unity	15	11	5	19
Developing the health care team	15	11	2	8
Third-party payments	10	7	—	—
Demise of independent pharmacies	6	4	—	—
Better pharmaceutical education	4	3	—	—
Peer review	3	2	—	—
Technicians	2	1	—	—
Economics	1	1	—	—
Too many pharmacists	1	1	—	—
Unenforcement of pharmacy laws	1	1	—	—
Holdups	1	1	—	—
Increased respect for hospital pharmacists	1	1	—	—
Failure to communicate with patients	1	1	—	—
Generic prescribing	1	1	—	—
Continuing education	1	1	—	—
Health care delivery	—	—	1	4
Lack of intellectual stimulation	—	—	1	4
Brand name drug marketing	—	—	1	4
No response	10	7	—	—
Total	134	100	26	100

on the merchant versus professional image of pharmacists. Governmental regulation, organizational unity and developing the health care team received equal percentages from the lawyers. The law students placed organizational unity second and governmental regulation third.

Discussion

Although 134 pharmacist-lawyers and pharmacist-law students were located for this survey, the total number is likely to be close to 200. Curran attributes the larger size of this group to the fact that "pharmacy is usually an undergraduate college-level degree while all of the other health-science degrees are at the masters or doctoral level."[9] While this is true to some extent, it must be considered in light of the findings here that 14 percent of the law graduates and 31 percent of the students hold degrees other than their basic degree in pharmacy or law.

The advantages of being a dual professional have been much touted. One author, speaking of the physician-lawyer, said that he "possesses several distinct advantages over individuals trained in only law or medicine. The dually trained individual is aware of many more facets of the problem that confronts his patient-client . . ." and "he is prepared to analyze a problem in greater depth and with a dual viewpoint."[10]

Shein, in a recent legal article, identified an area in which the dual expertise of the pharmacist-lawyer could be of great value— that of a civil action for damages against a drug manufacturer.[11] Stating that the first obstacle in such a case is to determine whether the drug caused or contributed to the injury alleged, he suggests contacting a pharmacist for a copy of the package insert and for comments concerning his experience with the drug involved. Adding further emphasis to the utility of a pharmacy background for such work is an advertisement for the *1973 Physician's Desk Reference* in *Case*

and Comment, a journal primarily for personal injury attorneys.[12]

In 1965, Woods[1] remarked that there is a "greater demand for the combination of law-medicine or law engineering than there is for the law-pharmacy background," and this was supported by a number of responses in this survey. One student who had written to several large pharmaceutical manufacturers for employment information submitted that the response was "our legal department has a slow turnover and we prefer attorneys with experience in a firm." Further, one attorney who graduated in the mid-fifties reported that he had been told "by the dean of pharmacy that pharmaceutical manufacturers were immensely interested in someone trained in law. I anticipated working into administrative or executive responsibilities with a drug manufacturer. When I graduated and contacted the manufacturers, only two were even remotely interested and the salary was no more than working as a community pharmacist."

Professor Curran also found disillusionment among physicians coming out of law school. Two-thirds of those in his study continued in the practice of medicine.[13]

As Steeves has emphasized, law graduates frequently start at a lower salary than a pharmacist and this may be a drawback. However, starting legal salaries are rising and over the long term the attorney may make more than the pharmacist, depending upon his reputation. Curran found that those holding the MD-JD combination do not have unusually large incomes as compared to others in their medical specialties at their ages and levels of activity.

In 1967 the APhA Committee on Legislation recommended formation of a legal section of APhA and the report was adopted by the House of Delegates.[14] With membership open to pharmacy association and state board attorneys, APhA members holding law degrees, and those actively engaged in teaching pharmaceutical law in accredited colleges of pharmacy, the legal section was seen as serving as a clearinghouse for legislative proposals and court cases of interest to pharmacy. Although the resources have never been available for establishing this subdivision, the 1971–72 Policy Committee on Organizational Affairs requested that the APhA Board of Trustees direct that preliminary steps be taken toward implementation of this proposal.[15] A number of those responding to this survey indicated an interest in just such an organization.

Evidence from this study seems to indicate that pharmacist-lawyers are a young group and that, although slightly over one-half practice law, many of those are still connected with pharmacy through teaching. Of those who do not practice law, many practice pharmacy or work in government service.

The group studied here has potential to be of great assistanc to the profession of pharmacy. The planning of an organization of pharmacist-lawyers should be supported.

References

1. Woods, William E., "Career Opportunities as a Pharmacist-Attorney," *The Squibb Review for Pharmacy Students*, IV, No. 1 (Oct. 1965)
2. Steeves, Robert F., "Legal Blotter: Pharmacist-Lawyers," *JAPhA*, NS7, No. 3, 145 (March 1967)
3. Curran, William J., "Cross-Professional Education in Law and Medicine: The Promise and the Conflict," *J. of Legal Educ.*, 24, 42 (1971)
4. "Letters from our Readers," *Pharmacy Times*, 37, 20 (Aug. 1971)
5. "Enrollment Falls at Schools of Law," *N.Y. Times*, Dec. 17, 1972, at 56, col. 1
6. Curran, *op. cit.*, p. 46
7. American Association of Colleges of Pharmacy, *Roster of Teaching Personnel in Colleges of Pharmacy, 1971–72* (Dec. 1971)
8. Letter from Ms. Ann Collins, American Bar Association Information Service (Nov. 1, 1972)
9. Curran, *op. cit.*, p. 44
10. Carter, Richard, "Ethical Considerations of Dual Practice by an Attorney-Physician," *Amer. Univ. Law Rev.*, 20, 151 (Aug. 1970)
11. Shein, Joseph D., "So You Want to Try a Civil Action against a Drug Company?" *Case and Comment*, 77, 16 (Nov.-Dec. 1972)
12. "Order Your 1973 PDR Now," *Case and Comment*, 77, 31 (Sept.-Oct. 1972)
13. Curran, *op. cit.*, p. 72
14. "APhA House of Delegates Actions—1967," *JAPhA*, NS7, No. 6, 317 (June 1967)
15. Memorandum to the APhA Board of Trustees from APhA Policy Committee on Organizational Affairs, April 17, 1972

Readings for a Broader Perspective

1. Fink, J. L. III, and Simonsmeier, L. M. "Legal Education of the Pharmacy Undergraduate," *American Journal of Pharmaceutical Education* (May 1977):89–91.

PHARMACY LIBRARIANSHIP

74—Pharmacy Librarianship

Virginia B. Hall

Considering the wide scientific base of the field of pharmacy, the person who chooses a career in pharmacy librarianship needs a degree in both pharmacy and library science. Who else but a pharmacist has a background in organic chemistry, physics, biology, mathematics, anatomy, physiology, microbiology coupled with the areas that are specifically pharmacy—pharmacology, pharmaceutics, medicinal chemistry, pharmacognosy and pharmacy administration? Yet little attention has been given to promoting pharmacy librarianship, even though it would be ideal for the person who is interested in the field, enjoys research, and wishes to pursue the theoretical rather than the practical aspects of pharmacy. The activities of a pharmacy librarian are closely related to the field of pharmacy, but much different from the activities of a practicing pharmacist.

Furthermore, librarians specializing in pharmacy are not confined to employment in academic pharmacy libraries, but are sought after for positions available in drug information centers, academic medical and chemistry libraries, and the pharmaceutical associations. Many pharmaceutical and chemical companies also employ librarians with special scientific backgrounds.

Perhaps the two greatest constraints in pursuing a career in pharmacy librarianship are the additional year of school beyond the five already spent acquiring the bachelor of science degree in pharmacy, and the fact that the beginning salary offered to pharmacy librarians is much lower than that offered to beginning pharmacists. However, the extra year of school does yield a masters degree, the salaries eventually even out (sooner in industrial libraries than in academic libraries), and there are other compensations.

The most obvious place for a pharmacy librarian to seek employment is in academic libraries associated with schools of pharmacy and schools of medicine. There are 83 accredited colleges of pharmacy in the United States, Canada, Puerto Rico, the Philippines and Australia, and more than 100 accredited colleges of medicine in the United States and Canada. All of these institutions support libraries in which one or more professional librarians are employed.

The duties of an academic librarian are to develop and keep current adequate holdings of books and journals suitable to the curriculum and research being done at the school. In addition, they may undertake reference work for students, faculty and occasionally for local pharmacists and physicians. The librarian also should be available to teach students the searching skills necessary to use the library literature. A library assistant usually will take charge of the actual running of the library and do the circulation work, check in the periodicals, get periodicals ready for the bindery, fill the interlibrary loan requests, and keep the closed reserve books current.

There are many advantages in academic librarianship. For the most part, librarians are given faculty status which has many responsibilities, opportunities and benefits associated with it. Faculty members are expected, in addition to their assigned work, to conduct research and to participate in professional organizations and community service. Rewards for achievement include advancement and tenure. Fringe benefits generally available to college faculty members include tuition-free education for children, group life insurance, major medical insurance, nearby dental and optometry clinics, excellent retirement programs, and four weeks annual vacation. Esthetically, a position as an academic librarian provides the intellectual stimulation of working with faculty and students who are involved in current research, the pleasant environment of a college campus, and the many cultural and sports events offered.

Another aspect of pharmacy librarianship is found in the scientific and technical libraries of the pharmaceutical and chemical companies. There are about sixty major pharmaceutical companies that have the capacity to do the research necessary to introduce new drugs. Most of these firms are concentrated in New York, New Jersey, Pennsylvania, Illinois, Indiana, Michigan, Massachusetts, Ohio, California, North Carolina, and Virginia. In addition to pharmaceutical firms, there are many chemical companies that have pharmaceutical operations. All of the pharmaceutical and chemical companies maintain libraries with considerably larger staff than in academic libraries.

Industrial libraries usually emphasize only the areas in which the company conducts research. Consequently, knowledge of the field is of primary importance, although a library science degree is usually also required. In addition, preference might be given to the person who, while studying for his library degree, specialized in computerized information retrieval systems, as companies need quick access to the most current information available. Unlike academic libraries, where completeness of collections including historical materials is important, industrial libraries emphasize current materials and utilize computerized data bases to a great extent. In an industrial library, the librarian does the searching, writes abstracts, and compiles bibliographies for the researchers as well as for other areas such as sales and advertising. The traditional tasks of collection development, reference work and cataloguing are part of the position duties.

Large companies usually have very good fringe benefits including retirement pensions, health care programs, and generous numbers of holidays and "roving holidays" to be taken at the employee's convenience. Vacations may be less for starting employees than in academic libraries, but lengthen and become equal as years of service increase. The salary is generally higher than for academic libraries, but there is no tenure. Although industrial librarians are encouraged to participate in professional meetings, there are no requirements to do so. There are no demands for publishing either, although many excellent articles that appear in the library journals have been written by librarians affiliated with industrial firms.

While academic and industrial pharmacy libraries seem to be the obvious source of employment for a librarian with a pharmaceutical background, there are other interesting possibilities. Hospital libraries require persons with a background in medicine and drugs. These libraries vary with the size of the institution, some employing several librarians, some only one. Most large hospitals have drug information centers that assist the doctors by providing information on drugs and drug choices. These centers would be delighted to find a librarian with a pharmaceutical background, since searching skills and thorough knowledge of retrieval methods and cataloguing would be very helpful.

There are also firms that provide smaller pharmaceutical and chemical companies with information retrieval services which would include literature searches, abstracts of journal articles and review articles in a specific field. Some of these companies require people with backgrounds in pharmacy and would be worth investigating. Another similar possibility exists among publishers of indexes in this field: i.e., American Chemical Society (publisher of *Chemical Abstracts*), American Society of Hospital Pharmacists (publisher of *International Pharmaceutical Abstracts*), or the U.S. National Institutes of Health (publisher of *Index Medicus*).

Book dealers that furnish large libraries with newly published books from all publishers in specific fields need people with special backgrounds also.

Since at this time there are very few people with pharmaceutical backgrounds who have entered these library-related fields, the possibility for future employment seems very good. There are enough challenges and diversity to make the work interesting and rewarding.

References

Andrews, T. "Pharmaceutical Libraries and Literature," in *Encyclopedia of Library and Information Science*, Vol. 22. New York: Marcel Dekker, 1977. pp. 158–78.

Zachert, M.J.K., ed., *Standards and Planning Guide for Pharmacy Library Service*, prepared for the Section of Librarians, American Association of Colleges of Pharmacy by the Committee on Standards, American Association of Colleges of Pharmacy, Washington, D.C., 1975.

Related Reading in This Volume

29. Drug Information

PROFESSIONAL ASSOCIATION EXECUTIVE .

75—Executive Director, The Ohio State Pharmaceutical Association

No job description ever could include the myriad of small details and individual functions that one is called upon to study and perform in the course of a "normal" working day. Nonetheless, the items listed below are illustrative of the major responsibilities of the Executive Director:

General Administration

Responsibility for the direction of the day-to-day functioning of the Association lodges with the Executive Director. His key role is that of leadership: To take the lead, to set the example, to show the direction—quickly, clearly, emphatically and with enthusiasm. He must have a broad, general understanding of all aspects of the Association and its activities. Among the most important general administrative tasks are:

- Reading, responding or routing of all written correspondence directed to the Association;
- Assignment of specific job functions to appropriate staff;
- Telephone contact with members, Association Officers and Directors;
- Special, personal tasks undertaken for officers, and agencies, other professional associations, etc.;

- Conferences with the Association President on specific programs;
- Financial Affairs—actually preparing, making and explaining the Association budget; and working closely with the Business Manager to assure a balanced budget and a good return on all Association expenditures and investments;
- Coordination of 25 Association Committees—planning agendae, scheduling meetings, notifying members, sending minutes, organizing projects, etc.;
- Planning and scheduling Executive Committee and Board of Directors Meetings;
- Setting agenda, scheduling meetings, notifying members, correcting minutes, etc.;
- Membership—Increasing both membership numbers and membership services must have a high priority at all times;
- Annual Meeting—Planning, programming, scheduling, organizing and directing all functions related to this event;
- Local Association Officers Conference—Planning, programming, scheduling, organizing and directing all LAO Conference activities;
- Overseas Convention—Planning, programming, working with travel agent, advertising, organizing continuing education (both obtaining lecturers and

working within IRS guidelines), organizing social activities, and directing the convention;

- Special Subject Continuing Education Seminars—Planning, coordinating and participating in special seminars, on specific subjects, i.e. "Drug Product Selection," presented in key cities around the state;
- Fund Raising—The contacting of pharmaceutical manufacturers, and other organizations doing business with pharmacy and with the Association for the purpose of raising funds for specific Association projects;
- Responding to information requests from members, Officers, Directors;
- Weekly staff meetings;
- Ideas—the constant search for new, and better, ways of doing the job.

Legislation

Today, the major decisions affecting all professions and business no longer are made within the professional or business associations themselves—regardless of whether local, state or national—but in the political arenas. This state of affairs probably is the result of business and professional neglect. Therefore, professional and business associations desiring some measure of control over their own destiny have no greater responsibility to their members than the establishing and maintaining of strong legislative relations. Among the most important legislative tasks are:

- Building personal relations with Legislators—This must be a constant activity—not just when favors are sought;
- Writing of legislation—If the profession wants to control its future the Association should actually write and seek the introduction of legislation in its own behalf;

- Attending Committee hearings on all legislation affecting pharmacy or pharmacy business;
- Lobbying—Both in favor of legislation desired by the Association and in opposition to potentially damaging legislation;
- Entertaining—Luncheon, cocktail and dinner meetings with key leaders, on a continuing basis;
- Legislative Reception—One annual major function, for all Legislators and Association leaders, to promote stronger individual contacts;
- Ideas—The constant creation of new programs, new approaches, new friends and greater awareness of the expanding role of the profession.

Publications

The publications of the Association are one of the most important tools of the Association. Publications are one of the few really tangible benefits of membership that the member can actually hold in his own hand—and see for himself what his Association is doing, and what kind of image it projects. Foremost among the publications responsibilities of the Executive Director are:

- Editor of the *Ohio Pharmacist*: (Journal of Ohio pharmacy). Establishing the over-all style for the magazine; setting the theme for each issue; writing monthly editorial; writing periodic special articles; designing cover (often drawn by hand, personally).
- Editor of "OSPA Newsletter"—(Newsletter for OSPA Officers, OSPA Directors, Past Presidents, Past Directors, Local Association Officers). Writing bimonthly newsletter outlining legislative and Association activities of importance to Local Associations.

- Editor of "Capital Comments"—Writing of periodic confidential "newsletter," available to all pharmacists in Ohio outlining Ohio pharmacy's concern about vital issues, such as pending legislation, directly affecting all pharmacy practitioners.
- Editor of "Pharmograms"—Writing of special appeals or notices to state pharmacy leaders and opinion makers.
- Ideas—The constant search for new approaches, new ways to tell the Association's story.

Public Relations

Good relations and mutual understanding, both within the Association—among the membership—and with the public—both general and specific groups—are vital to the vigor, health and growth of a strong professional Association. It is important that the Association present an accurate, attractive and active image to all its publics. Public Relations duties include:

- Active membership in Associations of other trade and professional Association Executives: American Society of Association Executives; The Ohio Trade Association Executives; The Distributive Services Committee; The Ohio Health Council; The Ohio Health Resources Committee; The Ohio Professions Council.
- "OSPA Nights"—presentations on

OSPA to all Local and Student Associations requesting a program.
- Personal contacts with: All State Administrative Agencies; Attorney General; Bureau of Workers' Compensation; Commission on Aging; Department of Public Welfare; Governor's Office; Industrial Commission; Insurance Commission; Labor Unions.
- Ideas—Creativity and new approaches must be a constant part of any public relations activity.

Special, Extra Duties

Some source of private income seems a prerequisite for serving as Executive Director of the Ohio State Pharmaceutical Association. Owing to the time-consuming procedure in obtaining OSPA cheques, personal funds must be used for many daily OSPA functions, which are only later reimbursed. In addition, the Executive Director is called upon to serve in the following capacities:

- Secretary-Treasurer: Ohio Pharmacy Political Action Committee. (Totally separate from, but serving, OSPA) Numerous telephone calls and constant fund-raising are unceasing requirements. . . .
- Overseas Convention Organizer. A great amount of personal time, effort, specialized overseas experience and contacts are required to sponsor first-class overseas programs. . . .

76—Field Secretary and Assistant to the Executive Director

General Introduction to Association Management

Desk Work with Executive Director
Staff Meetings
Specific Desk Assignments
Introduction to Legislature and Committees

Field Secretary

Planning and Executing of Membership Drives
Meetings, in field, with Local Associations
Share Responsibility for "OSPA Nights"

Staff Functions

Responsibility for Coordinating 8 of OSPA's 25 Committees

- Bail Bond Committee
- Consumer Affairs
- Education Conference
- Membership
- Ohio Historical Society Project
- Scholarship
- Third Party Commission
- Wholesaler-Retailer Relations

Serve as In-House Advisor to Continuing Education Committee

Planning and Executing In-Field Continuing Education Programs

Each OSPA staff member is expected to "pitch in" and help with special projects, publications, meetings [and so forth].

QUALITY ASSURANCE

77—PSRO—Participation Pathways for Pharmacists

Joseph L. Hirschman and Marc Laventurier

Introduction

. . . An earlier issue of *Drug Intelligence and Clinical Pharmacy*,[1] . . . provided a perceptive analysis of what Professional Standards Review Organizations are supposed to be doing, their structure, and some of their major problems. The main purpose of this article is to further delineate pathways by which pharmacists can participate in PSRO activities. [Table 77.1]

One would think that, with the enormous volumes of published literature that already exist on PSRO's, everything has been said already. Actually, this is probably true, at least when it comes to expressing opinions.

Table 77.1

Glossary of Acronyms

DUR	Drug Utilization Review
EMCRO	Experimental Medical Care Review Organization
FMC	Foundation for Medical Care
JCAH	Joint Commission on Accreditation of Hospitals
PSRO	Professional Standards Review Organization

It may be that all possible viewpoints on the potential virtues (or lack thereof) of PSRO's have been expressed. However, it is a matter of fact that very few PSRO's are actually operational ("conditional"). Most are in the "planning" and "provisional" stages. Consequently, little can be stated with the authority of experience. To be sure extrapolations can be inferred from the efforts of such PSRO prototypes as the EMCRO's and the FMC's, but there have been no attempts by these groups to review inpatient drug usage and prescribing habits. What it comes down to, presently, is that the impact of PSRO's on patient care, and more specifically, on rational drug therapy, has not been demonstrated one way or another.

For the purposes of this discussion, we can categorize all the "opinions" into two categories: positive and negative: (1) Positive: Those who support the notion that PSRO's are necessary and hope they can be made to succeed, and (2) Negative: Those who know that PSRO's are doomed to be an economic and patient care disaster. This discussion is based upon acceptance of the first opinion as being valid and will emphasize the ways in which they can be made to succeed.

The Need for PSRO's

PSRO's have many inherent "structural" defects because of the compromises that were made to assure passage of Public Law 92–603. There are also many deficiencies in the way we deliver health care in this country. Both of these inadequacies need remedial attention. The irony is that PSRO's were conceived as a response to the latter situation.

Pharmacists need to be hyperactive on both fronts but up to now those who were most concerned and willing to be involved in the planning for strong PSRO's have been kept out, as if by design. Yet it is apparent to any reasonable pharmacist that something must be done in the way of improving the general level of drug therapy practices as part of an overall effort to enhance the quality of patient care in the average community. In any case, the need for drug utilization review has been amply documented.[2-4] The need for pharmacists, actively involved in this process, is also clear. Drugs are the key to modern medicine. Surgery, radio-therapy, and diagnostic tests are important but the ability of health care providers to alter health outcomes [is] heavily dependent on drugs and the way they are distributed and controlled. If the rule were that rational drug usage generally prevailed, as claimed by those most influenced by the drug companies, there would be little need for pharmaceutical input in the management of PSRO's.

The key to rationalizing drug usage is the physician who, up to now, is the only person allowed to prescribe. Current efforts at motivating prescribers to become knowledgeable about drugs are thwarted by the vested interests of the physicians themselves—no one willingly gives up privileges. Part of the problem is the economic reality of the pharmaceutical market place, i.e., the need for drug companies to sell their products and return dividends to their stockholders. However, compounding the problem is that medical education is weak in pharmacology. But the solution does not lie in retraining physicians or intensifying the pharmacology sections of the medical school curriculum. Specialization in the health care profession is, by necessity, the rule. Attempts to reverse this trend will be futile for a multitude of reasons but especially because of the biomedical information explosion. The logical solution is to utilize existing expertise in a complementary fashion for the benefit of patients.

The "specialist" in drug therapy is the clinical pharmacist. He *has* been trained to contribute his valuable expertise in the analysis of appropriate drug therapy and the pitfalls of adverse drug reactions and interactions. The PSRO could offer one mechanism through which this expertise would be channeled into mainstream medical review. In sum, the prominence of the drug component in the medical record, the existing and expanding role of the pharmacist, and the specialized nature of drug therapy today, all dictate the need for the inclusion of the clinical pharmacist in the review process.

The Approaches

A PSRO offers a basic framework for the inclusion of DUR programs. Current forces, especially that of government, are not likely to sponsor redundant efforts so such activity on the part of the pharmacist is likely to be fruitless. There are, however, three basic approaches that can be pursued by pharmacists within the context of PSRO activity.

The first option, and the one most frequently cited, is through the avenue of the Advisory Groups that must be established to recommend policies governing nonphysician health care services to statewide PSRO Councils. (Figure 77.1)

A second approach is to work to get one's hospital designated as a "delegated review" facility and then to develop pharmacist-oriented concurrent review within the hospital.

Figure 77.1

PSRO schematic.*

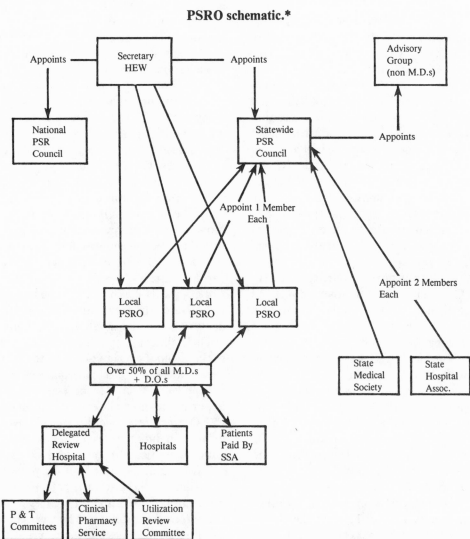

*Adapted from Welch, C.: Professional Standards Review Organizations—Problems and Prospects, *N. Engl. J. Med* 289:291–295 (Aug. 9) 1973.

Lastly, everyone within organized pharmacy should work to change the basic structure of PSRO's through political action.

These three basic approaches are more interdependent than one might think. There are some common denominator problems that must be worked on no matter what approach is opted for. In addition, it may prove too difficult to sustain meaningful activity solely through the first two approaches, unless there is some hope that the inborn errors in the legislatively dictated structure of PSRO's will not ultimately result in their being stillborn or crippled at birth. Thus, it is prudent that activity on all three fronts takes place simultaneously, but with due regard to current and local political considerations.

The Problems

There are two severe deficiencies legislated into the PSRO structure that will make it difficult for PSRO's to achieve their goals. These are immediately apparent to anyone who cares to objectively analyze the situation. The first and foremost problem is that of interdisciplinary review or, in the case of PSRO's, the lack thereof. The second is, to some extent, a corollary of the first problem: the physician-only structure of the PSRO is a classic example of a conflict of interest.

Since these situations have been built-in by Congress, it is going to take rather strong and sustained political action on the part of organized pharmacy to bring about appropriate alterations. This is our third listed option for pharmacist participation in PSRO's and it may seem rather indirect and not particularly professionally fulfilling. It is indirect but we think that is crucial to our professional future.

The current PSRO structure is more in line with the long gone age of the independent general practitioner with the image of the universal healer. Yet, the notion of utilizing formalized peer review bodies with the authority to act is a modern concept. The best health care has been delivered for some time now by multispecialists and interdisciplinary teams. In those team efforts the physician's primacy is being diffused to other health professionals as he yields his dominance with the many tasks he delegates. As a consequence, quality review and control mechanisms that utilize only the input of physicians will be increasingly ineffective as their "share" of the treatment program continues to diminish. It is probably inevitable that, as pharmacists increase their responsibility for health care, they will also increase their proportional representation on review boards. This is, the proportioned division of responsibility evident in the provision of care will also be apparent in the quality evaluation system. Just as rational therapeutic plans depend upon interdisciplinary inputs, so will their evaluation.

While the inevitability of all this seems apparent, the current reality is that the PSRO law is very explicit in reserving ultimate responsibility for review to physicians. It is the potential short-term consequences of this situation that are disturbing. If by some chance, PSRO's succeed in their present form, it will mean a perpetuation of the old encrusted hierarchies in the health care professions. This could, for example, retard the development of clinical pharmacy practice because control of review also means control of practices. If one group is able to monopolize all the review functions they will inevitably dictate patterns of practice to suit themselves. Obviously, pharmacists, health care organizations and consumers must work towards making review bodies more reflective of the true nature of health care delivery before the situation reverses itself.

The political process is such that it will probably not be reactive enough to neutralize adverse short-term consequences. Thus, advantage will have to be taken of what opportunities are allowed in the existing PSRO structure for interdisciplinary involvement to maintain at least a holding action until the political strategies produce results.

PSRO guidelines do encourage providers of ancillary services to participate. However, there can be substantial differences in how one perceives the difference between the letter of these guidelines and their spirit. Strict interpretation means that nonphysician health professionals will have their activity confined to that of an advisor via the statewide Advisory Groups called for by the guidelines. Advice tendered need not be heeded. On the other hand, a liberal view of the guidelines sees it as extending nonphysician activity into the actual review processes at a local level.

However, it will take more than the "moral support" expressed in the regulations to find an acceptable means of interdisciplinary review. The specter of a clinical pharmacist, for example, reviewing the prescribing habits of a physician is disconcerting to many of them. Interdisciplinary interaction within the context of a PSRO is going to require superior tact and diplomacy. Success is dependent on finding a common reference point upon which physicians can comfortably rationalize the attitudinal changes that are the basic prerequisite to establishing a functional and effective interdisciplinary review of health care. The common point of reference ought to be the patient's health status.

Some Solutions

Pharmacists cannot wait around to be invited to participate in the Advisory Group; they should actively seek it out. Pharmacy cannot afford to let nature take its course but must try to control it. Until such time as PSRO's are restructured by legislation, the impact of the nonphysician health professional at the PSRO level, local or statewide, is going to have an impact pretty much dependent upon the personalities of the individuals involved and their respective political skills.

At the institutional level there is reason to be more optimistic for earlier results. PSRO's can delegate review to the individual hospital. These so-called "delegated review" facilities presumably have demonstrated a capacity to conduct effective and timely review in such a way as to aid the PSRO in fulfilling its responsibilities. The theory is that the PSRO takes advantage and builds upon the existing capabilities of hospital review systems that are already operational including those required by the Joint

Commission for the Accreditation of Hospitals, Medicaid, and Medicare. However, if the delegation process is taken seriously by the PSRO and not used just to lessen their workload because of a lack of funding and other reasons, it is unlikely that we will see an overwhelming number of delegated review hospitals. This is so because, by and large, the utilization review programs extant are impotent shells, existing only to receive accreditation for the institution. At best, they have performed only in a perfunctory manner to comply with the letter of the law.*

The point here is that members of the pharmacy department in the hospital should play an aggressive role in working toward achieving delegated review status for their hospital. Increased local responsibility for review will provide increased opportunity for access to the reviewing process for pharmacists. A particularly useful vehicle for this purpose is the pharmacy and therapeutics [P & T] committee.

Traditionally, the primary responsibility of the P & T Committee is to provide guidance on policy matters for the operation of the pharmacy and in the maintenance of the drug formulary. More and more, these responsibilities are being interpreted to also embrace programs of drug utilization review and, in fact, have provided the only real mechanism in the hospital for this activity. Expansion of these activities is necessary. While highly developed in some hospitals, effective P & T Committees are still not the rule.

In addition to formulary control, P & T Committees do or should offer counsel on the appropriate use of drugs through newsletters and other communication techniques. Requiring compliance with this counsel and invoking remedial measures with those who

---

* AUTHORS' NOTE: Since the preparation of this article, there has been a disturbing trend toward designating facilities as "delegated review" without real evaluation as to whether they are actually qualified. This is because the federal funding for PSRO's is inadequate and so this is a way for them to continue operations. It is really a subversion of the whole process and a waste of money.

do not comply has not ordinarily been part of the committee's mandate. However, this is beginning to change and the role of the P & T Committee is expanding to assume more and broader authority in the area of drug utilization review and control. It is this broader view of the mission of the P & T Committee which pharmacists should pursue. This view offers an ideal starting place for bringing pharmacists into the mainstream of patient care review because, normally, interdisciplinary peer relationships have already been established and there are internal incentives for maintaining a viable P & T Committee since formularies represent direct cost savings to the hospital.

Clinical Pharmacy Service

There are, of course, currently available modalities in a hospital for making the presence of the pharmacist felt that offer more dramatic results than the P & T Committee. The general principle is that the closer you get to concurrent review the more likely you are to impact the quality of patient care directly and with positive outcome. The P & T Committee is a lot closer to the action than the area-wide PSRO. Clinical Pharmacy Service, in turn, is right there where the action is and thus nearer to the ideal, than the P & T Committee activities. The ideal review system is one where the system itself eliminates the need for retrospective review. This result occurs when the pharmacist through his clinical involvement and given the tools—probably computer-supported pharmacy and medical information system —works with the prescriber to promote rational drug therapy as part of the normal acceptable routine of the hospital. In these circumstances, the PSRO itself would serve more of an appeals function and as an arbiter of disputes that could not be solved by the delegated review hospital.

The term "clinical pharmacy service" is not meant to be synonymous with a particular drug distribution system, e.g., unit-dose. While good drug distribution systems are inherently a form of concurrent review of prescribing patterns, they are separable from clinical pharmacy services. Together, they are synergistic. Intensification of the clinical pharmacy movement is really what is called for as a primary pathway for pharmacist involvement in PSRO's.

Summary

Throughout this article, the general theme that recurs is one that stresses the importance of eventually resolving the basic flaws in the PSRO structure. No matter how valid, rational and necessary the need for Drug Utilization Review is in PSRO's, they will not work to the benefit of the patient if built-in insurmountable structural defects persist. The physician-only structure is an example of conflict of interest, does not reflect the real nature of health care delivery, and can serve only to perpetuate unreasonable and increasingly obsolete hierarchical structures in health care that do not serve the best interests of the patient.

The real problems all stem from this inherent conflict-of-interest situation. The only way PSRO's will ever work for the purpose for which they were intended is to alter their basic structure so that these conflicts are neutralized. The best approach is to build in the same checks and balances that are provided for and developing in the delivery of health care, not the least of which is the interdisciplinary team approach. Structured, equitable interdisciplinary representation in the PSRO by all members of the health team can and will reverse the "conflicts of interest" to one of interest in the quality of patient care.

References

1. Rucker, T. D.: PSRO: Current Issues—Future Trends, *Drug Intell. & Clin. Pharm.* 9:292–297 (June) 1975.
2. Silverman, M. and Lee, P.: *Pills, Profits, and Politics*, University of California Press, Berkeley, 1974, 403 pgs.
3. Brodie, Donald C.: Drug Utilization and Drug Utilization Review and Control, U.S. Department of Health, Education, and Welfare, National Center for Health Services Research and Development, Washington, D.C., 1970.
4. Rucker, T. Donald: The Need for Drug Utilization Review, *Am J. Hosp. Pharm.* 27:654 (Aug.) 1970.

Related Readings in This Volume

11. Drug Usage Review
57. Impact of Automated Drug Reviews in Clinical Practice

General References for Role Models as Non-Practitioners

1. Penna, R. P. "Pharmacists as Health Planners," *American Pharmacy* NS 19 (April 1979): 23–24.
2. Bush, P. J., and Johnson, K. W. "Where Is the Public Health Pharmacist?" *American Journal of Pharmaceutical Education* 43 (August 1979):249–52.

Chapter Six

Pharmacy Education

This chapter discusses the academic and practical experience requirements related to your objective of becoming a pharmacist. Once these requirements have been satisfied, you will be ready to sit for the State Board licensure examination, which is our subject for the next chapter.

Entrance Requirements

Since all pharmacy practitioners must have graduated from an accredited college of pharmacy, your first step is to gain admission to such an institution. In addition to receiving good grades in high school, it is essential that you take courses that are appropriate for the study of pharmacy. Although prerequisites vary from institution to institution, the most common minimum background is likely to include algebra, geometry, physical science(s), a biological science, a social science, and English. With the clinical pharmacist assuming an expanding role as a specialist in drug information, it should be apparent that written and verbal communication skills cannot be neglected in your preparatory work. For particular details, consult the official catalogues of those schools of major interest or write for *Pharmacy School Admission Requirements*, American Association of Colleges of Pharmacy, 4630 Montgomery Avenue, Bethesda, MD 20014 (payment of $5.00 must accompany your order).

The quality of high school education has been found to vary significantly between schools and over time. Consequently, many universities also require that a prospective student complete either the American College Test or the Scholastic Aptitude Test. While these indicators give a measure of an individual's ability to succeed in academic programs generally, they have not been reliable for predicting successful completion of pharmacy programs in particular. Therefore, more than 50 percent of the institutions now mandate or recommend that applicants take a specially designed examination, the Pharmacy College Admission Test. This instrument measures not only overall academic ability and reading comprehension, but proficiency in elementary mathematics, chemistry, and biology as well. Currently, this test is given three times a year, and deadlines for receiving completed applications are set in October, January, and April. The cost to the student for test administration is $20.00.

Considerations about preparatory studies for some individuals, however, will be significantly different if they already possess a baccalaureate degree in another field. For example, during the period from 1971 to 1978, 20 students with degrees in biology were admitted to the pharmacy program at The Ohio State University. A smaller number had backgrounds, in order of descending frequency, in zoology, chemistry, microbiology, education, mathematics, psychology, and science. This list also includes one student from each of the following fields: accounting, agriculture, French, geology, history, philosophy, radio/television, religion, and sociology.

The Academic Disciplines

Before reviewing the choices you will need to make when you select a college of pharmacy, we will pause for a brief overview of the content of pharmacy education. Table VI-1 summarizes the changing pattern of studies that you can expect during enrollment in a typical five-year program. You will observe that the early years are weighted heavily with the basic sciences (chemistry, biology, physiology, etc.) and other areas (the social sciences, the humanities, and liberal education electives). By the third year, however, the emphasis changes to the pharmaceutical sciences which are described below. Of course, clinical experience receives heavy emphasis during your final year.

Although the actual boundaries of certain disciplines are more flexible than fixed, the following descriptions suggest the academic domain of each of the disciplines that you may encounter as a pharmacy student.

Medicinal Chemistry. This area involves the study of the chemistry and pharmacy of inorganic and organic medicinal products, the biochemistry of medicinal preparations, the relationship of chemical structure to drug action in the body, and the qualitative and quantitative analysis of drugs.

Pharmacognosy and Natural Products. This special branch of medicinal chemistry has to do with those substances that are of biological origin—that is, they are derived from plants or animals. Students learn about the production, processing, identification, preservation, properties, and uses of such drug products.

Pharmacology. This discipline deals with the effects of drugs on living tissue. You will learn about the uses of drugs in diagnosis, treatment, and prevention of disease; their mechanisms of action, metabolism, toxicities, and side effects; and the relationship of their structures to physiological effects.

Pharmaceutics and Pharmaceutical Chemistry. Study in this field addresses the principles, processes, and techniques related to the fabrication of drugs and drug products. In addition to the manufacturing process, students learn how prescriptions are compounded, as well as dispensing fundamen-

Table VI–1

The Pharmacy Curriculum: Average Percent of Time Spent in Respective Disciplines, U.S.A., 1979

	Year in Five-Year Program				
	1	2	3	4	5
Basic Sciences	59.3%	60.2%	32.6%	12.9%	2.5%
Pre-Clinical Pharmaceutical Sciences	1.5	6.3	58.2	68.6	28.2
Clinical	0.6	0.8	5.1	11.6	55.1
Other	38.6	32.7	4.1	6.9	14.2
	100.0%	100.0%	100.0%	100.0%	100.0%

Source: President H. H. Wolf, AACP Legislative Conference, April 2, 1979.

tals. Further, technical knowledge covering areas such as drug nomenclature, calculations, and pharmacokinetics is acquired.

Administrative and Social Sciences. This area embraces a variety of applied subjects that are designed to help ensure that professional services are delivered efficiently within the practice setting. While the scope and content of these offerings have not been standardized in American schools of pharmacy, students may have an opportunity to take courses in one or more of the following areas: management, accounting, pharmaceutical marketing, jurisprudence, history of pharmacy, professional ethics, communication skills, the structure of our health care system, and social problems in drug use.

Pharmacy Practice. This area encompasses the applied disciplines pertaining to clinical proficiency. Here, all previous training involving laboratory and administrative sciences is focused on the provision of professional pharmacy services to patients and other health care specialists. In order to ensure their competence as practitioners, students receive instruction covering drug therapy related to patient disease, sterile products, applied pharmacotherapeutics, and dispensing procedures. In addition to gaining practical experience under preceptors, they learn about how pharmacists, physicians, and nurses work together as a team.

College Options

The potential pharmacy student is fortunate in that selection of a college can be made from among 72 accredited institutions in the United States today. Moreover, they are widely dispersed, being located in 43 states, the District of Columbia, and Puerto Rico. Only Alaska, Delaware, Hawaii, Maine, Nevada, New Hampshire, and Vermont lack a school of pharmacy. The largest number of institutions per state (four) are found in New York, Pennsylvania, and Ohio, while California, Michigan, and Texas each have three.

In reviewing your options for academic training, you should probably exclude foreign schools from consideration. Currently, most State Boards of pharmacy require that licensure applicants be graduates of institutions accredited by the American Council on Pharmaceutical Education. Since this body exercises jurisdiction over only domestic colleges, prospective practitioners are confined effectively to preparation offered by one of the American schools.

Some of you may still prefer to obtain your pharmacy education in a foreign country such as Canada, Italy, or New Zealand. Under these circumstances, your professional career in the United States would be limited to non-practitioner positions that do not depend on prior licensure (see Chapter Five.)

Let us now turn to the more realistic choices that are available for your pharmacy education. Table VI-2 lists the 72 American institutions by geographical region and ranks them according to the number of bachelor's degrees granted in the 1977–78 academic year. The regional basis for classification has been chosen because relatively few students seem interested, or perhaps financially able, to seek training which requires extended travel from their home. Further, the additional influence of preparation for licensure seems to produce a strong preference for education within the boundaries of the state of residence. In 1977, for the entire nation, less than 17 percent of all pharmacy students had crossed their state boundaries to obtain their professional training. Nevertheless, there are some colleges that seem to favor, or to be attractive to, out-of-state students. These institutions are ranked in Table VI-3.

In selecting the college that meets your needs best, you should consider many factors. Two of the most important, total

Table VI-2

Degrees Granted by American Colleges of Pharmacy Classified by Geographic Region and Ranked According to Number of Bachelor Graduates, 1977–78

College or School of Pharmacy	Number of Degrees Awarded			
	B.S.	Pharm.D.	M.S.	Ph.D.
NORTHEAST				
Massachusetts	240	3*	11	3
St. John's	226	—	49	8
Arnold & Marie Schwartz	225	—	30	—
Philadelphia CP&S	182	13*	11	3
Temple	122	—	15	5
Duquesne	120	10*	5	1
Northeastern[3]	111	—	27	1
Connecticut	110	—	2	5
Albany	109	—	—	—
Rutgers	103	—	5	6
Pittsburgh	93	—	3	6
Rhode Island	92	—	6	2
SUNY/Buffalo	72	7*	4	8
SOUTH				
Texas/Austin	197	10*	3	6
Northeast Louisiana	196	—	5	—
Puerto Rico	172	—	—	—
Georgia	163	—	8	3
North Carolina	143	—	5	3
Houston	138	—	9	—
Southwest Oklahoma	137	—	—	—
Tennessee[1]	119	15*	—	—
Samford	116	—	—	—
Oklahoma[4]	114	—	5	—
Auburn[4]	113	—	10	—
Florida[1]	111	4*	2	1
South Carolina	104	—	4	—
Mercer[1]	93	17*	—	—
Mississippi	92	—	21	4
Virginia	90	2*	—	2
Kentucky[1]	87	16*	1	—
Maryland	84	6*	4	2
Florida A & M[1]	84	—	—	—
West Virginia	65	—	1	—
Arkansas	64	2*	1	—
Medical University of South Carolina	62	15*	—	—
Howard[5]	51	—	—	—
Texas Southern	47	—	—	—
Xavier[3]	46	—	—	—
NORTH CENTRAL				
Illinois[3]	193	—	6	5
Ferris State[1]	161	—	—	—
Purdue[4]	155	8*	31	30
Wisconsin	153	—	19	8
Ohio Northern	137	—	—	—

Table VI-2 cont.

Degrees Granted by American Colleges of Pharmacy Classified by Geographic Region and Ranked According to Number of Bachelor Graduates, 1977-78

College or School of Pharmacy	Number of Degrees Awarded			
	B.S.	Pharm.D.	M.S.	Ph.D.
NORTH CENTRAL cont.				
St. Louis	129	—	—	—
North Dakota	117	—	8	1
Ohio State[6]	113	—	15	10
Minnesota[1]	110	16*	15	14
Wayne State	108	4*	8	2
Drake	93	—	—	—
Butler	92	—	3	—
Iowa	83	—	15	3
Toledo	79	—	1	—
Michigan[1]	78	19*	8	9
Wyoming	75	—	—	—
Kansas	73	—	18	14
Creighton	72	9*	—	—
Missouri/Kansas City	72	5*	2	1
Nebraska[1]	70	—	1	1
South Dakota	63	—	—	—
Cincinnati	57	4*	1	1
WEST				
Oregon State	103	—	2	—
Idaho State	81	—	1	—
Washington	78	—	3	—
Arizona[5]	75	—	2	—
Utah[2]	70	—	—	3
Washington State	67	—	2	1
Colorado	54	—	1	—
Pacific[1]	47	139†	3	3
New Mexico	47	—	—	—
Montana	32	—	—	—
Southern California	—	140†	13	3
California	—	88†	—	—

Source: Solander, Lars. *Degrees Conferred by Schools and Colleges of Pharmacy for the Academic Year of 1977-1978.* Bethesda, Maryland: American Association of Colleges of Pharmacy, 1978.

Note: In the first category, the Northeast, plans are underway for the merger of the two schools located on Long Island: St. John's and Arnold & Marie Schwartz.

* Number of Pharm.D. graduates secondary to B.S. graduates.
†Pharm.D. as the first professional degree dominates.

[1] College has terminated, or expects to discontinue, the B.S. program.
[2] Pharm.D. degree accredited, B.S. program to be maintained.
[3] Pharm.D. scheduled for review, B.S. program to be maintained.
[4] Pharm.D. only program anticipated by 1984.
[5] Pharm.D. only program anticipated by 1985.
[6] Pharm.D. authorized, B.S. program to be maintained.

Table VI–3

Thirteen Colleges of Pharmacy Where Out-of-State Enrollment in the Freshman Class Exceeded 30 Percent (Excludes Foreign Students)

Drake	72%
Mercer	67
Rhode Island	60
Samford	59
Idaho State	48
Wyoming	41
Philadelphia CP&S	41
Duquesne	37
Connecticut	34
Northeastern	34
Xavier	34
Massachusetts	32
Arnold & Marie Schwartz	30

Source: Peterson, Shailer. *Preparing To Enter Pharmacy School*. Englewood Cliffs, N.J.: Prentice-Hall, Inc., A Spectrum Book, 1979. pp.89–95.

Note: Thirteen institutions did not report data related to this classification.

annual cost and distance from home, depend on your personal resources and preferences. It is interesting to observe that Table VI–3 includes several of both the most expensive *and* the least expensive schools. (The annual charge for resident tuition and fees ranges from under $500 to over $3,000!) Further, you may favor a particular community or school because of its size or the proximity of friends.

There are additional criteria which, for many students, may be more critical. Perhaps the most logical place to begin is with the type of degree you desire. Your choice here is between the two professional degrees, the baccalaureate (B.S.) and the Doctor of Pharmacy (Pharm.D.). Approximately 90 percent of the schools of pharmacy offer the standard five-year program leading to the bachelor's degree. However, at least 24 institutions now confer a doctorate upon the satisfactory completion of the six-to-eight-year requirements. Eight of these colleges have terminated the baccalaureate plan in order to concentrate their resources exclusively on the professional doctoral program.

How can a college freshman or high school senior decide whether the bachelor's or the doctorate is the better route for supporting his professional career? Table VI-4 has been developed especially to help you resolve this complex question. As before, your Pharmacy Scorecard can be used to pinpoint the educational program that seems to correspond best with your current interests.

If this approach does not yield a firm answer, then it is recommended that you postpone this decision until your career objective in pharmacy can be formulated more clearly. As you ponder this question, the following choices should be kept in mind. If you think that you would like to become a practitioner, your options include the following. (1) Enroll in one of the schools that grant the bachelor's degree. This strategy may be the most appropriate if you are contemplating a career in community pharmacy. If it seems possible that your interests lie more in a hospital or nursing home setting, then one of the next alternatives might be superior. (2) Follow the first course, but plan to move on for further professional work at one of the 17 schools which award the Pharm.D. as a second degree. (3) Enroll in one of the eight schools that restrict their programs to training at the doctoral level. (4) Use any of the above options and later work for the M.S. degree or enter a hospital residency program as described below, or both.

If it appears that your pharmacy education will be the basis for a career as a non-practitioner, then your selection of a school should be tailored to suit this goal. For example, if you plan to become a college teacher, or a laboratory scientist employed by a pharmaceutical manufacturer or government agency, a decision of this nature implies additional training beyond the first degree in pharmacy. Under these circumstances, you will want to pursue work lead-

Table VI–4

How to Determine the Best Pharmacy
Degree for You

If these articles describe what you might like to do	The college degree that is most likely to help you achieve your career goal in pharmacy is
1, 2, 4, 5, 6, 7, 8, 9, 10, 12, 13, 14, 15, 16, 17, 20, 21, 22, 23, 24, 25, 31, 35, 39, 40, 41, 42, 43, 44, 45, 46, 47, 48, 49, 50, 51, 62, 65, 69, 70, 71, 72, 76	B.S. with judicious choice of electives.
5, 51, 62	Dual B.S. degree.
6, 8, 11, 20, 26, 27, 28, 29, 31, 32, 33, 34, 35, 36, 37, 38, 44, 45, 46, 48, 50, 57, 66, 68, 77	Pharm.D., or M.S. plus residency (clinical emphasis).
5, 29, 42, 45, 46, 51, 62, 75	M.S. (administrative emphasis).
70, 71, 72	M.S. (basic pharmacy science).
5, 29, 42, 51, 62, 70, 71, 72, 74, 77	M.S. in a non-pharmacy field (Statistics, Public Health, Preventive Medicine, etc.).
73	Graduate non-pharmacy professional degree.
27, 35, 70, 71, 72, 77	Ph.D.

ing to the doctor of philosophy degree (Ph.D.).* With this background, you will develop expertise in research methodology and become a specialist in a particular field. Since this decision will add an extra three to four years to the time required for a first degree, the five-year baccalaureate might be preferable to the professional doctorate.

It should be noted, though, that a few pharmacists with the highest professional degree (Pharm.D.) have also satisfied the requirements for the most advanced research degree (Ph.D.). This combined doctorate may be desired if you select career positions such as those of college instructors in clinical pharmacy or the specialists responsible for evaluating the prescribing and dispensing records in a drug insurance program.

If the type of degree represents your first level of evaluation, then the formula for determining the years of preprofessional education versus professional study might be the second. A majority of the schools operate on the 2-3 plan. Under this arrangement, your first two years of training are taken in an approved junior or liberal arts

* Stipends of $4,500 or more, which usually provide free tuition and fees, are available to a large number of students who are admitted to Graduate School. If you wish to compete for these awards, you should strive to obtain an average grade of "B" or better.

college. Upon your admission to pharmacy school, these credits will be transferred to the professional college you have selected. This procedure, of course, requires that your program be coordinated carefully with that of the institution where you intend to enroll.

The next most popular format, represented by 25 percent of the schools, is the 0-5, or integrated, plan. Under this system, entrance to the college of pharmacy is made directly from high school. Thus, a student spends five years taking courses that are controlled by the institution to which he or she has been admitted. The remaining schools offer a 1-4 or a 2-5 plan, while a few follow both the 1-4 and 2-3 plans simultaneously. Since you have already made a tentative decision about the degree that you desire, several of these choices may no longer be of concern.

This brief encounter with the pharmacy education maze may leave you still puzzled about how to cope with this question. Perhaps the next level of review, possible specialization within pharmacy, will serve to lead you out of the maze. Once this material has been reviewed, determination of the "best" degree and structure of the college program may be easier.

The type of program offered represents the third criterion that may be applied when you select a college of pharmacy. Most schools provide a balanced program, with no particular emphasis on specialization. While some of these colleges identify a track or option within pharmacy, the curriculum for specialized expertise is not highly developed. For those of you who contemplate a career as a staff pharmacist (a generalist without managerial or ownership responsibilities, and without specialized expertise), institutions of this sort could be your best choice for your pharmacy education.

However, some students may want to follow a specialized career in pharmacy. Under these circumstances, the availability of a strong track in your area of interest could be the reason you will prefer one college over another. Not all schools have the resources to provide a highly developed level of specialized training. Extra effort is thereby required to identify these institutions. Should you be willing to restrict your choice of colleges to those on a 2-3 plan, the question of selecting the best school for this particular purpose can be delayed for the maximum period of time.

What kinds of specialized training might warrant consideration as you try to differentiate between colleges? Four possibilities are outlined below.

Clinical Pharmacy. Does the school of pharmacy provide clinical training that is integrated with the total services of a large medical center? Or, does the school have a special clinical program that is oriented toward ambulatory care? If you believe that clinical pharmacy is important, then a good college should be able to develop your skills in this area. Alternatively, overlook this matter when selecting a baccalaureate program and plan to obtain clinical expertise via the Pharm.D. as a second degree.

Industrial Pharmacy. If you anticipate seeking employment in the manufacturing of drug products, your search should be confined to the dozen or so schools that furnish specialized training in this area. Alternatively, you can bypass this feature for the first degree and plan to follow the M.S. or Ph.D. program at one of the colleges with a specialty in industrial technology.

Pharmacy Management. If you expect to become the manager or owner of a pharmacy, or an executive in a chain store, the availability of an undergraduate track in pharmacy management may be a vital factor in your choice between schools. The number of colleges with a well developed program in this area, however, is less than 20. If making a selection within this relatively small group does not appear to be feasible, you could put this matter aside when choosing a school for the first degree. Since your undergraduate training will be based on a general pharmacy program, competence in the management sciences could be gained later via the M.S. in pharmacy administration or in business administration. Pursuit of these degrees will extend your training by an additional 15 to 24 months.

Pre-Graduate School. If you think your total educational program may include graduate training beyond the professional degree (B.S. or Pharm.D.), you might elect to take your first degree at one of the research-oriented schools of pharmacy. Upon completion of this program, you would apply for admission to graduate school at another institution within this same class. One method of identifying such a college is to calculate the total number of Ph.Ds granted over the past three years. If this figure is small—say, less than 15—it might signify inadequate commitment to graduate study. Given this criterion, the number of potential pharmacy schools of interest to you would fall from 72 to about 16.*

How can an individual with very little knowledge about pharmacy predict interest in one of the specialty tracks or options? First, look at the Pharmacy Scorecard and mark Table VI-5 in accordance with your summary evaluation of the readings. Second, examine the pattern of "0s" to determine if one of the tracks seems preferable to the others. Third, after enrolling in pharmacy school, but just before selecting an option, read the articles again and prepare a new Scorecard. Now transfer these ratings to Table VI-5 to determine whether your career goals in pharmacy have changed.

Instead of relying heavily on the type of degree or the availability of a particular program at a given college, you may wish to introduce a fourth measure: the overall reputation of the school. An ideal composite would include many variables such as the quality of the library, the competence of the faculty and their interest in teaching, research productivity of the staff, relevance of the curriculum, and so forth.

The major source of external control over undergraduate programs is accreditation of the school by ACPE, which takes place every six years. However, when all colleges are accredited, as they are today, none can be singled out as being superior. Since it is a mathematical impossibility that all 72 schools are equal, some students may wish to incorporate a recent comparative ranking in their evaluations. In 1974, the Deans of the Colleges of Pharmacy were requested to name the five best schools. While the criteria employed undoubtedly varied among these executive officers, and may reflect a bias toward known elements (such as publications by faculty members), the findings are reported in Table VI-6 for your consideration. In reviewing the ten "best" schools, you should note that not all of these have a strong graduate program (based upon the Ph.D. output level cited above). Moreover, four now offer only one professional degree, the Pharm.D. Further, school size does not seem to have much influence on qualification for this special listing. All but one receive financial support from the state in which they are located. If your previous efforts yield conflicting evidence about which college of pharmacy will meet your needs, the opinions reported in Table VI-6 might be used as a starting point for resolving this issue.

While the criteria outlined above should

---

* Another formula would limit selection to those schools that attract large amounts of funded research. The most recent rankings, based on awards for individual faculty members, indicate that ten schools attracted over 68 percent of the funds supplied by NIH-ADAMHA. These schools, in rank order, are: The University of California/San Francisco, Utah, Kansas, Purdue, SUNY/Buffalo, Wisconsin, Ohio State, Connecticut, Arizona, and Michigan. Since awards may fluctuate from year to year, a three-year average should be compiled.

Table VI-5

How to Identify Your Preferred Track
in Pharmacy Education

If these readings seem especially interesting	The best college for you should have a formal program, or adequate electives, in
1, 2, 4, 5, 6, 7, 10, 12, 13, 14, 15, 16, 20, 22, 23, 24, 39, 40, 41, 42, 62, 65	Professional practice/ community.
6, 8, 9, 10, 11, 13, 17, 20, 21, 22, 25, 26, 27, 28, 29, 31, 32, 33, 34, 35, 37, 38, 43, 45, 46, 47, 48	Professional practice/ institutional.
6, 11, 20, 21, 25, 26, 27, 28, 29, 31, 32, 33, 34, 35, 36, 37, 38, 44, 45, 46, 48, 49, 50, 66, 77	Clinical pharmacy (Pre-Pharm.D.or Pharm.D.).
5, 42, 62	Pharmacy Management.
70, 71, 72	Industrial Pharmacy.
27, 35, 70, 71, 72, 5, 29, 73, 74, 75, 77	Graduate school preparatory: Physical & Biological Sciences. Administrative & Social Sciences.

Table VI-6

Rankings of American Colleges of
Pharmacy by 48 Deans

Rank	Institution	Fraction of Votes
1	University of California/San Francisco	32/48
2	Purdue	27/48
3	Ohio State	25/48
4	Kentucky	19/48
5	Minnesota	15/48
6	State University of New York/Buffalo	14/48
7	Southern California	12/48
8	Wisconsin	12/48
9	Michigan	9/48
10	Illinois	8/48

Source: Change (Winter 1974–75).

suffice for some students, others may wish to follow a more personal formula in selecting a pharmacy school. Regardless of your pathway, it is probably unwise to make a determination without examining three or four college catalogues carefully and visiting, if possible, the campuses of at least two of your highly ranked institutions. These procedures are especially important if you are interested in a particular track in pharmacy.

This extended discussion should suggest that the selection of an appropriate school is a matter worthy of serious attention. The critical variable in determining your professional qualifications and performance, however, is likely to be within your control. The key factor to success as a pharmacist could be the effort which you apply to the academic and extracurricular programs available at the institution where you enroll. In summary, what you put into your educational experience will largely determine what you get out of it; selection of school A over B or C may be only secondary to meeting your career objective.

The Practical Experience Component

Once a student gains admission to a college of pharmacy and maintains a satisfactory record, he or she is on the way toward completion of the academic requirements for licensure as a practitioner. However, proficiency in practical experience represents an additional step necessary for becoming a registered pharmacist. Consequently, State Boards of Pharmacy establish conditions for practical training that must be completed before any candidate can be recognized as eligible to sit for the licensure examination.

At this writing, this requirement can be satisfied if you work a specified number of hours under the direction of a registered pharmacist who is licensed by the Board in the state where you intend to make applica-

tion. The traditional method of certification is called an internship and involves work experience based on the following characteristics:

1. Training is conducted before or after graduation but prior to Board licensing. Fortunately, most students are able to complete the 1,500-hour requirements by the time they graduate, through summer and part-time employment when school is in session (in the latter case, they are often limited to ten hours per week).

2. Training is under control of the State Board of Pharmacy. A major requirement here is that both the intern (pharmacy student) and the preceptor (registered pharmacist who certifies that your hours have been completed) fill out the appropriate forms in advance of employment activity.

3. No supervision of the practical experience is carried out by the faculty of the pharmacy school, nor is academic credit granted.

4. Students usually receive compensation for services provided. However, either because of poor planning or tight supply and demand conditions, especially in the community where the college is located, some individuals have been known to accept internship positions without pay. For example, if a student wishes to take the state licensure examination and is short 125 hours of practical experience, it is to his economic advantage to work during this brief period for nothing and thereby become eligible to take the test. Once this examination has been passed, the pharmacist can enter the labor market, where the opportunity to make $9 to $10 per hour should quickly offset the losses from unpaid employment.

The major weakness of internship programs has not been an economic one, but rather the shallow learning experience of some students. Interns have often spent a significant portion of their time performing clerical chores, rather than helping the pharmacist to carry out his professional duties. In order to better control this situation, the accrediting body of pharmacy schools now requires that each institution offer a structured externship. Although this new program may still leave the student with a certain number of hours to fill via the internship route, it should minimize the limitations noted above.

According to the American Association of Colleges of Pharmacy, an externship program exhibits the following characteristics:

(1) It is a component of a college-based program implemented prior to graduation.
(2) It is conducted outside the classroom in patient-care settings.
(3) Academic credit is granted to the extern whose experiences are
    (a) patient oriented, and
    (b) directly related to the distributive and management functions of the pharmacy,
    (c) supervised by a pharmacist preceptor, and
    (d) conducted under a 1:1 relationship between preceptor and extern.

The practical implication of the externship for the student is that (1) the college assumes the responsibility for placing externs in certified positions, (2) students no longer receive remuneration for their services, and (3) some academic component may be associated with the post.

Externship requirements also may be satisfied by a clerkship. Under a program of this type, the student becomes involved with clinical pharmacy services and only peripherally with distributive or management functions. Moreover, the preceptor may be either a physician or a pharmacist.

Practical experience also may be gained by a formal residency program* such as is operated in more than 100 hospitals in the United States. Ninety-six of these posts were officially approved by the American Society of Hospital Pharmacists, as reported in the May, 1979, issue of the Journal of the Association. While some residencies are conducted as an academic requirement under various Pharm.D. or M.S. programs, others are open only to graduates of these programs. Finally, the orientation of such training will usually focus on one of the following areas: administration, and clinical or specialized fellowships covering fields such as pediatric pharmacy, clinical pharmacokinetics, or drug information services.

Students contemplating pharmacy as a professional career may have difficulty thinking ahead to consider the desirability of these advanced programs. Such options reflect the specialization that characterizes the delivery of pharmacy services today. At the same time, they represent important opportunities for the provision of unique professional services on the part of those who are willing to plan their careers to satisfy society's needs.

Another type of internship program is sponsored by the National Pharmaceutical Council, a consortium supported by 26 of the largest pharmaceutical manufacturers. This summer internship program, which accommodates about 90 students with advanced standing, is designed to broaden the student's perception of various functions related to the development, production, and distribution of pharmaceutical products. An experience of this type could prove to be a valuable supplement to your classroom training. Moreover, such a program will not only generate funds from your summer's employment, it may yield credit for 200 to 400 hours of internship as well. Students who are interested in further information should write to the National Pharmaceutical Council, Inc., 1030 15th St. N.W., Washington, D.C. 20005.

Those of you who are willing to consider a

---

* Programs usually extend for one to two years and accept from one to six applicants per class. Although licensure usually is not required in order to qualify for these positions, many practitioners will achieve this status before completing their training.

unique practitioner-oriented extern experience may wish to examine the special program operated by the United States Public Health Service. Students who have completed at least two years of study in a professionally accredited college program may be eligible for assignments (one to three months in duration) in one of the following areas: (a) medical and hospital services, (b) research, and (c) public health practice. For details, write to the Director, Commissioned Personnel Operations - PHS, Room 4-35, Parklawn Building, Rockville, MD 20857.

Finally, certain State Boards of pharmacy permit a student to earn up to 300 hours of the total internship requirement by serving as a research assistant to a professor at the college where he is enrolled. Those who wish to explore innovative ways of applying their pharmacy training should not neglect this possibility.

Related Information Sources

If you are still perplexed as to which career in the health field may be attractive, put aside this volume temporarily and review the comprehensive survey of over 110 health occupations found in the U.S. Department of Labor *Health Careers Guidebook* (4th ed.), Washington, Government Printing Office, 1979, 221 pages. Moreover, pages 16–24 and 212–18 provide a current summary of financial aids that are available to students in all areas.

Should you desire a briefer and more elementary discussion of pharmacy as a career option, write to the American Association of Colleges of Pharmacy, at the above address, and request a copy of "Shall I Study Pharmacy?"

Perhaps you have already decided on pharmacy and wish to consider the options within the specialty area of pharmacology. Information on the nine subspecialties within this field can be obtained from the American Society for Pharmacology and Experimental Therapeutics, 9650 Rockville Pike, Bethesda, MD 20014. Unfortunately, similar information is not available for the other laboratory sciences—Medicinal Chemistry, Pharmaceutics, or Pharmacognosy.

Chapter Seven

State Licensure and Reciprocity

Frank Kunkel

One distinctive aspect of entrance into a profession such as pharmacy, one that sets it apart from the ordinary career occupation, is the requirement of successful completion of a comprehensive examination as the final condition for admission to active practice. All the concerns and considerations that have been discussed in previous chapters lead up to this final barrier to acceptance into the profession: the registration or licensure examination.

Historical Background

In the late 1800s, the legislatures of several of the most populous states, through the police powers vested in them by their state constitutions, began to set up minimum standards of qualification for pharmacists in the interest of protecting the public health of their citizens. As members of one of the most ancient professions, practitioners of pharmacy had traditionally been admitted through the apprenticeship system. Thus, the competency of the individual pharmacist was established by whatever satisfied his preceptor or employer. With the recognition by the state of the need for some minimal measure of safety and reliability in pharmacy practice, the first of a continuing and increasingly demanding set of educational and practical experience requirements was established. These rules were set up by the various State Boards or Commissions of Pharmacy, to which were delegated the legislative authority to construct, administer, and enforce them. The requirements for registration as a pharmacist have varied, and will probably always vary to some degree, from state to state. Basically, however, most of the necessary qualifications are uniform. The differences are found mainly in time and quantity of practical training or experience necessary for admission to the licensure examination.

Initially, these requirements included citizenship and a minimum age of 21 years, plus graduation from high school. This last requirement appeared in some states as early as 1910, but not generally until the 1920s. Then, following World War I, graduation from an accredited college of pharmacy program became an additional condition. Such programs in pharmacy began as one year of schooling and have advanced, with the progress in pharmaceutical knowledge and services, through successive requirements of two, three, four, and five years (with six years as an optional choice). Judging from historical experience and from the current concern expressed by the principal associations of organized pharmacy, it may be anticipated that the six-year program, as the minimum educational requirement, is inevitable.

In addition to the period covered by the four-year academic requirement, varying amounts of practical experience and training have been tied to the educational programs. Moreover, this component has differed according to variations in the individual state's internship and externship statutes and regulations. As a national guideline, the members of the National Association of Boards of Pharmacy have established the requirement of 1,500 hours of internship as a qualification for admittance to the licensure examination. A maximum of only 400 hours, however, may be obtained concurrently with attendance in a college of pharmacy. Since there is no single national set of standards for registration as a pharmacist, information about the prerequisites of a particular state should be obtained by contact with that State Board of Pharmacy.

The Licensure Examination

The first and principal responsibility of every State Board of Pharmacy historically has been to provide the public with assurance of the competency, safety, and reliability of pharmacists who are actively engaged in practice. This public assurance applies particularly to those involved with the compounding and dispensing of prescriptions.

The baccalaureate degree certifies the educational qualifications of a prospective pharmacist. Successful passage of the licensure examination certifies a candidate's ability to apply academic principles and information to everyday practical situations and circumstances which involve the safety of the patient.

Since 1967, an increasing number of states have required maintenance of practical competency by mandatory continuing education in pharmacy. Prior to the introduction of a standard examination by the National Association of Boards of Pharmacy (NABP) in 1970, licensure examinations were constructed by each state's pharmacy board members. The high standards of performance exhibited by practitioners during those years

usually served both the public and the profession very well.

In recent years, however, many Boards of Pharmacy have shown a concern over the use of modern testing methods and techniques in their licensure examinations. The question of how best to devise the test was especially problematic when the annual number of candidates was too small to permit a valid follow-up evaluation of the examination itself. Individual State Pharmacy Boards also recognized the inevitable limitations that would come from relying solely on the knowledge and experience of their respective members, and the potential advantages of sharing expertise among the member states of the NABP. Finally, members of the State Boards hoped that the important principle of reciprocity would be facilitated if the states could rely on a standardized examination, if it were one of high quality. The wisdom of this concern has also become more apparent in the light of increasing government interest in various kinds of barriers to employment in an occupation or profession.

The Nabplex Program

Initially, the NABP Advisory Committee on Examinations designed an outline of the most important qualifications and competencies of the modern pharmacist. This profile was derived from recommendations submitted by a panel of experts who were recognized for their knowledge and experience. The original group evolved into the Nabplex Review Committee, which represents, to the greatest extent possible, most geographic and occupational areas of the profession. The 1978–79 Nabplex Review Committee, which is representative of the usual complement of members, consists of 20 registered pharmacists who are currently actively employed in community or institutional pharmacies, as well as faculty members of schools of pharmacy. They are geographically distributed throughout 18 states, representing the nation from border to border and coast to coast. Further, 40 percent of these specialists are presently serving as members of their respective State Boards of Pharmacy.

This Committee screens and selects questions submitted by some 200 question writers with similar geographic and occupational backgrounds. These ad hoc participants are recognized professional pharmacists in their respective communities. The final pool of questions, which have been selected by these pharmacists for their relevance to contemporary pharmacy practice, eventually appear in licensure examinations in appropriate categories for testing. These categories include pharmacy theory and practice, chemistry, pharmacology, and mathematics.

Examinations are conducted throughout the country from two to four times a year, depending on the state. Each examination consists of approximately 500 questions that are presented under uniform conditions of administration, security, and grading. The Nabplex Examination is a content-valid, job-related, and objectively scored test of the knowledge, skills, and abilities that are necessary for the safe and competent practice of the profession of pharmacy. Each administrative unit employs a unique form of the various tests; these are made equivalent by the professional testing service which produces the Nabplex examinations in order to eliminate any variations in difficulty which may occur from test to test. This process assures each successive class of candidates for licensure fair and equal treatment.

The high quality of the Nabplex licensure examinations results from the marriage of three factors: (1) professional expertise, (2) the input of pharmacists with specialized skills, and (3) the test construction expertise that is provided by the Educational Testing Service (ETS) of Princeton, New Jersey. ETS specialists provide every material and service necessary to the production of the final examinations and they manage the entire Nabplex Program, beginning with the accumulation of raw test items and continuing through the processes of editing, printing, distributing, grading, and presenting final results to each participating pharmacy board. Special statistical reports of the performance of examination candidates in each of the test areas, grouped according to school of pharmacy, are also made available.

Whereas preparation and administration of these examinations is uniform, the Board of Pharmacy of each state may require additional tests that are unique. These are usually examinations in jurisprudence, with special emphasis on the state drug laws. In addition, a test may also include written or laboratory exercises on the manipulative skills necessary to the dispensing of prescriptions, oral interviews, and special tests on drug identification or the detection of errors or omissions in dispensed prescriptions. Each State Board of Pharmacy has sole responsibility for the standard of competency required for practice in its state.

The licensure examination, in effect, may test each candidate's knowledge of anything—or everything—about the profession of pharmacy to which he has been exposed during five years of education and one year of practice as an intern. To many, this appears to be an appalling task. In order to assist the pharmacy graduate to prepare for this important examination, the Nabplex Program provides the Candidate's Guide. This book contains lists of competency statements for each of the test areas upon which the questions are constructed, as well as a number of sample test questions for each competency. The Guide helps candidates to focus attention on those areas of pharmacy practice that are covered by the examinations. The failure rate for the licensure examination is relatively low: from 3 to 5 percent on any particular examination about 15 percent on the average for the entire test. Unsuccessful candidates may repeat the examination and, with further preparation, they usually pass on the second attempt.

Once registered as a pharmacist, a person may choose to practice in any of the United States except California, Florida, and Hawaii, without repeating the licensure examination. Transfer of qualifications and credentials can be arranged through procedures provided by the NABP at its Chicago office. The NABP was founded in 1904 for the express purpose of providing interstate reciprocity of pharmaceutical licensure and, although it has expanded its services into other areas, this continues to be the main benefit to its constituent members.

Most State Pharmacy Practice Acts have a permissive provision whereby the Pharmacy Board may register an individual as a pharmacist, without examination, if it can determine that (a) he holds a certificate in good standing as a pharmacist in another state, (b) he has successfully completed an examination for registration in the other state, and (c) such examination was at least as thorough as that required by the new state of registration at the particular time. This purpose is also served by the Nabplex Licensure Examination, since each participating State Pharmacy Board is administering the same test under uniform conditions and requirements. Applicants for registration by reciprocity, however, must meet all the same requirements as do the pharmacists who are registered in that state. Thus, the reciprocal procedure invariably includes some special feature such as examination on the state drug laws or any of the other add-on tests presented with that state's licensure examination.

Since registration as a pharmacist is an extremely desirable status, every possible effort is made to establish a candidate's qualification for the reciprocal position. As the national clearinghouse for the transfer of the credentials that are necessary to establish equality of qualification of reciprocity applicants, the NABP makes a painstaking check of a candidate's academic and practical experience records, moral and professional character, and legal background. It keeps

data about each state's requirements and performs a preliminary check to guarantee equality of qualification between the states concerned before issuing a formal application.

The lengths to which the NABP goes in order to provide the State Pharmacy Boards with accurate and detailed data on applicants for licensure by reciprocity may be seen in the following flow chart. (Figure VII-1). This diagram outlines the procedure from initiation of the application until final approval by the relevant pharmacy board. The benefits to the Boards of Pharmacy of one uniform scheme for transferring qualifications across state lines are obvious. Equally apparent is the facility with which pharmacists are enabled to move quickly from one occupational location to another. On the average, the paperwork for such a transmission may be completed in three to four weeks. Final approval of an application, together with the issuance of registration as a pharmacist, however, is always subject to the policies and procedures of a particular State Board of Pharmacy.

You may form some notion of the extent of the utilization of this service from the 1977 statistics, which show that more than 3,000 pharmacists became registered in states other than the state of licensure by examination, through the process of reciprocity. It is important to note that all reciprocity is based on the qualifications established by the original state of registration in its licensure examination. In no matter how many states a pharmacist may seek and obtain registration, each succeeding application follows the same path that begins at the Pharmacy Board which initially registered the applicant by licensure examination. For this reason, most pharmacists maintain their registration in that particular state whether they have any intention of practicing there or not.

While consistent in many respects, requirements for registration by reciprocity do vary from state to state. The fee for such registration may be any amount from $50 to

Figure VII–1

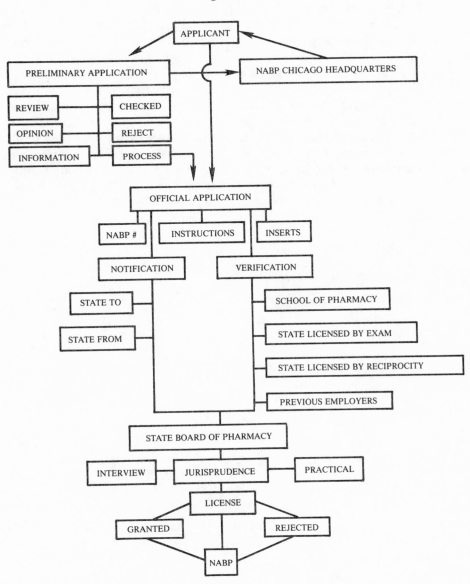

$150. Moreover, in some states applicants may be required to show evidence of residency or employment, as they are in Connecticut, Massachusetts, Michigan, New Jersey, and Rhode Island. Further, they may be required to show that they have practiced pharmacy for from 6 to 12 months in the original state of licensure before applying. In addition, they may have to appear for personal interviews with one or more board members, take the written or oral add-on examinations that are ordinarily used in that state and be required, almost without exception, to provide assurance of familiarity with the state's pharmacy and drug laws. Underlying the whole procedure must be a bilateral understanding between the states in question of acceptance of reciprocal candidates from

each other. Even though all prior requirements are fulfilled, applicants may find the
door to registration open only at certain
prescribed times. Thus, the processing of
reciprocal applications may be scheduled as
frequently as monthly or as seldom as once a
year.

The absence of any arbitrary, discrimina-
tory, or unreasonable barriers to registration
by reciprocity is due to voluntary agreement
among the active member states of the
National Association of Boards of Pharmacy. In order to maintain such active status, the constituent Boards agree to comply
with certain policies that are set forth in the
Association's constitution and by-laws. This
procedure means that any time a particular
Board denies registration by reciprocity for
any reason inconsistent with these policies,
future pharmacist candidates for reciprocal
registration from the state of denial may find
their applications rejected in any or all of the
46 other active membership states. The system has been in operation since 1904, and it
provides fair and equal treatment for pharmacists to the benefit of both the profession
and the public.

Chapter Eight

Finding a Job

The average total cost of completing the academic requirements in pharmacy soon will exceed $20,000. Indeed, attendance at some institutions already necessitates an expenditure of more than $30,000. Outlays of this magnitude can be justified, for student, family, and society, only if pharmacy graduates can find gainful employment within the health care industry.

It is appropriate, therefore, that we examine briefly some of the key factors pertaining to the job market. You may ask, "Will there be a demand for my services by the time I complete pharmacy training? What is the risk that the need for pharmacists may diminish during the middle of my professional career?" If this should occur, promotional opportunities or even job security could be jeopardized. These concerns are common to all who begin their college experience—the student who enrolls in a 4-year geology program as well as the person who initiates a 10- to 12-year course of study in medicine. Society, of course, would have neither geologists, physicians, nor pharmacists if all high school students refused to consider advanced training.

In any economy, career opportunities exist side by side in different areas that are simultaneously expanding, stable, and contracting. For example, employment in independent pharmacies has been falling for more than two decades while rising in hospitals, health maintenance, and chain organizations. Chapter Eight is designed to help you pinpoint your best chances for a job within the profession. However, there is no all-inclusive national list that covers either employed or unemployed persons with pharmacy backgrounds, and there is, therefore, no major foundation for developing accurate predictions about employment possibilities in the future. Due to this deficiency, and to the lack of a government policy on pharmacy, our view of the prospects for personnel with pharmacy training is subject to error.

Nevertheless, some opinions and evidence are available for your interpretation. The first section in this chapter describes general supply/demand conditions for pharmacists in the nation as a whole. This broad perspective is followed by specific recommendations that you can pursue in order to find a satisfactory position upon completion of formal study. The last section presents a number of observations about pharmacy as a profession which should help to make your ultimate choice more reliable.

A Social View of Employment Prospects

In May of 1978, the vice chancellor for health affairs at the University of North Carolina reported that " . . . the United States could face a serious oversupply of health professionals—including pharmacists—by 1980."* He noted that the pro-

* *apharmacy weekly* 17 (May 31, 1978):86. A subsequent issue (11 June, 1980) projected a potential surplus of 26,000 pharmacists by 1990.

jected supply of all highly trained practitioners into 1990 and beyond far outstrips any projected growth either in population or in demand for health care services. Further, the American Pharmaceutical Association supports this view "that the profession is threatened by a serious manpower oversupply that could radically alter the economic viability of all practitioners."* Finally, a Bureau of Health Manpower report noted in December of 1978 that "the supply of pharmacists may exceed the demand for their services, possibly in the mid-1980s." (You may wish to examine the section on pharmacy in this latest official report: "A Report to the President and Congress on the Status of Health Professions Personnel in the United States," Bureau of Health Manpower, PHS, DHEW Pub. No. (HRA) 78-93.)

This picture of a possible slowdown in the nation's demand for pharmacists, however, is not shared by all who have studied the problem. For example, *Money* magazine reported in November of 1977 that pharmacy was the 10th ranked profession with promise, and that the prospects for qualified job seekers were "average." This relative ranking seems especially favorable when compared with more than a dozen careers that were designated as having dismal employment potential. Finally, the Bureau of Health Manpower report cited above projects that the number of active pharmacists will grow from 117,000 in 1973 to 185,000 by 1990.

Since a number of factors are operative in the supply/demand equation, it is necessary to review selected components of the calculation. First, there are various forces that are leading to an increased use of drugs in our society. These include not only a growing population but also an increasing proportion of aged persons, who are usually heavy users. Further, weight must be given to expanded insurance coverage and the resulting rise in demand for prescriptions. More-

over, as the supply of physicians grows, the number of prescriptions written is likely to follow a similar trend. Thus, any oversupply of physicians will lead to a greater need for pharmacists, not a reduction.

While some increased demand for dispensing manpower seems assured, the role of the pharmacist as a drug consultant to both physicians and patients, especially in hospitals, should manifest significant growth. The trend toward an increase in quality assurance activities is supported not only by the current emphasis on clinical pharmacy in academic programs, but also by federal regulations under Medicare and Medicaid involving drugs used in nursing homes. Moreover, some states have mandated that community pharmacists maintain drug profiles and advise patients on the appropriate use of their prescription therapy.

While forces such as these are raising the demand for practitioner services, others are operating concurrently to decrease the available manpower. First, although the positions for non-practitioners still occupy less than 10 percent of all persons trained as pharmacists, this area alone, either directly or indirectly, is likely to provide jobs for about 4 percent of each graduating class. In addition, from 5 to 6 percent of the seniors who receive degrees go on to graduate school (and only a few of these ultimately become practitioners). Second, the number of students pursuing the Pharm.D. as an additional professional degree has risen sharply in the past two years; this pattern can be expected to continue for some time. Study at this level extends the duration of training by an extra year or two. Both these factors, of course, reduce the effective supply of applicants seeking practitioner positions in a given year.

Third, there has been a dramatic growth in the number of women entering pharmacy during the past decade. Since 1970, when female students accounted for only 22 per-

* *apharmacy weekly* 17 (May 31, 1978):86. A subsequent issue (11 June, 1980) projected a potential surplus of 26,000 pharmacists by 1990.

cent of all pharmacy students in their final three years of training, this figure has risen steadily, and it currently stands at 42 percent. Moreover, some experts feel that the national average will exceed 50 percent by 1990. As a result, the recent Bureau of Health Manpower report projects that the proportion of women practitioners will jump from 11 percent in 1973 to nearly 31 percent by 1990.

There are two major implications of this development that affect the job market for pharmacists. The first pertains to the type of special skills required. A recent survey indicates that 30 percent of the women prefer hospital practice, while only 16.6 percent of the men plan careers in this area.* Thus, relatively fewer women now seek positions in community practice. Since pharmacists employed in this setting usually become store managers by virtue of their superior educational level, career opportunities for males with additional training in administrative methods would seem to be very bright. At the same time, a larger proportion of the women entering institutional practice also may benefit from management training. Second, the assumption underlying the Bureau of Health Manpower report is that the hours of employment furnished by a female pharmacist over her lifetime are equal to approximately 50 percent of those provided by a male practitioner. This phenomenon is due to part-time and intermittent work patterns exhibited by women workers as a group.** Thus, according to 1977–78 data, a graduating class of 6,965 (which includes 2,510 women) will produce an effective addition to the labor force of about 5,710 persons. Therefore, current and future estimates of the supply of pharmacy graduates are overstated and should be adjusted to reflect these conditions.

The number of pharmacists is also influenced by federal capitation funds made available to the colleges annually since the early 1970s. This infusion of monies has stimulated the rise in pharmacy enrollments nationally from 15,326 in 1970 to 24,416 in 1975. Since that date, a slight decline has been reported. The predicted decrease in federal dollars is likely to accelerate this downward trend. Further, the transition from an academic emphasis on the baccalaureate to the professional doctoral program usually results in a reduction of class size by 40 to 50 percent; 20 schools have announced this change recently, and it seems likely that this number could rise to 25 or more by 1985. The cumulative impact of these forces, coupled with inflationary pressures in general, which will place the expense of a five-to six-year college education beyond the reach of a greater number of students, seems likely to bring pharmacy school registration down to around 21,000 within several years. In short, the possible oversupply of pharmacists already may be subject to self-correcting adjustments.

If we shift our attention to the practice setting, we find that the average community pharmacist works 46 hours a week. In addition, 15 percent of all pharmacists in 1973 had a secondary place of practice (moonlighting) where they worked an average of 15 additional hours. Moreover, two out of three pharmacists are salaried employees rather than proprietors. These factors indicate that many pharmacists manifest work patterns which are inconsistent with general trends toward increased leisure time. If an oversupply of pharmacists should develop, it can be anticipated that the average number of hours worked per week, and the number of secondary positions held, would fall and thus provide an important cushion for ab-

---

* *American Druggist* 177 (June 1978):62.

** The astute woman will also perceive that a pharmacy education may represent a very sound insurance policy.

sorbing any increase in the number of applicants.

There are offsetting factors within the practice setting which suggest that the supply of pharmacists could already be excessive. Several studies have shown that 10 to 20 percent of the community pharmacist's time was recorded as "idle." This problem could be aggravated if manufacturers increase the proportion of products that are packaged in "unit-of-use" containers. In addition, we have noted in Chapter One how practitioner productivity is impaired by the performance of many clerical functions. Moreover, the reading numbered 60 described some of the administrative chores imposed on the practitioner by drug insurance programs.

The problem of excess capacity (in positions where the pharmacist does not spend a high proportion of his time carrying out professional duties) might be reduced by better organization of pharmacy practice. Moreover, enhanced productivity might be pursued through the use of skilled technicians and computer technology designed especially to reflect both pharmacy and social needs. At this writing, though, no catalyst is on the horizon that might alter these conditions to any great extent.

While the foregoing analysis should be useful in helping you to understand pharmacy as a manpower problem, you will undoubtedly need some guidelines to help you decide whether you think the supply will exceed the demand. An oversupply may exist if two or more of the following conditions occur:

1. The average starting salary for pharmacists becomes equal to or falls below that offered to other students with five to six years of training. Since contemporary pharmacy graduates often receive a premium of between $2,000 and $5,000 over the salaries of graduates of comparable programs, it is difficult to sustain the oversupply argument until this gap is reduced. (The social justification for continuing to reward new pharmacists with a modest premium is a matter necessitating discussion elsewhere.)

2. The average number of hours worked per week falls below the comparable figure for professional workers in general or for those in competitive occupations.

3. The number of students participating in pharmacy programs remains above approximately 21,000. This figure, which reflects enrollment during the final three years of professional training, is compiled and released annually by the American Association of Colleges of Pharmacy.

Regardless of the employment outlook in pharmacy, either in comparison to alternative fields or in terms of prospects within the profession itself, these specialists retire, die, or otherwise leave their occupation for various reasons. Consequently, the replacement demand alone associated with some 185,000 practitioners, as predicted for 1990, could require nearly 7,500 new graduates per year.* When this sum is adjusted for those who are likely to become non-practitioners or enter graduate school, we obtain a reduced figure of under 6,800. This number represents less than 4 percent of the projected supply of active practitioners. If the professional responsibilities assumed by the modern pharmacist hold a challenge for you, it would seem essential that you examine those reasons that might keep your name from appearing on one of those diplomas.

Playing Probability

Although in 1973 the national average number of pharmacists per 100,000 population was 63, there was a wide variation among states with respect to this figure. Any

---

* A Public Health Service report, *Health, United States, 1979,* projects the number of pharmacy graduates at 7,455 in 1980 and 7,469 in 1990. These estimates are consistent with our conclusion that pharmacy represents a viable career option.

judgment about a possible under- or over-supply requires additional data involving factors such as the numbers of pharmacies, physicians, hospitals, etc. Nevertheless, from the point of view of job hunting, and all other things being equal, it is reasonable to assume that those areas with the highest ratios of pharmacists—Pennsylvania, Massachusetts, and Oklahoma—may not be the most likely places to initiate your search for a position. At the same time, areas with the lowest ratios—Alaska, Hawaii, Puerto Rico, West Virginia, North Carolina, and Virginia—could be the most desirable places to start your professional career.

Another basis for estimating job potential involves the relationship between prescribers and dispensers in metropolitan areas. Table VIII-1 presents data on practitioners for those communities in which the national averages were exceeded by the widest margins. Using probability as a guide for job seeking, you should first focus your attention on the 14 areas with an apparent undersupply of pharmacists. At the same time, it seems unlikely that the best employment prospects would lie in the 23 communities classified as having the greatest supply. It should be noted, though, that three metropolitan areas in Pennsylvania—the state with the largest supply of pharmacists per 100,000 population—were recorded as hav-

Table VIII-1

Standard Metropolitan Statistical Areas with a Possible Imbalance in the Ratio of Pharmacists to Physicians, U.S.A., 1973

Oversupply of Pharmacists	Undersupply of Pharmacists
Anderson, Indiana	Allentown, Pennsylvania
Bay City, Michigan	Anchorage, Alaska
Bloomington, Indiana	Augusta, Georgia
Burlington, North Carolina	Binghamton, New York
Davenport, Iowa	Harrisburg, Pennsylvania
Dubuque, Iowa	Honolulu, Hawaii
Evansville, Indiana	Killeen, Texas
Fayetteville, Arkansas	Lancaster, Pennsylvania
Gadsden, Alabama	Norfolk, Virginia
Gary, Indiana	Riverside, California
Huntsville, Alabama	Salinas, California
Lake Charles, Louisiana	San Jose, California
Laredo, Texas	Topeka, Kansas
McAllen, Texas	Vallejo, California
Owensboro, Kentucky	
Pine Bluff, Arkansas	
Racine, Wisconsin	
Richland, Washington	
St. Joseph, Missouri	
Sioux City, Iowa	
Steubenville, Ohio	
Texarkana, Texas	
Williamsport, Pennsylvania	

Note: Communities with medical and / or pharmacy schools, or large pharmaceutical manufactures, were deleted from the analysis.

Source: Ratios of pharmacists per 1,000 physicians were derived from *Health Manpower: A County & Metropolitan Area Data Book, 1972–75*. National Center for Health Statistics, DHEW Pub. No. (HRA) 76–1234. Rockville, Maryland, 1976.

ing the greatest relative shortage. This finding suggests that ratios based on state averages may not always reflect the most accurate index for estimating supply/demand ratios in particular communities. Finally, although the relative ranking of states in terms of pharmacists per 100,000 population is unlikely to change sharply over short periods of time, readers should consult the new Census statistics when they become available in 1982 or 1983.

A Public Health Service survey, conducted in 1979, reveals that a shortage of pharmacists existed in 133 counties (see Table VIII-2). While all these areas may not present a realistic employment opportunity, many could for those searching for a new frontier. In summary, the data presented in this section suggest that employment potential for practitioners may vary significantly between states, metropolitan areas, and even counties. Pharmacy graduates should not overlook these possibilities.

If geographic location represents one criterion that can be used in seeking employment, the type of position accounts for a second. No crystal ball has been invented, though, that will guarantee the supply/demand relationship that may exist for certain specialized skills by 1990, and certainly not for as far in the future as the year 2000. Nevertheless, there is a very high probability that manpower shortages are likely to persist in certain specialized fields for a number of years. Many of these positions call for advanced study beyond the B.S. in Pharmacy, while most fall in the non-practitioner category. This situation in pharmacy is similar to that in other vocational areas, where the complexity of modern life dictates both increased specialization and higher standards of professional performance. Some applicants for posts in hospital pharmacies are now required to give a lecture before the staff and answer questions concerning the particular subject which they have outlined.

The future seems especially promising for those pharmacists who are prepared to offer expertise that goes beyond the undifferentiated college degree and licensure certificate. Students who are willing to acquire advanced qualifications will not only fill an important social need but will probably maximize their earning power as well.

Areas with relatively high demand for personnel trained in pharmacy include the following:

- The recommendations presented in the latter part of Chapter Two.
- Many clinical positions defined at the beginning of Chapter Three under "Specialized Services/Medical Problems" (Also see the positions in Appendix A that are marked with an asterisk.)
- Health Care Administrator (These administrative posts are found in hospitals, clinics, and nursing homes; they require an M.S. degree from a program in this area.)
- "Drug Information Specialist" (Requires an M.S.* or a Ph.D. in Information Science and/or a hospital residency.)
- "Biostatistician" (Requires an M.S. in Applied Statistics.)
- "Data Systems or Computer Specialist" (Requires a B.S., an M.S., or a Ph.D. in Computer Science.)
- "Non-pharmacy Practitioner" (Requires a degree in Dentistry, Medicine, Podiatry, or Veterinary Medicine.)
- "Professor" (Faculty positions in Pharmacy Administration. Requires a Ph.D. in one of the following fields: Pharmacy Administration, Management, Marketing, Economics, Preventive Medicine, Social Psychology, or Medical Sociology. Academic requirements for a clinical instructor consist of a Pharm. D. degree plus an M.S. or a Ph.D. in an appropriate field.)
- "Scientific Writer" (Requires an M.S. in Communications or Journalism.)
- Specialized positions in the pharmaceutical manufacturing industry. According to a PMA report issued in December of 1978, the industry employs nearly 13,000 college graduates. Over 22 percent of these individuals hold a master's degree, while nearly 37 percent hold a doctorate. The need for scientific

---

* St. John's offers a dual master's degree in Library Science and Drug Information.

Table VIII-2

Pharmacy Manpower Shortage Areas, Classified by State and County, and Ranked According to Degree of Shortage, U.S.A., 1979

Code:
(1) No pharmacist
(2) Ratio of available pharmacists to required pharmacists is less than 0.5
(3) Ratio is between 0.5 and 1.0

Alabama
(2) Wilcox
(3) Greene, St. Clair, Washington

Arkansas
(1) Newton
(2) Lincoln
(3) Bradley, Lawrence, Perry, Sevier, Stone

Colorado
(1) Costilla, Elbert

Florida
(1) Glades, Lafayette, Liberty
(3) Sumter

Georgia
(1) Banks, Crawford, Glascock, Quitman
(3) Brantley, Oglethorpe, Wilkinson

Idaho
(3) Boundary, Madison

Illinois
(3) Clay, Marshall

Indiana
(1) Crawford
(3) Franklin, Switzerland, Washington

Kentucky
(1) Bracken
(2) Jackson, Lewis
(3) Breathitt, Casey, Knott, Pendleton

Michigan
(3) Leelanau

Minnesota
(3) Aitkin, Marshall

Mississippi
(1) Benton

Missouri
(1) Holt, Lewis, Maries, Hercer, Osage
(2) Caldwell, Miller, Shelby
(3) Chariton, Harrison, Hickory, Knox, Montgomery, Morgan, Reynolds, Ripley, Schuyler, Scotland, Sullivan

Montana
(1) McCone

Nevada
(1) Ormsby

New Mexico
(1) Catron, Mora

North Carolina
(1) Currituck, Hyde

North Dakota
(1) Oliver

Ohio
(1) Vinton

Oregon
(1) Wheeler

Pennsylvania
(1) Parts of Centre, Clearfield, Indiana, Lycoming, Mifflin, Northumberland, Schuylkill, Snyder and Tioga
(3) Fulton

South Dakota
(1) Dewey, Jerauld, Mellette
(3) Brule, Todd

Tennessee
(3) Bledsoe

Texas
(1) Crockett, Hudspeth, Jim Hogg, Kinney, Lipscom, Shackelford, Throckmorton, Zapata
(2) Dimmit
(3) Burnet, Hood, Jack, Lee, Refugio

Utah
(1) Emery
(2) San Juan

Virginia
(1) Bland, Charles City, Cumberland, King George, Rappahannock
(2) Buckingham, Floyd, Fluvanna, Greene, Madison, Powhattan
(3) Caroline, Richmond

West Virginia
(1) Clay, Hardy, Pendleton, Wirt
(2) Braxton, Lincoln, Webster
(3) Doddridge, Gilmer, Grant, Hampshire, Pocahontas, Ritchie, Roane, Wyoming

Wisconsin
(2) Buffalo
(3) Taylor

personnel seems especially strong in many of the areas enumerated in Table VIII-3. These estimates may be understated by more than 25 percent since some 300 smaller firms did not participate in the survey. The small numbers associated with the above posts should not deter you from considering these opportunities since the number of qualified applicants may be less than one-half of the need!

Table VIII–3

Estimates of Scientific Manpower Needed
by 34 Large Pharmaceutical Manufacturers, 1979

Area	Immediate Needs	Needs in Next 3–5 Years
Pharmacology; Toxicology*	56	178
Clinical Investigation	62	152
Analytical Chemistry*	59	154
Pharmaceutical; Medicinal Chemistry, Pharmacognosy	30	132
Pharmaceutics; Biopharmaceutics*	26	104
Pharmaceutical Biochemistry	19	93
Manufacturing, Ind. Pharmacy*	24	81
Marketing; Market Research	19	77
Pharmaceutical; Chemical Eng.	22	71
Pharmacokinetics	8	53
Physical Chemistry	9	41
Bionucleonics	1	32
Pharmacy; Health Care Adm.	5	18
Clinical Pharmacy	3	13
Other	27	97

* Additional stipends will be awarded to fellows in these areas.

Source: Report submitted by the 1979 Planning Committee of Scientific Manpower Needs in Industry, American Foundation for Pharmaceutical Education. *1979 Progress Report*. Fairlawn, N.J.

Preparing Your Strategy

Many students regard job hunting as a task requiring attention only during the latter part of their senior year in college. Such a strategy may suffice for some individuals, especially when applicants are in short supply. However, the last minute push may be neither the most efficient way to achieve your personal goals nor the most likely route to maximize job satisfaction or professional contribution. In addition, approaching job hunting as a single step, rather than as a continuing responsibility, could result in a lower level of income as well.

Consequently, the best match between pharmacy graduate and employer is likely to be made when this goal is viewed as a process. The process model for seeking a position requires that you systematically build a knowledge base about opportunities in pharmacy, accumulate technical skill qualifications to satisfy those possibilities, and pre-

pare a complete resume. Therefore, upon admission to professional school, you will want to raise the question, "Should I become a practitioner or a non-practitioner?" If you lean toward the practitioner role, it will be necessary to ask yourself, "Do I want to work as a staff pharmacist (generalist), or does some form of specialized training seem more desirable for my purposes?" However, if you are contemplating a career as a non-practitioner, preliminary identification of the appropriate auxiliary field will also be essential.

You will recognize that the procedures for deciding on pharmacy as a career, selecting a major within this area, and looking for a place of employment have many elements in common. Your first step in resolving this last issue should be to return to Chapter Two to determine whether several of the seven recommendations may help you in seeking a job or at least clarifying your career objectives. The second step requires that you verify your assessment of pharmacy by reading many of the selections in this volume again. Since your original Pharmacy Scorecard could have been prepared as many as four years ago, a new career profile can help you to confirm your original impression, or to record a shift in your interests. Third, prepare a list of all possible job titles that correspond with this evaluation.

Fourth, turn to Table VIII-4, which identifies the primary sources of job information. Review most of these references for several months but monitor on a continuing basis the four or five that seem most likely to generate vacancy notices consistent with your career aims. When an announcement is found that appears on your list, clip it, identify the source, and mount it in a notebook. Figure VIII-1 contains a number of sample announcements. Construct a separate classification file for each job category: hospital pharmacy, community pharmacy, etc. The sample announcements have not been classified and are merely illustrative of the various positions available to pharmacists. To gain the greatest amount of useful experience in probing the labor market, you can begin collecting notices during your next-to-last year in pharmacy school. By the beginning of your final nine months of training, you will have developed an efficient means of conducting your actual search for a position. You can use your senior year, therefore, to follow those sources that seemed to be of greatest value during the practice period and to submit applications when interesting notices appear.

As you review job announcements, retain those with the greatest appeal that call for 3 to 10 years of experience. This employment restriction on new graduates can be used to your advantage. (1) Write to the firm and inquire if the person who is hired will need an assistant. (2) Send in your application for consideration in the future. (3) Seek an entry-level post in another organization that will enable you to attain the desired experience. Within several years you will have accumulated the practical knowledge you will need for advancement either internally or externally.

Another technique that could facilitate your entry into the job market involves gaining an understanding of the various traits that employers seek in potential employees. For an important perspective from the other side of the interviewing table, you may wish to consult the following reference before starting your job search: Gumbhir, A.K.; "Prospecting for Pharmacy People," *American Pharmacy* NS 18 (February 1978): 47–49. In addition, the results of a survey of 183 companies conducted at Northeastern University should be of special value.* This study gives the following factors as the most frequent causes of applicant rejection by a potential employer: (1) inability to demonstrate self-confidence, (2) lack of enthusiasm, and (3) absence of a clear set of goals. Finally, more than two-thirds of all job openings are apparently not advertised. Therefore, if you can identify several employers who are high on your priority list, use personal contact or a letter to advise them of your availability.

There is an assumption that you will be entering the labor force with a degree from a college of pharmacy. Some readers, however, may still have difficulty determining whether this profession represents their best choice. One means of helping to resolve this question is to review alternative career opportunities. Students needing assistance in this matter should consult several of the references furnished in Table VIII-5. This brief list has been prepared especially for you by a professional career consultant who assessed over 50 sources in compiling these recommendations. After completing this exercise, your consideration of pharmacy can be resumed.

---

* "National Recruiting Survey," *New York Times*, October 14, 1979. p.73.

Table VIII-4

Major Sources of Employment Information
for Pharmacy Graduates

Type of Position		Source	Comment
Practioner	Non-Practitioner		
	X	1) *Academy Reporter*	Bimonthly, published by APhA Academy of Pharmaceutical Sciences
	X	2) *AACP News*	Monthly publication of the American Association of Colleges of Pharmacy
X	X	3) American Foundation for Pharmaceutical Education (Periodic Surveys)	Radburn Plaza Bldg. 14–25 Plaza Road Fairlawn, NJ 07410
X		4) *American Journal of Hospital Pharmacy*	Monthly published by ASHP, 4630 Montgomery Ave. Washington, DC 20014
X	X	5) *American Pharmacy*	Monthly publication of APhA, 2215 Constitution Ave., N.W. Washington, DC 20037
X	X	6) College placement office	Check with your local placement advisor
X	X	7) *Drug Intelligence & Clinical Pharmacy*	Monthly with student rate of $12 per year. Hamilton Press, Hamilton, IL 62341
X		8) Monthly journal of state pharmaceutical association	Many journals carry classified advertisements
X	X	9) National Registry for Pharmacists	Illinois Job Service 40 West Adams St. Chicago, IL 60603 (No fee is charged)
X		10) *New York Times*, Sunday sections "The Week in Review," "Business and Finance"	____
	X		A prime source for non-practitioner positions
X		11) *Pharmacy West*	Monthly published by Western Communications Ltd. 1741 Ivar Ave., Suite 116, Los Angeles, CA 90028
X	Seldom	12) Professional Pharmacy Meetings: National and State	____
	X	13) *Wall Street Journal*	Four regional editions are published

Figure VIII–1

Advertisements for Pharmacists*

PHARMACIST WANTED — R.Ph. for two community pharmacy practices in upper peninsula near Lake Superior. Blue Cross health insurance, two weeks paid vacation, MPA dues, liability insurance, paid holidays, opportunity to buy shares in corp.

DIRECTOR OF PHARMACY SERVICES. Challenging position for a Registered Pharmacist in a 580-bed teaching hospital located in central Illinois. Applicants must have experience with unit dose, I.V. admixtures and computer applications. Successful candidate must have completed an ASHP accredited residency and have 3-5 years recent managerial experience; Master's Degree preferred. Competitive salary and excellent benefits.

CLINICAL PHARMACIST, Drug Monitoring Project. Clinical Pharmacist to assist in the development of a computerized drug ordering/review system to be used in state facilities for the mentally ill and developmentally disabled. Duties will include: compiling and updating clinical guidelines for drug prescribing based on reviews of current literature; assisting in formulary and forms design. Possibility for independent research using large patient drug database. Masters degree in Pharmacy Science; experience as a Clinical Pharmacist in Mental Health, knowledge of and familiarity with computers.

PHARMACISTS WANTED. Outpatient clinic: Fast, high-volume dispensing experience in clinic or hospital required. Inpatient service: Must have experience in UD, IV ADs, TPN, 24-hour service pharmacy, 296 beds, JCAH-accredited. Must be self-motivated and or-iented towards progressive HMO institutional practice. Apply at Personnel. An equal employment opportunity, affirmative action employer.

CLINICAL RESEARCH ASSOCIATE. An expanding pharmaceutical manufacturing firm, has an immediate need for a fully experienced Clinical Research Associate.
Position requirements are a BS in Biological/Pharmaceutical Sciences, minimum of 3 years of clinical research experience within the pharmaceutical industry. Proven ability to plan, coordinate, and implement clinical research programs, and the capability to effectively interface with all levels of research organization.
Job scope includes implementing and managing programs for potential therapeutic agents.
This position offers an excellent salary and full benefits package.

PHARMACEUTICAL. Regulatory Affairs Assistant for rapidly expanding pharmaceutical company. BS/BA degree in one of the sciences and some exposure to Regulatory Affairs required. Salary commensurate with background and experience. Excellent benefit package in stimulating corporate atmosphere.

PHARMACIST—WRITER. Leading pharmacy business magazine seeks Pharmacist with interest in writing. Duties include writing, editing, developing stories and contacts. Some travel. High dollars and good benefit program. This is a "key" slot on a highly successful, retail-oriented publication.

*Names and addresses have been omitted from these otherwise actual advertisements from newspapers.

Earning Power

In Chapter Six we learned that the annual compensation of new pharmacy school graduates who enter community practice often reflects a premium of several thousand dollars over those with comparable training in another field. In an earlier section of this chapter, we noted the concern of some experts, who believe that too many pharmacists are being trained relative to the de-mand. If these predictions prove true, starting salaries can be expected to fall.

Nevertheless, in May of 1979, salaries of new graduates of one midwestern school ranged between $18,000 and $21,000 for those entering community practice.* For individuals taking positions in hospital pharmacies, the range was from $15,000 to $20,000. You will recall that less than one-half of the pharmacists in the 1977 survey remained as staff pharmacists within six

* A national survey, conducted in 1978 and measuring compensation based on a 40-hour work week, found a salary range of $11,340–$23,580 for new pharmacy graduates. Pharmacists already established in the labor force reported an annual income that ranged from $14,112–$29,676.

Table VIII–5

Career Guidance References

1. Moore, Charles Guy. *The Career Game* (*A Step by Step Guide Up the Ladder of Success*). New York: Ballantine Books, 1978 edition.

   • Excellent advice for college students and career changers.

2. Bolles, Richard N. *What Color Is Your Parachute?* (A Practical Manual for Job Hunters & Career Changers). Berkeley, California: Ten Speed Press, 1979.

   • A Bible in its field.

3. Lathrop, Richard. *Who's Hiring Who*. Reston, Virginia: Reston Publishing Company, Inc., 1976.

   • A complete overview of the job market that con-

tains succinct steps on how to 'crack' the employment field whatever your career area.

4. Buskirk, Richard H. *Your Career: How to Plan It, Manage It, Change It*. Boston: Cahners Books, Inc., 1976.

   • A professor of Business Management at Southern Methodist University provides sound, practical advice, illustrated by case studies, for persons seeking career improvement whether at the bottom, the middle, or top of their career ladders.

5. Bostwick, Burdette E. *Finding the Job You've Always Wanted*. New York: John Wiley & Sons, 1977.

   • Ten chapters packed with concise information which answers the questions of job hunter, job changer, and whatever-the-age career planner.

Compiled by Marion E. Rucker, Ph.D.

years of graduation. Consequently, it is instructive to consider the average earnings of the next largest occupational group, pharmacy managers. These data are provided by another 1977 survey covering the compensation of store managers employed by chain organizations (see table on this page). Data on the earning power of other occupational groups in pharmacy, such as supervisors and owners, are not readily available.

Number of Units in Chain	Annual Compensation of Pharmacy Manager		
	Salary	Bonus	Total
4–10	$21,950	$2,550	$24,500
11–30	25,654	4,120	29,774
31–100	26,364	5,706	32,070
101 and over	32,162	5,703	37,865

Source: *Drug Topics*, May 9, 1978, p. 25.

Your standard of living as a pharmacist will not be determined exclusively by your annual salary. It will be necessary to take into account fringe benefits—vacation allowance, coverage for retirement and health insurance, attendance at professional meetings—as well as number of hours per week and flexibility of work schedule. Moreover, it is unlikely that the higher salaries available in a metropolitan area can be obtained in a smaller community where the cost of living may be somewhat lower.

Further, the type of work environment may be of sufficient importance that you will want to take this factor into account in evaluating various salary levels. For example, one recent study found that job satisfaction and life happiness tend to be highest among pharmacists when they are employed in work settings that stress patient and professional orientation.* If the readings on clinical pharmacy have suggested the kind of role that you want as a practitioner, this factor

* Curtiss, F. R., *et al.*, "The Importance of Education . . . ," *Am. J. Pharmaceutical Education* 42 (May 1978):104–110.

could be a key one in your search for employment.

Pharmacy: A Summary View

Our extended study of pharmacy as a career possibility may seem unduly long and certainly far more complex than what you had anticipated. In order to provide an accurate overview of the many roles filled by pharmacists, I found that it was necessary to emphasize the diversity of these contributions. This foundation, of course, should be supplemented by a diligent follow-up to the recommendations provided throughout the text. Only such a total effort on your part can help you to establish whether pharmacy represents your best choice for a lifetime activity.

Pharmacy may be appealing because it offers the opportunity to become an expert in the chemical actions of drugs in the body, assist patients in improving their health, aid prescribers in getting the right drug to the right patient, hold a job that is largely insulated from the loss of employment due to business recessions, work in a pleasant environment, and even earn a comfortable living.

On the other hand, only above average students will be able to satisfy the rigorous academic requirements needed to master a great deal of technical information and to gain proficiency in clinical skills. Further, since the duration of training is at least five years, those who want instant success are likely to be disappointed in pharmacy as a career. Moreover, practitioners cannot escape value judgments about how to serve the needs of individuals who may need drug therapy. For example, if the patient presents a prescription which is incompatible with another medication he is using, would you be willing to advise him that his order should not be filled? Further, the pharmacist may be the only professional who is available to guide patients in the wise selection of over-the-counter remedies.

These two examples illustrate the importance of the responsibilities that are conferred on a pharmacist by society when a license to practice is granted. Our nation needs devoted young people who will enter the profession to improve the effectiveness and the efficiency with which prescribed drugs are used. If you are willing to view pharmacy as a profession dedicated as much to problem-solving as to dispensing, your career could be especially satisfying. Fortunately, you have an excellent base from which to begin this lifetime endeavor: a Trendex poll* ranked only one profession above pharmacy in terms of prestige and respect. The findings were as follows:

1) Clergy
2) Pharmacist
3) Police Officer
4) Lawyer
5) Public School Teacher
6) Accountant
7) Independent Supermarket Owner
8) State Legislator
9) Chain Market Manager
10) Appliance Store Owner
11) Factory Foreman
12) Grocery Wholesaler
13) Service Station Manager
14) Clothing Store Operator
15) Door-to-Door Salesman

In summary, pharmacy represents an occupation noteworthy for its diversity of opportunity as either practitioner or nonpractitioner. It also represents a profession with high social standing; this, I believe, reflects the role of pharmacists in helping patients to regain their well-being. If your interests lie in the health professions and your talents can satisfy the academic requirements associated with training in this scientific discipline, pharmacy could merit serious consideration as a career choice.

* *Changing Times* (January 1979).

Appendix A

Areas of Pharmacy Practice Not Treated

A. Areas with Illustrative Literature Citations

*1. *Allergy Clinic*

Hunter, R. B., and Osterberger, D. J. "Role of the Pharmacist in an Allergy Clinic," *Am. J. Hosp. Pharm.* 32 (April 1975):392–95.

2. *Burn Therapy*

Gee, S. "Topical Burn Agents: The Pharmacist's Role in Controlling Infections," *American Pharmacy* NS 19 (February 1979):30–33, 35.

3. *Cardiopulmonary Resuscitation*

Wooley, B. H. "Cardiopulmonary Resuscitation," *The Apothecary* 90 (September/October 1978):29–33.

4. *Clinical Laboratory Medicine*

Carlstedt, B. C. "The Clinical Lab," *U.S. Pharmacist* 42 (February 1977):20–22.

5. *Home Health Services*

"How Practitioners Perform in the Field," *American Pharmacy* NS 19 (Oct. 1979):52–53 (see also 50–51).

6. *Inventory Control*

Huffman, D. C. "Inventory Control for Maximum Profits," *NARD Journal* 99 (Dec. 1977):16–17, 27.

7. *Personnel Management*

Smith, H. A. "Building and Maintaining an Efficient and Happy Employee Team," *J. Am. Pharm. Assoc.* NS 15 (Nov. 1975):635–39.

*8. *Preparation and Maintenance of a Formulary*

Linkewich, J. A., and Prevoznik, S. J. "Guidelines on the Operation of the

---

* These functions represent areas where 50 or more pharmacists may be employed in a full-time capacity by 1990.

Pharmacy and Therapeutics Committee and Formulary," *Hospital Pharmacy* 14 (January 1979):7–22.

*9. *Sale of Medical Devices and Appliances*

Ruppersberger, J. "Rx's and Surgical Appliance: How to Promote Their Successful Marriage," *Pharmacy Times* 44 (February 1978):40–43.

McCormick, E. M. "Complete Stocks, Not Photos in a Catalog, Spark Sales of Surgical Appliances," *Pharmacy Times* 44 (August 1978):35–39.

*10. *Triage Function* (referring patients to an appropriate primary care resource)

Wilson, R. M. "A Broader Range of Services for the Community Pharmacist," *J. Am. Pharm. Assoc.* NS 14 (January 1974):24.

B. Fields or Functions but Literature Appropriate for This Guide Not Readily Available

*Clinical Pharmacology
*Clinical Toxicology
Extemporaneous Compounding
Hematology
Obstetrical Services
Ophthalmologic Pharmacy
Prescription Pricing
Veterinary Pharmacy

Appendix B

American Colleges of Pharmacy

ALABAMA
Auburn University
School of Pharmacy
Auburn, AL   36830

Samford University
School of Pharmacy
800 Lakeshore Drive
Birmingham, AL   35209

ARIZONA
University of Arizona
College of Pharmacy
Tucson, AZ   85721

ARKANSAS
University of Arkansas
School of Pharmacy
Medical Center
4301 W. Markham Street
Little Rock, AR   72201

CALIFORNIA
University of California
School of Pharmacy
San Francisco, CA   94143

University of the Pacific
School of Pharmacy
751 Brookside Road
Stockton, CA   95211

University of Southern California
School of Pharmacy
1985 Zonal Avenue
Los Angeles, CA   90033

COLORADO
University of Colorado
School of Pharmacy
Boulder, CO   80309

CONNECTICUT
University of Connecticut
School of Pharmacy
Storrs, CT   06268

DISTRICT OF COLUMBIA
Howard University
College of Pharmacy and Pharmacal
    Sciences
2300 4th Street, N.W.
Washington, DC   20059

FLORIDA
Florida A and M University
School of Pharmacy
Box 367
Tallahassee, FL   32307

University of Florida
College of Pharmacy
J. Hillis Miller Health Center
Gainesville, FL   32610

GEORGIA
Mercer University
Southern School of Pharmacy
345 Boulevard, N.E.
Atlanta, GA   30312

University of Georgia
School of Pharmacy
Athens, GA   30602

IDAHO
Idaho State University
College of Pharmacy
P.O. Box 8288
Pocatello, ID   83209

ILLINOIS
University of Illinois
College of Pharmacy
833 South Wood Street
Chicago, IL   60612

INDIANA
Butler University
College of Pharmacy
4600 Sunset Avenue
Indianapolis, IN   46208

Purdue University
School of Pharmacy and Pharmacal
   Sciences
West Lafayette, IN   47907

IOWA
Drake University
College of Pharmacy
25th and University Avenues
Des Moines, IA   50311

The University of Iowa
College of Pharmacy
Iowa City, IA   52242

KANSAS
University of Kansas
School of Pharmacy
327 Malott Hall
Lawrence, KS   66045

KENTUCKY
University of Kentucky
College of Pharmacy
Washington and Gladstone Streets
101 Pharmacy Building
Lexington, KY   40506

LOUISIANA
Northeast Louisiana University
School of Pharmacy and Allied Health
   Professions
Monroe, LA   71209

Xavier University of Louisiana
College of Pharmacy
7325 Palmetto Street
New Orleans, LA   70125

MARYLAND
University of Maryland
School of Pharmacy
636 W. Lombard Street
Baltimore, MD   21201

MASSACHUSETTS
Massachusetts College of Pharmacy
179 Longwood Avenue
Boston, MA   02115

Northeastern University
College of Pharmacy and Allied Health
   Professions
360 Huntington Avenue
Boston, MA   02115

MICHIGAN
Ferris State College
School of Pharmacy
901 S. State Street
Big Rapids, MI   49307

University of Michigan
College of Pharmacy
Ann Arbor, MI   48109

Wayne State University
College of Pharmacy and Allied
   Health Professions
Detroit, MI   48202

MINNESOTA
University of Minnesota
College of Pharmacy
Minneapolis, MN   55455

MISSISSIPPI
University of Mississippi
School of Pharmacy
Faser Hall
University, MS   38677

MISSOURI
St. Louis College of Pharmacy
4588 Parkview Place
St. Louis, MO   63110

University of Missouri-Kansas City
School of Pharmacy
5055 Rockhill Road
Kansas City, MO   64110

MONTANA
University of Montana
School of Pharmacy
Missoula, MT   59812

NEBRASKA
Creighton University
School of Pharmacy
2500 California Street
Omaha, NE   68178

University of Nebraska
College of Pharmacy
Omaha, NE   68105

NEW JERSEY
Rutgers, the State University of
New Jersey, College of Pharmacy
P.O. Box 789
Piscataway, NJ   08854

NEW MEXICO
University of New Mexico
College of Pharmacy
Albuquerque, NM   87131

NEW YORK
Arnold and Marie Schwartz College of
   Pharmacy and Health Sciences
75 DeKalb Avenue at University Plaza
Brooklyn, NY   11201

St. John's University
College of Pharmacy and Allied
   Health Professions
Grand Central and Utopia Parkways
Jamaica, NY   11439

State University of New York at Buffalo
School of Pharmacy
C126 Cooke-Hochstetter Complex
Amherst, NY   14260

Union University, Albany College of
   Pharmacy
106 New Scotland Avenue
Albany, NY   12208

NORTH CAROLINA
University of North Carolina
School of Pharmacy
Beard Hall
Chapel Hill, NC   27514

NORTH DAKOTA
North Dakota State University
College of Pharmacy
State University Station
Fargo, ND   58102

OHIO
Ohio Northern University
College of Pharmacy
Ada, OH   45810

Ohio State University
College of Pharmacy
500 W. 12th Avenue
Columbus, OH   43210

University of Cincinnati-
   Medical Center
College of Pharmacy
Health Professions Building
Cincinnati, OH   45267

University of Toledo
College of Pharmacy
2801 W. Bancroft Street
Toledo, OH   43606

OKLAHOMA
Southwestern Oklahoma State
   University
School of Pharmacy
Weatherford, OK   73096

University of Oklahoma
College of Pharmacy
644 N.E. 14th Street
Oklahoma City, OK   73104

OREGON
Oregon State University
School of Pharmacy
Corvallis, OR   97331

PENNSYLVANIA
Duquesne University
School of Pharmacy
Mellon Hall of Science
Pittsburgh, PA   15219

Philadelphia College of Pharmacy
   and Science
43rd Street and Kingsessing Avenue
Philadelphia, PA   19104

Temple University
School of Pharmacy
3307 N. Broad Street
Philadelphia, PA   19140

University of Pittsburgh
School of Pharmacy
1103 Salk Hall
Pittsburgh, PA   15261

PUERTO RICO
University of Puerto Rico
College of Pharmacy
G.P.O. Box 5067, University Station
Rio Piedras, PR   00936

RHODE ISLAND
University of Rhode Island
College of Pharmacy
Fogarty Hall
Kingston, RI   02881

SOUTH CAROLINA
Medical University of South Carolina
College of Pharmacy
171 Ashley Avenue
Charleston, SC   29403

University of South Carolina
College of Pharmacy
Columbia, SC   29208

SOUTH DAKOTA
South Dakota State University
College of Pharmacy
Brookings, SD   57007

TENNESSEE
University of Tennessee
College of Pharmacy
874 Union Avenue
Memphis, TN   38163

TEXAS
Texas Southern University
School of Pharmacy
3201 Wheeler Avenue
Houston, TX   77004

University of Houston
College of Pharmacy
4800 Calhoun Boulevard
Houston, TX   77004

University of Texas at Austin
College of Pharmacy
Austin, TX   78712

UTAH
University of Utah
College of Pharmacy
Salt Lake City, UT   84112

VIRGINIA
Virginia Commonwealth University
School of Pharmacy
Medical College of Virginia
Box 666
Richmond, VA   23298

WASHINGTON
University of Washington
School of Pharmacy
Seattle, WA   98195

Washington State University
College of Pharmacy
Pullman, WA   99164

WEST VIRGINIA
West Virginia University
School of Pharmacy
Medical Center
Morgantown, WV   26506

WISCONSIN
University of Wisconsin-Madison
School of Pharmacy
425 N. Charter Street
Madison, WI   53706

WYOMING
University of Wyoming
School of Pharmacy
Box 3375 University Station
Laramie, WY   82071

Index of Readings

Index